FUNDAMENTAL ASPECTS OF CANCER

Cancer Growth and Progression

SERIES EDITOR: HANS E. KAISER

Department of Pathology, University of Maryland, Baltimore, Md, U.S.A.

Scientific Advisors:

Kenneth W. Brunson / Harvey A. Gilbert / Ronald H. Goldfarb / Alfred L. Goldson / Elizier Gorelik / Anton Gregl / Ronald B. Herberman / James F. Holland / Ernst H. Krokowski [†] / Arthur S. Levine / Annabel G. Liebelt / Lance A. Liotta / Seoras D. Morrison / Takao Ohnuma / Richard L. Schilsky / Harold L. Stewart / Jerome A. Urban / Elizabeth K. Weisburger / Paul V. Woolley

Fundamental Aspects of Cancer

Edited by

RONALD H. GOLDFARB
Pittsburgh Cancer Institute
Pittsburgh, Pa., U.S.A.

Kluwer Academic Publishers

DORDRECHT / BOSTON / LONDON

Library of Congress Cataloging in Publication Data

Fundamental aspects of cancer.

   (Cancer growth and progression ; v. 1)
   Includes index.
   1. Cancer. 2. Cancer cells. 3. Metastasis.
I. Goldfarb, Ronald H. II. Series. [DNLM: 1. Cell
Transformation, Neoplastic. 2. Neoplasm Invasiveness.
3. Neoplasm Metastasis. QZ 200 C2151518 v.1]
RC262.F86 1988   616.99'4   87-24663

ISBN-13: 978-94-010-6980-9   e-ISBN-13: 978-94-009-1089-8
DOI:10.1007/ 978-94-009-1089-8

Published by Kluwer Academic Publishers,
P.O. Box 17, 3300 AA Dordrecht, The Netherlands.

Kluwer Academic Publishers incorporates
the publishing programmes of
Martinus Nijhoff, Dr W. Junk, D. Reidel, and MTP Press.

Sold and distributed in the U.S.A. and Canada
by Kluwer Academic Publishers,
101 Philip Drive, Norwell, MA 02061, U.S.A.

In all other countries, sold and distributed
by Kluwer Academic Publishers Group,
P.O. Box 322, 3300 AH Dordrecht, The Netherlands.

Cover design by Jos Vrolijk.

TABLE OF CONTENTS

INTRODUCTION

Individual neoplastic diseases often show discrete growth patterns subject to many modifications according to the stage of the disease, the species involved and the tumor type concerned. Primary neoplasms are less difficult to treat in contrast to secondary neoplasms. The chief type of secondary neoplastic growth, metastasis, is also comparatively less well understood. Phylogenetically, metastasis attains its highest level of development in the mammal and is best known in man, but is still far from being understood.

The process of cancer growth and progression, from the initiation of neoplastic transformation of normal cells to the selective development of subpopulations of invasive, metastatic (i.e. malignant) cells represents a time-dependent continuum of highly complex cellular and molecular events. These events include the properties of malignant cells and the properties of the host, including anti-tumor effects of the immune response. The ultimate development of metastases in patients with solid tumors yields the devastating clinical sequelae of treatment failure, morbidity and mortality. The life-threatening consequences of tumor progression to metastasis formation is underscored by the clinical reality that at the time of diagnosis of primary tumors, approximately fifty percent of patients with solid malignant tumors already harbor concealed, subclinical micrometastases. Indeed, the detection of a metastatic lesion may signify the presence of other occult micrometastases. The expansion of such micrometastatic lesions, composed of heterogeneous malignant subpopulations, and their disperse anatomic distribution may limit or prevent effective surgical or chemotherapeutic treatment. Although the treatment modalities of chemotherapy, radiotherapy and surgery effectively treat approximately fifty percent of patients who develop malignant tumors, the majority of patients who are refractive to these therapeutic modalities succumb to the direct or in-direct effect of tumor metastases or to adverse consequences associated with these therapeutic modes (e.g., complications of immunosuppression which can lead to mortality arising from infectious disease).

It is therefore quite clear that there is a crucial need for new methods for the detection of micrometastases and the development of new modalities for the treatment of established metastases. It is likely that such modalities must overcome tumor heterogeneity and drug resistance to yield new therapeutic modalities with improved margin of safety and efficacy over currently available anti-neoplastic drugs. This volume presents an overview of our current understanding of the biology of cancer in several species, including humans. Moreover, emphasis is placed on tumor heterogeneity and diversity as well as the biochemical and cellular characteristics of metastatic tumor cell subpopulations. Consideration is also given to the role of the immune response on the control of cancer progression and spread and the description of animal models of clinically relevant models of cancer metastasis. Multiple chapters in this volume discuss the diagnostic and therapeutic implications of understanding progressive stages of human malignant neoplastic growth.

In summary, this volume introduces the reader to themes that will be emphasized in subsequent volumes of this series: tumor biology in various species; tumor progression and metastatic spread, immune intervention, comparative tumor development, animal models of malignant diseases and the clinical relevance of cancer growth and progression to the diagnosis and treatment of human malignances.

Series Editor
Hans E. Kaiser

Volume Editor
Ronald H. Goldfarb

ACKNOWLEDGEMENT

Inspiration and encouragement for this wide ranging project on cancer distribution and dissemination from a comparative biological and clinical point of view, was given by my late friend E. H. Krokowski.

Those engaged on the project included 252 scientists, listed as contributors, volume editors and scientific advisors, and a dedicated staff. Special assistence was furnished by J. P. Dickson, J. A. Feulner, and I. Theloe.

I. Bauer, D. L. Fisher, S. Fleishman, K. Joshi, A. M. Lewis, J. Taylor and K. E. Yinug have provided additional assistence.

The firm support of the publisher, especially B. F. Commandeur, is deeply appreciated. The support of the University of Maryland throughout the preparation of the series is acknowledged.

To the completion of this undertaking my wife, Charlotte Kaiser, has devoted her unslagging energy and invaluable support.

CONTRIBUTORS

Dirk BERENS VON RAUTENFELD, M.D.
Functional and Applied Anatomy,
Medical Academy, 3000 Hannover,
P.O. Box 610180, FRG

Kenneth W. BRUNSON, Ph.D.
Cancer Metastasis Research Group
Pfizer Central Research,
Eastern Point Road,
Groton, Connecticut 06340, USA

Stephen K. CARTER, M.D.
Anti-Cancer Research,
Pharmaceutical Research and Development Division,
Bristol-Myers Company,
345 Park Ave., New York, New York 10140, USA

Bruce A. CHABNER, M.D.
National Cancer Institute/National Institutes of Health,
Bethesda, Maryland 20892, USA

John D. CRISSMAN, M.D.
Anatomic Pathology
Henry Ford Hospital
Detroit, Michigan 48202, USA

Isaiah J. FIDLER, D.V.M, Ph.D.
Department of Cell Biology,
The University of Texas System Cancer Center,
M.D. Anderson Hospital & Tumor Institute,
6723 Bertner Ave.,
Houston, Texas 77030, USA

Ronald H. GOLDFARB, Ph.D.
Pittsburgh Cancer Institute,
3343 Forbes Avenue,
Pittsburgh, Pennsylvania 15213, USA
and Department of Pathology,
University of Pittsburgh, School of Medicine

Eliezer L. GORELIK, M.D., Ph.D.
Pittsburgh Cancer Institute
3343 Forbes Avenue
Pittsburgh, Pennsylvania 15213, USA
and Department of Pathology,
University of Pittsburgh, School of Medicine

Ronald B. HERBERMAN, M.D.
Pittsburgh Cancer Institute
3343 Forbes Avenue
Pittsburgh, Pennsylvania 15213, USA
and Departments of Medicine and Pathology,
University of Pittsburgh, School of Medicine

James F. HOLLAND, M.D.
Department of Neoplastic Diseases,
The Mount Sinai Medical Center
of the City University of New York
One Gustave L. Levy Place
New York, New York 10029, USA

Carola HUNNESHAGEN, cand. vet. med.
Functional and Applied Anatomy,
Medical Academy, 3000 Hannover 1
P.O. Box 610180, FRG

Marvin L. JONES
Zoological Society of San Diego,
P.O. Box 551, San Diego, California 92112, USA

Hans E. KAISER, D.Sc.
Department of Pathology,
School of Medicine,
University of Maryland,
10 S. Pine Street,
Baltimore, Maryland 21201, USA

David G. KAUFMAN, M.D.
Department of Pathology,
University of North Carolina,
School of Medicine,
Chapel Hill,
North Carolina 27514, USA

Arthur S. LEVINE, M.D.
National Institute of Child Health & Human Development,
National Institutes of Health,
Bethesda, Maryland 20892, USA

Philip J. McCOY, Ph.D.
Pittsburgh Cancer Institute,
3343 Forbes Avenue,
Pittsburgh, Pennsylvania 15213, USA
and Department of Pathology,
University of Pittsburgh,
School of Medicine

Rajiv NAYAR, Ph.D.
Canadian Liposome Company
267 West Esplanade, Suite 308
North Vancouver, B.C.
Canada V7M 1A5

Peter A. NETLAND, M.D.
Department of Physiology and Biophysics,
Harvard Medical School,
Boston, Massachusetts 02115, USA

Takao OHNUMA, M.D., Ph.D.
Department of Neoplastic Diseases.
The Mount Sinai Medical Center of the City University of New
York,
One Gustave L. Levy Place,
New York, New York 10029, USA

John L. PARADISO, Ph.D.
Office of Endangered Species,
U.S. Fish and Wildlife Service,
Department of Interior,
Jacksonville, Florida 32216, USA

Monina D. PELINA, B.A.
118 Monroe Street,
Apt. 408, Rockville, Maryland, 20850, USA

Vincent A. POLLACK, Ph.D.
Cancer Metastasis Research Group
Pfizer Central Research
Eastern Point Road
Groton, Connecticut 06340, USA

Gene P. SIEGAL, M.D., Ph.D.
Division of Oncologic & Surgical Pathology,
Department of Pathology,
School of Medicine,
University of North Carolina at Chapel Hill,
Chapel Hill, North Carolina 27514, USA

James E. TALMADGE, Ph.D.
Smith Kline & French Laboratories
Research and Development Division
Immunology and Antiinfectives Therapy, L-101
P.O. Box 1539
King of Prussia, Pennsylvania 19406-0939, USA

James VARANI, Ph.D.
Department of Pathology,
University of Michigan,
Medical School,
1335 E. Catherine Street,
Ann Arbor, Michigan 48109, USA

Peter WARD, M.D.
Department of Pathology,
University of Michigan, Medical School
Ann Arbor, Michigan 48104, USA

Bruce R. ZETTER, M.D.
Departments of Physiology & Surgery,
Harvard Medical School,
Children's Hospital Medical Center,
300 Longwood Ave.,
Boston, Massachusetts 02115, USA

THE BIOLOGY OF HUMAN CANCER, AND THE DEVELOPMENT OF A RATIONAL BASIS FOR TREATMENT

ARTHUR S. LEVINE

Cancer biology: the evolution of modern concepts

Cancer is a very "old" disease, with the earliest recorded descriptions of tumors and their treatment found in Egyptian papyrie dating from 1600 B.C. (125). Nevertheless, little if any insight was brought to bear on the biology of cancer until the 19th century, with Schleiden and Schwann's discovery of the cellular nature of all organisms (140) and Muller's formulation of microscopic pathology as the foundation of our understanding of disease (99). Later in the 19th century, Virchow proposed that all cells arise from other cells, and that cancer reflected a constitutional predisposition together with an exciting cause, such as chronic irritation. Virchow also promulgated the notion of metastases (143), although he believed the metastatic process to have a "fluid" rather than a cellular basis. Modern cancer research began with Peyton Rous' demonstration in 1911 that sarcomas in the Plymouth Rock hen could be transmitted to normal hens by the injection of cell-free filtrates of the original tumor (117), suggesting the existence of identifiable cancer-causing agents.

The earliest attempts to formulate a therapeutic approach to cancer are attributed to Hippocrates (about 400 B.C.) who in addition to proposing that the disease resulted from a lack of proportion between the four humors, was the first to make the analogy to the crab (125). In 200 A.D., Galen appreciated that cancer might be a systemic illness, and consequently advocated systemic rather than local treatment (50). Curiously, the concept of cancer as a systemic disease was later abandoned and not truly resurrected until the recent advent of adjuvant chemotherapy.

Cancer epidemiology and ecogenetics

Shortly after Rous' landmark contribution to studies of cancer etiology, it became evident that population-based inquiry might illuminate the causes of cancer. The possible epidemiologic differences between tumors were not well appreciated until 1910–1930, when population-based and case-control investigations of cancer were first developed (30). In such studies, groups of patients with a specific tumor are compared to a control group lacking such a tumor. Among the most important studies in this regard were those of Haenszel and Smith (62, 130). They demonstrated clearly that migrants in many instances experience significantly different cancer rates than the populations in their countries of origin, thus stimulating much research on environmental

factors in cancer and generating a powerful distinction between nature and nurture in this disease.

The coal-tar cancers represent an excellent example of what Robert Miller has termed "bedside etiology" (96), in which clinical observations (e.g., scrotal cancer in chimney sweeps) have provided clues that led to the explication of causal factors in environmentally induced malignant diseases. Prospective (cohort) studies establishing an etiologic link between cigarette smoking and cancer (34), or asbestos exposure and cancer (93), are of exemplary value in this regard, just as the increased familial risk of breast cancer observed by many investigators in the 1940s and 1950s provided an important clue to the life-long influence of the genetic endowment (107). To the degree that environmentally induced cancers can only be avoided by minimizing exposure early on, knowledge in this area is as much the province of the pediatrician as the internist. Moreover, many workers have proposed that differences in the quality and quantity of food consumed may explain the marked variations in cancer rates often seen among various racial, religious, and geographic groups (133). While the possible link between nutrition and cancer enjoys a great vogue of current interest, the variables which confound studies in this area are legion. Whatever links are finally established, however, it seems likely that intervention must begin in childhood.

Clearly, the disciplines of epidemiology and ecogenetics are exceedingly important to cancer etiology and prevention – yet all too few investigators are trained in the methods of these disciplines, and fewer still are practitioners. One example of the possible yield from this area of study to our understanding of cancer etiology relates to the mammalian enzyme, aryl hydrocarbon hydroxylase (Ahh). The inducibility of this cytochrome P450 enzyme, which detoxifies benzene and other aryl hydrocarbons, has been reported to be abnormal (although not consistently so) in adults with lung cancer and other tumors apparently related to environmental carcinogens. Moreover, Nebert et al. have studied inbred rodents with abnormally high or low Ahh inducibility, and found that in "low Ahh" strains, hydrocarbon injection in weanlings leads consistently to leukemia, while in "high Ahh" strains, sarcomas are produced at the injection site (102). Rodents with normal Ahh inducibility remain disease-free after the same hydrocarbon exposure. These data suggest that ecogenetic studies of "cancer-prone" families may yield a greater dividend than studies of cancer patients *per se*, wherein the results may reflect the disease effect rather than the cause.

R. H. Goldfarb (ed.), Fundamental aspects of cancer.

The cytochrome P450 system has been the subject of intensive investigation; using modern molecular biologic techniques, cell receptors for hydrocarbons have been identified, as have the enzyme-encoding genes which are expressed as a consequence of ligand-receptor binding (103). Minor mutations in the genes underlying this system can be detected, and soon, molecular probes should become available for the detection of the individual risk of hydrocarbon-induced cancers. Such a development would, of course, revolutionize our approach to cancer prevention.

Although known ecogenetic correlations with cancer are rare, even in the aggregate, each new association is of great importance as still another insight into the oncogenic process is offered, e.g., the immunologic deficiency syndromes with their increased cancer risk, the concordance rates for malignancy in twins, the somatic genetics of bilateral retinoblastoma, associations between tumors and congenital defects, xeroderma pigmentosum and skin cancer, and the Purtilo syndrome (x-linked lymphoproliferative disease).

Experimental carcinogenesis

It is arguable as to which experimentally derived concepts of carcinogenesis moved the study of cancer forward by leaps, but the roster certainly includes the elucidation of the role of mutagenesis in the development of neoplasia (95). An appreciation of the cell cycle of DNA synthesis led to the identification of cycle-dependent and phase-specific therapeutic mechanisms (75). The demonstration of a graft rejection response to transplanted tumor cells in syngeneic mice paved the way for our extraordinary current interest in immunologic aspects of tumor biology (46, 111). Finally, the possibility that an abnormal chromosomal constitution might predispose to cancer originated with Boveri in 1907 (15). In this regard, the demonstration of a marker chromosome in chronic myelocytic leukemia was a seminal observation (106). With the development of recombinant DNA technology, experimental manipulations of "chromosomal constitution" to determine their effects on cell behavior are at hand. With further regard to experimental tumor biology, studies on chemical carcinogenesis are also of singular importance because they have suggested the multi-stage nature of cancer induction, i.e., the notion that the early event(s) of carcinogenesis are rapidly and irreversibly achieved, initiating a process which is responsible for the conversion of normal cells to latent tumor cells, followed by a promoting process which causes these "transformed" cells to progress slowly (and sometimes reversibly) toward a phenotype with oncogenic potential (10). These observations have provoked much interest in the possibility that the initial carcinogenic event may result from a unique, discrete genetic lesion followed by a great diversity of somatic mutations; whether these stages in any way correlate with the problem of transformation versus oncogenicity is of course a question (undoubtedly an immunological one) of profound importance. At the present time, the correlation between mutagenic and carcinogenic activities of chemicals is sufficiently good that a variety of mutagenic assays and DNA repair systems are employed to screen for the detection of potential carcinogens (3). Moreover, the correlation of mutagenic with carcinogenic activity certainly supports the notion that DNA is the primary target in carcinogenesis. This notion rests not only on the strong electrophillic reactivity of the ultimate reactive forms of virtually all carcinogens and of most chemical mutagens, but also on the recognition that tumor virus DNA is either integrated in host DNA per primum (in the case of DNA-containing oncogenic viruses) or after reverse transcription (in the case of RNA-containing oncogenic viruses).

Tumor virology

The work of Peyton Rous has already been characterized as having fathered modern cancer research. Since his experiments in 1911 (117), cancer virology has indeed proven to be one of the most valuable modern scientific disciplines, not only for explicating the possible relationship between viruses and human cancer, but also for exploring the molecular biology of eukaryotic cells (39). Since viruses that have the ability to transform cells *in vitro* or induce experimental tumors are known to play a role in the etiology of cancer in many animal species, exceptional effort has been invested in the past decade in investigating whether viruses are in fact agents of human cancer. This is an area of extraordinary complexity with many false leads and disappointments; however, the associations between viruses and human cancer remain sufficiently strong, i.e., EBV with Burkitt's lymphoma and nasopharyngeal carcinoma, hepatitis B virus with hepatoma, herpes simplex virus and papilloma viruses with cervical carcinoma, and human T-cell leukemia virus (HTLV-I, which is one of a family of human retroviruses) with adult T-cell leukemia/lymphoma (144), that complexity and disappointment must not inhibit our efforts to further explore this area. Moreover, animal tumor viruses provide simple, but extremely powerful experimental systems to manipulate and analyze the molecular biology of eukaryotic cells, and in particular, to study the molecular basis of cell transformation. Tumor viruses replicate, and their genomes are transcribed, in the nucleus of the infected cell, primarily utilizing host cell enzymes and mechanisms. Therefore, through an analysis of virus DNA replication, gene regulation, RNA transcription, and protein synthesis, the investigator has an elegantly narrow window through which to view these eukaryotic host processes in the otherwise exceedingly complex mammalian cell (39). Moreover, tumor viruses, unlike chemical carcinogens, are able to transform cells via a property which resides in only one or a very few viral-encoded proteins (124). By understanding the functions of these viral-encoded transforming proteins, we should be able to understand on a molecular level the basis of cell transformation and oncogenicity. In no other system is it possible to identify with such purity the critical event or molecular entity by which transformation is initiated in a normal cell.

Twenty years after Rous demonstrated that a tumor-producing agent could be transmitted to chickens in series by a cell-free filtrate, Shope showed that papillomata were transmissible to rabbits by cell-free filtrates, with the causative agent being the first known DNA-containing tumor virus (126). The first suggestion of the involvement of a virus in the induction of a carcinoma came from Bittner in 1936, who associated the "milk factor" with mammary cancer in mice (14). This factor was later identified as a retrovirus (MMTV). Other retroviruses, the study of which has played a central role in the field of tumor virology, include the avian sarcoma virus, the mammalian sarcoma viruses (which are defective and must be complimented for growth with a helper virus), and the defective and nondefective avian and murine leukemia viruses. In the 1950s and 60s, the very complex, but endlessly fascinating murine leukemia viruses (MULV) were discovered and studied by many investigators. The biologic expression of these retroviruses, some of which are endogenous to the host (i.e., in the germ line) and some exogenous, appears to be exquisitely dependent upon host genetics, immune regulation, the age of the host, and recombination of viral genes with one another as well as with host genes, providing a good indication of why it has been so difficult to associate retroviruses definitively with human cancer. The murine leukemia virus system is of particular importance because many of these viruses are naturally occurring: The genetics of their hosts can be defined and manipulated; the evolution of the viruses *pari passu* with that of the host can be delineated; the relationship of virus expression to the host's immune regulatory mechanisms and targets can be altered experimentally; and the genetic mechanisms of oncogenicity can in all likelihood be explored at a nucleotide level (118).

Of the DNA viruses, SV40, polyoma, and the human adenoviruses form especially powerful systems with which to analyze the molecular basis of cell transformation and oncogenicity. In addition to the introduction of DNA tumor virus systems as "windows" on the molecular biology of eukaryotic cells and their growth regulation, a number of further technical advances have made this area of biology explosive. These advances include the development and exploitation of restriction endonucleases and molecular cloning methods with which to dissect viral genomes (28); the development of efficient DNA transfection of the eukaryotic cell, employing defined genetic fragments of tumor viruses (54); the development of cell-free translation methods to identify gene products and map the genes for viral-encoded polypeptides; the development of highly sensitive molecular hybridization techniques with which to analyze viral DNA and RNA sequences in transformed cells; the development of rapid DNA sequencing procedures; and finally the use of recombinant DNA methods to alter the "viral" genome in a virtually infinite number of ways (26). The development of our appreciation for the molecular genetics of DNA tumor viruses has been matched by our acquisition of profoundly detailed knowledge on the structure on RNA viruses; the discovery of reverse transcriptase in 1970 by Temin and Baltimore (6, 137) provided further support for the unifying hypothesis of a DNA target for malignant transformation earlier discussed. More recently, the identification of the polypeptide product of the Rous sarcoma virus *sarc* gene, and the demonstration that the *sarc* gene product is a phosphoprotein with protein kinase activity (17), provides an important conceptual framework in which to examine how the interaction of a single gene product with membrane and other cellular components can induce the myriad of pleiotropic changes which occur in cells in association with transformation. This examination would appear to be one of the most fruitful studies to be undertaken in the next decade in attempting to answer the question: What is the molecular basis of cell transformation and oncogenicity?

Fruit flies and Oncogenes: development biology and cancer research come together

We do not yet have a theory of developmental biology, nor do we have a theory of oncogenesis, in the same sense that we have a theory of evolution or a theory of genetics. However, over the past few years, these seemingly quite unrelated areas of investigation, developmental biology and cancer research, have achieved some remarkable parallelisms, and the experiments done in one field are so quickly informing the experiments done in the other, that we no longer can overlook this extraordinary congruence (88).

There are many symmetries between the primary cell biological processes when one compares embryogenesis and early development with the formation of a tumor. In normal embryonic development, we see regulated cell growth and division, and in cancer, we have unregulated proliferation. Even in the early stages of development, we have orderly adhesion of cells to cells, but in cancer we have a disorderly cell mass with irregular adhesion. Normally, a cell recognizes its neighbor, and when, *in vitro*, these cells become confluent, they demonstrate a topo-inhibition; the growth and division of cancer cells is not inhibited by contact, and eventually such cells become invasive. In normal development, embryonic cells (both germ cells and somatic cells) migrate widely before homing toward and remaining in their correct domain, but in cancer, heterotopy and metastases occur. In normal development, cells are programmed to achieve a terminal differentiation, but in cancer the cells are driven toward a "dedifferentiated" or "undifferentiated" phenotype. Finally, normal development eventuates in senescence – the cells know when to age and when to die, even in tissue culture (64), but in cancer, the cells are "immortal," and most malignant cell lines will endure limitlessly in culture.

With these symmetries in mind, it will be useful to review the history of our present understanding of oncogenesis as a step-wise phenomenon, in some ways a slow reversal of normal development and differentiation. Epidemiological studies have long suggested that cancer usually occurs, at least in adults, many years after exposure to a carcinogen. A long latency is followed by an almost exponential cascade of clinically detectable malignant events. This long step-wise progression has a histologic parallel in tumors such as carcinoma of the uterine cervix, where an initial dysplasia is followed years later by metaplasia, then later still by anaplasia and finally, by metastatic disease. More than one hundred years ago, Broca observed that his wife's family had cancer in each generation for as many generations as he could trace; he postulated that there was a heritable mechanism to account for this pedigree, not manifest until adult life and not evident in other families that he studied in the same way (11). At the turn of the century, Boveri first suggested that chromosome abnormalities were the key to cancer (15). Only within the past several years have we come to realize that Broca and Boveri were prescient: They may indeed be "cancer genes." However, when Peyton Rous isolated a filterable agent from chickens with sarcomas, and induced sarcomas in healthy chickens by inoculating them with this agent, there seemed to arise two irreconcilable explanations for cancer, one related to genetics and one to environment.

How can we reconcile endogenous "cancer genes" with exogenous "cancer viruses"? To approach an answer to this question, it will be helpful to consider the classical ideas of chemical carcinogenesis: initiation and promotion. It is evident that after exposure to a carcinogen, cells *in vivo* are somehow initiated or prepared during early events to become malignant – already abnormal but not clearly cancerous – followed by another series of events, possibly promoted by a different group of chemicals, that eventuates in clinically detectable cancer. The notion of initiation and promotion may mirror the idea that there are both endogenous and exogenous, step-wise events underlying cancer, or at the least, multiple and inter-dependent events.

Analogous to these clinical, epidemiological, histological, and biological observations is the process of cellular transformation, an *in vitro* phenomenon (58). Whether induced by viruses, chemicals, or physical events, transformation also seems to reflect a step-wise progression. For example, soon after normal cells are infected with oncogenic viruses *in vitro*, the saturation density of the cells increases; they become overcrowded in culture, and fail to demonstrate topo-inhibition. Somewhat later, these transformed cells become increasingly autonomous, and are able, for example, to grow in a low concentration of serum; the cells appear to have become independent of the nutrients and growth factors in serum, and in this respect, their behavior is autocrine. The morphology of the transformed cells begins to change; cells that were initially flat and stellate become round and refractile as their cytoskeleton is disrupted. Along the route of this apparent dedifferentiation, the transformed cells become independent of their anchorage; whereas normal cells thrive in culture only if they can adhere to a surface, transformed cells remain fully viable and proliferative in soft agar or in liquid media. Finally, the cells become immortalized, and will undergo countless rounds of cell division in culture. Some, but not all, transformed cells will form tumors when the cells are inoculated in susceptible experimental animals, and many, but not all, tumor cells will eventually metastasize. Thus, *in vitro*, cellular transformation is a play-within-in-a-play, a recapitulation of the *in vivo* multi-stepped progression we have inferred from epidemiologic, clinical, histologic, and biological observations.

In 1967, Huebner and Todaro put forth their "oncogene hypothesis" (76). They postulated, on the basis of much information that had accumulated since the studies of Peyton Rous, that there were genes present in all animal cells ("proto-oncogenes"), normally not expressed, that might be activated to induce neoplasia if triggered in some way by the genes of an oncogenic virus ("virogenes"). Throughout the 1970s, many investigators tried to marshal evidence that would support or refute the oncogene hypothesis. Early studies indicated that the known RNA-containing oncogenic viruses (retroviruses) of mice, chickens and other animals each contained one (or rarely two) specific oncogenic genes (13); some 30 unique oncogenic genes were eventually identified among the different animal retroviruses, and their nucleotide anatomy and gene products analyzed. Importantly, by the mid-1970s it was apparent that normal, unin-fected and untransformed animal cells contained DNA sequences that demonstrated at least some homology (by nucleic acid hybridization techniques) to the known retrovirus oncogenic genes (141).

New techniques that for the first time permitted the transfer of large DNA fragments into animal cells enabled the search for further evidence of cancer genes in animal and human cells. In these experiments, gene-sized pieces of DNA were extracted from human tumor cells and transferred to indicator cells *in vitro* by transfection (27). In this method, total cell DNA is extracted, fragmented physically or with restriction enzymes, and then layered onto a sheet of indicator cells in a Petri dish. In early studies, the calcium phosphate precipitation technique was usd to promote cell uptake of the tumor cell DNA fragments. The indicator cells used were NIH-3T3 mouse fibroblasts, a commonly used continuous cell line. Subsequent studies employed cloned human tumor cell genes for transfection. When DNA from normal human cells was transferred into the test cells, the NIH-3T3 cells were unaffected, but when DNA from human tumor cells was employed, the 3T3 cells became fully transformed, formed morphologic "tumor-foci," and induced tumors when inoculated in nude mice (85). Thus, genes exist in at least some human tumor cells which, upon transfer, can induce neoplastic behavior in at least some mammalian indicator cells. If such genes exist in normal human cells, they must not be expressed or activated. However, it is important to note that NIH-3T3 cells are already a continuous line, i.e., immortalized, or "partly transformed." NIH-3T3 cells do not form tumors when inoculated into nude mice, but morphologically and functionally, they behave as if in the early path toward full transformation. Thus, they are given a "coup de grace" by transfection with DNA taken from human tumor cells.

With the new and powerful techniques of molecular biology, one can analyze the human tumor DNA sequences that were transferred into NIH-3T3 cells, eventuating in their neoplastic transformation. With these methods, total DNA was extracted from the transformed mouse cells and digested with restriction endonucleases. The DNA fragments were separated by gel electrophoresis, cloned, transferred to nitrocellulose filters, and the human sequences hybridized to radioactive DNA or RNA probes of known origin. Autoradiography was then employed to determine if nucleic acid hybrids had in fact formed, i.e., if the human DNA extracted from the transformed mouse cells was homologous to any particular probe.

Investigators in several laboratories sought to learn if the transformation-inducing DNA sequences from human tumor cells, now called oncogenes, might correspond to the oncogenic genes of known retroviruses, and very quickly, it was found that indeed, this was the case – human oncogenes are homologous to genes present in the fast-transforming retroviruses of animals (38). However, most retroviruses found in nature are not fast-transforming viruses. Their linear genomes contain long repeated sequences of nucleotides at both termini which influence the mechanisms by which the DNA provirus is integrated into host chromosomal DNA and then expressed following infection. The rest of the genome contains genes that encode the proteins necessary for the virus to replicate itself: The *gag* gene which encodes internal, packaging proteins; the *pol* gene which encodes the reverse transcriptase with which the RNA genome synthesizes a DNA provirus copy of itself, and the *env* gene which encodes the viral envelope protein. The retroviruses which lack the capacity to rapidly transform animal cells contain no counterparts to cellular *onc* genes, but surprisingly, the genes in fast-transforming retroviruses which correspond to the oncogenes from human tumor cells also show extensive homology to genes cloned from normal cells (38). Of course, for some years prior to the human tumor DNA transfection experiments described above, it was known that normal animal cells contained DNA sequences with at least some homology to sequences in avian and murine oncogenic retroviruses (141).

From all of these data, the following picture has emerged: When retroviruses infect eukaryotic cells, they occasionally incorporate certain normal genes from these normal cells; these are the genes which are now termed "proto-oncogenes". In other words, the virus transduces the normal cell gene, analogous to the mechanism by which phage transduce genes from bacteria. After the normal *onc* gene is recombined into the viral genome, it may become altered structurally (by a base-pair change, addition, deletion, or inversion) such that it is still homologous, but no longer identical to the normal proto-oncogene. It appears that such alterations in the v(viral)-*onc* genes are necessary for "activation," i.e., for rapid transformation (38). In the course of transduction, the retrovirus has lost some of the genetic material responsible for the virus' ability to replicate itself, and in place of this material, the *onc* gene transduced from a normal animal cell has been inserted. When this retrovirus infects fresh cells, it transforms them rapidly, but cannot replicate without the presence of a "helper" virus, limiting its existence in nature (12). Thus, it appears that both in evolution and in contemporary events, retroviruses have been able to "fish" throughout the large and complex human genome and incorporate a small number of normal cellular genes which, when altered structurally and then reintroduced by the virus into fresh cells, rapidly induce malignant transformation. The retroviruses have thus spared us a "needle-in-the-haystack" search which might have taken us countless years to accomplish; the viruses have identified for us just those normal cell genes which when "activated" seem to be necessary, if not sufficient, for oncogenesis. Such a result must surely reflect the fact that oncogenes endow the virus with a tremendous survival advantage since the virus is now able to immortalize the cells that have been infected, permitting endless and economical replication (at least in the presence of helper virus).

The oncogenes which are expressed in human tumor cells did not arise from an exogenous retroviral infection, but were normal, unexpressed proto-onc cell genes initially. Later in the cell's lifespan, these genes may have suffered alterations similar to those found in the v-*onc* genes of fast-transforming retroviruses, but the activated oncogenes demonstrable in tumor cells may also simply be hyper-expressed without being mutated (27, 38). On the other hand, a common mechanism of oncogene activation may be chemical or physical carcinogen-induced mutations of the proto-oncogene or its regulatory sequences.

To summarize, activated *onc* genes are found in fast-transforming retro-viruses (v-*onc* genes) and in tumor cells, including human cancer (c-*onc* genes, or oncogenes). In both settings, activation implies that the genes are altered with respect to the structure and/or the expression of the same genes as they are found in normal cells, but where there are structural changes in the c-*onc* genes, these changes may not be identical to those found in v-*onc* genes. *Onc* genes in an active form have now been demonstrated, using the NIH-3T3 assay, in at least some samples (50–80%) from a wide diversity of primary human tumors and cell lines, including carcinomas of the bladder, lung, colon, pancreas, breast, and ovary; B and T cell lymphomas; acute lymphocytic and myelocytic leukemias; and neuroblastoma, sarcomas, melanomas, and gliomas (129). However, there are few specific correlations between any one c-*onc* gene and the type of malignancy with which it is associated. Virtually all of these tumor samples, if they do contain a detectably activated *onc* gene, reveal at least one particular family of *onc* genes, *ras*. The *ras* gene family is found in retroviruses isolated from rodent sarcomas, e.g., the Harvey, Kirsten, and Balb/c sarcoma viruses. Many human tumor samples reveal additional activated *onc* genes found in other animal retroviruses, e.g., the *myc* gene present in the chicken myelocytomatosis virus; the *src* gene present in the Rous chicken sarcoma virus; and the *mos* gene present in the Moloney murine sarcoma virus (129). Importantly, all normal vertebrate and invertebrate cells so far studied – including yeasts, sponges, fish, frogs, and drosophila – contain *onc* genes (11), as detected with appropriate probes. These genes, which reveal a high degree of homology even between totally unrelated species and are generally present in one copy per cell, are normally not consistently expressed and can not be detected in the NIH-3T3 test. However, it appears that they are transcribed transiently during normal embryogenesis (100), and in proliferative processes such as hematopoiesis, wound healing, and liver regeneration. All of these results are consistent with the hypothesis that these genes have evolved from a small number of critically important, and therefore highly conserved, ancestral sequences. Thus it seems likely that *onc* genes are necessarily, but transiently, expressed during cell differentiation, and/or cell proliferation; indeed, the term *onc* may be a misnomer for the normal and usual form of the gene, a historical accident merely reflecting the fact that such genes were first discovered in oncogenic viruses and cancer cells. Only when *onc* genes become constitutively activated, i.e., expressed in the wrong amount, at the wrong time, and/or in the wrong cell, are they associated with oncogenesis.

What mechanisms might permit expression of the *onc* gene excessively, at the wrong time, and/or in the wrong cell? One answer has become apparent with the demonstration of the human chromosomal loci of *onc* genes. More than 30 *onc* genes have been detected in transforming retroviruses and their homologues in animal or human cells. (With another 30 oncogenes found in cells but not in retroviruses, a total of 60 discrete oncogenes have been identified.) The c-*onc* genes in human tumor cells have been detected using the NIH-3T3 assay, so it is possible that with another indicator test, still more c-*onc* genes, not transduced by known retroviruses, might be found. Moreover, the *in vitro* assay detects "dominant-acting" genes, so that activated *onc* genes operating "recessively" would not be detectable. Nonetheless, a large amount of experimental data has accumulated within the past several years with very few new *onc* genes becoming apparent, so it seems likely that the total number of *onc* genes will remain limited. The known *onc* genes have often been named after the animal tumor-associated retroviruses with which they are homologous. All of the known *onc* genes have now been mapped to their chromosomal loci in various animal cells, including human chromosomal loci for those *onc* genes detectable in human cells (145). For example, the *src* gene has been mapped to human chromosome 20, the Ha-*ras*-1 gene to chromosome 11, the *myc* gene to chromosome 8, the *fes* gene to chromosome 15, etc. With this information in mind, the chromosomal sites of various activated c-*onc* genes have been determined in several human tumors (145). Many patients with Burkitt's lymphoma have a reciprocal chromosome translocation in their tumor cells, t8:14 (82). As discussed previously, the *myc* gene has been mapped to chromosome 8. A most extraordinary discovery was the finding that the fragment of chromosome 8 containing *myc* is the very fragment translocated to chromosome 14, and as a consequence of this reciprocal translocation, the *myc* gene is inserted within the Cμ immunoglobulin gene region of chromosome 14 (136). This is an area which is constantly being rearranged with respect to nucleotide architecture and is highly expressed virtually throughout the life of the B-lymphocyte, since this is the gene coding region responsible for the elaboration of antibody diversity. Thus, the normally unexpressed *myc* gene has now been moved into a highly expressed and highly rearranged gene region, and most investigators believe that this translocation and the consequent near-constitutive expression of the *myc* gene is associated intimately with the etiology and/or evolution of this lymphoma. The translocation itself may be a consequence of EBV infection, which might induce chromosome breakage and recombination. The *abl* and *sis* genes (Abelson murine leukemia virus and simian sarcoma virus) also have homologs in normal human DNA; they have been mapped to chromosomes 9 and 22, respectively (56). Since some patients with chronic myelocytic leukemia have a reciprocal 9:22 translocation, it is likely that these *onc* genes have been activated by translocation from normally quiet areas of one chromosome to highly active areas of the other. In some patients with acute myelocytic leukemia, an 8:21 translocation has occurred in the leukemic cells; the c-*mos* gene is normally found on chromosome 8. In Wilm's tumor, there is an especially interesting case, because the portion of chromosome 11 which is deleted consistently in this tumor is proximate to the Ha-*ras*-1 gene. However, while *ras* is very close to the deletion, it is not within it. A genetic element which normally suppresses *ras* may have been deleted, i.e., Wilms' tumor (and hereditary retinoblastoma) may result from homozygous ("two-step") deletion of "anti-*onc*" genes (101). Recently, other human tumors have been found to have deletions of "anti-oncogenes," genes which normally suppress oncogenes.

The frequent translocation of c-*myc* into the immunoglobulin loci in tumors of B-lymphocytes (and an analogous translocation in murine plasmocytomas) prompted Kirsch, et al. (81) to determine whether cancer-associated translocations in other cell types would also involve regions of the genome that encode important differentiation-specific products made by these cells. Indeed, cytogenetic analyses of human erythroleukemia cells revealed translocations within the regions where the genes that encode alpha- and beta-

globin reside. Yunis has published a human chromosome map (145), compiled from many sources, which demonstrates the chromosomal defects that are regularly associated with human tumors; the areas that are transcriptionally very active, e.g., those associated with immunoglobulin coding; "hot spots," i.e., regions that are unusually fragile and can easily be recombined or translocated to other chromosomes; and the loci of known *onc* genes. Although these map features are still preliminary, it is obvious that a synthesis of the data will reveal likely scenarios by which some external event – viral infection, a familial chromosome breakage syndrome (e.g., ataxia-telangiectasia, Bloom's syndrome or xeroderma pigmentosum), radiation, or a chemical carcinogen – might produce a genetic rearrangement or mutation which would activate an *onc* gene and yield a consistent association with a tumor.

Translocation into a highly active region of the genome is not, however, the only alteration that can activate an endogenous proto-*onc* gene. As noted previously, these genes can be activated in nature by incorporation between the controlling elements of a retrovirus and mutation, producing a highly oncogenic virus. Moreover, a normally unexpressed *onc* gene can be activated by inserting a retrovirus into the proximate cellular DNA: The controlling elements of the retrovirus can then promote *onc* gene expression, overriding the normal cell regulatory gene elements (65). Thus, mutations and other structural alterations are not the only route to *onc* gene activation: Expression of the normal gene in the wrong amount, at the wrong time, and/or in the wrong cell may suffice. It is even possible to activate an *onc* gene by ligating to it (*in vitro*) just the long terminal repeat sequences (containing transcription promotor elements) of a retroviral genome. C-*onc* genes may be mutated within the cell, as well as within a retrovirus, by a spontaneous base-pair mutation; in the case of the E-J human bladder cancer, the *ras* gene present in cells of that tumor has a single base substitution (usually at amino acid position 12, glycine $\rightarrow$ valine), but cells from uninvolved tissue of the same patient reveal no mutation in the *ras* gene (112). This single point mutation yields a gene product with a greatly altered steric configuration (108). Moreover, this same proto-*onc* gene mutation results from exposure to a chemical carcinogen (7). Therefore, specific somatic cell mutations (and possibly other structural alterations in the substance of the normal *onc* gene or its regulatory region) are sufficient to activate c-*onc* genes and endow them with transforming potential (i.e., a positive NIH-3T3 transfection assay). The same end may be achieved by gene amplification: The insertion of multiple copies of a normal proto-*onc* gene within an expressed region of the chromosome may lead to cellular transformation. The leukemia in Down's syndrome (trisomy 21) may reflect such an event. Thus, activation of a c-*onc* gene may occur because its expression is driven abnormally, or because DNA alterations have yielded an abnormal gene which is no longer responsive to normal transcription stop signals (and a gene product which may not function in an end-product inhibition pathway). Once again, activation implies that the *onc* gene product is made at the wrong time, in the wrong amount, and/or in the wrong cell. Whether the *onc* gene product is normal or abnormal, we should not necessarily anticipate a general hyper-expression in tumor cells, but rather a subtle activation on a cell-by-cell basis.

The intersection between normal growth and cancer

What are the products of *onc* genes? Here too, the preliminary answers are spectacular. The various *onc* genes so far identified, whether in cells or retroviruses, differ with respect to their products. The *ras* family of *onc* genes encodes a 21,000 dalton phosphorylated protein (on a threonine residue) that binds to trinucleotides (i.e., GTP), has phosphatase activity, and is located on the inner surface of the transformed cell membrane (p21) (12). In that location, it appears that these *onc* gene proteins influence the signal resulting from the binding of a growth-promoting ligand (e.g., growth factors or hormones) with its cell surface receptor. Another family of *onc* genes is represented by *src*; *src* products appear to be 60,000 dalton proteins (pp60^{src}) with an ATP-utilizing protein kinase activity (78); these enzymes phosphorylate tyrosine residues on other proteins, including other protein kinases, as well as autophosphorylate their own tyrosine residues. For example, these enzymes have been found to phosphorylate tyrosine residues within cyclic AMP. The *src* product is also located on the inner cell membrane. This biochemical and topographical description is very consistent with the possibility that these *onc* gene products may be associated with specific activation or inactivation of substrates, e.g., phospholipase A2, that have an essential role in promoting normal growth and division of cells and an anabolic cellular metabolism. The *myc* gene product, unlike the products of *ras* and *src*, is found within the nuclear matrix; the *myc* protein binds to DNA, and in this location, it may alter the configuration of the DNA and promote inappropriate and/or excessive transcription of proximate genes (including other *onc* genes) involved in cell growth and division (35). Alternatively, *myc* could influence DNA synthesis directly. Thus, *onc* gene products are of at least two broad types, some found at the cell surface, and some found within the nucleus.

Recently, it has been reported that the v-*sis* gene (the simian sarcoma virus *onc* gene) encodes a 20,000 dalton phosphorylated glycoprotein which is almost identical to one polypeptide chain of human platelet-derived growth factor (PDGF) (142). This important factor, which is normally elaborated during wound repair and stimulates fibroblast proliferation at the site of the wound, may thus be the specific product of the *sis* gene. With respect to human tumors, activated c-*sis* genes have been found in sarcomas and gliomas, tumors that contain cells of fibroblastic and other reticular origin. The normal homologues of such cells might be expected to elaborate PDGF. This factor binds to its receptor, and the ligand binding event activates the receptors's protein kinase domain, probably triggering a further phosphorylation cascade. In this regard, PDGF is similar to epidermal growth factor, insulin, transferrin, and the phorbol ester tumor promoters (which bind to and activate protein kinase C). All of these hormones, growth factors, and promoters affect cell shape, growth, and proliferation. The finding that the *sis* product is similar if not identical to PDGF is extraordinary, but consistent with the notion that c-*onc* genes are normal regulatory genes that transiently promote cell-cycle specific growth and proliferation as well as differentiation.

Finally, a recent report indicates that the v-*erb* B gene (present in the avian erythroblastosis virus) product is highly homologous to the inner (tyrosine kinase) domain of the EGF (epidermal growth factor) receptor (36). Thus, the truncated *erb* B product, inserted in the cell membrane just like the normal EGF receptor, probably deceives the cell into believing it is under constant stimulation by EGF, yet the cell does not respond to normal controls generated by ligand binding and release due to the absence of the receptor's outer ligand-binding domain. These results suggest strongly that the normal EGF receptor gene (i.e., the c-*erb B* or proto-oncogene) gave rise to v-*erb* B, and may be activated in some human tumors.

DNA oncogenic viruses probably also contain *onc*-like genes. Polyoma, SV40, and adenoviruses all have DNA sequences that may be the functional equivalent of the *onc* genes incorporated in retroviruses, but through millions of years of evolution, the oncogenic sequences in DNA viruses may have lost the same high degree of homology that retrovirus *onc* genes share with normal cellular *onc* genes. Transforming retroviruses survive only if accompanied in the infected cell by helper viruses since they are missing the gene products necessary to replicate themselves. However, DNA oncogenic viruses may have incorporated normal cell DNA sequences which then evolved *pari passu* with the viral genes proper. Moreover, most DNA oncogenic viruses are not defective and they are able to reproduce themselves in the absence of helper viruses. Thus, they are genetically stable and we cannot distinguish the cell sequence within DNA viral genomes in the same sense that we can distinguish sequences with homology to cellular sequences in the more recently and continuously arising transforming retroviruses. Despite this lack of significant homology, there is an interesting observation: The polyoma virus genome encodes a transforming, membrane-bound protein termed "middle T" antigen, and the middle T antigen protein appears to have homology with gastrin, the intestinal secretagogue. Gastrin is mitogenic for intestinal epithelial cells, and induces protein kinase C activity; polyoma middle-T also induces cellular protein kinase C activity, apparently to enable final virus protein modifications necessary for correct capsid geometry (5). Taking all of these data together, and mindful of the fact that all organisms from metazoa onward in the evolutionary scheme require external growth signals, a picture is emerging that both RNA and DNA viruses have incorporated normal eukaryotic gene sequences during infection; in the cell, these sequences may normally encode growth factors, growth factor receptor components (with or without kinase activity), "G" proteins (signal coupling molecules), DNA binding proteins or other proteins that regulate gene expression and DNA synthesis, and ultimately cell growth, proliferation and differentiation. When these gene products cannot be turned off, they may induce continuous cellular proliferation followed by transformation, and after subsequent stages in which further DNA lesions are sustained, eventuating in cancer.

In the NIH-3T3 transfection assay, one possible complication relates to the fact that these particular cells are already partially transformed. They grow in a low serum concentration and are immortalized, but do not induce tumors when inoculated in nude mice and are not anchorage-independent (85). Most investigators believe that this ambiguity may have clouded the interpretation of *onc* gene transfection experiments: Why is it not possible to transform primary cells, in addition to immortalized cells, with DNA from human tumors? In an attempt to address this question, several laboratories considered the notion that more than one *onc* gene may be needed for full transformation and tumorigenesis (86, 104). Perhaps *onc* genes complement one another. The NIH-3T3 cell line might already contain one activated *onc* gene, but a second *onc* gene, transferred from the human tumor cell, would be necessary to bring the mouse cell to a fully transformed oncogenic phenotype. A primary rodent cell, as opposed to a continuous cell line, would lack the first activated *onc* gene. To test this notion, transfection experiments were undertaken using different mix-and-match combinations of the various *onc* genes. Instead of using NIH-3T3, the cells used in these assays were primary cells, e.g., baby rat kidney cells which are not immortalized and which would ordinarily die out after just a few passages in tissue culture. These experiments revealed that when the primary rodent cells were transfected with only one activated c-*onc* gene, e.g., *ras*, no tumorigenic foci appeared. However, when a second activated c-*onc* gene, e.g., *myc*, was transferred to the primary cell, full transformation and tumorigenesis was obtained. Thus, normal primary cells that have not been "established" or "initiated" require two activated *onc* genes to induce the tumorigenic phenotype, in many ways analogous to the initiation and promotion steps of chemical carcinogenesis.

In studies on oncogene complementation, the indicator cell may be exposed to various representatives of the two complementation groups in any temporal order, unlike the initiator and promoter experiments of classical chemical carcinogenesis studies. However, it appears that representatives of one complementation group immortalize the cell (the "establishment" function) and representatives of the other complementation group then induce the full tumorigenic phenotype. Most of the human solid tumors so far tested contain an activated *onc* gene of the *ras* family (129), and we would put this gene in the second complementation group. In the first complementation group are the genes necessary for establishing the cells such that they are primed for the tumorigenic event; the *myc* gene (found in B-cell lymphomas) may be placed in this group. Moreover, other genes have been used in the mix-and-match experiments, including DNA virus sequences. For example, human adenovirus has an early region (transcribed from the viral genome immediately after the virus has infected a cell but prior to viral DNA replication), termed E1, which is necessary and sufficient for transformation (58). This early region comprises about 11% of the viral genome, and is subdivided into an A and a B region. Tumorigenic transformation of primary rodent cells is obtained by complementing the E1a region (related to *myc* structurally and probably sharing a common ancestral sequence) of the adenovirus genome with the E1b region (related to *ras*) of the same virus. Moreover, we can complement the large T antigen-coding region of the polyoma virus with the middle T antigen region of the same viral genome. We can complement certain *onc* genes that appear to encode growth factors (e.g., *sis* and PDGF) with physical or chemical carcinogens. We can even complement the N-terminal of the large T antigen-coding region of SV40 with the C-terminal coding region of the same gene. Genes and their products in the "establishment" complementation group appear to mediate events at the level of cellular DNA,

probably altering the configuration of DNA by binding to it and influencing DNA synthesis or activating enhancers of transcription (35). Cells transfected by genes in this group still look basically normal, i.e., flat and spindly, even though they have early stigmata of transformation, grow in soft agar, and have been immortalized (119). On the other hand, when we now add the second class of *onc* genes, which encode products located at the cell surface and appear to mediate signal transduction events, we obtain round, anchorage-independent, fully transformed and tumorigenic cells (104, 119). Genes of the *ras* type are mainly activated as a result of structural alterations; genes of the *myc* type may be activated as a result of inappropriate expression of the normal gene (84).

Onc genes appear to be activated transiently in certain normal cellular events. Several recent studies using nucleic acid hybridization analyses have revealed the expression of these genes during prenatal development of the mouse (100). Moreover, various *onc* genes appear to be turned on at different times and in different tissues during the developmental sequence. For example, the *fos* gene is expressed as a detectable mRNA transcript in embryonic tissues (especially bone) during the first week of development, but this mRNA is not detectable again until the third week. In contrast, the *abl* gene transcript is barely detectable in the first week, peaks at 10 or 11 days (especially in testis), and is barely detectable in the third week. The c-*ras* gene is strongly expressed throughout the first 3 weeks of development in all tissues. However, while there is some evidence of tissue specificity, there has as yet been no exclusive association between the expression of one *onc* gene and a specific cell type at a specific time, possibly due to the technical problems inherent in studying a homogeneous cell type during early embryonic development. A more selective model is the development of the neural retina. Here, the expression of c-*src* has been shown to be developmentally regulated, with expression increased in highly specific neuronal subsets during differentiation, but not proliferation (131). These data suggest very strongly that *onc* genes have a normal and specific role in cell differentiation and development. As noted earlier, the c-*ras* gene is also expressed during regenerative liver growth following hepatectomy, with the peak expression of c-*ras* mRNA occurring at about the time of peak DNA synthesis.

How might all of these data concerning *onc* gene expression in cancer and in normal development be synthesized so as to construct a reasonable model of oncogenesis? A facile scheme begins with a mature, terminally differentiated "inert" cell. This cell is flat and adherent, does not proliferate, and is on the pathway toward senescence and death. However, if *onc* genes of the c-*myc* complementation group are activated, e.g., by the t8:14 translocation in Burkitt's lymphoma, then a *myc*-like protein will be expressed which binds to the cell's DNA such that its conformation is changed and the cell is released from the DNA conformation and/or transcriptional regulation that normally characterizes end-stage differentiation. The cell may not demonstrate any detectable change in its differentiated phenotype morphologically, yet it can now proliferate once again. Such a cell is probably minimally dedifferentiated, since the evidence is strong that differentiation and proliferation are tightly and inversely linked cell processes –

terminally differentiated cells don't proliferate and proliferating cells are not terminally differentiated (9). Following the expression of the genes in group I, the cell is established (immortalized). Under the influence of the second complementation group (represented by the *ras* gene product), growth factors, growth factor receptor domains, coupling factors (e.g., the *ras*-regulated "G" proteins) and activated protein kinases further stimulate the cell to proliferate and to dedifferentiate. Again, reversal of the differentiated state is a necessary correlate of proliferative self-renewal. Since the expression of *onc* genes has been detected in normal developmental processes, the transient expression of these genes is not sufficient for oncogenesis, and we would anticipate their expression in the right cell, at the right time, and in the correct amount during normal embryogenesis, hematopoiesis, wound healing, and other events – at whatever age cell proliferation (and the appropriate differentiation stage) is required. In cancer however, these activated genes are expressed constitutively, i.e., they are expressed excessively, in the wrong cell, and/or at the wrong time. Their constitutive expression now promotes a continuing series of interdependent events, mediated by various *onc* products that together increasingly alter the control of the normal cell cycle at a biochemical level. Phosphorylation of the protein kinase domain of a growth factor receptor, as induced by ligand binding (or simulation of binding in the case of a truncated receptor), may well be the key lesion in the process, with the activated receptor kinase then phosphorylating a second kinase, etc., until a cascade of enzymatic (phosphorylation) perturbations occurs which lead to the cell becoming increasingly transformed and increasingly automitogenic – the cell acts as if it is elaborating its own growth factors, becoming independent of its environment, and not responding to the topoinhibitory stimuli of neighboring cells. It should be noted that phosphorylation by kinases is perhaps the cell's most common method for controlling the activities of many enzymes.

While the kinase phosphorylation cascade seems to have a critical role in the regulation of cell division and differentiation, the tyrosine kinase products of *ros* and *src* can phosphorylate membrane phosphatidyl inositol, thus increasing the formation of polyphosphoinositide and its hydrolysates that mediate signal transmission from several hormones, growth factors, and tumor promoters. Other kinases do not catalyze this reaction. Since there is a strong correlation between inositol lipid turnover and cell division, this association with *onc* genes is especially exciting, if proven to have a physiological role.

Following the initial biochemical changes in the cell, the cytoskeleton is disrupted, probably also by phosphorylation – dephosphorylation changes, and the cell, which was initially flat and stellate, now becomes round, refractile, and non-adherent. (In this regard, it is of interest that the products of two *onc* genes, *fms* and *fgr*, show some homology with cytoskeletal components.) At this point the cell is undifferentiated, and proliferates without control. In such a setting, the statistical likelihood of further DNA alterations becomes very high, and secondary, tertiary, and quaternary alterations and rearrangements of DNA – inversions, deletions, additions, point mutations, and translocations – become the rule. Other *onc* genes may be activated. The cells become invasive, there may be gene amplification (a

phenomenon often associated with tumor progression and drug resistance) and interestingly, down-regulation of various cellular immune targets may occur (e.g., certain domains of the MHC complex that ordinarily serve as the targets for immune surveillance and the host's rejection of transformed cells). In the absence of cell targets for immune surveillance, metastases may ensue.

In this facile scheme, it is again important to recognize that the processes of cell proliferation and differentiation are, in all likelihood, tightly linked, i.e., when the cell reaches its terminally differentiated phenotype, it ceases to proliferate, and when the cell becomes subtly dedifferentiated, it may proliferate once again. All of the steps discussed here are proposed to be interdependent, each step committing the next one, with most if not all of these differentiation-proliferation decisions mediated by *onc* gene products. Once again, the initial lesion may not only be a qualitatively abnormal *onc* gene product which precludes feed-back inhibition or yields an altered function, but may be a quantitative lesion that permits override of normal cell regulatory mechanisms, with the normal *onc* gene product then synthesized excessively, in the wrong cell, and/or at the wrong time. Finally, oncogenesis may not only reflect an *onc* gene dosage anomaly, but the loss of normal *onc* gene suppressor sequences. Indeed, both phenomena may be necessary.

Schrier and his colleagues (121) have shown that the non-oncogenic serotypes of adenovirus appear to up-regulate immune target structures, whereas SV40 and the highly oncogenic serotypes of adenovirus seem to down-regulate these immune targets. These data suggest strongly that the products of specific transforming virus genes may or may not promote the expression of host MHC molecules, and that cells transformed by viruses which do induce such MHC expression are not tumorigenic in immunologically competent hosts. This conclusion is especially interesting in view of the fact that morphologically, the non-oncogenic hamster cells transformed by adenovirus 2 appear to be very undifferentiated (90), whereas the highly oncogenic cells transformed by SV40 appear morphologically to be almost normally differentiated! This result suggests still another complex relationship between the state of cell differentiation, cell proliferation, immune surveillance, and tumorigenesis *in vivo*.

Thus, we have at hand the molecular tools to identify a presumably limited number of cell control genes which function in normal embryonic development and restorative processes later in life (88). We are developing a robust notion that when these genes are altered structurally, or the expression of their normal gene products is turned on inappropriately, they induce the steps that lead to cancer. We are beginning to identify the structure and function of *onc* gene products (growth factors, growth factor receptor components, DNA binding proteins, etc.), and can speculate as to how the various *onc* gene products may interrelate and interdepend on one another. Nonetheless, the true relationships and precise mechanisms are still obscure. Within the *onc* gene paradigm, there remain inconsistencies and themes which are not yet unified. The function of *onc* gene products within the cell and in the animal may prove far less tractable to study than the molecular genetics of the *onc* genes themselves. Even when we are able to illuminate the pathway of oncogenesis *per se*, we shall still require a far more profound understanding of immune surveillance and other mechanisms that govern tumor behavior, and we shall still need other model systems that will permit us to understand why tumor cells do or do not metastasize, or spontaneously regress.

As discussed previously, retroviruses, through evolutionary serendipity, have saved us uncountable years of "needle-in-the-haystack" searching for the few cellular genes that appear to be intimately associated with normal development and oncogenesis. Still, mammalian cells, with all of their genomic extent and complexity, may not be the most appropriate window for the views we now require. Recent studies in much simpler forms of life may be as, or more revealing, than studies in mammalian cells, at least with currently available techniques. For example, *Drosophila melanogaster*, the common fruit fly, has been of intense interest to geneticists since the classic experiments reported by Thomas Morgan and his colleagues on eye color. Studies on *Drosophila* were, of course, essential to developing the foundation for our modern understanding of genetics. Over the last several years, we have seen that *Drosophila* is also a very useful model for studies of normal growth and development at the level of molecular genetics. This fly has a limited number of chromosomes, and a comprehensible number of genes. We can identify the genetics of specific, complex, and spatial-temporal development patterns. All of these developmental programs have been mapped with respect to their genetic and molecular loci, and it will not be long before the genes and their products which regulate these complex developmental pathways are analyzed with respect to structure and function. How might one employ *Drosophila* further to define relationships between normal development and cancer? There are 5, 000 genes in the four polytene chromosomes of this organism. The genes are easily studied, since one chromosome band (as demonstrated by cytogenetic techniques) corresponds to one gene. Moreover, the generation time of *Drosophila* is ten days, and mutants are created readily. In another dramatic chapter of the rapidly unfolding *onc* gene story, Hoffman-Falk and her colleagues (74) discovered that the *Drosophila* genome contains *onc* genes (e.g., *src*, *ras*, *abl*) which are closely homologous to the *onc* genes found in human cells, appear to be necessary for early stages of fly embryogenesis, and may underlie *Drosophila* tumors. These genes have thus been conserved through 160–180 million years of evolution, and they seem to have the same critical role in the normal development of *Drosophila* that we believe they have in mammals, including humans – thus accounting for their extraordinary conservation. In *Drosophila* and its mutants however, we have a model that will undoubtedly permit far more rapid and incisive study of the complex relationships between *onc* genes, tyrosine-specific kinases, growth factors, growth factor receptors, etc., which we must understand if we are to make further progress in relating oncogenesis to developmental biology.

Several laboratories have now reported that yeasts (e.g., *S. cerevisiae*) also contain *onc* genes which are closely homologous to those found in retroviruses and in human cells (110), taking the evolutionary conservation of these genes even further backward in time. For example, the product of

one such yeast gene is 90% homologous to the human p21 *ras* protein between positions 3 and 183, which includes the region involved in tumorigenesis. Several of these genes have been shown to encode products with protein kinase activity which influence cell division and viability at a specific stage of the replicative and growth cycles of this organism, and yeasts have an exceptional attraction as a powerful genetic model, since genes can readily and precisely be inserted into (or deleted from) specific chromosomal loci of this organism (insertional mutagenesis). Thus, several classical and simple animal models, well-studied by developmental biologists and geneticists, now promise to reveal to us at an incisive and analytical level how *onc* genes may function in human cells with respect both to normal development and to oncogenesis.

Finally, the trans-genic mouse model has allowed an elegant proof of the role of oncogenes in cancer. In this model, a cloned gene, with the gene's regulatory sequence (transcription promoter) attached, is micro-injected into a fertilized mouse egg and the egg is implanted in a surrogate mother. The progeny have the foreign gene integrated in all cells, somatic and germ, and the gene is passed on in classical mendelian fashion. Using this method, the *myc* oncogene has been inserted with either an MMTV promoter (132) or an immunoglobulin promoter (1). The progeny develop breast cancer during pregnancy (i.e., the MMTV promoter is turned on by hormones) in the first case, and B-cell lymphomas in the second – demonstrating not only that cancer results from over-expression of a normal proto-oncogene, but that the cell factors that bind to and turn on the promoter sequences are cell-specific.

The origins of cancer treatment

Together with attempts to describe and explicate cancer, there occurred an evolution in the treatment of evident tumors (87), surgery of course being the oldest therapy. Until the late 18th century, surgical techniques in cancer patients reflected the limitations of descriptive anatomy and physiology. The concept of the wide if not radical resection – which was the cornerstone of surgical therapy for cancer until recent developments in radiation therapy and chemotherapy appeared to lessen the need for radical operations – was first articulated in the late 19th century by Moore and Halsted (63). The present century has been characterized by increasingly sophisticated organ specific cancer operations which respect the known biology and natural history of malignant disease in those sites. Moreover, modern surgical oncology has emphasized the preservation of function and, in young patients, normal growth, with an extraordinary diversity of "high technology" prostheses now available, and considerable attention paid to postsurgical metabolism and the influence of chemotherapy on wound healing. Historically, the management of cancer was in the hands of surgeons, and even within this generation, one of the most important contributions to modern cancer treatment was that of a British surgeon, Dennis Burkitt, who in 1952, perceiving an "experiment of nature," described and defined the most common cancer of African children, demonstrated its unique geographic distribution (with important etiologic implications), and became one of the first to cure patients with an advanced cancer using drugs (cyclophosphamide) alone (18).

Radiation therapy is a far more recent development in the history of cancer treatment than surgery. Its entire history, beginning with the discoveries of Roentgen, Bequerel, and Curies, does not extend for much more than 80 years. The earliest radiation therapists were, in fact, dermatologists and surgeons and they employed this treatment in single massive exposures analogous to surgical extirpation. As a consequence, the benefits of this therapy were often nullified by its major complications, and there was little understanding of the physical nature of irradiation. Dose fractionation was described in 1920 by Regaud and Coutard; these workers reported durable relapse-free survival in patients with tumors that had never before been cured (113). The development of the kilovoltage apparatus led to still greater success, at least in the treatment of superficial tumors. However, it was not until after World War II, with the development of megavoltage equipment such as the linear electron accelerator, that it became relatively easy to deliver tumoricidal doses to neoplasms deep within the body (122). Megavoltage equipment also circumvented the severe skin reactions induced by low energy beams, but at the same time permitted large fields to be treated, as in the management of malignant lymphomas. As with Halsted's linking of his insight regarding the biology of carcinoma of the breast to his development of radical mastectomy, so did the radiotherapist link his new understanding of the natural history of malignant lymphomas to the conceptual development of extended field or total lymphoid radiotherapy (79). A wide variety of radiation sources are currently employed and with this armamentarium, there is little question that the role of radiotherapy is as established as that of surgery as a curative treatment for many tumors. Radiotherapy appears to hold still further promise as studies at the molecular level improve our understanding of the biology of this modality. In particular, recognition that the radiosensitivity of mammalian cells depends on their state of oxygenation (55) has suggested the possibility that the ratio of tumor to normal cell injury can be increased importantly with radiosensitizers and/or radioprotectors. Modified fractionation schemes, total body or total nodal radiation, hyperthermia, and intraoperative radiation therapy are all new techniques (or new applications of established techniques) likely to enhance the utility of radiotherapy to a still greater degree. Deep lesions (e.g., gliomas, truncal sarcomas, retinoblastoma) should be more approachable with less toxicity using new particle beam equipment (neutrons, heavy ions, protons, negative pi mesons). Moreover, the integration of CT scanning with simulation permits treatment planning in three dimensions and optimal joining of fields, increasing the antitumor benefit while minimizing irreversible sequellae. PET (positron-emission tomography) scanning, which assesses metabolic activity as well as anatomy, offers even more precision regarding identity of the tumor target, especially in the central nervous system. NMR (nuclear-magnetic resonance) imaging is the most recent development for whole-body definition of the tissue to be radiated, and its resolution is so extraordinary that the use of invasive diagnostic tests is rapidly declining. In most circumstances, however, the ultimate utility of radiotherapy, as with surgery,

will be in conjunction with adjuvant chemotherapy, which is implicit in Galen's concept that cancer is a systemic disease.

The development of effective drugs

Since it has become clear that cancer is often a systemic disease at the time of diagnosis, with clinically undetectable micrometastases already present at the time of local treatment, it is evident that systemic chemotherapy should have a profound role in cancer treatment. Of all patients with cancer, surgery and/or radiation are curative in 30%, but with the advent of systemic chemotherapy in addition to local treatment, the cure rate has risen to more than 40% and promises to reach 50% shortly (31). These data, of course, include patients of all ages and with all tumor types.

The first antitumor drug to be described in the literature was colchicine (125) and, while it was not curative, the fact that it did cause tumors to regress was commented on repeatedly from the first century through the 1930s. Between 1850 and 1950, a number of benzol and arsenic-containing compounds were studied, particularly in chronic myelocytic leukemia (CML). Arsenicals indeed appeared to have some tumoristatic effect but, perhaps prematurely, arsenic-containing drugs fell into disuse. Benzol was abandoned because of its toxicity. Shortly after the beginning of World War II, Haddow and his colleagues discovered the antitumor effects of urethane, particularly (as with benzol and arsenicals) in CML (61). At about the same time, it became clear that several hormones played a role in the therapy of breast and prostate carcinoma (77), but the only hormones shown to be useful in the treatment of cancer in childhood were the corticosteroids (45). Thus, by the end of World War II, it was apparent that a variety of drugs, chemicals and hormones could cause regression of human cancer. Moreover, by this time, the availability of inbred strains of mice with implanted tumors permitted the development of predictive preclinical screening systems of clinically active agents (148).

During and after World War II, drugs with truly curative potential were discovered. The first of these drugs was the alkylating agent, nitrogen mustard, the antitumor properties of which were noted by investigators at Yale, first in mice and then in patients with lymphomas (51). Many other alkylating agents have subsequently been developed, but nitrogen mustard is still used. The other major alkylating agent which can be defined as a curative drug is cyclophosphamide, developed in 1958 (31, 87). This drug is particularly important in the treatment of childhood cancer.

A second class of curative drugs comprises the folate antagonists. The development of these drugs followed upon the observations that folic acid accelerated the leukemic process. Metabolic antagonists to folic acid were developed at Lederle as a consequence of these and other observations, and in 1947, Farber reported temporary remissions in acute childhood leukemia produced by aminopterin (44). In 1949, methotrexate (amethopterin) was developed and replaced aminopterin because of its better therapeutic index. In the mid 1950s, methotrexate was shown to be exceptionally effective (and often curative) in a solid tumor, choriocarcinoma (91), and ten years later, a great wave of interest in high-dose methotrexate therapy for other solid tumors occurred after Djerassi introduced the notion of leukovorin rescue (33). For reasons that are still not entirely clear, normal cells can more readily be "rescued" from the lethal effects of high-dose methotrexate by folates than can tumor tissue, and the optimal methotrexate dose can be adjusted individually on the basis of blood levels. Unfortunately, many tumors become resistant to methotrexate, and this resistance has stimulated much recent work on general mechanisms of drug resistance, e.g., gene amplification (in the case of methotrexate, the gene encoding dihydrofolate reductase is amplified under selective pressure, and the excess enzyme rapidly inactivates the drug) (2).

Another of the important discoveries of curative drugs is that of the purine antimetabolite, 6-mercaptopurine (6-MP). This drug was specifically designed by Hitchings and Elion as a result of their biochemical reasoning relating the structure of compounds in the purine and pyrimidine pathways to the potential of antagonists for antitumor activity (73). Following the synthesis of a number of such compounds and their testing in animal tumor models, Burchenal in 1953 established the clinical activity of 6-MP in acute lymphocytic leukemia (21).

A final class of the "pioneer" chemotherapeutic agents is that of the antibiotics, the first of which to be described was actinomycin D. A series of actinomycins was first prepared by Waxman and Woodruff in 1940 and the clinical activity of actinomycin D was demonstrated in children with metastatic Wilms' tumor by Farber in 1956 (43). It is currently used not only in Wilms' tumor but in Ewing's tumor and rhabdomyosarcoma as well.

Following the demonstration that guinea pig serum (known to contain L-asparaginase) caused mouse tumors to regress, this enzyme became the first of a class of curative enzymes to be used in the clinic. The effectiveness of *E. coli* L-asparaginase in man was shown first by Hill and his colleagues in 1967 (72), and it is among the most useful drugs at present for the treatment of acute lymphocytic leukemia.

Between 1945 and 1955, much interest in and enthusiasm for cancer chemotherapy developed, although skepticism and hostility to what was then considered such therapeutic venturism prevailed. Organized drug development programs were initiated at a number of institutions throughout the world, and rodent tumor systems were widely employed to assess drug activity. In 1955, the National Cancer Institute (NCI) created the Cancer Chemotherapy National Service Center which, for the first time, reflected the elements of a national program in chemotherapy development. At about this time as well, there developed the notion of large, highly organized clinical trials in cancer treatment, particularly with respect to the infrequently occurring tumors of the young. It was soon appreciated that there would be need for considerable cooperation between institutions in order to generate meaningful drug response data in children. The first such collaboration was formed between Roswell Park and the NCI in 1954, which later developed into Leukemia Group B. Cooperative groups have, since 1960, carried out the majority of clinical trials in cancer patients in the United States and elsewhere. The success of the cooperative group approach has occurred *pari passu* with the emergence of the statistician/biometrician as an integral member of the clinical research team. The contribution of this investigator to our understanding of the necessity for rigorous study design, feasibility studies, and validation tests cannot be questioned. The large cooperative trials that require such an important analytic contribution indeed complement other studies undertaken in single institutions with access to special expertise or resources or to a unique patient population.

Over the past 30 years, additional classes of drugs, each having some importance in the treatment of cancer patients, have been described with an accelerating frequency. The vinca alkaloids were described and assessed by a number of workers in 1955–1960; vincristine was shown to have marked activity in acute lymphocytic leukemia in 1962 by Karon et al. (80). In 1964, Selawry and Frei found that the combination of vincristine and prednisone produced a very high and rapid induction of complete remission in ALL (123); the therapeutic effect was clearly additive, with no increment in the independent toxicities of the two drugs. This was a singularly important observation in the history of cancer chemotherapy, because it provided the rational basis for all future curative combination chemotherapy regimens.

Among the lymphomas and solid tumors, Hodgkin's disease has shown a useful response to procarbazine, a monoamine oxidase inhibitor discovered in 1963 (147), CNS tumors to nitrosoureas (e.g., BCNU), and sarcomas to DTIC, an imidazole carboxamide. More recently developed and widely used drugs include cytosine arabinoside, daunomycin, adriamycin, and cis-platinum diamminedichloride. The most important activity of cytosine arabinoside is in acute myelocytic leukemia (42); its use in that disease, together with an anthracycline, is responsible for the fact that a rapidly increasing number of patients with this disease are being cured (41). It is also of great interest because of its very specific killing effect upon cells in the S phase of DNA synthesis. Because of this phase-specific activity, it is of particular importance in cell kinetic studies. Daunorubicin was discovered in 1963 as a result of the interest of pharmaceutical companies in *Streptomyces* antibiotics (37). It was shown to be effective in childhood leukemia by Tan et al. in 1965 (135); subsequently, a congener of daunorubicin, adriamycin (4), was shown to have a much broader spectrum of activity, including solid tumors as well as hematologic neoplasia. Regrettably, the anthracyclines are cardiotoxic, possibly due to their generation of free radicals in the heart tissue (which lacks a free radical defense system); in an NCI study, 50% of patients receiving adriamycin as an adjuvant for sarcoma treatment later developed significant electrocardiographic abnormalities (53). Noncardiotoxic congeners or "rescue" agents are clearly needed before the full potential of this class of drugs can be realized.

Rosenberg and his colleagues discovered cis-platinum diamminedichloride in 1965 while studying the effects of electric fields on bacteria – an object lesson in the proximity of basic research to the bedside (115)! Testicular tumors are now largely curable because of cis-platinum (31, 87), and neuroblastoma, brain tumors, and osteosarcoma have shown significant response rates to this agent. It is likely that new combinations, e.g., cytosine arabinoside and cis-platinum, will yield synergistic activity, and a platinum "rescue" agent could improve the therapeutic ratio.

Other important antitumor agents include 5-fluorouracil, bleomycin, 5-azacytidine and the more recently described m-AMSA (31, 87). The first of these drugs is important in the treatment (although non-curative) of gastrointestinal malignancies, the second in lymphomas, and the latter two are still undergoing clinical study. 5-azacytidine and m-AMSA are effective in relapsed AML; whether their use in premier regimens will significantly enhance the duration of first remission is not yet known.

While evidence was clear from the 1940s onward that systemic chemotherapy would induce tumor regression, the first proof that chemotherapy could cure metastatic disease came when Li and Hertz, employing an intermittent schedule of methotrexate, were able to cure patients with metastatic choriocarcinoma (70). The next proof of cure of metastatic disease occurred in Burkitt's lymphoma. This tumor, as noted previously, is of singular interest in oncology because of the extraordinary opportunities it offers to students of tumor etiology, biology, epidemiology, immunology, and therapy. In the 1960s, Burkitt and his colleagues reported on the remarkable sensitivity of this tumor to cyclophosphamide (19). Ziegler, and later Magrath, continued the studies initiated by Burkitt; in a follow-up report, Ziegler et al. reported that 40% of 200 Ugandan patients were cured of Burkitt's lymphoma with chemotherapy, the minimum follow-up being 10 years (146). Results in American patients are at least this good and rapidly improving.

Combinations of drugs

The role of single agents in inducing transient remission in acute lymphocytic leukemia (ALL) has already been described. However, cures of disseminated malignancy with single agents have only been possible in choriocarcinoma and Burkitt's tumor. In fact, childhood ALL has been the single most important model in the development of new principles leading to the cure of cancer, not only with respect to remission-inducing chemotherapy regimens, but with regard to the mathematic implications of the difference between remission induction and remission maintenance, the role of pharmacologic sanctuaries as a nidus for relapse, and the importance of prolonged maintenance treatment. Although these principles were inferred from the results of clinical trials, the appropriate inferences probably could not have been made had there not been developing, at the same time, a body of information generated in murine leukemia (and mammary carcinoma) by Skipper, Schabel, Mendelsohn, Bruce and others regarding the relation of cell kinetics to curability (31, 87). With respect to acute lymphocytic leukemia, the notion arose that single drugs were bringing about only a few logs of cell kill, whereas 12 logs of leukemic cells would have to be killed if, in fact, one remaining viable cell could eventuate in relapse. Such observations as those of Frei et al. that 6-MP plus methotrexate produced a greater percentage of complete remission than either drug alone (47), and Selawry and Frei that vincristine and prednisone was a very active combination for remission induction (123), led to the concept that drugs may have differing molecular targets and differing toxicities and that two drugs could, therefore, be combined to give twice the tumor cell kill with less than twice the damage to bone marrow and other normal tissues. The first multiagent chemotherapy regimen tried in ALL was VAMP (vincristine, amethopterin, mercaptopurine, and prednisone) which, because of the high

rates and prolonged durations of complete remissions achieved, demonstrated in the early 1960s that total cell kill had for the first time been approached (48). The biggest obstacle in the treatment of childhood ALL remaining after the development of systemic combination chemotherapy was the occurrence of meningeal relapse, apparently resulting from the fact that the drugs employed for systemic treatment did not achieve tumoricidal concentrations in the central nervous system, with the result that residual meningeal foci induced many late relapses. With the evidence that irradiation of the cranial-spinal axis, as well as intrathecal methotrexate, had some efficacy in overt meningeal leukemia, it was not long before "prophylaxis" of CNS leukemia was introduced as a consistent part of the initial treatment of this disease (109). The remarkable cure rate resulting from the use of systemic combination chemotherapy and "prophylactic" treatment of the central nervous system is one of the great dramas of modern medicine (87).

Early treatment successes with the VAMP regimen in childhood leukemia led quickly to the exploration of drug combinations in adult lymphomas. Frei and his colleagues began to study drug combinations in Hodgkin's disease in 1963. The MOPP regimen, consisting of nitrogen mustard, vincristine, prednisone, and procarbazine, was the result of these efforts; as reported by DeVita, Serpick and Carbone, this regimen produced an exceptionally high complete remission rate in patients with advanced stages of Hodgkin's disease (32). Ten-year follow-up leaves no doubt that in 70–80% of patients, the MOPP regimen has achieved cure of this disease; a considerable number have been cured even with the most advanced stages.

The curative results of nonlymphomatous solid tumors by chemotherapy alone have not been as impressive as the results in the hematologic neoplasms. The leukemias and lymphomas are usually rapidly growing tumors with large growth fractions, whereas nonlymphomatous solid tumors usually are slowly growing and have small growth fractions. However, in those solid tumors that do have large growth fractions, cure has been possible in children as well as in adults. Choriocarcinoma has already been mentioned in this regard, and a very significant number of patients with metastatic testicular carcinoma are now being cured with chemotherapy alone (40). In the case of the metastatic solid tumors of young patients, there are some data that drugs alone may be curative. However, the majority of clinical trials have employed treatment of the primary tumor and metastases with surgery and/or radiation followed by chemotherapy. Important results in this regard include the cure of metastatic Wilms' tumor by Farber using drugs plus radiation (43), and the cure (albeit rare) of patients with metastatic Ewing's sarcoma using high doses of chemotherapy and total body irradiation (87). This approach, i.e., supra-intensive chemoradiotherapy with maximum supportive care (e.g., autologous or allogeneic marrow "rescue") for tumors that are resistant to standard doses of treatment but may show a linear dose-response curve, is now being tested rather widely in pediatric and adult malignancies, including those of brain, testes, ovary, and lung, as well as lymphoma. Even with more conventional chemotherapy regimens, a significant number of patients with disseminated ovarian carcinoma experience long-term survival with combination chemotherapy and local treatment, as do a significant number of patients with metastatic embryonal rhab-domyosarcoma (87). However, the evidence that available chemotherapy has an important role in inducing long-term survival of adults with other metastatic solid tumors, especially the most common ones (e.g., lung, breast, gastrointestinal), or of young patients with metastatic osteosarcoma, metastatic neuroblastoma (beyond infancy), or CNS tumors is lacking.

The combination of chemotherapy with surgery and radiotherapy: adjuvant treatment

One of the most important conceptual developments in the history of cancer treatment is that of adjuvant chemotherapy (20). In the adjuvant setting, chemotherapy is not only used to kill any residual tumor cells at the primary site, but metastases that are clinically undetectable (micrometastases) as well. In other words, the rationale of adjuvant therapy is based on the assumption that a given tumor has already metastasized when the primary site first becomes apparent. This assumption follows from what is known of the natural history of specific tumor types. For practical purposes, this development can be said to have taken on a clinical reality when children with Wilms' tumor were given actinomycin D as well as local treatment (43). In 1967, Burgert et al. showed in a randomized trial that patients receiving this drug and irradiation after surgery for the primary tumor had a 2-year survival rate of 90% compared to 45% among those receiving surgery and irradiation only (22). In 1969, the National Wilms' Tumor Study Group was formed and has, since its inception, authored studies which continue to be among the most elegantly designed cooperative clinical trials. In 1976, D'Angio et al., reporting for this group, demonstrated the superiority of actinomycin D plus vincristine as an adjuvant compared to either alone, thus extending the concept of combination chemotherapy to the adjuvant setting (29). The notion of adjuvant chemotherapy given at the earliest possible time after, or in tandem with local treatment, is extremely important for kinetic reasons as well as for reasons of drug resistance: Micrometastases are younger than the primary tumor and usually have larger proliferative fractions, both of which phenomena possibly make them more sensitive to chemotherapy than the primary tumor and more susceptible to complete cell kill.

Other tumors shown to enjoy high cure rates through the use of combined modality treatment and adjuvant regimens include embryonal rhabdomyosarcoma, Ewing's sarcoma, and ovarian carcinoma. Moreover, osteogenic sarcoma, a particularly lethal tumor of young people, with less than a 20% survival rate historically, is increasingly curable with surgery and adjuvant chemotherapy (87). The great success of the adjuvant approach in the treatment of pediatric malignancies has led directly to the use of such regimens in the common adult malignancies, e.g., carcinoma of the breast with early node involvement (i.e., micrometastases to one or two proximal lymph nodes), and results to date indicate that the lives of many thousands of women with disseminated breast cancer are being saved with adjuvant regimens (31).

The era of chemotherapy is still very new, and we have a still imperfect understanding of when and how to use the available drugs to maximum advantage. The concept of dose to the tumor, rather than systemic dose, is only now being reflected in clinical trials (e.g., intraperitoneal chemotherapy for ovarian carcinoma). Moreover it is only very recently that *in vitro* assay of fresh tumor for drug sensitivity (analogous to antibiotic sensitivity testing) has become a possibility (120). Also recently developed are human tumor xenografts in nude mice, and the rodent renal capsule assay for human tumors, both yielding information of possibly greater clinical relevance than that of rodent tumor screens. The new science of "molecular pharmacology" can also be expected to contribute in a major way to further advances, with its synthesis of molecular biology (e.g., alkaline elution, dichroism of DNA, and other methods that examine DNA-drug interactions directly) and classical pharmacologic methods. Since most cancer therapy works at the level of macromolecular events and targets (e.g., DNA and RNA synthesis), this methodologic synthesis is particularly germane to the rational design of structural analogs and to the discovery of primary mechanisms of action. As the reader explores those chapters of this text which describe newer concepts of drug sensitivity and resistance, as well as conceptual advances in the explication of cell kinetics and tumor cell biology in general, it will be apparent that we are in fact still at the beginning of the chemotherapy era, and the full potential of this era seems yet to be realized.

Drug resistance

Whatever the etiologic agent of malignant transformation, it is clear that a single viable cancer cell may give rise to a fatal cancer cell population in an appropriate host. The observation by Furth and Kahn in this regard, using murine leukemia as a model, represents a milestone in the evolution of our understanding of cancer biology and treatment (49). The knowledge that survival of one or a few neoplastic cells may result in treatment failure was part of the evidence that led to the development of the concept that a given dose of drug will kill the same fraction, but not the same number, of tumor cells in populations with widely varying size – assuming that the dose concentration within the tumor, the growth fraction, and the ratio of drug sensitive to drug resistant cells in these variously sized populations remain the same. The growth fraction concept derives in large part from the work of Mendelsohn (94), with this fraction simply defined as the proportion of proliferating cells within a population.

Since one viable tumor cell remaining after remission induction may eventuate in relapse, it is essential that an understanding be gained as to why such cells survive. In some situations, e.g., large masses of solid tumor, only a relatively small percentage of the cells are in the mitotic cycle at any given time, as recently confirmed by flow microfluorometry studies. Clearly, cells that are not in cycle will be refractory to alkylating agents and will remain viable so long as the cells do not attempt DNA replication. While rapidly growing neoplasms have higher growth fractions than slowly growing neoplasms, this is not uniformly the case; however, the growth fraction of the tumor (as well as that of normal stem cells) can be altered – often favorably – by prior treatment with radiation or cytotoxic drugs (16). Moreover, tumor cell loss may have a profound effect on tumor growth rate and potential doubling time of the remaining tumor cells, whatever the cause. Thus, drug resistance for reasons of cell kinetics may be reversible. On the other hand, it has become increasingly apparent that drug-resistant cancer cells continually arise (with selective pressure) from mutations, much as in phage-resistant and drug-resistant bacterial cell populations. Indeed, selection and overgrowth of such drug-resistant cells appears to be a major cause of chemotherapeutic failure in cancers that initially respond to drugs but later resume growth in the face of continuing treatment with the same drugs. Therefore, drug resistance can occur for at least two reasons: Tumor cells may be refractory to many drugs while resting, but when they revert to the cycle of DNA replication, they again become drug-sensitive. In contrast, the biochemical variants of tumor cells which are selected and overgrow during treatment are heritably resistant and usually retain this specific resistance for the life of the cell (and all of its progeny) with no further drug exposure. This type of resistance usually occurs only to the drug or drugs that selected such mutants, although in the case of some drug properties, e.g. lipophilia, the resistance spectra may include drugs with widely varying structures, e.g., adriamycin and the vinca alkaloids, both of which are lipophilic but otherwise unrelated. With regard to biochemical resistance, these notions imply that treatment failure begins very much in advance of the clinically apparent selection of a subline that is composed solely of drug-resistant tumor cells. Evidence supports the idea that when as little as 10% of the tumor cell mass has become resistant, i.e., while the bulk of the tumor may still be responding, treatment failure is already at hand (128). Such notions may explain early relapse after seemingly complete remission; however, if chemotherapy is switched at a propitious time, a significant number of "near cures" might be converted to a significant number of "cures."

Several new and interesting refinements are at hand, both with respect to "kinetic" resistance and "genetic" resistance. It has long been intriguing that certain tumors, e.g., the lymphomas, may be treated to the point of complete remissions yet recur in the same site with retained sensitivity to the initial therapy. This observation is not consistent with the concept that small tumors are more sensitive to treatment and, in fact, suggests that as the tumor bulk is decreased by the initial therapy, the tumor may become more resistant to treatment with respect to the dose-response relationship. Norton and Simon (105) have proposed an alternative view of the relation between drug dosage and tumor size using the following equation to describe the general case of growth rate for an untreated tumor: $GR = GF \times V$, where GR is the growth rate, V is the tumor volume at any given time, and GF is the instantaneous growth fraction. These authors use GF to mean the total number of cells in mitosis, but incorporate in the term the cell loss associated with cell death or other removal processes. Most tumors grow exponentially but, as their size increases, growth decreases exponentially (due to insufficient supply of nutrients, etc.) so that a plateau size is reached. In this "Gompertzian" pattern of growth, GF is not constant but is proportional to the logarithm of the ratio of ideal plateau size to tumor volume at a given time. In the Gompertzian growth pattern, the growth rate is smallest both for very small and very large tumors, and is maximum at an inflection point when the tumor is approximately one-third of its maximum size. It should be emphasized that for this type of growth, a large GF does not necessarily imply a high GR. The log-kill

hypothesis of Skipper et al., previously detailed, is certainly applicable to exponential tumor growth, with a given dose of drug killing the same percentage of cells no matter the tumor size. However the alternative view of Norton and Simon is that the growth-inhibiting effect of the treatment is proportional to the growth rate of an untreated tumor, with the growth rate approaching zero when the tumor is either very large or very small. These authors thus propose that sensitivity to therapy, in terms of rate of regression for a given dosage, would decrease with decreasing tumor size, even though GF may be increasing. This does not necessarily mean that a small tumor is less curable than a large one; although its rate of regression may be smaller, it is also closer to the limiting volume beyond which regrowth cannot occur. This view suggests that a drug dose which may cause a dramatic rate of regression in an intermediate-size tumor may be insufficient to cure a very small tumor, and leads to the proposal that therapy should remain intensive when remission is achieved – exactly the converse of many current chemotherapy regimens.

With respect to the relationship between the drug sensitivity of tumors and mutations toward phenotypic drug resistance, new concepts are also evolving. The development of resistance mutants within a tumor is surely as important as the kinetic processes previously detailed. Although we have earlier discussed the selection of resistant mutants as a consequence of drug exposure, there is substantial evidence suggesting that drug-resistant mutants in mammalian tumor cells may also arise by a process analogous to that seen in microbial populations, i.e., drug-resistant phenotypes arise spontaneously (with no selective pressure) and with a definite frequency independent of any potential selecting agent. The mean size of the resistant population relates to the total tumor size; this relationship was first derived by Luria and Delbruck in their classic paper on mutations to resistance in bacterial populations (92). Goldie and Coldman have developed a compelling mathematic model which suggests that as tumor size increases, the probability of resistant clones increases (52), and thus for reasons quite independent of growth kinetics, we would expect increasing resistance to treatment with increasing tumor size. The development of a resistant clone by any group of tumors is a random event and the time for it to occur will be a function of the growth curve of the tumor and the mutation rate. However, the required log increase in growth is independent of the growth curve, indicating that at certain times in the growth of a tumor population, there is a period in which its susceptibility to chemotherapy changes rapidly. The higher the mutation rate, the earlier in the growth of the tumor this transition will occur. Since this interval constitutes a relatively brief proportion of the tumor's total growth history, brief delays in institution of therapy during this critical transition time may seriously compromise the efficacy of the therapy. Thus, in the model of Goldie and Coldman, the expectation of cure of cancer is a function of the spontaneous mutation rate toward resistance – an intrinsic property of the tumor – and the size the tumor has reached from the initial transformation to the time when therapy begins. Tumors early in their growth history can be expected, on stochastic grounds alone, to have a much better likelihood of cure than tumors which have reached an advanced stage.

A therapeutic paradigm which would synthesize the concepts derived from the reasoning of cell kinetics, as well as those derived from models of mutational drug resistance, suggests the importance of (a) switching chemotherapeutic agents at an early point in time in the hope that resistance, if it has begun to develop, remains narrow, and (b) the use of maximally tolerable doses of drugs, particularly as the tumor mass become very small. The early use of sequential, alternating high-dose combinations of non-crossresistant agents should have the effect of reducing the unfavorable impact of both kinetic and mutational phenomena.

Tumor immunology and immunotherapy

The previous discussion of tumor biology and strategies for treatment has largely been taken up with the notions of cell "kinetic" resistance and primary (heritable) biochemical drug resistance. However, even cells that have become resistant to drugs might be damaged or killed by the immune system. While interest in tumor immunology has been explosive in recent times, the ultimate contributions of this field to tumor treatment can be only vaguely perceived at the moment. The concept that tumors possess antigens not found on normal cells was advanced by Gross in 1943, who found that tumors failed to develop following intradermal injection of a small number of tumor cells into mice of the strain in which the tumor had arisen (60). Those injected mice could thenceforth reject a much larger tumor cell inoculum, one usually lethal in normal, unprotected mice. Thus, it was established that tumors could immunize the host in which they arose, and the unique antigens responsible for such immunity came to be known as tumor-specific transplantation antigens (TSTA). In these and other mouse experiments, normal tissues of the primary tumor host could not induce the immunity, and tumor-immune mice could not reject normal tissues of the donor, i.e., the responsible antigens did not appear to be detectable on normal tissues.

Subsequent study has indicated that tumor immunity is a type of cell-mediated immunity in most cases, similar to the phenomenon involved in rejection of genetically incompatible normal tissues (83). Another area of similarity between allograft immunity and tumor immunity involves the phenomenon of immunologic enhancement, i.e., the process by which, in some circumstances, pre-immunization with tumor tissue eventuates in enhanced tumor growth (8). The possibility of enhancement has, in fact, caused a continuing apprehension that efforts to practice immunotherapy against tumors might actually lead to immunologic acceleration of tumor growth. In any event, the concept that cell transformation is not identical to oncogenicity accords well with the concept of immunologic surveillance, i.e., the notion that homograft immunity might represent a primary mechanism for natural defense against neoplasia based biologically on the need to control abnormal cells continually arising in the body as a consequence of somatic mutation (111). The "experiments of nature" provided by immunodeficient and immunosuppressed patients, with their greatly increased risk of developing malignancy, may be of singular importance in regard to this concept. Patients with AIDS (the acquired immunodeficiency syndrome), in which depletion of critical immune cells by infection with HIV eventuates in Kaposi's sarcoma and lymphomas, is the latest

and most dramatic chapter in this story (57, 89). It should be noted that much of the risk for patients with defective immunity lies in the development of lymphoid neoplasia *per se*, and the role of defective immunity in the pathogenesis of these tumors is a very complex one, with tenable (but less likely) alternatives to the surveillance hypothesis.

The advent of *in vitro* tests for tumor immunity has clearly increased the sophistication of tumor immunology, but these tests have generated data that are not readily interpretable in terms of clinically obvious resistance. For example, *in vitro* cytotoxicity assays may detect tumor antigens that do not induce tumor immunity *in vivo*; they may define antigenic relationships among tumors that are not evident using tumor rejection tests *in vivo*; and the results for each of several in vitro assays may differ one from the other and be entirely different from the situation of host resistance *in vivo*. Ultimately, the only meaningful test for tumor immunity is *in vivo* tumor rejection.

The possibility has already been discussed that some elements of the host's immune system could enhance rather than suppress the growth of tumors. Indeed, earlier experiments suggested that the sera of some tumor-bearing animals might actually protect the tumor cells from the cytotoxic effect of sensitized lymphocytes, i.e., that cell-mediated immunity was beneficial but that some antibodies were detrimental. Further work has implicated suppressor cells, antigen-antibody complexes, and /or circulating soluble antigens in the "blocking" phenomenon (66). A still experimental clinical method, "immunopheresis," developed by Terman et al. (138) and employing filtration of the patients's plasma through filters loaded with protein A from the Cowan strain of staphylococcus, is designed to purify the plasma of such "blocking" factors, but it is not clear that the phenomenon is clinically useful, nor if so what its mechanism of action may be. Moreover, other studies have suggested that certain antibodies from tumor-free individuals may counteract the "blocking" factors, and potentiate the cytotoxic effects of sensitized lymphocytes or even induce nonsensitized lymphocytes to become specifically cytotoxic (antibody-dependent cell-mediated cytotoxicity) (67).

As noted above, mechanisms of tumor escape from immune effector function must exist in humans, since many cancer patients do demonstrate cellular and humoral immunity at the time of diagnosis. In addition to the activity of suppressor lymphocytes and antibody or immune complex-mediated immunological enhancement, these escape mechanisms may include tumor growth-enhancing T lymphocytes, clonal deletion of immune response genes, immunological tolerance, and antigenic modulation (the "masking" or "down-regulation" of surface antigens).

Recent work has shown that lymphocytes of normal, presumably nonimmune individuals can show significant levels of cytotoxicity for tumor cells *in vitro*, and that the level of cytotoxicity can be augmented by a variety of cytokines, functionally and biochemically unique soluble proteins synthesized by lymphoid and nonlymphoid cells. This effect is due to a population of lymphocytes lacking the surface markers of either T or B cells, and such natural killer (NK) cells may constitute an alternative form of lymphocyte differentiation (68). Since NK cells are present in nude mice (congenitally athymic), it seems likely that they account for the resistance of those animals to a variety of transplanted or primary tumors. In contrast, beige mice, which have a defective NK population, are usually susceptible to tumorigenesis (98). Another form of tumor resistance appears to reside in the macrophage-monocyte series; macrophages activated by suitable agents become cytotoxic for certain tumor cells *in vitro*, but such macrophages spare normal cells or other transformed cells even though the latter may carry strong alloantigens foreign to the macrophages (71).

Observations on rodent tumor-immunity and the concept of immune surveillance have led to much interest in the possibility of immunotherapy of cancer as well as immunoprophylaxis. However, the diversity and unpredictability of antigens on chemically or physically induced tumors, and the absence of effective TSTA on autochthonous tumors, seem important obstacles to practical immunoprophylaxis of nonvirus-induced cancer. With respect to virally induced cancers, immunoprophylaxis of naturally occurring neoplasia in animals has been demonstrated to be feasible; the routine administration of a herpes viral vaccine to hatchlings has eliminated Marek's disease (a lymphoma-like proliferative disorder) from the poultry industry. With regard to immunotherapy, the major problem has been that tumor immunity is relatively weak, even against laboratory animal tumors which usually are known to be virus-induced and/or which bear strong transplantation antigens as well as histocompatibility antigens – all quite unlike the probable situation with the autochthonous tumors of man which have a long latency, slow growth, and low immunogenicity. The immunotherapy regimens that have so far been employed in the clinic have been derived quite empirically, with only a limited understanding of the nature of the tumor antigens involved, the complexity of the natural host response to the tumor, and the mechanisms of nonspecific immune stimulation. The failure of these adjuvant immunotherapy regimens in the treatment of human cancer suggests that success is likely to remain limited until rational treatment can be based upon a more profound understanding of the biology and chemistry of tumor antigens, the regulation and balance of tumor immunity, and the mechanism of action of immune adjuvants. Nonetheless, immunological methods hold abundant promise for identifying and defining cancer cells, detecting cancer in its earliest stages, and for yielding new means to prevent and treat the disease.

The tumor-specific transplantation antigens found in both virus-induced and chemically induced malignancies are not the only antigenic determinants of importance in or on malignant cells. A diversity of tumor-associated antigens which do not appear to function in tumor rejection also obtain, including illegitimate blood group antigens, differentiation antigens, carcinoembryonic, and oncofetal antigens. These proteins may be as useful as TSTA in our understanding of tumor biology and diagnosis.

The introduction of resistance genes by transplantation of allogeneic bone marrow has permitted the prevention of genetically determined malignancies in rodents. Since new methods have been developed recently which may permit transplantation of hematopoietic or lymphoid cells across the major histocompatibility barriers without producing lethal graft-versus-host reactions (e.g., depletion of T cells within donor marrow using monoclonal antibody), the prospects are good for applying a variant of this approach to the treatment of malignancy in humans. Two other phenomena must be considered here: First, marrow transplantation (whether autologous or allogeneic), employed as a means to "rescue" the patient from the effects of intensive chemoradiotherapy regimens, is a method of supportive care and will be no more effective than the tumor therapy per primum. If this therapy is not applied at certain critical kinetic and biochemical points in the natural history of the cancer (as discussed above), then many tumor cells will not be killed no matter how great the treatment dose. Transplantation in this circumstance, no matter how refined, will not ultimately be useful. Secondly, much current work in clinical immunology devolves about eliminating GVHD while practicing the widest possible histoincompatibility with the use of various physical and immunological methods to rid the donor marrow of GVH-inducing cells. However, recent evidence suggests that in humans, as earlier shown in rodents, some degree of GVHD may be beneficial in that there appears to be a graft-versus-tumor as well as graft-versus-host effect (134). Thus, the immunological balance clearly has a critical importance.

The production of monoclonal antibody using hybridomas (97) is another development of great importance; in all probability, one of the two recent technical advances in biology – the second being recombinant DNA methodology – which will most influence cancer research in the forseeable future. The development of monoclonal antibody directed against tumor-specific antigens and/or tumor-associated antigens should not only facilitate diagnosis and staging, but should have an important role in treatment as well, either by direct cytotoxicity or by specifically directing the "homing" of a drug, toxin, or radio-emitter. Moreover, monoclonal antibody might be employed to expunge autologous marrow of residual tumor cells in the case of leukemia and lymphoma and possibly solid tumors as well, thus broadening the possibilities for stem cell rescue with autologous marrow reinfusion.

Finally, much is being learned about the cytokines (lymphokines and monokines) and their possible role in inducing tumor regression. These peptides affect inflammation, cell proliferation, cell cytotoxicity, cell activation, and cell mobility, and include the interleukins, tumor necrosing factor, interferon, macrophage activation factor, colony stimulating factor, transfer factor, products of suppressor and helper T cells, and a number of other related molecules, all of which can potentially be produced in microbial systems in great abundance and with profound specificity by molecular cloning and recombinant DNA technology. While clinical results of interferon have been disappointing, studies of the cytokines in tumor therapy – first in animal tumor model systems and then clinically – hold much promise, as does the possibility of practicing adoptive immunotherapy by "educating" the T cells of a tumor-bearing host or donor and facilitating their *in vitro* amplification through the use of T-cell growth factor. The power of this educated cytotoxicity will be enhanced by increasing the abundance of such cells at the tumor site; the cells may derive from the host's or donor's peripheral blood or, in fact, they may be removed from the tumor itself and then expanded *in vitro*. It has already been shown that cytotoxic T lymphocytes obtained in this way are capable of curing mice bearing syngeneic lymphoid tumors, and recently, Rosenberg et al. have obtained preliminary evidence that this approach (i.e., treatment with "killer" lymphocytes plus lymphokine) may cause durable tumor regression in a small but meaningful percentage of some human tumors, e.g., melanoma and renal cancer (116).

Unique biologic and therapeutic aspects of cancer – prospects and challenges

Finally, a few summary comments are in order on the "state of the art"; once again, pediatric tumors offer helpful clues. As a generality, cancer in the young is characterized kinetically by rapid growth with a large growth fraction. For this and probably other biologic reasons, the "pediatric" tumors have more often than not demonstrated great sensitivity to chemotherapy – thorough and complete clinical responses, but also early relapses. As discussed previously, they have thus served as paradigms for the explication of new treatment concepts later successfully applied in the less tractible, but far more common adult malignancies such as carcinoma of the breast, small-cell carcinoma of the lung, testicular and ovarian carcinoma, aggressive lymphomas, and soft tissue sarcomas.

The differences between cancer in young people (i.e., those tumors occurring in the first three decades of life) and cancer in older patients have not only to do with growth kinetics, but with the fact that these tumors are unique in their germ-layer(s) of embryologic origin, and therefore the tissues in which they occur; in their proximity to germ and somatic cell genetic events and aberrations of differentiation; and in embryogenetic and possibly immunologic or virologic phenomena that are age-dependent (and for which good animal models appear to exist). Finally, it seems likely that environmental carcinogenesis, with respect to life-long exposure to endogenous and exogenous carcinogens, is more relevant to the etiology of the tumors of older patients than to those of younger ones; such environmental associations as that between maternal exposure to diethylstilbesterol and subsequent gynecologic malignancy in the daughter seem to be exceptional (69).

Remarkable improvements in the outcome of therapy for acute lymphocytic leukemia over the past 30 years have already been described, as have the reasons for the progressive improvement: The rational and empiric development of specific chemotherapeutic agents with sufficient selectivity for the leukemic cell population versus normal cells to permit clinical application; the realization that combinations of these agents can provide additive and possibly synergistic antileukemic effects while not producing an intolerable increment in toxicity; the concept of maintenance chemotherapy in the face of continued disease remission (i.e., the necessity to continue treatment until all remaining cancer cells have been destroyed, which may be many logs below the level of clinical remission); and the notion that sites which are "protected" from systemic chemotherapy, e.g., the CNS "sanctuary," are often responsible for ultimate relapse and treatment failure.

The major avenues of future clinical research in ALL are already apparent at this time. The observation that approximately 15% of males remaining in continuous remission for 3–5 years will relapse in another sanctuary, the

testes, when taken off chemotherapy (127) should lead to close and early monitoring of potential testicular involvement and suggests selective prophylaxis. Furthermore, it has been known for some time that certain patient characteristics which are present at diagnosis, such as age, sex, and initial white blood cell count, have an important prognostic value for remission duration and survival (25). This information permits the design of clinical trials for "good-prognosis" patients which seek to reduce the amount (or alter the type) of therapy, and hence the side-effects and long-term sequelae encountered. This objective is critical to the production of the "truly cured" patient, particularly with respect to CNS function. At the same time, we must evaluate either more intensive therapy or new therapeutic approaches altogether for "poor-prognosis" patients. Our ability to understand the prognostic implications of much more subtle characteristics of leukemic cells, such as the unique biochemical pathways corresponding to their differentiated anlage, should facilitate the process of segregating good-prognosis from poor-prognosis patients and designing their therapy accordingly. Clearly, the avenues of future research in acute myelocytic leukemia are similar, with a mandate to determine whether bone marrow transplantation in this disease, as increasingly practiced, does truly provide a major survival advantage not possible with optimum current chemotherapy.

These concepts in acute leukemia are also relevant to the management of cancer in general, particularly the identification of clinical and laboratory prognostic factors, the improvement of therapeutic ratios in good-prognosis patients, and the intensification of therapy and/or development of new therapeutic approaches altogether for poor-prognosis patients. The most notable example of progress in the treatment of non-lymphomatous solid tumors has, of course, occurred in Wilms' tumor – an object lesson in "fine-tuning" – with the progress occurring in incremental steps: Surgical removal of the primary tumor resulted in a 10–20% cure rate, with the remainder dying of local recurrence and systemic metastases. The introduction of radiotherapy to the tumor bed reduced the risk of local recurrence, and the introduction of actinomycin D produced a major improvement in survival by reducing the likelihood of systemic metastases. Finally, the use of the adjuvant combination of vincristine and actinomycin D, in conjunction with surgery and radiotherapy, has produced apparent cure rates of greater than 90% for localized disease, and a 5-year disease-free survival of 50% for patients presenting with distant metastases at diagnosis (87). Progress, for similar reasons, has been similarly heartening in patients with advanced stages of rhabdomyosarcoma, Ewing's sarcoma, and lymphomas; in the latter case, much biological work is still required to provide an adequate nosology, beyond morphology, so that treatment can be appropriately individualized. Such a nosology will undoubtedly be based on specific DNA rearrangements in lymphocyte classes. Only two settings in young patients are marked by their almost abject lack of durable chemotherapeutic responsiveness, i.e., many brain tumors and most metastatic neuroblastomas.

As the therapy for cancer has become increasingly effective, it has become mandatory to extend widely the concept of individualizing treatment as a function of site-specific staging, pathologic grading, histotypical, and other prognostic variables. The new radiologic and nuclear medicine methods, as well as biologic marker and ultrastructure studies, are powerful aids to increasing our therapeutic selectivity. Moreover, we are just beginning to perceive the contributions to diagnosis and selection of treatment which will be made by molecular genetic studies of individual tumors. Staging has been advanced remarkably by nuclear magnetic resonance imaging and positron-emission tomography, in addition to CT scanning, ultrasound, and the diversity of scintiscans now available. Finally, complications of the diseases and their treatments have acquired greater importance in determining the outcome of each disease episode. These side effects may be of immediate or late onset (87). While the immediate effects are generally transient and reversible, life-threatening complications may result. Therefore, much attention has been paid to sophisticated supportive care technologies dealing with the infectious (e.g., laminar air flow isolation) and hematologic (e.g., granulocyte transfusion, bone marrow transplantation) complications of malignancy and its treatment, and more recently, the nutritional concomitants of cancer (87). However, carefully designed and well-controlled (usually randomized) clinical trials of these technologies are as important in validating our principles of management in the area of supportive care as in the treatment of the tumor per primum. By and large, these technologies are demanding and costly and are only halfway methods, bearing the same relationship to our ultimate understanding of the biology and manipulation of cancer as "the iron lung does to the poliovirus vaccine" (139). Study of the long-term sequelae of cancer is, of course, a recent luxury, the importance of which grows by the day, not only with respect to the somatic and psychosocial concomitants of the illness and its impact on patient, family, community, and clinicians, but also with regard to the possibility of morbidity years after cancer cure – e.g., lowered IQ after CNS prophlaxis in childhood ALL and cardiomyopathy after adjuvant treatment of breast cancer with anthracyclines. Equally important are the potential delayed adversities of cancer treatment on the function of the gonads (with respect to fertility and fetal anomalies), the liver, and the lungs, as well as the development of second malignancies as a mutagenic consequence of cancer treatment (23, 113).

Certainly with regard to the basic sciences, the study of the leukemias, lymphomas, sarcomas, and neural crest tumors is rich and rewarding, with the gap between our appreciation of the basic mechanisms of disease and the expression of clinical illness far more narrow than appears to obtain with the common "adult" malignancies which occur after a life time of "wear and tear." The influence of recombinant DNA and hybridoma technologies on such studies is at its very beginning. Other new methods and reagents that are immediately applicable to this area of medical investigation include the development and manipulation of neoplastic tissue culture lines which undergo spontaneous or induced differentiation, e.g., HL-60, a human promyelocytic leukemia line which can be induced to differentiate along the myeloid or macrophage pathways depending on the chemical used for induction. Relevant to this field also is the "cataloging" of all of the genes of the human genome, and all of the proteins synthesized by the genome at any given time (approximately 3000–10,000, with

the total potential number of expressed genes and unique proteins in human cells being 20,000–50,000), so as to create a human gene and protein map. Such a library could identify all human proteins, their functions and locations, the genes that direct their synthesis, and the location of these genes on the chromosomes. A gene and protein index, which would be linked to the human gene map and would also depend on recombinant DNA methods, DNA sequencing, monoclonal antibody, and image analysis/data reduction, might ultimately permit us to understand the entire human genetic program for differentiation and differential gene expression, to associate specific tumors with specific mutations, and to monitor or predict the efficacy of a specific therapy, assuming that "new" proteins are associated with development of drug resistance (59).

It is evident that the molecular genetics of individual human cancer risk, as well as the genetics underlying individual human sensitivity or resistance to treatment, are both at hand. Whether we shall be equally adroit at illuminating the cell biology of cancer remains to be seen. In any event, we now know how to prevent the great majority of human cancers with simple maneuvers, such as not smoking, and the elegance and power of modern molecular and cell biologic techniques should not and can not replace the social imperatives of classical preventive medicine and public health.

REFERENCES

1. Adams JM et al: C-Myc oncogene driven by immunoglobulin enhancer induces lymphoid malignancy in trans-genic mice. *Nature* 318:533–5, 1985

2. Ah FW, Kellems RE, Bertino JR, Schimke RT: Selective multiplication of dihydrofolate reductase genes in methotrexate-resistant variants of cultured murine cells. *J Biol Chem* 253:1357–70, 1978

3. Ames RN, Durston WE, Yamasaki E et al: Carcinogens are mutagens: A simple test system combining liver homogenates for activation and bacteria for detection. *Proc Natl Acad Sci USA* 70:2281–5, 1973

4. Arcamone F, Cassinelli G, Fantini G et al: Adriamycin. 14-hydroxydaunomycin, a new antitumor antibiotic from *S. peucetius* var. *caesius. Biotechnol Biochem* 11:1101, 1969

5. Ballmer-Hofer K, Benjamin T: Modulation of phosphorylation of plasma membrane proteins in polyma virus infected cells by the HR-T gene of polyoma virus (abstract). *J Cell Biochem Suppl* 8A:253, 1984

6. Baltimore D: Viral RNA-dependent DNA polymerase. *Nature* 226:1209–11, 1970

7. Barbacid M: Oncogenes in human cancers and in chemically induced animal tumors. *Prog Med Virol* 32.86–100, 1985

8. Bartlett GI, Kreider JW, Purnell DM: Immunotherapy of cancer in animals: Models or muddles? *J Natl Cancer Inst* 56:207–10, 1976

9. Bell E, Marek LF, Levinstone DS et al: Loss of division potential *in vitro*: Aging or differentiation? *Science* 202:1158–63, 1978

10. Berenblum I: The cocarcinogenic action of croton resin. *Cancer Res* 1:44–9, 1941

11. Bishop JM: Cancer genes come of age. *Cell* 32:1018–20, 1983

12. Bishop JM: Retroviruses and cancer genes. In: Klein G, Weinhouse S (eds) *Advances in Cancer Research.* vol. 37, New York: Academic Press, pp. 1–32, 1982

13. Bishop JM, Varmus H: Functions and origins of retroviral transforming genes. In: Weiss R, Teich N, Varmus H, Coffin

J (eds). *RNA Tumor Viruses.* New York: Cold Spring Laboratory, pp. 99–1109, 1982

14. Bittner JJ: Some possible effects of nursing on mammary gland tumor incidence in mice. *Science* 84: 162–3, 1936

15. Boveri T: Zellenstudien VI. Die Entwicklung dispermer Seeigeleier. Ein Beitrag zur Befruchtungslehre und zur Theorie des Kerns. *Z Naturwiss* 43:1, 1907

16. Bruce WR, Meeker BE, Valeriote FA: Comparison of the sensitivity of normal hematopoietic and transplanted lymphoma colony forming cells to chemotherapeutic agents administered *in vivo. J Natl Cancer Inst* 37:233–245, 1966

17. Brugge JS, Erickson RL: Identification of a transformation-specific antigen induced by an avian sarcoma virus. *Nature* 269:346–8, 1977

18. Burkitt D: A sarcoma involving the jaws in African children. *Br J Surg* 46: 218–23, 1958

19. Burkitt D, Hutt MSR, Wright DH: The African lymphoma. Preliminary observations on response to therapy. *Cancer* 18:399–410, 1965

20. Burchenal JH: Adjuvant therapy-theory, practice, and potential. The James Ewing Lecture. *Cancer* 37: 46–57,1976

21. Burchenal JH, Murphy MI, Ellison RR et al: Clinical evaluation of a new antimetabolite in the treatment of leukemia and allied diseases. *Blood* 8:964–999, 1953

22. Burgert EO, Glidewell O: Dactinomycin in Wilms' tumor. *JAMA* 199:464–8, 1967

23. Canellos GP, DeVita VT Jr, Arseneau JC et al: Second malignancies complicating Hodgkin's disease in remission. *Lancet* 1:947, 1975

24. Chermann JC, Barre-Sinoussi F, Montagnier L: A new human retrovirus associated with acquired immunodeficiency syndrome (AIDS) or AIDS-related complex. *Prog Clin Biol Res* 182:329-42, 1985

25. Coccia P, Sather H, Nesbit M et al: Inter-relationship of initial WBC, age and sex in predicting prognosis in childhood acute lymphoblastic leukemia. *Am Soc Hematology Meeting* (abstract), 1976

26. Cohen SN, Chang ACY, Boyer HW et al: Construction of biologically functional plasmids *in vitro. Proc Natl Acad Sci USA* 70:3240–4, 1973

27. Cooper GM, Lane M-A, Krontiris TG, Goubin G: Analysis of cellular transforming genes by transfection. In: Klein G (ed) *Advances in Viral Oncology*, Vol. 1, New York: Raven Press, pp. 243–59, 1982

28. Danna KJ, Nathans D: Bidirectional replication of simian virus 40 DNA. *Proc Natl Acad Sci USA* 69:3097–3100, 1972

29. D'Angio GJ, Evans AE, Breslow N et al: The treatment of Wilms' tumor – results of the National Wilms' Tumor Study. *Cancer* 38:633–46, 1976

30. Davis WH: The relation of the foreign population to the mortality rates of Boston. *Bull Am Acad Med* 14:19–54, 1913

31. DeVita VT, Jr, Hellman S, Rosenberg SA (eds): *Cancer: Principles and Practice of Oncology.* Philadelphia, PA: JB Lippincott Company, 1986

32. DeVita VT, Jr, Serpick A, Carbon PP: Combination chemotherapy in the treatment of advanced Hodgkin's disease. *Ann Intern Med* 73:881–95, 1970

33. Djerassi I, Boyer G, Treat C et al: Management of childhood lymphosarcoma and reticulum cell sarcoma with high dose methotrexate and vitrovorum factor. *Proc Am Assoc Cancer Res* 9:18 (abstract), 1968

34. Doll R, Hill AB: Smoking and cancer of the lung. *Br Med J* 2:739–48, 1950

35. Donner P, Greiser-Wilke R, Moelling K: Nuclear localization and DNA binding of the transforming gene product of avian myelocytomatosis virus. *Nature* 296:262–6, 1982

36. Downward J, Yarden Y, Mayes E et al: Close similarity of epidermal growth factor receptor and v-erb-B oncogene protein sequences. *Nature* 307:521-7, 1984

37. Dubost M, Gauter P, Maral R et al: Un nouvel antibiotique a proprietes antitumorales. *CR Acad Sci Paris* 257:1813–20, 1963

38. Duesberg PH: Retroviral transforming genes in normal cells? *Nature* 304:219–26, 1983

39. Dulbecco R: Cell transformation by viruses. *Science* 166:962–8, 1969

40. Einhorn LH, Furnas BF, Powell N: Combination chemotherapy of disseminated testicular carcinoma with cis-platinum diammine dichloride (CPDD), vinblastine (VLB) and bleomycin (BLEO) *Prod Am Soc Clin Oncol* 17:240, 1976

41. Ellison RR, Glidewell O: Improved survival in adults with acute myelocytic leukemia. *Proc Am Assoc Cancer Res* 20:161, 1979

42. Ellison RR, Holland JF, Weil M et al: Arabinosyl cytosine. A useful agent in the treatment of acute leukemia in adults. *Blood* 32:507–23, 1968

43. Farber S, D'Angio G, Evans A et al: Clinical studies of actinomycin D with special reference to Wilms' tumor in children. *Ann NY Acad Sci* 89:421–5, 1960

44. Farber S, Diamond LK, Mercer RD et al: Temporary remissions in acute leukemia in children produced by folic acid antagonist, 4-aminopteroylglutamic acid (Aminopterin). *N Eng J Med* 238:787, 1948

45. Farber S: The effect of ACTH in acute leukemia in childhood. In: Mote JR (ed) Proc of the First Clinical ACTH Conference New York: Blakiston p. 328, 1950

46. Foley EJ: Antigenic properties of methylcholanthrene-induced tumors in mice of the strain of origin. *Cancer Res* 13:835, 1953

47. Frei E, III, Freireich ET, Gehan E et al: Studies of sequential and combination antimetabolite therapy in acute leukemia, 6-mercaptopurine and methotrexate. *Blood* 18:431–545, 1961

48. Freireich EJ, Karon M, Frei E, III: Quadruple combination therapy (VAMP) for acute lymphocytic leukemia of childhood. *Proc Am Assoc Cancer Res* 5:20, 1964

49. Forth J, Kahn MC: The transmission of leukemia of mice with a single cell. *Am J Cancer* 31:276–82, 1937

50. Galen: On Anatomical Procedures, the Later Books (Duckworth, WLH, trans). Cambridge: Cambridge University Press. 1962

51. Gilman A: The initial clinical trial of nitrogen mustard. *Am J Surg* 105:574–5, 1963

52. Goldie JH, Coldman AJ: A mathematic model for relating the drug sensitivity of tumors to their spontaneous mutation rate. *Cancer Treat Rep* 63:1727–33, 1979

53. Gottdiener JS, Mathisen DJ, Borer JS et al: Doxorubin cardiotoxicity: Assessment of the late left ventricular dysfunction by radionuclide cineangiography. *Ann Intern Med* 94:430–5, 1951

54. Graham FL, Abrahams PJ, Mulder C et al: Studies on *in vitro* transformation by DNA and DNA fragments of human adenoviruses and Simian virus 40. *Cold Spring Harbor Symp Quant Biol* 39:637–50, 1974

55. Gray LH: Oxygenation in radiotherapy. 1. Radiobiological considerations. *Br J Radiol* 30:403–6, 1957

56. Groffen J, Heisterkamp N, Stephenson JR et al: C-sis is translocated from chromosome 22 to chromosome 9 in chronic myelocytic leukemia. *J Exp Med* 158:9–15, 1983

57. Groopman JE, Hartzband PI, Shulman L et al: Antibody seronegative human T-lymphotropic virus type III (HTLV-III)-infected patients with acquired immunodeficiency syndrome or related disorders. *Blood* 66(3):742–4, 1985

58. Grodzicker T, Hopkins N: Origins of contemporary DNA tumor virus research. In: Tooze, J (ed). "DNA Tumor Viruses." New York: Cold Spring Laboratory, pp. 1–61, 1981

59. Gros P, Croop J, Roninson I et al: Isolation and characterization of DNA sequences amplified in multidrug-resistant hamster cells. *Proc Natl Acad Sci USA* 83:337–41, 1986

60. Gross L: Intradermal immunization of C3H mice against a sarcoma that originated in an animal of the same line. *Cancer Res* 3:326–33, 1943

61. Haddow A, Sexton WA: Influence of carbamic esters (urethanes) on experimental animal tumors. *Nature* 157:500–03, 1946

62. Haenszel W: Cancer mortality among the foreign-born in the United States. *J Natl Cancer Inst* 26:37–132, 1961

63. Halsted WS: Surgical Papers. Baltimore: Johns Hopkins, 1924

64. Hayflick L, Moorehead P: The serial cultivation of human diploid cell strains. In: Pollack, R (ed), *Readings in Mammalian Cell Culture*. New York: Cold Spring Laboratory, pp. 27–64, 1981

65. Hayward WS, Neel B, Astrin S: Activation of a cellular *onc* gene by promoter insertion in ALV-induced lymphoid leukosis. *Nature* 290:475–80, 1981

66. Hellstrom I, Hellstrom KE, Evans CA et al: Serum mediated protection of neoplastic cells from inhibition by lymphocytes immune to their tumor-specific antigens. *Proc Natl Acad Sci USA* 62:362–8, 1969

67. Hellstrom I, Hellstrom KF, Sjogren HO et al: Serum factors in tumor-free patients cancelling the blocking of cell-mediated tumour immunity. *Int J Cancer* 8,185–91, 1971

68. Herberman RB. Natural cell-mediated cytotoxicity in male mice. In: Fogh J; Giovanella BC (eds). *The Nude Mouse in Experimental and Clinical Research*. New York: Academic Press, pp. 135–66, 1978

69. Herbst AL, Code P, Colton T et al: Age-incidence and risk of diethylstilbestrol-related clear cell adenocarcinoma of the vagina and cervix. *Am J Obstet Gynecol* 125:43–50, 1977

70. Hertz R, Lewis J, Lipsett MB: Five Years' experience with the chemotherapy of metastatic trophoblastic diseases in women. *Am J Obstet Gynecol* 86:805–14, 1963

71. Hibbs JB, Jr, Lambert LH, Jr, Remington JS: Possible role of macrophage mediated nonspecific cytotoxicityrin tumour resistance. *Nature New Biol* 235:45–50, 1972

72. Hill JM, Roberts J, Loch E et al: L-asparaginase therapy for leukemia and other malignant neoplasms. *JAMA* 202:882–8, 1967

73. Hitchings GH, Elion GB: The chemistry and biochemistry of purine analogs. *Ann NY Acad Sci* 60:195–9, 1954

74. Hoffman-Falk H, Einat P, Shilo B-Z: *Drosophila melanogaster* DNA clones homologous to vertebrate oncogenes: Evidence for a common ancestor to the src and abl cellular genes. *Cell* 32:589–98, 1983

75. Howard A, Pele SR: Synthesis of deoxyribonucleic acid and nuclear incorporation of S/35 as shown by autoradiographs. In: Wolstenholme GFW (ed). *Isotopes in Biochemistry*. London: Churchill, pp. 138+, 1951

76. Huebner RJ, Todaro GI: Oncogenes of RNA tumor viruses as determinants of cancer. *Proc Natl Acad Sci USA* 64:1087–94, 1969

77. Huggins C, Hodges CV: Studies on prostatic cancer I. The effect of castration, of estrogen and of androgen injection on serum phosphatase in metastatic carcinoma of the prostate. *Cancer Res* 1:293–7, 1941

78. Hunter T, Sefton BM: The transforming gene product of Rous sarcoma virus phosphorylates tyrosine. *Proc Natl Acad Sci USA* 77:1311–15, 1980

79. Kaplan HS: Fundamental mechanisms in combined modality therapy of cancer. Janeway lecture, 1977. *Am J Roentgenol* 129:383–93, 1977

80. Karon MR, Freireich EJ, Frei F, III: A preliminary report on vincristine sulfate – a new agent for the treatment of acute leukemia. *Pediatrics* 30:791–6, 1962

81. Kirsch IB, Morton C, Korsmeyer S et al: Translocations that highlight chromosomal regions of differentiated activity. *J Cell Biochem Suppl* 8A:88 (abstract), 1984

82. Klein G: Specific chromosomal translocations and the genesis of B-cell derived tumors in mice and men. *Cell* 32:311–5. 1983

83. Klein G: Tumor antigens. *Ann Rev Microbiol* 20:223-52, 1966

84. Kontiris TG: The emerging genetics of human cancer. *New Engl J Med* 309:404–09, 1983

85. Land H, Parada LF, Weinberg RA: Cellular oncogenes and multistep carcinogenesis. *Science* 22:771–78, 1983

86. Land H, Parada LF, Weinberg RA: Tumorigenic conversion of primary embryo fibroblasts requires at least two cooperating oncogenes. *Nature* 304:596–602, 1983

87. Levine AS: Cancer in the Young. Masson Publishing, Inc. USA, 767 pp, 1982

88. Levine AS: Fruit flies, yeasts and onc genes: Developmental biology and cancer research come together. *Med Ped Oncol* 12:357–74, 1984

89. Levine AS: Viruses, immune dysregulation, and oncogenesis: inferences regarding the cause and evolution of AIDS. In: AIDS: The Epidemic of Kaposi's Sarcoma and Opportunistic Infections. Friedman-Kien, AE; LJ Laubenstein (eds). Masson Publishing, Inc. USA, pp. 7–21, 1984

90. Levine AS, Cook JL, Patch CT et al: Adenovirus 2 early gene expression suppresses the tumorigenicity of hybrids formed between hamster cells transformed by adenovirus 2 and simian virus 40. In: Bishop, JM; Graves, M; Rowley, JD (eds) *Genes and Cancer*. New York: A.R. Liss, pp. 621–38, 1984

91. Li MC, Hertz R, Spencer DH: Effect of methotrexate upon choriocarcinoma and chorioadenoma. *Proc Soc Exp Biol Med* 93:361–6, 1956

92. Luria SF, Delbruck M: Mutations of bacteria from virus sensitivity to virus resistance. *Genetics* 28:491–511, 1943

93. Lynch K, Smith W: Pulmonary asbestosis in carcinoma of the lung in asbesto-silicosis. *Am J Cancer* 24:56–64, 1935

94. Mendelsohn MI: Autoradiographic analysis of cell proliferation in spontaneous breast cancer of c3H mouse III. The growth fraction. *J Natl Cancer Inst* 28:1015–29, 1962

95. Miller JA: Carcinogenesis by chemicals: An overview GHA Clowes Memorial Lecture. *Cancer Res* 30:559–76, 1970

96. Miller RW: The discovery of human teratogens, carcinogens and mutagens. Lessons for the future. In: Hollaender A, deSerres RJ (eds) *Chemical Mutagens*. vol. 5. New York: Plenum, 1978

97. Milstein C, Kohler G: Continuous cultures of fused cells secreting antibody of predefined specificity. *Nature* 256:495–7, 1975

98. Mitchison NA, Kinlen IJ: Present concepts in immune surveillance, in; Fougereau, M; Daussel, J (eds) *Progress in Immunology 1980*. London: Academic Press, pp. 641–50, 1980

99. Muller J: Classics in oncology. *CA* 21:305–12, 1971

100. Muller R, Slamon DJ, Tremblay JM et al: Differential expression of cellular oncogenes during pre- and postnatal development of the mouse. *Nature* 299:640–4, 1982

101. Murphree Al, Benedict WF: Retinoblastoma: Clues to human oncogenesis. *Science* 223:1028–33, 1984

102. Nebert DW: Genetic differences in susceptibility to chemically induced myelotoxicity and leukemia. *Environ Health Prospect* 39:11–22, 1981

103. Nebert DW, Gonzalez FJ: Cytochrome P-450 gene expression and regulation. *Trends in Pharmacol Sci* 6:160–4, 1985

104. Newbold R, Overell RW: Fibroblast immortality is a prerequisite for transformation by EJ c-Ha-ras oncogene. *Nature* 304:648–51, 1983

105. Norton L, Simon R: Tumor size, sensitivity to therapy, and design of treatment schedules. *Cancer Treat Rep* 61:1307–17, 1977

106. Nowell PC, Hungerford DA: A unique chromosome in granulocytic leukemia. *Science* 132:1492, 1960

107. Penrose LS, Mackenzie HJ, Korn MN: A genetical study of mammary cancer. *Br J Cancer* 2:168–76, 1948

108. Pincus MR, van Renswoude J, Harford JB et al: Prediction of the three-dimensional structure of the transforming region of the human bladder oncogene product and its normal cellular homologue. *Proc Natl Acad Sci USA* 80:5253–5257, 1983

109. Pinkel D: Five-year follow-up of "total therapy" of childhood lymphocytic leukemia. *JAMA* 216:648–52, 1971

110. Powers S, Kataoka T, Fasano O et al: Genes in *S. cerevisiae* encoding proteins with domains homologous to the mammalian ras proteins. *Cell* 36:607–12, 1984

111. Prehn RT: Immunological surveillance: Pro and con. In: Bach, FH; Good, RA (eds) *Clinical Immunobiology*, vol. 2. New York: Academic Press, pp. 191–203, 1974

112. Reddy EP, Reynolds RK, Santos E, Barbacid M: A point mutation is responsible for the acquisition of transforming properties by the T24 human bladder carcinoma oncogene. *Nature* 300:149–52, 1982

113. Regaud C, Coutard H, Hautant A: Contribution au traitement des cancers endolarynges par les rayons. Tenth Internat'l Congress of Otolaryngology, pp. 19–22, 1922

114. Reimer RR, Hoover R, Fraumeni JF, Jr, Young RC: Acute leukemia after alkylating-agent therapy of ovarian cancer. *N Engl J Med.* 297:177, 1977

115. Rosenberg B, Van Camp I, Krigas T: Inhibition of cell division in Escherichia coli by electrolysis products from a platinum electrode. *Nature* 205:698–9, 1965

116. Rosenberg S: Lymphokine-activated killer cells: a new approach to immunotherapy of cancer. *JNCI* 75(4):595–603, 1985

117. Rous P: Transmission of a malignant new growth by means of a cell-free filtrate. *J Am Med Assoc* 50:198, 1911

118. Rowe WP: Leukemia virus genomes in the chromosomal DNA of the mouse. In: Harvey Lecture Series 71. New York: Academic Press, pp. 173–92, 1976

119. Ruley HE: Adenovirus early region 1A enables viral and cellular transforming genes to transform primary cells in culture. *Nature* 304:602–6, 1983

120. Salmon SE, Hamburger AW et al: Quantitation of differential sensitivity of human tumor cells to anticancer agents. *New Engl J Med* 298:1321–7, 1978

121. Schrier PI, Bernards R, Vaessen RTMJ et al: Expression of class I major histocompatibility antigens switched off by highly oncogenic adenovirus 12 in transformed rat cells. *Nature* 305:771–84, 1983

122. Schultz MD: The supervoltage story. Janeway lecture, 1974. *Am J Roentgenol* 124:541–59, 1975

123. Selawry OS, Frei E, III: Prolongation of remission in acute lymphocytic leukemia by alteration in dose, schedule and route of administration of methotrexate. *Clin Res* 12:231 (abstract), 1964

124. Sharp PA: Molecular biology of viral oncogenes. *Cold Spring Harb Symp Quant Biol* 44:1305–22, 1980

125. Shimkin MB: Contrary to Nature. DHEW Publication No. NIII 76–720. Washington, DC: Government Printing Office, 1977

126. Shope RF: Infectious papillomatosis of rabbits. *J Exp Med* 58:607–24, 1933

127. Simone JV, Verzosa MS et al: Initial features and prognosis in 363 children with acute lymphocytic leukemia. *Cancer* 36:2099, 1975

128. Skipper HE: Reasons for success and failure in treatment of murine leukemia with the drugs now employed in treating human leukemias. Cancer Chemotherapy (vol. 1). Ann Arbor, Michigan: University Microfilms Internatl, 1978

129. Slamon DJ, deKernion JB, Verma IM, Cline MJ: Expression of cellular oncogenes in human malignancies. *Science* 224:256–62, 1984

130. Smith RL: Recorded and expected mortality among the Japanese of the United States and Hawaii, with special reference to cancer. *J Natl Cancer Inst* 17:459–73, 1956

131. Sorge LK, Levy BT, Maness PF: pp60/c-src is developmentally regulated in the neural retina. *Cell* 36:249–57, 1984

132. Stewart TA, Pattengale PK, Leder P: Spontaneous mammary adenocarcinomas in transgenic mice that carry and express MTV/myc fusion genes. *Cell* 38(3):627–37, 1984

133. Stocks P, Korn MN: A cooperative study of the habits, home life, dietary and family histories of 450 cancer patients and of an equal number of control patients. *Ann Eugen (Lond)* 5:237–80, 1933

134. Storb R, Weiden PL, Sullivan KM et al: Antileukemic effect of chronic graft-versus-host disease: Contribution to improved survival after allogeneic marrow transplantation. *N Engl J Med* 304:1529–33, 1981

135. Tan C, Tasaka H, DiMarco A: Clinical studies of daunomycin. *Proc Am Assoc Cancer Res* 6:64 (abstract), 1965

136. Taub R, Moulding C, Battey J et al: Activation and somatic mutation of the translocated *c-myc* in Burkitt lymphoma cells. *Cell* 36:339–48, 1984

137. Temin HM, Mizutani S: RNA-dependent DNA polymerase in virions of Rous sarcoma virus. *Nature* 226:1211–13, 1970

138. Terman DS, Young JB, Shearer WT et al: Preliminary observations of the effects on breast adenocarcinoma of plasma perfused over immobilized protein A. *N Engl J Med* 305:1195–99, 1981

139. Thomas L: The lives of a cell. New York: Viking, 1974

140. Triolo VA: Nineteenth century foundations of cancer research: Advances in tumor pathology, nomenclature, and theories of oncogenesis. *Cancer Res* 25:75–106, 1965

141. Varmus HE: Form and function of retroviral proviruses. *Science* 216:812, 1982

142. Waterfield MD, Scarce FT, Whittle N et al: Platelet-derived growth factor is structurally related to the putative transforming protein P28/sis of simian sarcoma virus. *Nature* 304:35–9, 1983

143. Wilder RJ: The historical development of the concept of metastasis. *J Mt Sinai Hosp* 23:729–34, 1956

144. Wong-Staal F, Ratner L, Shaw G et al: Molecular biology of human T-lymphotropic retroviruses. *Cancer Res* 45(9 Suppl):4539s–44s, 1985

145. Yunis JJ: The chromosomal basis of human neoplasia. *Science* 221:227–365, 1983

146. Zeigler JL, Magrath IT, Olweny CLM: Long survival of Burkitt's Lymphoma in Uganda. *Proc Am Soc Clin Oncol* 20:430 (abstract), 1979

147. Zeller, P, Gutmann II., Hegedus B et al: Methylhydrazine derivatives, a new class of cytotoxic agents. *Experientia* 19:129, 1963

148. Zubrod CG, Schepartz S, Leiter J et al: The chemotherapy program of the National Cancer Institute. History, analysis and plans. *Cancer Chemother Rep* 50:349–540, 1966

ORGAN CULTURE: USE IN EXPERIMENTAL ONCOLOGY FOR COMPARISONS AMONG SPECIES

DAVID G. KAUFMAN and GENE P. SIEGAL

ORGAN CULTURE

Organ culture has been defined as "The maintenance or growth of organ primordia or the whole or parts of an organ *in vitro* in a way that may allow differentiation and preservation of the architecture and/or function." (63). During the past two decades organ culture has become a valued technique in many areas of modern biology and medicine. Everything from fetal guinea pig inner ear (18) to adult mouse intestine (23) have been successfully maintained or propagated as organ cultures outside the body of the donor animal. Although organ culture has been used most extensively in recent years, its history as a valuable scientific technique goes back much farther. During a Festschrift in her honor (7), Dame Honor Fell traced the early history of organ culture to the period before the First World War. Although some work was reported in the late 1800's, she credited the pioneering experiments of Thompson (69) and Maximow (46) and, especially between the two world wars, the Strangeways Research Laboratory at Cambridge, Pieter Gallgard's group in the Netherlands and the French under Professor Etienne Wolff (22) with maintaining the momentum of this science. In her opinion, many in the United States turned their attention to tissue rather than organ culture due to the strong influence of Carrel's work at the Rockefeller Institute (14) during these early years.

Although some work has been done with lower vertebrate species such as urodele and anuran amphibians (15), in order to better draw species comparisons with man, much work had been done with organ cultures of mammals including humans. An even casual perusal of the biomedical literature will reward one with a myriad of papers on organ culture of fetal, neonatal, and adult tissues, including eye (10, 51, 52), ear (2), periodontum and teeth (58, 78), pituitary (3), thyroid and parathyroid (5, 50, 68), trachea and lung (25, 42, 61, 75, 76, 79), alimentary canal (9, 12, 19, 23, 29, 54, 56, 62, 74), pancreas (32, 40, 41, 47), breast (28, 57), prostate and genitourinary tract (36, 45, 53), and nerve (33) and other messenchyme-derived organs such as cartilage, and blood vessels (48, 73). Today, organ culture is being used in toxicology testing (6, 24), for evaluation of teratogenic agents (8), in studies of effects of infectious agents on mammalian tissues (70, 72, 77), and in carcinogensis (38, 49). This list is in no way complete and could include the many studies of the effect of physical and chemical agents, including drugs and vitamins on organs *in vitro* as well as tumor development, cancer chemotherapy, embryomorphogenesis, and organ metabolism.

It is also known that the human placenta (65) as well as its component parts including the amniotic membranes (11) can be maintained in organ culture. The amnion has a number of potential and real uses including surgical (burn) dressings and immunologic studies. We have used this as a model system for studying tumor invasion *in vitro* (39). The usefulness of this technique has been demonstrated in a study of polymorphonuclear leukocyte migration (60), in a study of the effects of protease inhibitors on a well characterized reticulum cell sarcoma tumor cell line (71) and by us in a study of the invasive capacity of Ewing's sarcoma cells in the presence of human interferons (64). Currently, we are using this organ culture system to measure the effect of a novel esteroprotease inhibitor on tumor cell invasion of human bone sarcoma cells (17). Our own major interest has been in the field of organ culture as it relates to the female genital tract system, especially the uterus. We shall briefly discuss the results of some of these studies in the following sections to offer an example of the application of organ culture methods to research on disease pathogenesis.

HUMAN ENDOMETRIAL ORGAN CULTURE

In biological sciences, the goals of obtaining essential data or answering basic questions, may be restricted or precluded for ethical but occasionally also for financial or other reasons, particularly as these studies concern the use of living whole animals including humans. For humans, this difficulty often can be overcome by the culture of human cells, tissues and organs obtained from surgical specimens or from immediate autopsy. Harris and Trump (26) have reviewed the use of human cells and tissue in biomedical experimentation. As discussed by them, many normal human tissues have now been grown in culture. Multiple factors impact on the use of model systems in scientific experimentation. The difficulty of growing and maintaining mammalian tissue as organ cultures is often notably greater than for single cells. In these studies one attempts to closely duplicate the *in vivo* state. This becomes progressively more difficult as the complexity of the model becomes multidimensional. Despite the difficulty, the potential payoff is enhanced as one can begin to be able to understand the complex interrelationships within and between different tissues as well as with their supporting extracellular matrices.

The endometrial lining of the uterus is a complicated tissue to study. First, this is because it is an organ that passes through three major postfetal functional and morphologic

R. H. Goldfarb (ed.), Fundamental aspects of cancer.

stages of development during the host's passage from premenarche to postmenopause. Second, during the central phase, the endometrium regularly cycles itself with repetitious programmed self-destruction and renewal in the absence of pregnancy. Third, it is exceedingly sensitive to external stimuli, especially steroid hormones. Fourth, the endometrium is composed of multiple cell types which change both qualitatively and quantitatively in relation to each of the above mentioned factors (13, 34).

For more than 50 years attempts have been made to study the human endometrium with *in vitro* techniques. Beginning with menstrual effluents, attempts at tissue growth progressed to examine outgrowths of endometrial curretting fragments and eventually biopsy specimens in fluid media (both by hanging drop and by roller bottle techniques) (55, 66). Manipulation of the physiologic conditions, including pH levels and atmospheric gas composition, allowed growth for approximately one month *in vitro* (55). Changes in biochemical pathways including glycolysis and cellular respiration were examined during stages of the menstrual cycle (67). The beneficial effects of estrogen and progesterone on the maintenance of the two major cell types, glandular epithelium and stromal cells, were studied in culture (21, 30). More recently, short term (1-2 weeks) cultures have been used in studies of hormone receptor levels and macromolecular synthesis in the endometrium (59).

We have described methods for the obtainment, sampling and transport of the endometrial tissue as well as the long-term maintenance of human endometrium after optimization of organ culture conditions (34, 35). Because our aim was to use organ cultures to study various aspects of chemical carcinogenesis, our goals were to maintain the tissue for extended periods of time and to preserve the unique organotypic relationship of the cellular components by achieving a high level of differentiation in the cultures. As we could maintain the endometrium for greater than 200 days we also were able to perform long-term biochemical and morphologic analysis of these tissues. The light microscopic and ultrastructural features, macromolecular synthesis of nucleic acids and proteins, and responsiveness to hormonal challenge were qualitatively similar, after long-term culture, to that seen in fresh tissue.

SPECIES COMPARISON OF UTERINE TISSUES

Endometrial organ cultures subsequently have been used to study a number of questions dealing with chemical carcinogenesis which, for obvious reasons, can not be performed *in vivo*. These include studies which show that organ cultures of human endometrial tissue can metabolize the model polycyclic aromatic hydrocarbon benzo(a)pyrene (BP) and that the proportions of various metabolic products are influenced by the estrogen status of this tissue. For example, in the absence of an estrogenic stimulus, such as in a postmenopausal state, there is a greatly reduced proportion of BP-phenol sulfate conjugates (44). Additionally, it has been shown that radiolabelled BP binds to the DNA of endometrium (20). The range of binding was large with increased levels occurring during the proliferative phase of the menstrual cycle when estrogen levels are high. Since it was possible to measure the metabolic capacity and DNA

binding in human endometrium, it seemed reasonable to examine the endometrium from other mammalian species. We prepared endometrial organ cultures from appropriate experimental animals in an effort to compare factors in the etiology of endometrial cancer in these various species, as we have previously suggested (35). This information could contribute to more reliable extrapolations to endometrial cancer risks in humans from data regarding compounds shown to be carcinogenic in experimental animals.

Initially we selected the uterine horns of Fischer 344 rats and Syrian golden hamsters to compare with human endometrial tissues. We developed efficient methods for demarcating and separating rodent endometrial tissues from the surrounding cervical and myometrial tissue and for determining estrus-cycle status through vaginal cell cytology. Next, methods were developed for maintaining rodent endometrial tissue in organ (as well as tissue) culture in order to perform identical carcinogen metabolism studies to those with the human tissue. Because our earlier studies used BP as the carcinogen, we began comparative studies by examining BP metabolism in rats and hamster endometrial tissue by the same methods (44). In contrast to our observations with liver in similar studies (43) a minor fraction (1-5%) of the BP substrate was consumed during the 18 hour incubation period. Despite the low level of metabolite activity both rat and hamster endometrium produced detectable quantities of BP metabolites. These results resembled the differences in the spectrum of metabolites previously observed for rat and hamster tracheas (42). We also observed that both rat and hamster endometrium produced large proportions of glucuronide- and sulfate-conjugated 1,6-, 3,6-, and 6,12-quinone and 7,8-diol BP metabolites. BP metabolite profiles for endometrium of rat or hamster did not vary as a function of the phase of the estrus cycle. Interestingly, treatment of rats and hamsters intraperitoneally with B-naphthoflavone (BNF) resulted in increased BP metabolism in endometrium of both species as evidenced by 10-20% of the parent compound recovered as oxidized metabolites. Although organic soluble metabolites produced by BNF-pretreated and control animals were similar in both groups, pretreatment with BNF resulted in the production of increased quantities of conjugated quinone (water soluble) metabolites by endometrium of both species. These results indicate pretreatment of rats and hamsters with BNF increases conjugation of oxygenated metabolites of BP, which is thought to be a detoxification pathway in vertebrate species.

Methods have also been developed to study carcinogen binding to DNA in small quantities of rodent endometrial tissue using methods similar to those we used earlier to study binding in human endometrial tissue (20). Our developmental studies employed BP as the carcinogen. In our efforts to demonstrate carcinogen binding to DNA, we initially worked with hamster endometrium as we had shown that there was a greater extent of metabolism in hamster as compared to rat endometrium. Hamster endometrial tissue was placed in organ culture with ^{3}H-BP and maintained for 18 hr. After incubation, DNA was extracted and purified by hydroxyapatite chromatography (1, 37) and the specific activity of BP binding was determined. Binding levels were comparable to our earlier observations of BP binding in human endometrial tissue.

We further pursued the issue of carcinogen binding by

examining the adducts of BP formed in the DNA of hamster, rat, mouse and human endometrial tissue. Following treatment of endometrium with ^{3}H-BP in culture, DNA was purified and enzymatically digested to deoxyribonucleosides. The digest was loaded onto a C_{18}-reverse phase HPLC column and chromatographed. The column was initially washed with water which removes polar materials including uncharacterized radioactive products. Two DNA adduct peaks which eluted with a linear water-methanol gradient were identified as BPDEI-deoxyguanosine and BPDEII-deoxyguanosine adducts, based on the elution of BP-metabolite-deoxyguanosine and BPDEII-deoxyguanosine adduct reference standards. The major adduct was BPDEI-deoxyguanosine and it was present at twice the quantity of the BPDEII-deoxyguanosine adduct. Among the three animal species examined the level of BPDEI adduct was highest in hamster and lowest in rat. The BPDEII adduct was present in human, hamster, and rat but not in mouse endometrium. There was an additional unidentified adduct present only in rat tissue. These results indicate that there are potentially significant differences between organ cultures of endometrial tissues from humans and from the three rodent species.

DISCUSSION AND PERSPECTIVES

In our own studies we have attempted to develop techniques which could be applied to answering fundamental questions of uterine carcinogenesis. The underlying rational for this is as follows: Depending on whether dietary factors, endogenously generated carcinogens, hormones, and lifestyle factors are excluded or included, from 50 to 90% of human cancer in industrialized, socially and economically advanced countries like the United States, has been attributed to environmental exposures (27). Recognition of this association has led to the passage of laws and acts in the U.S. which attempt to protect persons against exposure to human cancer hazards of environmental origin. Recently it has become less satisfactory to merely demonstrate qualitatively that a substance has carcinogenic activity and thus poses a potentially increased risk for cancer in the human population. Now, an effort must be made in many cases to estimate quantitatively how large this risk is in terms of probable increases in the number of cases of cancer in the exposed population. Both qualitative and quantitative estimates of human cancer risk are best made from sound epidemiologic data. Unfortunately, this type of data is unavailable for most substances. In the absence of epidemiologic data, most substances are evaluated in bioassays using animals to determine whether they are carcinogenic. The qualitative determination that a substance exhibits carcinogenic activity is a rather well defined process (31). If a statistically significant excess of tumors is found in a test group, and if this is verified in a second species, and, further, if the tumor response occurs in relation to dose in a multi-dose study, then it can be asserted with high probability that the substance is carcinogenic. The quantitative assessment of human cancer risk is far more difficult (16, 31). Assessments of human cancer risks have been made with extrapolations to correct for differences in total dose and dose rate, route of exposure

and species (4). This is an intelligent and conscientious effort to solve an important practical problem with the insufficient information available. Unfortunately, it is largely untested in a critical scientific manner, and the error in the estimates of human cancer risks generated in extrapolations from animal studies may be multiple orders of magnitude. The underlying problem causing the imprecision of these estimates is the virtual absence of critical knowledge of the important factors contributing to carcinogenesis in both humans and animals that would be necessary to make more accurate estimates. The studies reported above illustrate a way that one may attempt to obtain some of this critically needed information so that more scientifically sound extrapolations may be achieved, through the use of organ culture, both with human tissues and other animal's organs and tissues.

ACKNOWLEDGEMENTS

Supported by grants CA32239 and CA31733 from the National Cancer Institute. GPS is a Junior Faculty Clinical Fellow of the American Cancer Society (#JFCF739). The authors thank Dr. Hans Kaiser for advice in preparation of this manuscript. The authors also acknowledge the following individuals for their efforts in the primary research studies: Thomas A. Adamec, Robert L. Becker, Jr., Karen Calloway, Charles N. Carney, Iris E. Dominy, B. Hugh Dorman, Bonnie B. Furlong, Valerio M. Genta, Lynell Grosso, Joe W. Grisham, Marcos Irigaray, Mahmooda Kulkarni, Lisa Lombard, Marc J. Mass, Susan A. Melin, Karen G. Nelson, N. Terry Rodgers-Neame, Jill M. Siegfried, and Leslie A. Walton.

REFERENCES

1. Adriaenssens PI, Bixler CJ, Anderson MW: Isolation and quantitation of DNA-bound benzo(a)pyrene metabolites: comparison of hydroxyapatite and precipitation procedures. *Anal Biochem* 123:162–169, 1982
2. Anniko M: Extracorporeal preservation. Organ culture of the postnatal mammalian inner ear. *Acta Otolaryngol (Stockh)* 88:211–219, 1979
3. Anniko M, Eneroth P, Werner S, Wersall J: *In vitro* preservation of human pituitary tumours in organotypic differentiation. *Acta. Otolaryngol (Stockh)* 88:424–431, 1979
4. Albert RE, Train RE, Anderson E: Rationale developed by the Environmental Protection Agency for the assessment of carcinogen risks. *J Natl Cancer Inst* 58:1537–1541, 1977
5. Au W: Inhibition by 1,25 dihydroxycholecalciferol of hormonal secretion of rat parathyroid-gland in organ-culture. *Calcif Tiss* 36:384–391, 1984
6. Balls M, Clothier R: Differentiated cell and organ culture in toxicity testing. *Acta Pharmacol Toxicol (Copenh)* 52:115–137, 1983
7. Balls M, Monnickendam MA eds: *Organ Culture in Biomedical Research* Cambridge, Cambridge University Press, 1976
8. Barrach HJ, Neubert D: Significance of organ culture techniques for evaluation of prenatal toxicity. *Arch Toxicol* 45:161–187, 1980
9. Berteloot A, Chabot JG, Menard D, Hugson JS: Organ culture of adult mouse intestine. III. Behavior of proteins, DNA content and brush border membrane enzymatic activities. *In Vitro* 15:294–299, 1979
10. Bourne WM, Doughman DJ, Lindstrom RL, Kolb MJ, Mindrup E, Skelnik D: Increased endothelial cell loss after transplantation of corneas preserved by a modified organ-culture technique. *Ophthalmology* 91:285–289, 1984

11. Burgos H, Faulk WP: The maintenance of human amniotic membranes in culture. *Br J Obstet Gynaecol* 88:294–300, 1981

12. Calvert R, Micheletti PA: Selection of chemically defined medium for culturing fetal mouse small intestine. *In Vitro* 17:331–344, 1981

13. Cane EM, Villee CA: Synthesis of prostaglandin-F by human endometrium in organ culture. *Prostagland* 9:281–288, 1975

14. Carrel A: Rejuvenation of cultures of tissues. *J Amer Med Assoc* 57:1611, 1911

15. Clothier RH, Dewar JR, Santos MA, North AD, Foster S, Balls M: A comparative study of the deacetylation of para-cetamol by urodele and anuran amphibian organ cultures. *Xenobiotica* 11:149-157, 1981

16. Committee on Prototype Explicit Analyses for Pesticides: *Regulating Pesticides*, Washington, D.C., National Academy of Sciences, 1980

17. Cresson DH, Beckman WC Jr, Tidwell RR, Geratz JD, Siegal GP: *In vitro* inhibition of human sarcoma cells' invasive ability by Bis(5-amidino-2-benzimidazolyl)methane – A novel esteroprotease inhibitor. *Am J Pathol* 123: 46–56, 1986

18. Davis GL, Hawrisiak MM: *In vitro* cultivation of the fetal guinea pig inner ear. *Ann Otol Rhinol Laryngol* 90:246–250, 1981

19. Donaldson RM Jr, Kapadia CR: Organ culture of gastric mucosa: Advantages and limitations. *Methods Cell Biol* 21:349–363, 1980

20. Dorman BH, Genta VM, Mass MJ, Kaufman DG: Benzo(a)-pyrene binding to DNA in organ culture of human endometrium. *Cancer Res* 41:2718–2722, 1981

21. Ehrmann RL, McKelvey HA, Hertig AT: Secretory behavior of endometrium in tissue culture. *Obstet Gynecol* 17:416–433, 1961

22. Fell HB: *The Development of Organ Culture*. In: Balls M, Monnickendam MA, eds: *Organ Culture in Biomedical Research*, Cambridge, Cambridge University Press, pp. 1–14, 1976

23. Ferland S, Hugon JS: Organ culture of adult mouse intestine. I. morphological results after 24 and 48 hours of culture. *In Vitro*, 15:278–287, 1979

24. Gabridge MG: Hamster tracheal organ cultures as models for infection and toxicology studies. *Prog Exp Tumor Res* 24:85–95, 1979

25. Gross I, Freedman RM, Wilson CM, Lindsey S: Organotypic culture of fetal rat lung: Evaluation and comparison with organ culture. *Am Rev Resp Dis* 123:313–319, 1981

26. Harris CC, Trump BF: Human tissues and cells in biomedical research. *Surv Synth Pathol Res* 1:165–171, 1983

27. Higginson J, Muir CS: Environmental carcinogenesis: misconceptions and limitations to cancer control. *J Natl Cancer Inst* 63:1291–1298, 1979

28. Hillman EA, Vocci MJ, Combs JM, Sanefuji H, Robbins T, Janss DH, Harris CC, Trump BF: Human breast organ culture studies. *Methods Cell Biol* 21:79–106, 1980a

29. Hillman EA, Vocci MJ, Schurch W, Harris CC, Trump BF: Human esophageal organ culture studies. *Methods Cell Biol* 21:331–348, 1980b

30. Hughes EC, Demers LM, Csermely T, Jones DB: Organ culture of human endometrium. *Am J Obstet Gynecol* 105:707–720, 1969

31. Interagency Regulatory Liaison Group, Work Group on Risk Assessment: Scientific bases for identification of potential carcinogens and estimation of risks. *J Natl Cancer Inst* 63:241–268, 1979

32. Jones RT, Hudson EA, Resau JH: A review of *in vitro* and *in vivo* culture techniques for the study of pancreatic carcinogenesis. *Cancer* 47:1490-1496, 1981

33. Juurlink BH, Fedoroff S: The development of mouse spinal cord in tissue culture. I. Cultures of whole mouse embryos and spinal cord primordia. *In Vitro* 15:86–94, 1979

34. Kaufman DG, Adamec TA, Walton LA, Carney CN, Melin SA, Genta VM, Mass MJ, Dorman BH, Rodgers NT, Photopolous GJ, Powell J, Grisham JW: Studies of human endometrium in organ culture. *Methods Cell Biol* 21b:1–27, 1980

35. Kaufman DG, Siegfried JM, Dorman BH, Nelson KG, Walton LA: Carcinogen-induced changes in cultured human endometrial cells. In: Harris CC, Autrup H, eds, *Human Carcinogenesis*, Academic Press, New York, 1984

36. Knowles MD, Hicks RM, Berry JR, Milroy E: Organ culture of normal human bladder: Choice of starting material and culture characteristics. *Methods Cell Biol* 21:257–285, 1980

37. Kulkarni MS, Anderson MW: Persistence of benzo(a)pyrene metabolite: DNA adducts in lung and liver of mice. *Cancer Res* 44:97–101, 1984

38. Langenbach R, Nesnow S, Rice JM: *Organ and Species Specificity in Chemical Carcinogenesis*. Plenum Press, New York, 1983

39. Liotta LA, Lee CW, Morakis DG: New method for preparing whole intact surfaces of human basement membrane for tumor invasion studies. *Cancer Lett* 11:141–152, 1980

40. Mandel TE, Collier S, Hoffman L, Pyke K, Carter WM, Koulmanda M: Isotransplantation of fetal mouse pancreas in experimental diabetes. Effect of gestational age and organ culture. *Lab Invest* 47:477–483, 1982

41. Mandel TE, Hoffman (Higginbotham) L, Collier S, Carter WM, DeMoore G, Martin FIR, Campbell D: Organ cultured fetal pancreas: A source of islets for transplantation in diabetic mice. *Transplant Proc* 13:832–836, 1981

42. Mass MJ, Kaufman DG: A comparison between the activation of benzo(a)pyrene in organ cultures and microsomes from the tracheal epithelium of rats and hamsters. *Carcinogenesis* 4:297–303, 1983

43. Mass MJ, Kaufman DG: (^{3}H) benzo(a)pyrene metabolism in tracheal epithelial microsomes and tracheal organ culture of Syrian golden hamsters. *Cancer Res* 38:3861–3866, 1978

44. Mass MJ, Rodgers NT, Kaufman DG: Benzo(a)pyrene metabolism in organ cultures of human endometrium. *Chem Biol Interactions* 33:195–205, 1981

45. Masters JR, Krishnaswamy A, Rigby CC, O'Donoghue EP: Quantitative organ culture: An approach to prediction of tumour response. *Br J Cancer (Sup)* 41:199–202, 1980

46. Maximow A: Tissue Cultures of young mammalian embryos. *Contributions to Embryology*. Carnegie Inst. 16:47–113, 1925

47. McAteer JA, Hegre OD: A continuous flow method of organ culture. *In Vitro* 14:795–803, 1978

48. McDonagh MJN: Mechanical-properties of muscles from xenopus-borealis following maintenance in organ culture. *Comp Bioc A* 77:377–382, 1984

49. Mossman BT, Craighead JE, MacPherson BV: Induced epithelial changes in organ cultures of hamster trachea: inhibition of retinyl methyl ether. *Science* 207:311–313, 1980

50. Naji A, Barker CF, Silvers WK: Relative vulnerability of isolated pancreatic islets, parathyroid and skin allografts to cellular and humoral immunity. *Transplant Proc* 11:560–562, 1979

51. Nelson JD, Lange DB, Lindstrom RL, Doughman DJ, Hatchell DL: McCarey-Kaufman (MK) organ culture and MK medium-shifted corneas. *Arch Ophthalmol* 102:308–311, 1984

52. Nelson JD, Mindrup EA, Chung CK, Lindstrom RL, Doughman DJ: Fungal contamination in organ culture. *Arch Ophthalmol* 101: 280–283, 1983

53. Preminger GM, Koch WE, Fried FA, Mandell J: Utilization of chick chorioallantoic membrane for *in vitro* growth of the embryonic murine kidney. *Am J Anat* 159:17–24, 1980

54. Pritchett CJ, Senior PV, Sunter JP, Watson AJ, Appleton DR, Wilson RG: Human colorectal tumours in short term organ culture. A stathmokinetic study. *Cell Tissue Kinet* 15:555–564, 1982

55. Randall JH, Stein RJ, Stuermer NM: Cytodynamic properties

of human endometrium. I. Cultivation in fluid media; effects of different oxygen tensions, hydrogen ion concentrations and temperatures. *Am J Obstet Gynecol* 60:711–720, 1950

56. Reiss B, Williams GH: Conditions affecting prolonged maintenance of mouse and rat colon in organ culture. *In Vitro* 15:877–890, 1979

57. Rivera EM, Hill SD, Taylor H: Organ culture passage enhances the oncogenicity of carinogen-induced hyperplastic mammary nodules. *In Vitro* 17: 159–166, 1981

58. Riviere GR, Tarbox GS, Bringas P Jr, Slavkin HC: Murine tooth organ transplantation after *in vitro* culture. *J Dent Res* 62:980–984, 1983

59. Rodgers NT, Kaufman DG: The measurement of cytosolic estrogen receptors in human endometrial tissue and organ cultures. *J Steroid Biochem* 14:801–806, 1981

60. Russo RG, Liotta LA, Thorgeirsson UP, Brundage R, Schiffmann E: Polymorphonuclear leukocyte migration through human amnion membrane. *J Cell Biol* 91:459–467, 1981

61. Saffiotti U, Harris CC: Carcinogenesis studies on organ cultures of animal and human respiratory tissues. In: Griffin AC, Shaw CR, eds: *Carcinogens: Identification and Mechanisms of Action* Raven Press, New York, 65–82, 1979

62. Schiff LJ, Moore SJ, Ketels K M: Surface characteristics of cultured adult rat colon using scanning electron microscopy. *Scan Elec Microscopy* II:201–204, 1980

63. Schaeffer WI: Proposed usage of animal tissue culture terms (revised 1978). Usage of vertebrate cell, tissue and organ culture terminology. *In Vitro* 15:649–653, 1979

64. Siegal GP, Thorgeirsson UP, Russo RG, Wallace DM, Liotta LA, Berger SL: Interferon enhancement of the invasive capacity of Ewing sarcoma cells *in vitro*. *Proc Natl Acad Sci USA* 79:4064–4068, 1982

65. Stromberg K: The human placenta in cell and organ culture. *Methods Cell Biol* 21:227–252, 1980

66. Stuermer VM, Stein RJ: Cytodynamic properties of human endometrium. II. Cultivation and behavior of stromal cells of human decidua *in vitro*. *Am J Obstet Gynecol* 60:1332–1338, 1950

67. Stuermer VM, Stein RJ: Cytodynamic properties of the human endometrium. V. Metabolism and the enzymatic activity of the human endometrium during the menstrual cycle. *Am J Obstet Gynecol* 63:359–370, 1952

68. Talmage DM, Dart G: A search for the optimum conditions for culturing allografts before transplantation. *Clin Immunol Immunopathol* 15:314–317, 1980

69. Thompson D: Some further researches on the cultivation of tissues *in vitro*. *Proc Royal Soc Med* 7:21–46, 1914

70. Thompson KG, Little PB: Effect of haemophilus somnus on bovine endothelial cell in organ culture. *Am J Vet Res* 42:748–754, 1981

71. Thorgeirsson UP, Liotta LA, Kalebic T, Margulies IM, Thomas K, Rios-Candelore M, Russo RG: Effect of natural protease inhibitors and a chemoattractant on tumor cell invasion *in vitro*. *J Natl Can Inst* 69:1049–1054, 1982

72. Tobin SM, Fish EN, Wilson WD, Papsin FR: Organ culture model for the study of HVH-II infections in carcinoma of the cervix. *Obstet Gynecol* 53: 559–564, 1979

73. Todd ME, Friedman SM: The rat tail artery maintained in culture: An experimental model. *In Vitro* 14: 757–770, 1978

74. Usugane M, Fujita M, Lipkin M, Palmer R, Friedman E, Augenlicht L: Cell proliferation in explant cultures of human colon. *Digestion* 24: 225–233, 1982

75. Weinhold PA, Burkel WE, Fischer TV, Kahn RH: Adult rat lung in organ culture: Maintenance of histotypic structure and ability to synthesize phospholipid. *In Vitro* 15: 1023–1031, 1979

76. Williams PP, Gallagher JE: Cytopathogenicity of mycoplasma hypopneumoniae in porcine tracheal ring and lung explant organ cultures alone and in combination with monolayer cultures of fetal lung fibroblasts. *Infect Immun* 20: 495–502, 1978

77. Wolffing BK, Gabridge MG: Effect of *in vitro* cultivation and mycoplasma pneumoniae infection on intracellular cyclic AMP levels in hamster tracheal organ cultures. *In Vitro* 15: 308–314, 1979

78. Yen EH, Melcher AH: A continuous-flow culture system for organ culture of large explants of adult tissue: Effect of oxygen tension on mouse molar periodontium. *In Vitro* 14: 811–818, 1978

79. Yoshida Y, Hilborne V, Freeman AE: Fine structural identification of organoid mouse lung cells cultured on a pig skin substrate. *In Vitro* 16: 994–1006, 1980

OVERVIEW OF CURRENT UNDERSTANDING
OF TUMOR SPREAD*

RONALD H. GOLDFARB and KENNETH W. BRUNSON

INTRODUCTION

Progressive stages of malignant neoplastic growth can lead to cancer metastasis which is the major cause of treatment failure, moribidity, and death for patients with solid malignant tumors (5, 12, 33, 44, 45, 51, 56, 58, 59). Although the treatment modalities of radiotherapy, chemotherapy, and surgery effectively treat approximately 50 per cent of patients who develop malignant tumors, the majority of patients who are refractile to these therapeutic modalities succumb to the direct or indirect effect of tumor metastases or to adverse consequences associated with these therapeutic approaches (5, 33). At the time of diagnosis of primary tumors, approximately 50 per cent of patients with solid malignant tumors already host subclinical micrometastases, which may subsequently expand and contribute to direct anatomical compromise. In fact, a detected metastatic lesion in a particular organ may indicate the presence of other occult micrometastases. The heterogeneity of metastatic subpopulations and their scattered anatomic distribution may indeed limit or prevent effective surgical or chemotherapeutic intervention (5, 33). Furthermore, some of these treatment modalities may lead to adverse complications of immunosuppression which can lead to mortality arising from infectious disease.

The investigation of progressive stages of malignant neoplastic growth, and particularly tumor invasion and metastasis, is therefore the current focus of intense efforts in basic research in cancer molecular biology, cell biology, biochemistry and immunology and therapeutic intervention by pharmacologists and clinical oncologists (2–4, 8, 12, 16–20, 23, 30, 33–35, 40–43, 45, 48, 51–54, 57). This overview will provide highlights of contemporary insights into the mechanisms of tumor progression to metastasis from the perspectives of: biochemical mechanisms in tumor invasion and metastasis; modes of tumor spread; and tumor cell heterogeneity. We also review the potential clinical significance of these findings for the diagnosis and therapy of human malignant neoplastic disease.

BIOCHEMICAL MECHANISMS IN TUMOR INVASION AND METASTASIS

During tumor invasion malignant cells penetrate a number of barriers for metastatic spread including extracellular ma-

trices (19, 31, 33, 43). Extracellular matrices include dense lattice meshworks of collagen and elastin embedded within ground substances consisting of glycoproteins and proteoglycans (19). The matrix can function as a supporting scaffold which can mediate cell attachment events, delineate tissue compartment boundaries, and influence tissue architecture (33–35, 45). The matrix plays important functional roles in morphogenesis, mitogenesis, and differentiation and can also function as a filter for macromolecules (33, 34). In neoplasia, the interactions between normal cells and the matrix are modified and also contribute to tumor proliferation and invasion. The various extracellular matrices, such as basement membranes, interstitial stroma, bone and cartilage may differ from each other in the content and amount of matrix components. The basement membrane, for example, is composed of type IV collagen, specific glycoproteins including laminin and entactin, and heparan sulfate proteoglycans. Interstitial stroma and basement membranes separate tissue compartments from each other. During metastatic tumor invasion malignant tumor cells must penetrate these barriers as they cross tissue boundaries. Following expansion from the boundaries of the primary tumor, invasive tumor cells interact with basement membranes at a variety of steps in the metastatic process including: tumor cell entry or exit from blood vessels, the invasion of nerve and muscle, and during the penetration of epithelial boundaries (33, 34). In addition, tumor cells penetrate the epithelial basement membrane to enter the underlying interstitial stroma during the transition from *in situ* to invasive carcinoma. During intravasation or extravasation, invasive malignant cells penetrate through the wall of a capillary or venule and must traverse the perivascular interstitial stroma prior to the growth of metastatic foci in the target organ parenchyma. It has therefore been documented, by a large number of research groups, that penetration of extracellular matrices take place at multiple steps in the metastatic cascade.

A three-step hypothesis has been proposed to describe the sequence of biochemical steps involved in the invasion of extracellular matrices by invasive cancer cells (33, 34). The first step is tumor cell attachment to the extracellular matrix by cell surface receptors which specifically bind to components of the extracellular matrix. Laminin, a major glycoprotein of the basement membrane, plays an important role in the interaction of tumor cells and the basement membrane since it can form a bridge between the cell surface laminin receptor and type IV collagen in the basement membrane. The second step of tumor cell invasion of the matrix is local degradation of the matrix by tumor cell-associated

*This chapter is dedicated to the late Jørgen Fogh, M.D., who was associated for many years with the Sloan-Kettering Institute for Cancer Research, Rye, New York.

R. H. Goldfarb (ed.), Fundamental aspects of cancer.

proteolytic enzymes (19, 23, 33). In addition to the production of degradative enzymes, malignant cells may also recruit adjacent host cells to release hydrolytic enzymes. Metastatic tumor cells produce a battery of degradative proteases that contribute to tumor invasion including: type IV collagenase; plasminogen activator (which generates plasmin by plasminogen activation); heparanase (endoglucoronidase); cathepsin B; procoagulants; and additional neutral serine proteases (19, 23, 33). In addition, the proteolytic activity of lymphoid effector cells infiltrating metastatic deposits in situ may also contribute to proteolysis operative in invasion and metastasis (18–20, 23). The third step in the three-step hypothesis of metastatic tumor cell invasion of the matrix is tumor cell locomotion into the domain of matrix locally degraded by proteolysis. The direction of locomotion may be regulated by chemotactic factors (33, 36, 53). Continued invasion of the extracellular matrix may take place by cyclic repetition of these three sequential steps. For a more comprehensive biochemical description of these events the reader is directed to more detailed chapters in subsequent volumes in this series.

MODES OF TUMOR SPREAD

Tumors with moderate metastatic potential appear to spread initially to regional lymphatic and/or additional regional sites than to distant sites (44). It is likely that the regional location of metastases can be largely explained by mechanical and anatomical architecture including efferent venous circulation and/or lymphatic drainage to regional lymph nodes (44). The most frequent organ site of blood-borne metastatic involvement is the first organ that these cells encounter. Nevertheless, metastasis formation often occurs in distant organs and many tumors may tend to display relatively specific patterns of organ distribution sites (for more detailed description see volumes III, VII and VIII in this series). A number of explanations have been proposed to explain the formation of distant secondary metastatic lesions independent of lodgement in initial blood draining capillaries or draining regional lymph nodes. The 'seed and soil' hypothesis proposed by Paget in 1889 stated that the microenvironment of particular organs constituted the "soil" which can influence the implantation, growth, and survival of particular "seeds", i.e. tumor cells (26, 44). Alternatively, mechanical-anatomical entrapment, hypothesized by Ewing in 1928, has been suggested as a means to explain cancer invasion and metastasis. In addition, recognition by metastatic tumor cells of organ capillary endothelial cells in target organs may be modulated by specific cell surface molecules (16). Tumor cell binding studies in cryostat sections have been shown to correlate with their *in vivo* organ-specific adhesive patterns (38, 39). Indeed, cells selected for organ-specific adhesion *in vitro* have displayed changes in organ-specific formation of metastases providing additional evidence for a role of specific metastatic tumor cell-tissue adhesion interactions in organ-specific metastasis (139) chapter 11, this volume). In summary, it may be unlikely that any one mechanism for determination of patterns of metastases is the same for all tumor systems. It is likely that the different mechanisms will not be proven to be mutually exclusive (26).

LYMPHATIC AND HEMATOGENOUS TUMOR SPREAD

It has been suggested that the division of tumor spread into lymphatic and hematogenous modes is rather arbitrary since disseminating tumor cells may pass from one system to the other through numerous interconnections (12).

Disseminating tumor cell emboli can penetrate small lymphatic vessels and may be trapped by the first encountered lymph node (12, 26). Alternatively, tumor cells may traverse initially encountered lymph nodes or bypass them to form distant metastases. It has been suggested that lymph nodes can act as a filter for disseminating cancer cells. Indeed, lymph nodes of normal animals can effectively, albeit temporarily, block tumor dissemination in some systems (60). Nevertheless, most tumor cells that reach the draining lymph node rapidly enter the efferent lymphatics and subsequently the blood stream (13). Potential diagnostic significance of these observations is that lymph nodes draining the primary tumor lesion may be enlarged and clinically detectable.

Widespread tumor dissemination may result from the penetration of blood vessels, lymphatics, or both (12). Invasive cells of malignant neoplasms frequently penetrate thin-walled capillaries or venules but rarely invade arteriole walls or arteries. This resistance to invasion appears to be linked to the presence of protease inhibitors within connective tissues or smooth muscle cells (32, 47). The sequence of steps involved in hematogenous metastasis is reviewed below.

SEQUENTIAL STEPS IN HEMATOGENOUS METASTASIS

The process of metastasis is recognized as being a complex and dynamic interplay between the biochemical and cellular properties of invasive tumor cells and the properties of the host including anti-tumor immune reactivity (11). Degradative processes related to penetration of extracellular matrices also appear to contribute to early events in the formation of new blood vessels by tumor cells during neovascularization (15). Following initial growth, malignant tumor cells induce the ingrowth of new capillaries from host tissues by the release of tumor angiogenesis factors, thereby providing a new blood supply for tumor expansion (14). Following progressive local growth and vascularization of the primary neoplasm, metastatic cells must penetrate surrounding tissue and penetrate through blood vessels and/or lymphatic channels in order to disseminate. Subsequent to invasive penetration of vessel walls, metastatic cells detach, are released into the circulation, and some of the tumor cells form emboli.

The process of cancer metastasis is also highly selective and only subpopulations of tumor cells derived from the primary neoplasms can complete all of the steps needed to successfully form secondary metastatic colonies (11). In the circulation, tumor cells must survive mechanical trauma of blood flow and the reactivity of lymphoid effector cells including the lytic capacity of natural killer cells (18, 20). Tumor cells can then attach to blood vessel endothelium by a variety of non-specific or specific mechanisms including:

mechanical wedging, entrapment with platelets and fibrin, or attachment to target organ endothelium by specific cell surface recognition molecules (16, 38, 43). Invasive tumor cells must then penetrate through the subendothelial extracellular matrix and extravasate to invade the perivascular stroma of the target organ and subsequently form secondary metastatic colonies (33, 34, 45). During the events of this metastatic cascade, metastatic cells must overcome or evade systemic and local (i.e. lymphoid effector cells infiltrating the microenvironment of metastatic lesions) host immune responses as well as other host defenses (9, 24, 25, 29, 49). This sequence of cascading events may then be repeated to give rise to local invasion of secondary tumors and ultimately metastases from metastases (7, chapter 15, this volume).

TUMOR CELL HETEROGENEITY

A critical advance in the understanding of progressive neoplastic malignant growth has been the observation that tumor cells within a malignant tumor have differing metastatic propensities (50, 51). Indeed, the discovery that phenotypically heterogeneous subpopulations have differing properties, including metastatic potential, is of major significance for elucidating the biochemical and molecular properties of metastatic tumor cells, and for potential therapeutic implications for eventual clinical control over tumor metastases. Tumor cell heterogeneity has been revealed for numerous phenotypic properties in both primary and metastatic tumors including differences in: karyotype, antigenicity, immunogenicity, biochemical properties, growth behavior and susceptibility to chemotherapeutic drugs, radiation, hyperthermia, and recognition and destruction by humoral and/or cell-mediated cytotoxicity (50, 51).

It has been suggested that tumor cell heterogeneity, and consequent tumor progression with time are key reasons for treatment failure and recurrence of human malignant tumors (10, 12, 28, 51). The term "tumor heterogeneity" has been thought of by many as the presence of multiple tumor cell subpopulations within single tumors arising within a single host (28, 46). Additional aspects of tumor heterogeneity ("secular heterogeneity") including variation in: inflammatory infiltrates, vasculature, supporting tissue, tumor necrosis, nutrients, and pH gradients (46). These "secular" changes are in contrast to those that can be distinguished from transmitted genetic and epigenetic differences which determine cell lineages (27).

Ample evidence has been accumulated to demonstrate that malignant tumors contain multiple subpopulations of cells with a variety of metastatic capabilities and with a variety of differing sensitivities to anti-neoplastic agents (10). The demonstration of tumor heterogeneity is therefore of key importance in understanding progressive stages of neoplastic malignant growth leading to widespread metastatic disease (41, 46, 50, 55). Indeed, the demonstration of heterogeneous capabilities of distinct cellular subpopulations within the same tumor has led to major research efforts to elucidate this generation of cellular diversity and its regulation (50, 51). Recent studies probing these issues have indicated that the rate of formation of new tumor cell populations with novel phenotypes is influenced by interactions among subpopulations within the same tumor.

It is apparent that a thorough understanding of tumor heterogeneity and cellular diversity will provide important insights for an understanding of tumor progression and metastatic spread, and ultimately contribute to advances in diagnosis and more effective therapeutic intervention (12, 28, 40, 50, 51).

CLINICAL SIGNIFICANCE; DIAGNOSIS AND THERAPEUTIC STRATEGIES

Recent advances in elucidating the biochemical and cellular basis for progressive stages of neoplastic malignant growth, including tumor invasion and dissemination, have identified important targets for improved diagnosis and potential therapeutic intervention in malignant disease. Our current understanding of the biochemical mechanisms of tumor invasion and metastasis have already identified methods with clinical utility for the diagnosis of tumor pathology (23, 34). For example, reagents that detect either the degradation of basement membranes and/or basement membrane components such as type IV collagen or laminin, or reagents that detect degradative enzymes such as type IV collagenase and plasminogen activator, appear to be useful probes to identify or confirm the diagnosis of invasive malignancies (23, 34).

Recent studies implicating a role for degradative enzymes in tumor invasion and metastatic spread have stimulated a large number of research groups to seek inhibitors of particular classes of proteolytic enzymes for the prevention or treatment of metastases (30, 45). Indeed, prodrugs have already been designed as substrates for tumor cell-derived proteolytic enzymes, and protease inhibitors have already been employed in clinical trials (1, 6). To fully determine whether inhibitors of proteolytic enzymes may be useful for the prevention or therapy of metastases there is a need for the development of pharmacokinetically suitable and bioavailable, non-toxic, efficient, specific in vivo-active agents (37). Insights and understanding of cell surface adhesive properties of metastatic cells (43), and understanding of the cellular diversity and tumor heterogeneity within malignant tumors also provide essential information for the design of more effective therapeutic modalities for the control of cancer metastases (27, 28, 50, 51). It is indeed likely that the successful therapy of multiple metastases composed of tumor cell subpopulations heterogeneous for responsiveness to anti-tumor drugs, as well as metastatic propensities, will require regimens that can overcome such heterogeneity (50, 51).

It is intriguing to speculate that selective inhibition of degradative enzymes that play a role in local tumor invasion of primary tumors or established micrometastases might lead to therapy of disseminated cancer (23). It is equally intriguing to speculate that enhancement of host anti-tumor cell-mediated cytotoxic mechanisms might lead to enhanced therapy of established micrometastases (10, 20–22, 43, 49). Non-toxic protease inhibitors, or immune-response modifiers, might indeed have the capacity to overcome problems associated with tumor heterogeneity and drug resistance, and thereby contribute to therapeutic modalities with improved margin of safety and efficacy over many currently available anti-neoplastic agents. Disease targeting based on the understanding of tumor progression in cellular and molecular terms may indeed provide new avenues for: the maintenance of clinically dormant micrometastases; the prevention of the invasive outgrowth of these metastases; the prevention of local tumor invasion of clinically detectable primary tumors and their metastases, the prevention of metastases from metastases; and ultimately, the elimination of micrometastases.

CONCLUSIONS

Recent research and clinical advances have provided insights into the molecular biology, biochemistry, cell biology and immunology of neoplastic progression, including tumor invasion and metastasis. These advances have provided impetus for the exploration of urgently needed new approaches for the diagnosis and therapy of malignant disease. It is clear from the more detailed chapters in this series that the crucial insights that have been elucidated in the study of progressive stages of malignant neoplastic growth have identified a broad array of approaches which should now be exploited to rapidly reduce to clinical implementation new diagnostic techniques and novel modalities for the efficacious therapy of human metastatic cancer.

REFERENCES

1. Astedt B, Glifberg I, Mattsson W, Trope T: Arrest of growth of ovarian tumor by tranexamic acid. *J. American Med. Assoc.* 238:154–155, 1977
2. Brunson KW, Joshi SS: Properties of malignant lymphosarcoma variant cell lines associated with enhanced liver metastasis. In K Lapis, A Jeney and MR Price, Eds. *Tumour Progression and Markers.* Kugler Pub., Amsterdam, pp. 137–143, 1982
3. Brunson KW, Nicolson GL: Selection of malignant melanoma variant cell lines for ovary colonization. In RO Hynes and CF Fox, Eds. Prog in Clin and Biol Res (*Tumor Cell Surfaces and Malignancy*) 41:359–370, 1980
4. Brunson KW, Nicolson GL: Experimental brain metastasis. In L Weiss, HA Gilbert, JB Posner, Eds. *Brain Metastasis.* GK Hall and Co., Boston, pp. 50–65, 1980
5. Chabner BA: Present status and future prospects for treatment of metastatic cancer. In KV Honn, WE Powers, BF Sloane, Eds. *Mechanisms of Cancer Metastasis.* Potential Therapeutic Implications. Martinus Nijhoff, Boston, pp. 15–22, 1986
6. Chakravarty PK, Carl PL, Weber MJ, Katznellenbogen JA: Plasmin-activated prodrugs for cancer chemotherapy. 2. Synthesis and biological activity of peptidyl derivatives of doxorubicin. *J Med Chem* 26:638–644, 1983
7. Crissman JD, Honn KV: Applications for antimetastatic therapies. In KV Honn, WE Powers, BF Sloane, Eds. *Mechanisms of Cancer Metastasis. Potential Therapeutic Implications.* Martinus Nijhoff, Boston, pp. 399–417, 1986
8. DeVita Jr VT, Hellman S, Rosenberg SA Eds. *Cancer. Principles and Practice of Oncology.* J.B. Lippincott Co., Philadelphia, 1985
9. Evans R, Haskill S: Activities of macrophages within and peripheral to the tumor mass. In RB Herberman, H Friedman, Eds. *The Reticuloendothelial System. A Comprehensive Treatise.* Volume 5, Cancer. Plenum Press, New York, pp. 155–176, 1983
10. Fidler IJ, Berendt MJ: The biological diversity of malignant neoplasms. In E Mihich, Ed. *Biological Responses in Cancer.* Vol. 1, Plenum, New York. pp. 269–299, 1982
11. Fidler IJ, Gersten DM, Hart IR: The biology of cancer invasion and metastasis. *Adv Cancer Res* 28:149–250, 1978
12. Fidler IJ, Hart IR: Principles of cancer biology: Cancer metastasis. In VT DeVita Jr, S Hellman, SA Rosenberg, Eds. J.B. Lippincott Co., Philadelphia, pp. 113–124, 1985
13. Fisher B, Fisher ER: The Interrelationship of hematogenous and lymphatic tumor cell dissemination. *Surg Gynecol Obstet* 122:791–798, 1966
14. Folkman J: How is blood vessel growth regulated in normal and neoplastic tissue? G.H.A. Clowes Memorial Award Lecture. *Cancer Res* 46:467–473, 1986
15. Glaser BM, Kalebic T, Garbisa S, Connor TB, Liotta LA: Degradation of basement membrane components by vascular endothelial cells: Role in neovascularization. In *Development of the Vascular System* (Ciba Foundation Symposium 100), Pitman, London. pp. 150–162, 1983
16. Goldfarb RH: Proteases in tumor invasion and metastasis. In LA Liotta, IR Hart, Eds. *Tumor Invasion and Metastasis.* Martinus Nijhoff, The Hague. pp. 375–390, 1982
17. Goldfarb RH: Plasminogen activators. In H-J Hess, Edit, *Ann. Rep. Med Chem.*, Volume 18, Academic Press, New York, pp. 257–264, 1983
18. Goldfarb RH: Biochemistry of NK cytotoxicity. In RB Herberman, DM Callewaert, Eds. *Mechanisms of Cytotoxicity by NK Cells.* Academic Press, New York, pp. 137–153, 1985
19. Goldfarb RH: Proteolytic enzymes in tumor invasion and degradation of host extracellular matrices. In KV Honn, WE Powers, BF Sloane, Eds. *Mechanisms of Cancer Metastasis. Potential Therapeutic Implications.* Martinus Nijhoff, Boston, pp. 341–375, 1986a
20. Goldfarb RH: Cell-mediated cytotoxic reactions. *Human Pathology.* 17:138–145, 1986
21. Goldfarb RH, Berendt MJ: Natural killer cells: Role in cell-mediated immunity. In HJ Hess, Ed., *Ann Rep Med Chem*, Volume 18, Academic Press, New York. pp. 265–273, 1983
22. Goldfarb RH, Herberman RB: Characteristics of natural killer cells and possible mechanisms for their cytotoxic activity. In G Weissman, Ed. *Adv. Inflammation Res*, Volume 4, Academic Press, New York. pp. 45–72, 1982
23. Goldfarb RH, Liotta LA: Proteolytic enzymes in cancer invasion and metastasis. Seminars in Thrombosis and Hemostasis. 12:294–307, 1986
24. Golub SH, Moy PM, Gray JD, Karavodin LM, Kawate N, Niitsuma M, Burk MW: Systemic and local regulation of human natural killer cytotoxicity. In M Torisu, T Yoshida, Eds. *Basic Mechanisms and Clinical Treatment of Tumor Metastasis.* Academic Press, Orlando, pp. 123–161, 1985
25. Hanna MG, Bucana CD, Pollack VA: Immunological stimulation *in situ*: The acute and chronic inflammatory responses in the induction of tumor immunity. In IP Witz, MG Hanna, Eds. *Contemp Topics Immunobiol*, Volume 10, Plenum, New York, pp. 267–296, 1980
26. Hart IR: "Seed and soil" revisited: mechanisms of site-specific metastasis. *Cancer Metastasis Rev* 1:5–16, 1982
27. Heppner GH: Tumor heterogeneity. *Cancer Res* 44:2259–2265, 1984
28. Heppner GH: Problems posed for cancer treatment by tumor cell heterogeneity. In KV Honn, WE Powers, BF Sloane, Eds. *Mechanisms of Cancer Metastasis. Potential Therapeutic Implications.* Martinus Nijhoff, Boston, pp. 69–79, 1986
29. Herberman RB, Ed: *NK Cells and Other Natural Effector Cells.* Academic Press, New York, 1982
30. Honn KV, Powers WE, Sloane BF, Eds: *Mechanisms of Cancer Metastasis. Potential Therapeutic Implications.* Martinus Nijhoff, Boston, 1986

31. Jones PA, De Clerck YA: Extracellular matrix destruction by invasive tumor cells. *Cancer Metastasis Rev* 1:289–317, 1982

32. Laug WE: Inhibition of tumor cell-associated fibrinolysis by vascular bovine smooth muscle cells. *J Natl Cancer Inst* 75:345–352, 1985

33. Liotta LA: Tumor invasion and metastasis-role of the extracellular matrix: Rhoads Memorial Award Lecture. *Cancer Res* 4:1–7, 1986

34. Liotta LA, Goldfarb RH: Interaction of tumor cells with the basement membrane of endothelium. In KV Honn and BF Sloane, Eds. *Hemostatic Mechanisms and Metastasis.* Martinus Nijhoff, Boston, 319–336, 1984

35. Liotta LA, Hart IR, Eds: *Tumor Invasion and Metastasis.* Martinus Nijhoff, The Hague, 1982

36. McCarthy JB, Basara ML, Palm SL, Sas DF, Furcht LT: The role of cell adhesion proteins-laminin and fibronectin-in the movement of malignant and metastatic cells. *Cancer and Metastasis Rev* 4:125–152, 1985

37. Nelles LP, Schnebli HP: Are proteinase inhibitors potentially useful in tumor therapy? *Invasion and Metastasis.* 2:113–124, 1982

38. Netland PA, Zetter BR: Organ-specific adhesion of metastatic tumor cells *in vitro. Science.* 224:1113–1115, 1984

39. Netland PA, Zetter BR: Metastatic potential of B16 melanoma cells after *in vitro* selection of organ-specific adherence. *J Cell Biol* 101:720–724, 1985

40. Nicolson GL: Generation of phenotype diversity and progression in metastatic tumor cells. *Cancer Metastasis Rev* 3:25–42, 1984a

41. Nicolson GL: Tumor progression, oncogenes and the evolution of metastatic phenotypic diversity. *Clin Expl Metastasis* 2:85–105, 1984b

42. Nicolson GL, Brunson KW: Organ specificity of malignant B16 melanomas: *In vivo* selection for organ preference of blood-borne metastasis. In PG Stansly, H Sato, Eds. Gann. Monographs, 20 (*Cancer Metastasis. Approaches to the mechanism, prevention, and treatment*): 15–24, 1977

43. Nicolson GL, Brunson KW, Fidler IJ: Specificity of arrest, survival and growth of selected metastatic variant cell lines. *Cancer Res* 38:4105–4111, 1978

44. Nicolson GL, Poste G: Tumor implantation and invasion at metastatic sites. *Int Rev Exp Path* 25:77–181, 1983

45. Nicolson GL, Milas L, Eds: *Cancer Invasion and Metastasis: Biologic and Therapeutic Aspects.* Raven Press, New York, 1984

46. Owens AH, Coffey DS, Baylin SB, Eds: *Tumor Cell Heterogeneity: Origins and Implications.* Academic Press, New York, 1982

47. Pauli BU, Schwartz DE, Thonar EJM, Kuttner KE: Tumor invasion and host extracellular matrix. *Cancer Metastasis Rev* 2:129–153, 1983

48. Pollack VA, Fidler IJ: Use of young nude mice for selection of cells with increased metastatic potential from non-syngeneic neoplasms. *J Natl Cancer Inst* 69:137–141, 1982

49. Pollack VA, Fidler IJ: Stimulation of the RES and control of cancer metastasis. In RB Herberman, H Friedman, Eds. *The Reticuloendothelial System. A Comprehensive Treatise.* Volume 5, Cancer. Plenum, New York. pp. 177–191, 1983

50. Poste G: Tumor cell heterogeneity and the pathogenesis of cancer metastasis. In M Torisu, T Yoshida, Eds. *Basic Mechanisms and Clinical Treatment of Tumor Metastasis.* Academic Press, Orlando, pp. 79–100, 1985

51. Poste G: Pathogenesis of metastatic disease: Implications for current therapy and for the development of new therapeutic strategies. *Cancer Treat Rep* 70:183–199, 1986

52. Quigley JP, Goldfarb RH, Scheiner CJ, O'Donnel-Tormey J, Yeo T: Plasminogen activator and the membrane of transformed cells. In RO Hynes and CF Fox, Eds. Prog Clin Biol Res (*Tumor Cell Surfaces and Malignancy*) 41:773–796, 1980

53. Quigley JP, Cramer E, Fairbairn S, Gilbert R, Lacovara J, Ojakian G, Schwimmer R: Interaction of malignant cells with substrata: Adhesion, degradation and migration. In KV Honn, WE Powers, BF Sloane, Eds. *Mechanisms of Cancer Metastasis. Potential Therapeutic Implications.* Martinus Nijhoff, Boston, pp. 309–340, 1986

54. Schirrmacher V: Cancer Metastasis: Experimental approaches, theoretical concepts, and impacts for treatment strategies. *Adv Cancer Res* 43:1–73, 1985

55. Stackpole CW: Generation of phenotypic diversity in the B16 mouse melanoma relative to spontaneous metastasis. *Cancer Res* 43:3057–3065, 1983

56. Sugarbaker EV, Weingrad DN, Roseman JM: Observations on cancer metastasis in man. In LA Liotta, IR Hart, Eds: *Tumor Invasion and Metastasis.* Martinus Nijhoff, The Hague, pp. 427–465, 1982

57. Torisu M, Yoshida T, Eds: *Basic Mechanisms and Clinical Treatment of Tumor Metastasis,* Academic Press, Orlando, 1985

58. Weiss L: A critical overview of the metastatic process. In KV Honn, WE Powers, BF Sloane, Eds. *Mechanisms of Cancer Metastasis. Potential Therapeutic Implications.* Martinus Nijhoff, Boston, pp. 23–40, 1986

59. Welch DR, Tomasovic SP: Implications of tumor progression on clinical oncology. *Clin Expl Metastasis* 3:151–188, 1985

60. Zeidman I, Buss JM: Experimental studies on the spread of cancer in the lymphatic system: I. Effectiveness of the lymph node as a barrier to the passage of embolic tumor cells. *Cancer Res* 14:403–410, 1954

61. Auerbach, R; Lu, WC; Pardon, E et al.: Specificity of adhesion between murine tumor cells and capillary endothelium: An *in vitro* correlate of preferential metastasis *in vivo. Cancer Research* 47:1492–96, 1987

4

INTRASPECIES AND INTERSPECIES COMPARISON

H.E. KAISER

INTRODUCTION: THE ENHANCEMENT OF KNOWLEDGE BY THE COMPARATIVE METHOD

Knowledge can be enhanced by comparisons. This holds especially true in such a basic problem as that of growth and its most important abnormal variation: neoplastic growth. As one of the characteristics of life, growth is a very complex phenomenon, with its variations in many species, including 1,250,000 species of animals, to which the number of 5 to 7 million of undetected species, especially of insects, may be added. Some 300,000 vascular plants must also be included. But growth varies not only in the species as such, it varies also in different developmental phases of the individual of a particular species; it varies sexually, under the influence of nutrition, or, very importantly, as regards the different tissues in various species and in the same species. The different growth processes cannot be adequately examined here. Abnormal growth processes can be divided according to (1) into non-neoplastic and neoplastic ones. Non-neoplastic growth processes can appear, such as acquired atrophy or congenital diminished growth, such as hypoplasia, aplasia,

or agenesis; excessive growth cells (hypertrophy, hyperplasia); disturbances of cellular differentiation, such as metaplasia; and development of tumor-like masses, such as hamartomas and heterotopias (see (2)). Neoplastic diseases of man can be divided into neoplasms deriving from mesenchymal tissues; neoplasms from epithelial tissues; and mixed neoplasms, especially teratomas. All three groups exhibit benign and malignant forms. Different types of development complicate the picture of neoplastic development within the framework of abnormal growth. We observe neoplastic growth in vascular plants with their very important meristematic tissues (which retain their embryonal potential) or the catastrophic development of holometabolic insects which are in sharp contrast to the continued development in the mammal. These findings strongly suggest that comparison of these different processes will enhance our understanding of the diseases subsumed under "cancer". It should be noted that all neoplastic diseases are diseases in their own right, so that the term "cancer", lately extended to include the malignant mesenchymal tumors, is misleading. In research, the comparative approach offers two avenues: (1) the intraspe-

Table 1. Intraspecies comparison of human neoplasms.

Aspects	Comments
Histology	Prognoses of cutaneous malignant melanoma and basal cell carcinoma of the skin are remarkably different with regard to progression.
Differentiation	Anaplastic carcinomas support a worse prognosis than those which are well-differentiated paralleling a similar distribution and aggressiveness.
Age	Why different tumors of man exhibit such a great age variation, also affecting prognosis, is not fully understood.
Sex	Not only do sex-related neoplasms vary, such as in mammary cancer, but also certain solid neoplasms show a sex variation (see (2)).
Topography	Cutaneous malignant melanoma is more aggressive at the extremities than on the ventral area (trunk). Metastatic neoplasms are very dangerous depending on the topography which they invade. The direction of spreading depends on the location of the primary neoplasm in many, but not all cases (soil theory).
Stage	Stage development of neoplasms varies.
Race	The element of race, or better, populations resulting from intermarriage, varies markedly in number and type of neoplasms. For example, Burkitt's lymphoma is well known from Uganda and other African countries, while mammary cancer, very common in the USA and western Europe, is uncommon in Japan and Singapore, among other nations.
Behavior of host	Occupational and social behavior of the host exhibits remarkable intraspecific variations. Smoking may be cited as a well-known example; also (possibly) coffee drinking.
Nutritional condition	Obesity is considered breast-cancer promoting in women, fatty diet is suspected of promoting colon cancer in both sexes.
Metabolism	Interference with entire body metabolism varies in different types of neoplasms (see Chapter 1/III).
Immunological condition	Interference by malignant tumors with immunological functions in man.
External environment	External environment exercises a variable influence on human neoplastic development, especially at the beginning of the development of neoplastic diseases, but is not equally important for all cases.

33

R. H. Goldfarb (ed.), Fundamental aspects of cancer.
© 1989, Kluwer Academic Publishers, Dordrecht. ISBN 978-94-010-6980-9

cies comparison; and (2) the interspecies comparison. This sequence is based on self-evident logical considerations.

INTRASPECIES COMPARISON WITH SELECTED EXAMPLES

The intraspecies comparison is concerned with different processes in individuals of only one species. The species of greatest interest to us, of course, is man himself. In Table 1, a selection of tumor-differentiating characteristics of various human neoplasms is presented.

A review of the findings cited in the above table, limited perforce in scope, offers material for fruitful comparison, but many questions remain to be answered. Why do some tumors exhibit one age peak in adolescents but another in those of older age? Can we determine what are the tumor-promoting elements at this or that particular age? What is the reason for the rare occurrence of certain neoplasms at specific ages?

ILLUSION OF THE LOSS OF THE WAR "AGAINST CANCER" (3)

Modern therapy has made marked progress in the treatment of certain neoplasms (see Chapter 16/I), including youthful nephroblastoma, and acute leukemias of the young (7), but has remained virtually at a standstill in other neoplasms, such as certain types of lung cancer, colon cancer and, in general, the solid tumors of adults in the middle-age bracket. Two routes toward further progress could be taken. A more extensive investigation of the very common neoplasms might shed new light on the problem; or, a similarly intensive study of the more rarely seen neoplasms. The most promising route would be, of course, a combination of both. It has been suggested that cancer research should shift from a therapeutic approach to a preventive one. Perhaps a scientific approach directed toward an understanding of a specific neoplasm or group of neoplasms is needed. The comparative approach appears to offer greater chances of success.

INTERSPECIES COMPARISON WITH SELECTED EXAMPLES

In contrast to the intraspecies comparison, the interspecies comparison deals with individuals of different species. The latter forms the backbone of the testing of chemical compounds for carcinogenic activity and related investigations.

In interspecies comparison, the same problems as in the intraspecies comparison are investigated, but naturally broaden the framework of comparative oncology. The basis for such a view lies in the comparative approach to different mammals. The mammal must provide the central focus of our investigation for two reasons: (1) the mammal is the class to which we ourselves belong and (2) the mammal

exhibits the culmination, meaning the highest development of neoplastic growth.

A few examples only may suffice: melanoma occurs especially in gray horses; ocular melanoma is seen in cattle in Australia; mammary cancer is common in the mouse (see Chapter 19/V) and in the bitch but is uncommon in cattle, pig, sheep and goat (see Chapter 20/V). There also exist, of course, significant differences in metastatic neoplasms among the different species. We know, for example, that mammary carcinoma in the mouse spreads, in general, directly to the lung and not first to the regional lymph nodes, as in the human female. These comparisons could be extended and are further discussed elsewhere (see (6), pp. 649–721).

SUMMARY AND CONCLUSION

The adoption of the comparative method as a means toward enhancement of knowledge so useful to scientific investigation, is a choice open to oncology today. The focal point of the comparison is constituted by the human body. It is naturally our greatest concern. Furthermore, neoplastic disorders of man are the most extensively studied; the histological types of neoplasms, the best known. Intraspecies comparison can be extended through interspecies comparison and offers a promising approach to the successful execution of essential studies in both clinical and experimental pathology.

REFERENCES

1. Anderson WAD, Scotti TM: *Synopsis of Pathology* (9th edition). St. Louis, Missouri: C.V. Mosby Company, 1976
2. Ashley DJB (ed): *Evans' Histological Appearances of Tumours* (3rd edition). Vols. 1 and 2. Edinburgh–London–New York: Churchill Livingstone, 1978
3. Bailar JC III, Smith EM: Progress against cancer? *New Engl J Med* 314(19):1226–32, 1986
4. Kaestner A (H-E Gruner, ed.): Lehrbuch der speziellen Zoologie. vol. 1: Wirbellose Tiere. Pt. 1 (1980), pt. 2 (1984), pt. 3 (1982). Stuttgart–New York: Gustav Fischer Verlag, 1980
5. Kaiser HE: *Species-specific Potential of Invertebrates for Toxicological Research.* Baltimore: University Park Press, 1980
6. Kaiser HE (ed.): *Neoplasms – Comparative Pathology of Growth in Animals, Plants, and Man.* Baltimore: Williams & Wilkins, 1981
7. Levine AS: *Cancer of the Young.* New York: Masson Cie, 1983
8. Nowak RM, Paradiso JL: *Walker's Mammals of the World* (4th edition). Vols. 1 and 2. Baltime–London: The Johns Hopkins University Press, 1983
9. Remane A, Storch V, Welsch U: *Kurzes Lehrbuch der Zoologie* (5th edition). Stuttgart–New York: Gustav Fischer Verlag, 1985
10. Remane A, Storch V, Welsch U: *Systematische Zoologie* (2nd edition). Stuttgart–New York: Gustav Fischer Verlag, 1985
11. von Denffer D, Ehrendorfer F, Maegdefrau K, Ziegler H (eds): Strasburger – *Lehrbuch der Botanik.* Jena: VEB Gustav Fischer Verlag, 1978

THE LIFE SPAN OF MAMMALS: A COMPARISON

H.E. KAISER, J. PARADISO and M. JONES

INTRODUCTION

Mammals are an extremely diverse group, and it is important to take into account this great diversity in any comparative studies of neoplastic diseases in this group. This chapter discusses some of this diversity, and its relation to the study of neoplastic diseases.

Neoplasms are best known in mammals, the group to which human beings also belong. Most data on spontaneous neoplasms have been obtained from humans, and most experimental data are obtained from inbred strains of mice and rats. These are followed in importance by hamsters, guinea pigs, and certain primates. The maximum life span of a feral house mouse (*Mus musculus*) is thought to be about three years, but in the laboratory it usually lives only a year or less. The longevity difference between these mice and human beings, who may have a potential life span of 70 + years, is important to take into consideration in studying progressive stages of neoplastic growth. An extensive knowledge of primary tumors exists for such domestic animals as dogs and cats, which are advantageous to study in that various breeds of these animals exhibit different tumor patterns. However, data on secondary tumors in dogs and cats are scarce since most specimens are valued pets and hence die not available for research purposes. For a proper understanding of tumor spread, these different tumor patterns need to be studied.

LIFE SPAN AND THE ENVIRONMENT

The life span of an individual of any species is greatly influenced by the environment under which the individual lives. A fox, in the hazardous environment of the wilderness, may live three to four years, but in a zoological garden, under the protection and care of a veterinarian, the same fox may live 12 or 14 years. In domesticated animals, there are species which are usually allowed to live out their full lives, such as dogs, cats, and horses. Other species, such as pigs, are generally slaughtered for meat production at different ages of their lives as dictated by the economy. Various breeds or strains of domestic animals, such as dogs and mice, may exhibit differing life spans. For example, it is well known that large breeds of dogs, such as Irish wolfhounds, are often shorter-lived than smaller breeds such as beagles or terriers.

LIFE SPAN AND PHYLOGENY

Phylogeny is the accumulation of many ontogenies in the sense of hologeny. A short-lived species, such as a small rodent, may produce a sequence of many ontogenies in contrast to a long-lived mammal, such as man or the blue whale, which may have undergone only two ontogenies during the same time period. The first type is considered a fast phylogeny, and the second a slow phylogeny. This is an important principle that must be recognized in any research project in comparative oncology.

CHRONOBIOLOGICAL DATA

The chronobiological activity of mammals varies also, and needs to be considered in selecting mammals for use in research projects. This can be readily demonstrated by looking at circadian rhythms in different species. Best known are the nocturnal mammals, such as mice and raccoons, or daylight animals, such as horses, or cattle. These species have different peaks in their metabolic activity on which their other activities, such as psychological or behavioral, are based. But there are also animals which are active mainly at dawn, such as white-tailed deer, and these species have different circadian rhythms. Beside the circadian rhythms, there are other rhythms, such as yearly rhythms, to which certain mammals in the arctic, walruses for example, are adapted.

COMPARISON OF LIFE SPAN IN WILD, CAPTIVE (ZOO), DOMESTIC AND LABORATORY MAMMALS

It is necessary to distinguish between three basic types of mammals in comparative oncology. These are the wild, the domestic and the laboratory mammals. It should be noted, however, that due to environmental destruction, and other threats, some mammals, such as Pere David's deer, have become extinct in the wild and today are found only in captivity (Table 1).

In domestic animals there are those types that generally are allowed to live out their full lives, as has been noted with the dog and cat, and those that are brought to a premature end by slaughtering for economic purposes. But even in the latter species many individuals are kept for breeding pur-

R. H. Goldfarb (ed.), Fundamental aspects of cancer.

Table 1. Selected mammalian longevities

Species	Maximum known longevity in captivity	Maximum known or estimated longevity in wild
Order: Marsupialia		
Didelphis virginiana, Northern opossum	4 yrs, 10 mos	few survive 3rd yr in wild
Phascolarctos cinereus, Koala	17 yrs	exceeds 10 yrs
Trichosurus vulpecula, Gray brush-tailed possum	14 yrs, 8 mos	generally 6 to 7 yrs, but occasionally up to 13 yrs
Pseudocheirus peregrinus Ring-tailed possum	5 yrs, 8 mos	4 to 5 yrs
Order: Insectivora		
Sorex sp. Long-tailed shrews	3 mos[1]	1 to 2 yrs
Blarina brevicauda Short-tailed shrew	2 yrs, 3 mos	2 yrs, 6 mos
Scalopus aquaticus Eastern mole	1 yr, 11 mos	3 yrs
Rhynchocyon chrysopygus Yellow-backed elephant shrew	9 yr, 2 mo	4 to 5 yrs
Order: Dermoptera		
Cynocephalus variegatus Colugo	1 mo	one kept as pet under semi-wild conditions 17 yrs, 6 mos
Order: Chiroptera		
Rhinolophus sp. Horseshoe bats	1 mo[2]	generally 6–7 yrs; max. record 24 yrs
Artibeus jamaicensis Jamaican fruit bat	10 yrs	at least 7 yrs
Desmodus rotundus Vampire bat	13 yrs, 2 mos	9 yrs
Myotis sp. Little brown bats	6 mos[3]	30 yrs[4]
Lasionycteris noctivagans	1 mo	at least 12 yrs
Eptesicus fuscus Big brown bat	11 mos	at least 19 yrs
Plecotus sp. Big-eared bats	2 mos[5]	10 yrs, 1 mo[6]
Tadarida brasiliensis Free-tailed bat	1 yr, 6 mos	8 yrs
Order: Primates		
Galago sp. Galago	16 yrs, 6 mos[7]	8 yrs[8]
Callithrix sp. Marmosets	12 yrs, 6 mos[9]	10 yrs
Macaca sp. Macaques	37 yrs, 1 mo[10]	less than 5 yrs[11]
Hylobates concolor Gibbon	44 yrs, 1 mo	
Hylobates syndactylus Siamang	28 yrs	25 yrs
Pongo pygmaeus Orang-utan	59 yrs est.	–
Pan troglodytes Chimpanzee	53 yrs est.	about 60 yrs
Gorilla gorilla Gorilla	52 yrs, 4 mos	up to 50 + yrs
Order: Lagomorpha		
Ochotona princeps Pika	3 yrs, 1 mo	average 5 yrs, 7 yrs max
Sylvilagus sp. Cottontails	2 yrs[12]	average 15 mos; 1 lived 9 yrs[13]
Lepus sp. Rabbits	7 yrs, 5 mos[14]	estimated 5 yrs[15]

Table 1. Selected mammalian longevities (continued)

Species	Maximum known longevity in captivity	Maximum known or estimated longevity in wild
Order: Rodentia		
Aplodontia rufa Mountain beaver	3 yrs, 6 mos	5–6 yrs not uncommon
Tamias striatus Eastern chipmunk	7 yrs	2–3 yrs
Eutamias sp. Western chipmunks	8 yrs, 4 mos[16]	few live more than 64 mos; max. known 8 yrs[17]
Marmota marmota Marmot	12 yrs	13–15 yrs
Ammospermophilus leucurus White-tailed antelope squirrel	5 yrs, 10 mos	most die in first year
Sciurus carolinensis Eastern gray squirrel	23 yrs, 6 mos	12.52 yrs
Tamiasciurus hudsonicus Red squirrel	9 yrs, 10 mos	7 yrs
Geomys sp. Pocket gophers	7 yrs, 2 mos[18]	5 yrs or more
Perognathus sp. Pocket mice	8 yrs, 4 mos[19]	most die in first year; some live to 4 yrs
Castor canadensis Beaver	15 yrs, 10 mos	24 yrs (max record)
Oryzomys sp. Rice rats	2 yrs, 10 mos[20]	few live more than 1 year
Reithrodontomys sp. Harvest mice	1 yr, 9 mos[21]	few live as long as 1 yr; record 18 mos
Peromyscus sp. White-footed mice	7 yrs, 8 mos[22]	less than 2 yrs
Rhyzomys sumatrensis Sumatran bamboo rat	3 yrs, 6 mos	about 4 yrs
Tachyoryctes splendens Mole rat	1 yr, 10 mos	average 1 yr; max known 3.1 yrs
Arvicola terrestris European water mole	2 yrs, 5 mos	mean longevity 5.4 mos
Microtus sp. Meadow mice	3 yrs, 11 mos[23]	less than 1 mo, but some may live up to 1 yr[24]
Ondatra zibethicus Muskrat	5 yrs, 6 mos	3 yrs
Apodemus sp. Common field mice	4 yrs, 5 mos[25]	1 yr or less
Glis glis Fat dormouse	8 yrs, 8 mos	more than 4 yrs
Muscardinus avellanarius Hazel dormouse	2 yrs, 6 mos	4 yrs
Zapus hudsonius Meadow jumping mouse	5 yrs	4 yrs
Napaeozopus insignis Woodland jumping mouse	3 mos	4 yrs
Hystrix sp. Old world porcupines	27 yrs, 3 mos[26]	12–15 yrs
Erethizon dorsatum New world porcupine	8 yrs, 5 mos	10 yrs
Hydrochaeris hydrochaeris Capybara	11 yrs, 11 mos	8–10 yrs
Chinchilla laniger Chinchilla	11 yrs, 4 mos	10 yrs
Order: Cetacea		
Delphinus delphis Common dolphin	4 mos	over 20 yrs
Globicephala sp. Pilot whales	11 yrs[27]	est 50 yrs
Orcinus orca Killer whale	12 yrs, 2 mos	at least 50 yrs
Neophocaena phocaenoides Harbor porpoise	3 yrs, est 23 yrs	

Table 1. Selected mammalian longevities (continued)

Species	Maximum known longevity in captivity	Maximum known or estimated longevity in wild
Monodon monoceros Narwhal	4 mos	est 40 yrs
Order: Carnivora		
Canis latrans Coyote	21 yrs, 10 mos	$14\frac{1}{2}$ yrs max known
Canis lupus Gray wolf		10 yrs considered old
Lycaon pictus African wild dog	10 yrs, 1 mo	14 yrs
Ursus americanus Black bear	26 yrs, 4 mos	26 yrs
Ursus arctos Brown bear	26 yrs, 10 mos	at least 25 yrs
Ursus maritimus Polar bear	39 yrs	25–30 yrs
Procyon lotor Raccoon	20 yrs, 7 mos	few more than 5 yrs; some est at 13–16 yrs
Taxidea taxus Badger	26 yrs	14 yrs
Felis rufus Bobcat	32 yrs, 4 mos	12 yrs
Panthera tigris Tiger	26 yrs, 3 mos	est 26 yrs
Order: Pinnipedia		
Otaria flavescens South American sea lion	22 yrs, 10 mos	est 20 yrs
Callorhinus ursinus Northern fur seal	12 yrs	females 22 yrs; males 15 yrs
Hydrurga leptonyx Leopard seal	6 yrs, 11 mos	potential 26 yrs
Leptonychotes weddelli Weddell seal	7 mos	at least 20 yrs
Order: Proboscidea		
Elephas maximus Asian elephant	est 69 yrs	–
Loxodonta africana African elephant	48 yrs	50–70 yrs
Order: Sirenia		
Dugong dugon Dugong	8 yrs	as much as 40 yrs
Order: Perissodactyla		
Rhinoceroses (all species)	31–45 yrs	about 50 yrs
Order: Artiodactyla		
Sus scrofa Wild boar	21 yrs	about 10 yrs average
Hippopotamus amphibius Hippopotamus	54 yrs, 4 mos	41 yrs in protected population
Odocoileus sp. North American deer	18 yrs, 6 mos[28]	rarely more than 10 years
Alces alces Moose	17 yrs, 11 mos	27 yrs
Rangifer tarandus Caribou	20 yrs, 2 mos	average $4\frac{1}{2}$ yrs; max 13 yrs
Capreolus capreolus Roe deer	8 yrs, 6 mos	average 10–12 yrs; max 17 yrs
Giraffa camelopardalis Giraffe	36 yrs, 2 mos	26 yrs
Syncerus caffer African buffalo	29 yrs, 6 mos	18 yrs
Bison bison Bison	33 yrs	20 yres

Table 1. Selected mammalian longevities (continued)

Species	Maximum known longevity in captivity	Maximum known or estimated longevity in wild
Litocranius walleri Gerenuk	11 yrs, 5 mos	8 yrs
Saiga tatarica Saiga	8 yrs	10–12 yrs
Oreamnos americanus Mountain goat	13 yrs, 8 mos	18 yrs
Ovibos moschatus Muskox	16 yrs, 8 mos	23 yrs

[1]*S. araneus,* [2]*R. ferrumequinum,* [3]*M. daubentoni,* [4]*M. lucifugus,* [5]*P. auritus,* [6]*P. rafinesquei,* [7]*G. senegalensis,* [8]*G. alleni,* [9]*C. jacchus,* [10]*M. fascicularis,* [11]*M. sinica,* [12]*S. idahoensis,* [13]*S. floridanus,* [14]*L. europaeus,* [15]*L. americanus,* [16]*E. dorsalis,* [17]*E. ruficaudatus,* [18]*G. bursarius,* [19]*P. fallax,* [20]*O. longicaudatus,* [21]*R. fulvescens,* [22]*P. crinitus,* [23]*M. guentheri,* [24]*M. pennsylvanicus,* [25]*A. sylvaticus,* [26]*H. brachyura,* [27]*G. melaena,* [28]*O. virginianus.*

poses and hence have a longer life potential. Similar conditions occur in laboratory mammals. All of these factors need to be taken into consideration in any investigation of neoplastic diseases in mammals. There are some mammalian orders the longevity of whose members is known only from animals in captivity. Some data are summarized in Table 2.

IMPLICATION FOR THE LIFE SPAN OF MAN

From the examples given above, it may be seen that the life span of any particular species of mammal is variable and dependent on a number of factors; it may be considerably extended if the conditions for a particular individual are good. The data on life span in man given in the chapter on ageing show that in some countries humans have only a life span of 36 to 39 years, whereas in other countries the average life span is as high as 70 years or more. Research on ageing must have as its special goal the encouragement of health conditions that will allow an extended life span for man. Conclusions based on available data from mammals in the wild and in zoos are that man's life span is similarly flexible and that man can reach greater ages under healthy conditions without signs of senility such as exhibited in Alzheimer's disease or dementia senilisis. It is also important

to remember this when treating neoplasms in children or young adults with chemotherapy. In such cases, it is necessary to take precautions, for example by protecting the gonads, as outlined in the chapter 20/VII, or to consider the possibility of therapy induced, second cancers outlined in the chapter 21/VI.

OUTLOOK FOR THE FUTURE

Only a relatively few species of mammals have been utilized in research of neoplastic disease. There are approximately 6000 mammalian species in the world, and many more may be able to contribute in one way or another to our knowledge in oncology. But for any value to be derived from a study of these various mammals, it is essential to take into account the life span and other factors discussed in this chapter. Comparison of neoplasms in mammals should always be expressed in terms of a percentage, taking the age at onset of the neoplastic disease and dividing by the potential life span of the species involved. Only in this way can the time of dissemination of a cancer in one species validly be compared to the time of dissemination in another species. Each stage of cancer progression should also be treated as a percentage of the potential life span of the species involved.

Table 2. Longevity of selected mammals. Known in these orders only from captivity

Order	Family	Species	Life span
MONOTREMATA	Tachyglossidae	*Tachyglossus aculeatus,* Australian echidna	49 yrs, 5 mo
	Ornithorhynchidae	*Ornithorhynchus anatinus,* platypus	17 yrs
EDENTATA	Bradypodidae	*Choloepus hoffmanni,* Hoffmann's two-toed sloth	34 yrs, 3 mo
	Dasypodidae	*Burmeisteria retusa,* pigmy armadillo	0 yr, 2 mo
PHOLIDOTA	Manidae	*Manis crassicaudata,* Indian pangolin	19 yrs, 3 mo
TUBULIDENTATA	Orycteropodidae	*Orycteropus afer.* aardvark	23 yr, 0 mo
HYRACOIDEA	Procaviidae	*Dendrohyrax arboreus,* hyrax	12 yr, 3 o
		Heterohyrax syriaca, Syrian hyrax	8 yr, 10 mo

SUMMARY AND CONCLUSION

The life span of the different mammalian species varies and is an important parameter in comparative oncology; it should be always expressed as a percentage in relation to the potential life span of each species investigated. Many mammal species that have hitherto not been used in research may contribute additional sources of importat information in comparative oncology.

Some of the findings and data have been brought up to date during the period of proofreading.

REFERENCES

1. Jones ML: *Longevity of captive mammals*. Zool Garden NF Jena 52 2, pp. 113–128, 1982
2. Kaiser HE: *Neoplasms – Comparative Pathology of Growth in Animals, Plants and Man*. Chapter 13: "Ontogenetic and complementary aspects of neoplastic growth", pp. 243–66; chapter 43: "Species specific spectrum of neoplasms", pp. 649–721; Chapter 48: "Animal neoplasms – a systemic review", pp. 747–812. Baltimore: Williams & Wilkins, 1981
3. Nowak RM, Paradiso JL: *Walker's Mammals of the World*, 4th edition, vols. 1 and 2, Baltimore–London: The Johns Hopkins University Press, 1983

THE CULMINATION OF NEOPLASTIC DEVELOPMENT IN THE MAMMAL

H.E. KAISER

DOMINATION OF THE MAMMAL SINCE THE OLIGOCENE EPOCH

Comparative pathology and oncology must raise the question, where is the culmination of neoplastic growth to be found? Where are the neoplastic diseases most highly diversified and specialized? What role is played by the body plan (morphology, physiology and biochemistry)? What is the influence of the ecology of the particular organism? The different population groups of mammals, including man himself and perhaps the dog, may afford us answers, if the conditions are compared with other appropriate organisms. It is worthwhile to look at the situation of the mammal, since it arose with three-rooted teeth as unambiguous marker in the upper Triassic period of the earth history.

Since the Oligocene epoch the mammals became the dominating and most highly developed organismic class. They are far outnumbered by such animals as insects but developed nevertheless the largest diversity of body structures with the most extensive span of size and body weight and a long life span and adaptation to air (chiroptera or bats are the second largest order of mammals with 942 species), water (with the cetacea or whales, of which the blue whale is the largest animal which ever lived, pinnipeds and sirenia) and the many terrestrial species to which man belongs are typical. The mammals have a very well-developed sense or care for the young which is evident from the nourishment of those with the breast glands. These organs gave the class the name mammals. The breast gland in man is one of the most tumor-prone organs, also it is, perhaps, one of the youngest types of tissues.

THE TWO PEAKS OF MAMMALIAN DEVELOPMENT

The intensified development of the mammals since the Oligocene epoch exhibits two points of culmination: one comprising the whole mammalian group on the one hand, and the rise of man on the other. The development of the basic plan of the mammalian type shows real variation, if compared with the two other major types of recent vertebrates, the fishes and birds, which both exhibit an undivided body plan. The amphibians and reptiles should not be considered here because a mere remnant of them was left after the Mesozoic. The characteristics of the mammalian body plan in relation to neoplastic development are described in the following chapters on body structure and the comparative importance of the lymphatic system.

CONTINUED DEVELOPMENT IN MAMMALS: COMPARISON TO CATASTROPHIC DEVELOPMENT

Mammals exhibit continued development. The young resemble the parents, but are smaller. Roundabouts of aberrant development are present only in the form of the placenta and in some evolutionary remnants, such as branchial arches or the teeth in whalebone whales. Continued development is hence readily distinguishable from catastrophic development, as seen in the case of holometabolic insects, where tissues and even organs are histolyzed when redundant. In later chapters, this type of organ histolysis is compared with tumor regression (in Volume IV).

VARIATIONS IN THE CARE OF OFFSPRING

Care for the offspring varies among different phyla of the animal kingdom. Insects, which are generally bisexual, as well as many other invertebrates, produce a large number of offspring, while in contrast the mammals evince care for their relatively small number of offspring. We see the same principle in small mammals, such as mouse and rat which have a larger number of offspring than large species. In the mammals, placental neoplasms appear; also, the transmission of neoplastic cells from fetus to mother via the placenta, and vice versa. Placental neoplasms among nonmammalian vertebrates and invertebrates have not been observed.

THE LEVEL OF THE OTHER HIGHEST NONVERTEBRATE ANIMAL ORGANISMS: CEPHALOPOD MOLLUSCS, DECAPOD CRUSTACEANS AND HOLOMETABOLIC INSECTS

These organisms, that develop advanced structures of the senses, circulatory systems and endocrine glands, among other structures, if compared to vertebrates, reach in their development only the level of the fishes.

STRUCTURAL SUPERIORITY OF THE MAMMALS IN RELATION TO NEOPLASTIC GROWTH

In comparison to other organisms, the structure of the mammal attains the highest degree of development as a basis

R. H. Goldfarb (ed.), Fundamental aspects of cancer.
© 1989, Kluwer Academic Publishers, Dordrecht. ISBN 978-94-010-6980-9

for neoplastic development and progression. This is due to the fact that bone, with its many typical neoplasms, is a characteristic of most vertebrates; that the breast gland and the hairs also develop several characteristic tumor types; and the stratified epithelia reach their highest degree of development. According to comparative findings plant tissues, the endocrine structures of invertebrates, and oblique striated musculature are all of no great importance in neoplastic development.

THE SUPERIORITY OF BODY STRUCTURE AS BASIS FOR THE MOST DIVERSIFIED NEOPLASTIC DEVELOPMENT

The body structure of the mammal is greatly diversified with regard to the function of the various cellular complexes united to form a large number of tissue combinations, themselves with diversified functions. The possibility of neoplastic development and progression is enhanced by the high development of the system of body fluids, of the immune system and of the endocrine system. The equally high development of man's central nervous system, especially of the human brain, has been incidentally a contribution to the development of human neoplasms.

The brain of man can be said to be the initiator of pollution of much of the world's water, soil and air. In turn, this pollution, becomes the initiator of carcinogenesis, along with many social habits which may pose carcinogenic risks. The human brain is also the source of therapies devised to combat neoplastic disorders. Man remains the best subject in our continuing search for progress in oncological science.

SUPERIORITY OF THE SYSTEM OF BODY FLUIDS, TOGETHER WITH A HIGHLY DEVELOPED IMMUNE SYSTEM

The mammal exhibits the most highly developed system of body fluids, a system which interacts with an equally highly developed immune system. The blood circulation is connected with a well-developed lymphatic system which does not penetrate the central nervous system as an exception but exhibits also the highest developed lymphatic system with lymph nodes and lymph organs (see Chapter 12/I). The immune system exhibits humoral and structural defense.

HIGHEST DEVELOPMENT OF THE CENTRAL NERVOUS SYSTEM

The CNS in the mammal and especially man has reached its highest development. If we compare the vertebrates with the invertebrates we wil see that the highest development of the CNS in the most advanced invertebrates, such as cephalopod molluscs, decapod crustaceans, and best developed insects reaches a condition not higher than in fishes. One possible exception is the eye in cephalopod molluscs which resembles our own eye, but the ontogenetic development differs. It must be noted that the eye is only partially (retina) a portion of the CNS and is otherwise a sense organ.

HIGH DEVELOPMENT OF THE ENDOCRINE SYSTEM

Endocrine glands reach a developmental peak in the mammal. But the whole endocrine system of cephalopod molluscs and arthropods is comparable in its complexity to the endocrine system in vertebrates. Endocrine comparable glands occur in the form of the optic glands in cephalopod molluscs; Y-organs, and in the male androgen glands in crustaceans; and corpora allata, thoracic glands, and in some insects, ventral glands, are all epithelial endocrine glands.

REFERENCES

1. Bailar JC III, Smith EM: Progress against cancer? *New Engl J of Med* 314 (19):1226–32, 1986
2. Highman KC, Hill L: *The Comparative Endocrinology of the Invertebrates.* (2nd edition). Baltimore: University Park Press, 1977
3. Kaiser HE: *Species-specific Potential of Invertebrates for Toxicological Research.* Baltimore: University Park Press, 1980
4. Kaiser HE: Distribution of true (real) tissues in organisms: a preliminary condition of neoplastic growth. In: *Neoplasms – Comparative Pathology of Growth in Animals, Plants, and Man,* HE Kaiser (ed.). Baltimore: Williams & Wilkins, 1981

THE INFLUENCE OF THE BODY STRUCTURE ON TUMOR DEVELOPMENT

H.E. KAISER

Neoplastic cells originate from normal cells of the organism undergoing neoplastic transformation. Cells are cells but their specializations culminating in the formation of tissues vary according to the taxonomic position of the organism. In general, considering organisms with true tissues (animals, plants and higher fungi) three tissue types can be distinguished. These are the tissues of animals and man, the tissues of vascular plants and the plectenchymata of fungi. The first two groups develop by cell division whereas the last group develops by cell clogging up, interweaving or coalescing. The tissues of the highest algae, especially pheophyta and rhodophyta, can be considered comparable to true tissues but of a low level and are known as pseudoparenchymata. Mosses also have tissues that are similar in general too but differ in particular, from the true tissues of higher life forms. A short table summarizes the most important facts (1)(3).

Neoplasms can be seen as caricatures, inferior in character to the normal tissue or tissues from which they derive. They never reach a higher level of differentiation than the tissue from which they derive. The normal tissue spectrum of the healthy organism is the basis for the possible neoplastic spectrum (3). The appearance of neoplasms depends on the normal body structure. It does not matter if we see the neoplastic growth in relation to its site, as many pathologists prefer, or if we see the neoplasms in relation to the tissues. Neoplasms of the breast can only be found in man and other mammalian species. The same is true of neoplasms developing from the hair – anlage. Chordomas, benign or malignant, can only develop in those organisms which exhibit chorda tissue. They are therefore restricted to the chordate phyla. Table 2 offers a few selected examples of the theoretical tumor spectrum based on the normal distribution spectrum of tissues.

It is instructive to look at the different types of breast cancer as shown in Table 3. The epithelial neoplasms are of interest because they can be seen interacting with the other nonepithelial neoplasms and with the healthy and neoplastic breast tissues where the neoplasms develop. This results in a whole specific picture of the "organ" breast with neoplas-

Table 1. Tissue types of the organisms.

A. *Tissues below the level of or on the border to true tissues*
1. Plectenchymata of fungi
2. Pseudoparenchymata of algae
3. Tissue-thalli of phaeophyceae (brown algae) –
   (already true tissues)
4. Tissues of mosses (bryophyta)

B. *True Tissues of vascular plants*
1. Meristemic tissues
   Apical meristems
   Lateral meristem
   Meristemoids
   Succeeding meristems
   Phellogen
2. Fully differentiated tissues
   Phytoepidermis
   Rhizodermis
   Collenchyma
   Sclerenchyma
   Xylem
   Phloem
   Periderm
   Secretory structures

C. *True tissues of animals*
1. Epithelial tissues
   Simple lining membranes
   Stratified lining membranes
   Excretory glands
   Incretory glands, including those of invertebrates

2. Connective, hematopoietic and supporting tissues
   Mesenchyme
   Spinocellular connective tissue
   Reticular connective tissue
   Gelatinous connective tissue
   Loose connective tissue
   Fibrous connective tissue
   Melanogenic system
   Adipose tissue
   Chordal tissue
   Chondroid tissue
   Cartilage
   Bone
3. Muscular tissue
   Myoepithelial tissue
   Smooth musculature
   Helically striated musculature
   Transverse striated musculature
   Cardiac musculature
4. Nervous tissue and glia
   Neurons of the central nervous system
   Neurons of the peripheral nervous system
   Autonomous nervous system and chromaffin tissue
   Meninges
   Choroid tissue
   Central glia
   Peripheral glia
   Neurosecretory cells/tissue

43

R. H. Goldfarb (ed.), Fundamental aspects of cancer.
© 1989, Kluwer Academic Publishers, Dordrecht. ISBN 978-94-010-6980-9

Table 2. Selected cases of the comparative tissue/tumor spectrum.

Tissue	No. of phyla	Est. no. of species
Simple columnar epithelium	26	1 203 000
Stratified columnar epithelium	1	45 000
Mammary glands	1	5 000
Chordal tissue	4	50 000
Bone	1	45 000
Transverse striated musculature	7	1 000 000–7 000 000

tic disease (see Chapters V17–20, VI7, IX7, 20). Cuboidal ductular epithelium, from which intraductal carcinoma of the breast may arise, is interwoven with the other tissues differently than the same type of epithelium, as for example in the case of squamous cell and basal cell carcinoma of the conjunctiva.

The same picture results if we investigate the lungs as breathing organs. Each gaseous exchange which takes place in the various organs of animals and plants and serves this function acts as a gaseous transport from one location (medium) to another via a separating membrane. Table 4 lists the organs of gaseous exchange in the organisms. Table 5 offers a tubular review of the human lung. Again, we observe neoplasms of epithelial and mesenchymal tissues which are of primary origin and those which are of secondary. From both types of tumor it is possible to draw conclusions on the tissue of origin. Exceptions are highly undifferentiated neoplasms, epithelial and mesenchymal.

The tissue spectrum and the organ spectrum of neoplasms

The various organisms with true tissue exhibit a variation of tissue distribution which results at site in a different interaction of tissues. Neoplasms in organisms below the level of true tissues (including plectenchymata and pseudoparenchymata in fungi and algae and tissues of mosses are problematic) are an illusion (unicells are only able to exhibit comparable cell abnormalities to single neoplastic cells). The combination of a characteristic tissue arrangement with functional interaction and distribution is an organ. The tissues are comparable if they show similar morphology, of which the functional state may vary in different locations, for example a squamous or basal cell carcinoma of the

Table 3. Neoplasms of the human breast.

Fibro-adenoma
Giant fibroadenoma
Cystic hyperplasia
Adenoma or florid papillomatosis of the nipple
Intraduct-papilloma + cystadenoma
Lobular carcinoma
Extraduct carcinoma
Medullary carcinoma
Colloid carcinoma
Adenoid cystic carcinoma
Paget's disease of the nipple
Cancer of the male breast

Secondary tumors are rare in the breast, except the metastasis of a tumor of one breast to the contralateral breast

conjunctiva and a squamous cell carcinoma of the urethra. A mediastinal teratoma may develop from different cells with varying pluripotentiality, an osteogenic sarcoma of soft tissues as well as an osteochondroma from the pluripotential mesenchymal stem cell or its derivatives. This tissue interrelationship may also be an explanation for dissimilar aggressiveness of human malignant cutaneous melanoma of the back or the trunk in contrast to the skin of the lower leg.

The tissue spectrum of neoplasms is of great comparative importance because it is the only possible means of comparing structures, i.e., tissues of similar form and function in different species. The organ arrangement in the organisms is much more variable than that of the tissues. In different individuals of the same species, the tissue is a good indicator of tumor growth.

The formation of organs to be used for tumor characterization is another effective method, especially in one species or in a few related species, with the exception of species

Table 4. Structures of gaseous exchange.

1. Animals
a. No respiratory structures: Bentastomida, Tardigrada, Phoronida (perhaps lophophor tentacles
b. Surface epithelia act as respiratory structures in: Cnidaria, Ctenophora, Platyhelminthes, Nemertinea, Gnathostomulida, Entoprocta, Acanthocephala, Rotifera, Gastrotricha, Kinorhyncha, Nematoda, Nematomorpha, Priapulida, Pentastomida, and Tardigrada, Mollusca, Echiurida, Annelida, Echinodermata (papulae and tube feet).
c. Specialized body surface underlined with blood vessels act as respiratory structures:
    Sipunculida, Ectoprocta
d. Body appendages and tentacular crowns act as respiratory structures in Annelida
e. Gills act as respiratory structures in Mollusca, Annelida, Echinodermata (Echinoidea), Cephalochordata and Vertebrata
f. Tracheids act as respiratory structures in Onychophora and Arthropoda.
g. Booklungs act as respiratory structures in arachnid Arthropods.
h. Tracheid gills act as respiratory structures in larval Arthropoda.
i. Lophophore (mantle) acts as respiratory structures in Brachiopoda.
j. Branchial apparatus and/or gill intestine act as respiratory structures in Chaaetognatha and Tunicata.
k. Lungs act as respiratory structures in Pulmonata (Mollusca) and Vertebrata.
2. Plants
    The leaf acts as respiratory structure in vascular plants.

Table 5. Neoplasms of the lung in man.

I. Epithelial Neoplasms

Primary Epithelial Neoplasms

1. Epidermoid carcinomas
2. Small cell anaplastic carcinomas
3. Adenocarcinomas
4. Large cell carcinomas
5. Combined epidermoid and adenocarcinomas
6. Bronchial gland tumors
7. Papillary tumors of the surface epithelium

Secondary Epithelial Neoplasms
(blood borne metastases)

1. Oral and pharyngeal carcinomas
2. Carcinoma of esophagus
3. Carcinoma of stomach
4. Carcinoma of intestine
5. Carcinoma of liver
6. Carcinoma of pancreas
7. Carcinoma of breast
8. Carcinoma of uterus
9. Carcinoma of ovary
10. Carcinoma of prostate
11. Carcinoma of thyroid gland
12. Carcinoma of kidney
13. Malignant melanoma
14. Chorion epithelioma
(Systemic dissemination of secondary
neoplasms of the lung is common
via small venules)

II. Mesenchymal Neoplasms

Primary Mesenchymal Neoplasms
1. Fibroma
2. Myoma
3. Lipoma
4. Angioma
5. Chondroma
6. Osteoma
7. Lymphoblastoma
8. Sarcomas
3. Mixed Neoplasms
1. "Mixed" tumors and carcinosarcomas
2. Mesotheliomas
3. Melanomas
4. Unclassified

Secondary Mesenchymal Neoplasms
1. Osteosarcoma
2. Other sarcomas

which have catastrophic development. It is not effective in some species because the organs in the organisms have a much wider variety than tissues. In a single species such as man the determination of a neoplasm is first made by most pathologists in relation to the site and second in relation to tissue. Certain sarcomas in one organ may also differ from those in another organ. These facts result in the behavioral tumor background of tissue interaction of neoplasma composed of the same tissues at different site in one organism of the same species.

Not only variations of cells and tissues, but also of the structures of the body plan can restrict tumor distribution. Eumetazoans can be divided into acoelomate animals such as flatworms in which the organs are embedded in connective tissue and no body cavity exists. The second group of animals are the pseudocoelomates in which a body cavity surrounding the organs is present but not covered with a lining membrane. The third group of animals are the coelomates, to which man belongs, and which is characterized by a body cavity (divided during later development) which is lined by an endothelium. Therefore mesotheliomas can only be expected in coelomate species. Endotheliomas, hemangiotnelioma or angiosarcoma can only be found in organisms with a closed circulatory system.

The development of an organism, however, can give rise to a variation of neoplasms which differ in various develop-

mental stages. This is the case in continued development as can be seen in the age distribution of man, or in catastrophic development as observed in *Drosophila*. These developmental variations complicate the theoretical picture of tumor development. Certain cells of earlier developmental stages are able to remain in a dormant stage up to later stages of development of an organisms and are then able to give rise to tumors to be expected at an earlier age.

REFERENCES

1. Highnam KC, Hill L: *The Comparative Endocrinology of the Invertebrates.* 2nd edition. Baltimore: University Park Press, 1977

2. Kaiser HE: *Species-Specific Potential of Invertebrates for Toxicological Research.* Baltimore: University Park Press, 1980

3. Kaiser HE: *Distribution of True (Real) Tissues in Organisms: A preliminary Condition of Neoplastic Growth* in *Neoplasms – Comparative Pathology of Growth in Animals, Plants and Man,* edited by Kaiser HE, pp. 43–88, Baltimore: Williams & Wilkins, 1981

4. Kaiser HE: *Species-Specific Spectrum of Neoplasms,* in *Neoplasms – Comparative Pathology of Growth in Animals, Plants and Man,* edited by Kaiser HE, pp. 649–724, Baltimore: Williams & Wilins, 1981

5. Kaiser HE: *Principles of a Comparative Functional Histology*, *Gegenbaurs morph Jahrb*, Leipzig 129 2, pp. 137–180, 1983
6. Kreyberg L: *Histological Typing of Lung Tumours*, WHO, Geneva, pp. 9–26, 1967
7. Strasburger E, Noll F, Schenck H, Schimper AFW (eds): 31st edition, *Lehrbuch der Botanik*, Jena: Gustav Fischer Verlag, 1978
8. von Albertini A: *Histologische Geschwulstdiagnostik*, 2nd edition, Stuttgart: Georg Thieme Verlag, 1974
9. Willis RA, *The Spread of Tumours in the Human Body*, 3rd edition, London: Butterworth 1973

THE EVOLUTION OF DIVERSITY WITHIN TUMORS AND METASTASES

JAMES E. TALMADGE

INTRODUCTION

Despite advances in the use of aggressive adjuvant chemotherapy and radiotherapy, which in combination with surgery are often successful in the eradication of the primary
tumor, most deaths in cancer patients result from metastasis. This chapter reviews the process of metastasis on a
cellular basis and is approached using as a goal the improvement of therapeutic protocols. Excellent reviews on the
mechanism of metastasis and the characteristics of metastatic cells are provided by L.A. Liotta elsewhere in this series.

A question important to our understanding of the pathogenesis of metastasis and to the improvement of cancer
therapy is whether tumor cells that give rise to metastatic
foci are random survivors of the cells within the primary
tumor or represent a select subpopulation of tumor cells that
preexists within the primary tumor population. If the metastatic process is selective, then the cells within a metastatic
foci represent an enlarged pool of tumor cells endowed with
specialized characteristics and it may be possible to develop
therapeutic modalities directed against the unique
phenotype. The development of novel therapeutic modalities is important since tumor cells within primary tumors are
heterogeneous with regard to their metastatic potential and
their response to most therapeutic modalities, including
chemotherapy, radiotherapy, and specific immunotherapy.
This phenotypic heterogeneity is not unique to the primary
tumor but is also observed among metastases (interlesional)
as well as within metastases (intralesional). Clearly the only
successful treatment of disseminated cancer will be one
capable of overcoming the problems associated with the
heterogeneity of the tumor cells. The development of screening protocols to identify novel anticancer agents must not
only monitor the response of the primary tumor to therapy
but also examine the efficiency of such agents or protocols
against the metastatic subpopulations within the primary
tumor.

Recent studies of metastasis have increased our understanding of the metastatic process as it is influenced by both
tumor cell properties and host-tumor cell interactions.
Many of these studies have challenged established beliefs,
resulting in the modification of experimental techniques and
models that are used to study metastasis as well as alter our
outlook on therapeutic protocols designed to treat established secondary tumor foci. Therefore, the goal of this chapter
is to provide an overview of these studies.

THE HETEROGENEOUS NATURE OF NEOPLASMS

Histological studies have long demonstrated morphologic
differences among cells within the same tumor. For this
reason, pathologists routinely examine several sections of a
tumor to determine whether a tumor is benign or whether it
contains nests of invasive and malignant cells. Dunn (38)
examined the histology of numerous primary murine mammary tumors and concluded that cancer does not represent
a single alteration of one cell that reproduces itself without
change. Foulds (56–59) also noted that murine mammary
tumors are composed of zones of tumor cells with different
morphologies and that within each zone the cells appear
homogeneous. To study this zonal heterogeneity,
Henderson and Rous (80) fragmented tumors of mixed
morphology, which, after transplantation as individual fragments, tended to develop into tumors with a uniform morphology. Other more recent studies have described differences in cellular morphology (35) and tumor histopathology
(71, 99, 124, 145) within primary tumors of various his-
totype. The coexistence of multiple subpopulations of tumor
cells within single neoplasms has been repeatedly demonstrated in animal tumors of diverse etiology and histological
type. These include melanoma (49, 53, 70, 131), lymphoma-
leukemia (23, 124, 139), sarcomas (102, 123, 130, 159, 190,
212, 218), and carcinomas (31, 35, 37, 71, 80, 119, 125, 129,
145, 196, 204, 209, 227). Heterogeneity in tumors induced by
chemical agents (196, 218), physical agents (102), steroids
(37), or viruses (30, 31, 35, 119, 124, 125) have been described. Long-term passaged tumors (53, 134), tumors of
recent origin (49, 102), as well as autochthonous tumors (35,
139) have also been found to contain multiple subpopulations. At the time of diagnosis, most neoplasms are populated by cellular subpopulations with diverse phenotypes.

Tumors are composed of cells that are heterogeneous with
regard to their antigenicity (1, 24, 30, 32, 72, 89, 95, 129, 146,
147, 156, 168, 188) and immunogenicity (16, 17, 55, 64, 65,
69, 94, 116, 128, 129, 131, 133, 140, 169, 202). These variations in antigenicity and immunogenicity are important
since they can profoundly influence the success of specific
immunotherapy. In another study, Olsson and Ebbesen
(139), using a number of AKR mouse lymphomas, found
that vaccination procedures against polyclonal tumors
failed to prevent tumor growth following challenge since
only the dominant subclone was restricted in growth. The
minor subpopulations, which did not constitute a sufficient

R. H. Goldfarb (ed.), Fundamental aspects of cancer.
© 1989, Kluwer Academic Publishers, Dordrecht. ISBN 978-94-010-6980-9

mass in the vaccine to stimulate the immune response, were able to proliferate following the vaccination and eventually became the dominant population. In certain tumor systems, a successful host immune response to tumor cells bearing strong antigens may result in the emergence of tumor cell variants lacking the antigen. For example, Reading and co-workers (163) analyzed a number of *in vivo* and *in vitro* selected murine RAW117 lymphosarcoma cell lines (and clones derived from these cell lines) for their metastatic properties and cell surface antigen expression. They found that the ability to metastasize to the liver was inversely correlated with the expression of the antigenic RNA tumor virus envelope glycoprotein gp70, as determined by competitive radioimmune assay. In this system, successful metastasis apparently requires escape from host immune surveillance via antigen deletion on the highly metastatic lymphosarcoma cells. However, in other metastatic systems such as the B16 melanoma there is no relationship between metastasis and viral antigens such as gp70 (54). In contrast, other tumors express antigens that may be increased on metastatic cells. Shearman and Longenecker (176) reported an increase in cellular antigen content that correlated with the ability of Marek's disease virus-transformed chick lymphoma cells to metastasize to the liver. In this system, the amount of cell surface antigen detectable with monoclonal antibody increased concomitantly with the ability to colonize the liver. Thus, there appears to be no simple relationship between the display of cell surface antigens, immunogenicity, and metastasis.

Tumor cell populations residing within a parent neoplasm can also be heterogenous with regard to drug sensitivity. Cells isolated from rat hepatomas (6), methylcholanthrene-induced mouse sarcomas (73, 74), murine lung cancers (165, 205), a murine melanoma (115, 209), and a mouse mammary tumor (81) have different *in vitro* and *in vivo* sensitivities to various cytotoxic agents and radiation therapy (13, 73, 74, 81, 83, 107–109, 185, 204–207). During an extensive study, Tsuruo and colleagues (209) examined the *in vitro* sensitivity to various chemotherapeutic agents of tumor cells from parent tumors (rodent and human), their *in vitro* cloned populations, and spontaneous metastases from these tumor lines. Their findings demonstrated that differences in drug responsiveness exist among cells populating parent tumors (*in vitro* clones), as well as between the parent line and its metastatic subpopulations. These differences in drug sensitivity between the primary and secondary tumors obviously have profound implications for the treatment of metastases with cytotoxic drugs.

Cells within individual tumors have also been shown to differ with regard to their growth rate both *in vitro* and *in vivo* (21, 28, 31, 34, 35, 70, 127, 181, 197, 227). Tumor subpopulations can differ in expression or production of "markers" of differentiation, including appropriate pigments (49, 52, 70, 136), receptors (179), cell products (124), and specialized biosynthetic enzymes (37). The subpopulations also differ on the basis of DNA content (14, 184), karyotype (12, 35, 86, 87, 103, 111, 122, 130, 137, 138, 157, 173, 174, 187, 213–215) as well as the presence or absence of marker chromosomes in different tumor subpopulations (174). Tumor cells also express various cell surface receptors for lectins (23, 161, 162, 198, 200), hormone receptors (19, 60, 84, 85, 179), and metabolic characteristics (2, 9, 10, 96,

104, 173). Using murine mammary tumor virus (MuMTV) DNA as a probe, cellular heterogeneity in the location and copy number of a specific gene has been demonstrated in the GR mouse mammary tumors (119, 125). This is in accordance with the heterogeneity observed in the expression of MuMTV-coded antigens within individual mammary tumors (30). Studies on the differential response of BALB/cf and C_3H mammary tumor subpopulations to inducers of MuMTV gene expression suggest that the differences in regulation of MuMTV genes also correlate with tumor subpopulation heterogeneity (72).

There is considerable evidence to suggest that human tumors are also composed of heterogeneous subpopulations. Heterogeneous histological patterns have been observed in multiple samples of breast carcinoma (66, 142) and oat cell carcinoma (43) as well as from a histological and ultrastructural study of the tumor cells in a bronchial carcinoid (117). As discussed earlier human tumors also exhibit marked intralesional heterogeneity in antigenicity and immunogenicity (1, 24, 116, 121, 199). It was reported recently (118) that Ca antigen (3) may be detected in some areas of a carcinoma but not in others, even in those cells that were obviously malignant by morphological criteria. This suggests the possibility that the cells from a tumor differ in the expression of the Ca antigen, either on the cell membrane or in the cytoplasm.

Intratumor heterogeneity in tumor cell DNA content or ploidy levels has been reported for small cell carcinoma of the lung (186, 214) and colon carcinoma (215, 216). Tumors have also been shown to be heterogeneous for markers that may be associated with the degree of differentiation, including β2-microglobulin (223), estrogen receptors in breast cancer (19, 106, 144), steroid receptors in prostatic cancer (40, 216), and calcitonin levels in small cell carcinoma of the lung (10). Tumor cell heterogeneity for calcitonin has also been described in virulent medullary carcinoma (112). This is especially interesting in that the heterogeneity for calcitonin staining was seen in medullary carcinomas with a high likelihood of metastatic spread, whereas uniform staining was observed in tumors with a small chance of recurrence.

Histological examination of tumor samples generally reveals differences in the morphology of tumor cancer cells within the same lesion. In addition, host infiltrating and connective tissues are not evenly distributed in tumors, and areas of necrosis may be present. Depending upon tumor size, marked disturbances in vasculature can occur, leading to focal differences in oxygen tension, pH, substrate supply, and waste drainage (212). The cells within a tumor may be cycling or noncycling, quiescent or reproductively dead (33). Cells may be at any stage of the cell cycle. The stage of cell cycle may influence cellular properties such as membrane biochemistry (15, 143), antigen expression (29, 42, 141), sensitivity to immune killing (110, 177), drug cytotoxicity (210), and ability to metastasize (191, 220), resulting in the appearance of tumors that are heterogeneous with regard to all these properties. Therefore, the *in situ* demonstration of tumor heterogeneity cannot constitute proof of a stable phenotypic heterogeneity. However, formal proof vis-á-vis isolation and characterization has been presented for a number of human tumors.

Tumor lines that differ in drug sensitivity (5, 7), antigenicity (1), or tumorigenicity in nude mice (4) have been isolated from individual melanomas, both from primary lesions (4, 5, 7) or multiple metastases of the same patient (1, 4) as well as from tumor subpopulations isolated from primary human colon carcinomas (18, 36). Certain of these subpopulations differ in karyotype (18), *in vitro* growth properties (18, 36), tumorigenicity (18), and tumor histology in nude mice (14, 187). Similar isolations of tumor subpopulations have been reported for lung (25), ovarian (120), and bladder (79) cancer. Other human neoplasms, including melanoma (5, 7, 114), colon adenocarcinoma and gastric carcinoma (205, 207), ovarian carcinoma (206), breast carcinoma (8, 114, 178), lymphoma-leukemias (13, 105), and lung cancer (19), also contain different subpopulations of cells with different drug sensitivities.

Shirpo and co-workers (174) studied the karyotypic heterogeneity within human tumors by karyotyping tumor cells from fresh samples of human gliomas within six to 72 hr after surgery. An array of unique karyotypes was found in each tumor. Simultaneously, dissociated tumor cells were cloned by dilution plating and the clones were karyotyped. By matching karyotypes of the clones with those in the fresh sample, it was possible to show that the clones were present at the time of resection. Each of eight gliomas were found in this way to have from three to 21 subpopulations – a minimal estimate since different subpopulations can have similar karyotypes. Different clones from the same tumor also differed in morphology and growth kinetics. A recent report from this laboratory also demonstrated the heterogeneity of the cloned subpopulations to chemotherapeutic agents (226).

TUMOR HETEROGENEITY FOR INVASION AND METASTASIS

The possibility that cells with differing metastatic capabilities might coexist within the same tumor was first suggested in 1939 by Koch (100), who isolated a highly metastatic subline from the Ehrlich carcinoma tumor by serially transplanting lymph node metastases. In 1955, Klein (97, 98) demonstrated that the gradual conversion of solid murine neoplasms into ascites variants was due to the selective overgrowth of a small number of cells that differed from the parent population in their ability to proliferate in the peritoneal cavity and metastasize to the lungs. Since the change was stable and heritable, Klein concluded that the gradual conversion of the solid tumor to the ascites form involved mutation and selection and was not attributable to adaptation.

Three different experimental approaches can be used to isolate tumor cell subpopulations with differing invasive and/or metastatic abilities. The first involves enrichment of the fraction of invasive-metastatic subpopulations in heterogeneous tumor cell populations. This uses the technique of repeated cycling to gradually enrich for a subpopulation with a desired metastatic phenotype. Spontaneous metastasis or an analogous model is allowed to occur and the metastatic population is recovered and recycled. The biological behavior of the selected cells is then compared with that of the cells of the parent tumor to determine whether there is now enhanced metastatic capacity. This

procedure was used to obtain the B16-F10 line from the unselected B16 melanoma (46). In these investigations, tumor cells were injected intravenously, lung tumor nodules were excised three weeks later, and the recovered tumor cells were established in culture and then reinjected into new mice. After ten such cycles, a tumor line emerged that showed a marked increase in its ability to produce pulmonary tumor colonies (46). Recent studies from several laboratories, using similar strategies with animal tumors of diverse histologic origin, have also revealed significant variations in the metastatic capabilities of cells isolated from the same tumor (23, 31, 35, 152, 181, 192, 201, 227). Nonetheless, these selected tumor lines may still be heterogeneous and contain multiple subpopulations with differing metastatic potentials as well as other phenotypes. The selection pressures serve only to enrich for a general tumor population with subpopulations of tumor cells that may express differing invasive and metastatic properties.

The second and related method to isolate sublines with differing metastatic properties from a common parent tumor line is to select for (or against) properties considered important for successful metastasis. As in the enrichment method, variants displaying (or lacking) the property of interest are recovered and tested to determine whether their metastatic behavior is altered. This method has been used to examine whether properties as diverse as adhesive characteristics (20), lectin resistance (162, 200), invasive capacity (77, 153), resistance to cytotoxic T lymphocytes (47, 62, 167), and resistance or sensitivity to natural killer (NK) cells (68, 75) influence the ability of tumor cells to metastasize.

The third approach to demonstrate that malignant primary tumors contain subpopulations of cells with differing metastatic capabilities involves cloning tumor cell populations. The clones can be compared within the same population to determine if a defined propriety affects the process of metastasis. Obviously the phenotypic analysis of tumor cell clones is the most direct and satisfactory of the three techniques to demonstrate cellular heterogeneity as well as to determine if a unique phenotype is important to metastasis.

The demonstration of metastatic heterogeneity within a primary tumor was first reported in 1977 by Fidler and Kripke (53) using the B16 melanoma. To investigate whether primary tumors contained cells of differing or uniform metastatic potential, they prepared a cell suspension from a subcutaneous primary tumor and divided it into two parts. One part was immediately assayed for its ability to form experimental pulmonary metastases after intravenous injection into mice. From the other part of the original suspension, 17 clones were isolated (each one was established from an individual cell). After incubation for the same period of time, equal numbers of tumor cells in suspension from each of the cloned lines and from the parent tumor were injected into syngeneic mice. It was reasoned that if the tumor contained cells of uniform metastatic potential, then the cloned sublines should each produce the same number of pulmonary colonies as the uncloned parent population. This was not the case. The original uncloned parent tumor cell population produced similar numbers of metastases when injected into different animals, but the cloned sublines differed markedly in their metastatic potential. Control subcloning experiments showed that this variability was not introduced by the process of cloning, since groups of animals injected with a cloned parent tumor or subcloned lines all had a similar range and distribution of metastases (53). They concluded, therefore, that tumors contained cellular subpopulations that were heterogeneous in their metastatic potential.

The B16 melanoma is an established tumor line that has been maintained by repeated passage in animals or cell culture for many times the life span of its natural host. Thus, the metastatic diversity in this tumor line could have been an artifact caused by its longevity. However, comparable data were observed with another murine melanoma of recent origin (49). This tumor arose in a C3H mouse that had been subjected to ten one-hr exposures of UV radiation followed by the application of 2.5% croton oil in acetone to the skin of the scapular region for two years. The primary tumor that developed was removed, and fragments were transplanted into immunodeficient animals to circumvent the possibility of immune selection. Several weeks later, a tissue culture line was established; during the fifth passage, the cell line was cloned. Analysis of the metastatic capacity of the parent tumor (K-1735) and its cloned lines was performed in a manner similar to the original study. The clones differed dramatically from each other and from the parent line in their production of lung tumor colonies with regard to their size, number, and pigmentation. Within each injected clone, however, these three characteristics were expressed uniformly. Thus, lung colonies produced by one clone could be distinguished readily from those produced by another on the basis of size and pigmentation. Statistical analysis of the results indicated that only two of 22 K-1735 clones were indistinguishable from the parent tumor (49). With these figures as an indication of the degree of metastatic heterogeneity for metastasis, the K-1735 melanoma was shown to be no less heterogeneous than the B16 melanoma. These results indicate that longevity of neoplasms is not the sole arbiter of metastatic heterogeneity.

Clonal variation in metastatic properties is not peculiar to melanomas. Comparable extensive heterogeneity with regard to malignant-metastatic properties has been described in clones isolated from tumors of diverse histologic origin from the mouse (35, 101, 172, 182, 190), the rat (196), the chicken (175), and the hamster (41). In those studies, tumor cell subpopulations with differing metastatic phenotypes isolated from primary tumors or cultured tumor cell lines were as heterogeneous as those reported previously.

The value of tumor cell clones in analyzing any aspect of tumor cell behavior requires that the phenotypic characteristic(s) of interest remain stable during serial passage of the clones whether *in vivo* or *in vitro*. Poorly metastatic and highly metastatic clones were isolated from the UV-2237 fibrosarcoma (101) and were cultivated *in vitro* for 72 or 60 days, respectively (27). Simultaneously, both clones were also grown subcutaneously in syngeneic mice. Then, cell cultures were established from these solid tumors: one week later, subclones were isolated from both the *in vitro* and the *in vivo* passaged tumor lines. The ability of the subclones to form experimental metastases was compared between the subclones derived from clones grown in culture or *in vivo* and subclones isolated and frozen when the parent clones were initially established. The patterns of behavior of all the subclones derived from the poorly metastatic clone were remarkably similar to that of the parent clone, regardless of whether the subclones were derived at the time of isolation or after 72 days of continuous growth *in vitro* or *in vivo*. In contrast, after 60 days of cultivation *in vitro* or *in vivo*, the metastatic behavior of the subclones derived from the highly metastatic clone differed considerably from that of the parent clone, suggesting that the metastatic phenotype of the highly metastatic clone is unstable (27). The authors suggested that this rapid generation of diversity may have been caused in part by increased genetic instability.

Recent studies using the B16 melanoma have also demonstrated that the invasive and metastatic properties of clones from this tumor are highly unstable during serial passage and that subclones with different invasive and metastatic properties are generated rapidly on serial passage either *in vitro* or *in vivo* (17, 76, 85, 151, 158, 183). Observation of individual B16 clones carrying a variety of stable biochemical markers has revealed that, whereas the metastatic phenotype is unstable when clones are grown singly, mixing and cocultivation of clones eliminate this phenotypic instability, and the formation of variant subclones with altered metastatic properties is reduced dramatically (151). This suggests that some form of "interaction" is occurring between the various cellular subpopulations in polyclonal populations, which somehow "stabilizes" not only their invasive-metastatic properties but also their relative proportions within the total populations (151). This type of interaction would conserve clonal diversity within a tumor cell population and prevent domination of the population by a few subpopulations, or even a single subpopulation. This "stabilizing" effect produced by mixing clones is, however, specific for cells from the same tumor. Single clones of B16 melanoma cocultivated with clones from the Lewis lung carcinoma or UV-2237 fibrosarcoma show marked phenotypic instability and rapidly generate subclones with widely differing metastatic properties (151).

The role of clonal interactions in regulating the stability of the metastatic phenotype is not unique to the B16 melanoma. Similar instability of the metastatic phenotype has been found in the mouse UV2237 fibrosarcoma (27), mouse RAW117 lymphosarcoma (23), mouse KHT sarcoma (76), and rat 1AR6 hepatocarcinoma (196).

METASTASIS AS A SELECTIVE OR RANDOM PROCESS

The preexistence of metastatic variation within the parent tumor does not answer the question of whether the cells that ultimately form metastatic foci possess a greater metastatic potential than the cells that populate the parent neoplasm. We recently examined the issue of whether metastases result from the random survival of cells released from the primary tumor or from the selective growth of cells with specialized properties that allow them to complete the metastatic process. If the process of metastasis is selective, as suggested by previous studies, direct evidence to support this hypothesis would be the demonstration that cells populating spontaneous metastases should be demonstrably more metastatic than the cells within the heterogeneous parent neoplasm as long as 1) the starting tumor population was unselected and heterogeneous with respect to metastatic potential and 2) the metastatic process *per se* exerted selective pressures upon the tumor cells.

The initial studies from our laboratory to address this question used three metastatic variants of the B16 melanoma, thus minimizing variables that would be introduced by using tumor models with varying biological characteristics. The malignant melanoma, B16-F1 (46), is an unselected tumor cell line that metastasizes poorly after intravenous injection (experimental metastasis) or footpad injection (spontaneous metastasis). The B16-F10 tumor was selected ten times for its ability to colonize the lungs after intravenous injection (46) and has a high rate of experimental metastasis. The B16-BL6 tumor line was selected *in vitro* for its invasive ability and demonstrates a high incidence of spontaneous metastasis following intrafootpad implantation (77).

The experimental design was as follows: the tumor lines were implanted into the footpads of syngeneic mice (Figure 1). When the tumors reached a diameter of 1 to 1.2 cm, the tumor-bearing leg, including the popliteal lymph node, was resected. Several weeks later, when a few mice in each group appeared listless, the entire group was killed. From each group, well-isolated pulmonary metastases were surgically excised and established in culture as individual cell lines. The metastatic potential of cells from the parent tumor and their respective spontaneous metastases was then examined using assays of experimental and spontaneous metastasis.

We found that tumor cells harvested from spontaneous metastases of the poorly metastatic B16-F1 tumor line produced significantly more lung tumor colonies after intravenous injection than an equal number of cells from the parent line. Tumor cell lines from spontaneous metastases of the B16-BL6 tumor variant also produced significantly more lung colonies than the parent (B16-BL6) tumor line. However, the increase in metastatic potential of cell lines from spontaneous metastases of the B16-BL6 tumors was less than that observed with tumor cells from spontaneous metastases of B16-F1. Tumor cells from spontaneous metastases of the B16-F10 variant line, which was previously selected for the ability to form lung colonies, did not exhibit any increased lung-colonizing potential compared with the parent tumor. This latter observation was not attributable to the number of lung colonies involved since the injection of fivefold fewer tumor cells gave similar results, i.e., the lung-colonizing potential of the tumor cells from spontaneous metastases was comparable to that of tumor cells from the parent tumor, although the total numbers of tumor foci were lower (192).

The spontaneous metastatic potential of these same tumor variants and their respective spontaneous metastases were studied, with results that were different overall from the results of the studies of lung-colonizing potential. As was found in the lung colony assays, tumor cells from spontaneous metastases of the B16-F1 tumor were significantly more spontaneously metastatic than the tumor cells from the parent tumor ($P = 0.007$), but tumor cells harvested from spontaneous metastases of the B16-F10 tumor also exhibited an increased propensity for spontaneous metastasis ($P = 0.004$), whereas they did not express an increased lung-colonizing potential. Similar studies with metastases of the B16-BL6 tumor did not demonstrate a statistical difference ($P = 0.22$) in spontaneous metastases ability compared with that seen with the parent B16-BL6 tumor. The B10-BL6 tumor variant had been previously selected for an invasive phenotype and therefore was already highly spontaneously metastatic, thus, the tumor cells from spontaneous metastases did not differ from the parent tumor with regard to their metastatic properties. We concluded from this study that metastases obtained from an unselected, heterogeneous, and poorly metastatic cell line (B16-F1) contained tumor cells with enhanced metastatic potential. In contrast, when the parent population was previously selected and was already near peak metastatic predilection (B16-F10 for lung colonization or B16-BL6 for spontaneous metastasis), further selection for the particular metastatic phenotype could not be achieved.

To rule out the possibility that these results were unique to the B16 melanoma tumor system, we repeated this study with four other tumor cell populations (194) in a manner similar to the original study. These tumors included a malignant melanoma of recent origin (K-1735); an ultraviolet-radiation-induced fibrosarcoma (UV-2237) and a cloned subline (clone 40); the Lewis lung carcinoma (3LL); and the reticulum cell sarcoma of histiocytic origin (M5076). We found in each of these tumor models that cells from spontaneous metastases of heterogeneous parent tumors always expressed a greater propensity to metastasize than tumor

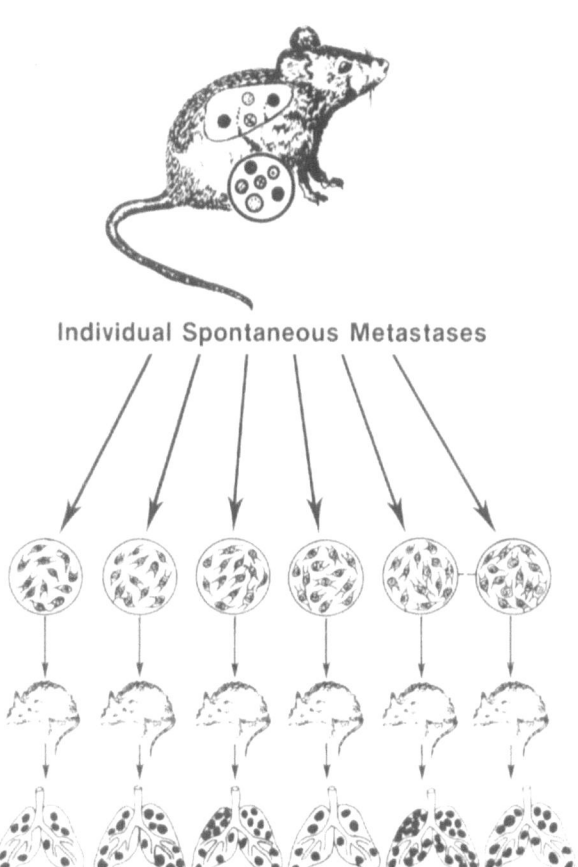

Individual Spontaneous Metastases

Figure 1. Procedure used to compare the metastatic potential of tumor cells from spontaneous metastases to the metastatic ability of tumor cells from their parent tumor, i.e. whether metastasis is a selective or random process.

cells from the parent tumor. However, cells from spontaneous metastases of a cloned parent tumor (UV-2237, clone 40), presumably a homogeneous tumor population, did not differ significantly in potential for experimental metastasis from the parent (cloned) tumor population. The metastatic homogeneity of clone 40 was not unique to this tumor since spontaneous metastases from the heterogeneous parent tumor population (UV-2237), from which the clone was obtained, exhibited a greater metastatic potential than the heterogeneous parent tumor line.

Studies using the reticulum cell sarcoma, M5076 (194), demonstrated that the increased metastatic potential of tumor cells from spontaneous metastases was not affected by the anatomical location of the metastases. The M5076 tumor consistently metastasizes to the liver and only rarely to the lungs (and then late in the course of tumor growth) (78). Thus, we found that spontaneous hepatic metastases from the M5076 tumor exhibited an increased propensity to metastasize to the liver compared with the parent M5076 line (193). This increase in metastatic potential occurred not only during experimental metastasis but also in mice bearing unresected primary tumors.

We conclude from these studies that tumor cells from spontaneous metastases of unselected tumors, which are heterogeneous with regard to a metastatic phenotype, have an increased metastatic potential compared with the present tumor. In contrast, metastases from homogeneous (clonal) tumors or tumors previously selected for a metastatic phenotype vary only slightly from the parent tumor in their ability to metastasize. Therefore, although the process of metastasis is generally selective, it may give the appearance of being random if artifactually homogeneous tumors are examined.

These studies have been extended to other models. Pollack and Fidler (148) utilized young nude mice to investigate whether these animals, which lack functional T lymphocytes and express low levels of NK cells, could provide a model to select for metastatic subpopulations from heterogeneous allogeneic melanoma. Three-week-old nudes received a single cell suspension of either B16 or K-1735 melanoma tumor cells injected intravenously. Individual pulmonary metastases were harvested three weeks later and their metastatic potential was assessed in both nude mice and normal syngeneic mice. In all cases, the cells from the metastases colonized the lungs with significantly higher efficiency than did cells from the parent tumors. Kozlowski (unpublished results), using a similar stratagem, found that lung colonies from the human malignant melanoma A-375 in nude mice contained a select subpopulation of tumor cells of high metastatic potential compared with the parent tumor cell populations.

Raz and colleagues (159) have shown that mouse UV-2237 fibrosarcoma cells recovered from lung metastases produced by a cloned parental cell line with low lung colonization potential do not express an increased capacity to colonize the lung when injected intravenously. This indicates that growth in the lung is not sufficient to augment the ability of cells from this tumor to localize and grow in the lung. Additional evidence indicating that growth in the lung is not required for tumor cells to localize selectively in the lung was presented by the same authors who found that an uncloned UV-2237 cell line grown in the peritoneal cavity

contained multiple clonal subpopulations, including clones with a high capacity to colonize the lung. This observation is in agreement with that previously described by Klein (97, 98): that adaptation to peritoneal growth resulted in cell lines with a high lung-colonizing potential.

Comparable findings investigating tumor adaption have been obtained by Nicolson and Custead (135). Mice were given intravenous injections of 120–180-μm diameter plastic microbeads coated with B16-F1 melanoma cells, which have a low lung colonization capacity. Entrapment of the beads within the pulmonary microcirculation serves to artificially enhance the localization of these cells within the lung. When visible lung colonies had formed, they were excised and dispersed to yield tumor cells that were grown *in vitro* for a brief period, reattached to new beads, and reinjected intravenously. After nine such cycles of *in vivo-in vitro* transfer employing carrier beads, cells recovered from lung colonies were reinjected into mice without beads and their metastatic ability was compared with the B16-F10 subline. The latter was isolated after an identical number of *in vivo-in vitro* transfers, but cells were injected as single cell suspensions rather than attached to beads. Nicolson and Custead found that even after ten cycles of growth in the lung, B16-F1 cells attached to beads (B16-F1A10) were no more metastatic than parental B16-F1 cells. In contrast, the B16-F10 cell line was highly efficient in colonizing the lung, producing between five and 13 times more lung metastases than the parental B16-F1 cell line. In a series of elegant studies, Poste and co-workers (150, 155) examined the metastatic properties of tumor cell clones isolated from individual metastatic lesions obtained following the intravenous injection of various B16 melanoma variants. The individual metastatic lesions were examined at different stages in the evolution of metastasis (i.e., larger or smaller pulmonary nodules). They found that the progressive growth of metastatic lesions was accompanied by the emergence of variant tumor cellular subpopulations with altered metastatic properties within the lesion. They investigated the experimental metastatic potential of the clones obtained from the different metastases and found that the cells populating the individual metastases were inevitably metastatic. In contrast, the tumor cells within the parent tumor included nonmetastatic variants. Poste and co-workers (150, 155) concluded that subpopulations isolated from different metastases in the same host differ markedly in their metastatic ability and that cells with both high and low, but not nonmetastatic, metastatic capacities can be recovered from metastases.

Neri and colleagues (132), in a study similar to ours (192, 193), using the rat 13762 mammary adenocarcinoma, examined the selective or random nature of metastases. They reported that the unresected parental mammary adenocarcinoma, following subcutaneous implantation into the mammary footpad of syngeneic rats, metastasizes at a low frequency to the lymph nodes and lungs. Cell lines adapted to tissue culture from individual secondary sites were, in contrast to the parent tumor, inevitably metastatic (without resection) from a subcutaneous site within 23 days of transplantation, confirming the selective nature of metastasis in a rat mammary tumor model. Another study using a Herpesvirus hominis type 2 induced tumor line from a Syrian hamster (217) also demonstrated the selective nature of metastasis. The parent tumor exhibited a low level of spontaneous metastases from the primary subcutaneous tumor site. However, tumor lines established from lung foci showed an elevated metastatic potential compared with the parent cell line such that all animals injected with cells from the metastases developed secondary foci within 40 days following resection of the primary tumor.

Despite the experimental evidence supporting the selective process of metastasis, the conclusion that metastatic cells arise by a selective process has not been universal. Mantovani and co-workers (123) and Giaviazzi and co-workers (67) reported that cells with high and low metastatic potential gave rise to metastases and that the metastases were not always formed by cells with the highest metastatic potential. The selection hypothesis is outlined in this review states that in order for tumor cells to form metastases, they must express a phenotype that allows them to complete all the steps in the metastatic process as well as avoid destruction during metastasis. Tumor cells that lack any of these attributes will be unable to produce metastases, an observation supported by our studies (192, 193); in every case in our studies, the tumor cells within metastases were metastatic. However, metastases are not necessarily composed of cellular subpopulations with the greatest metastatic potential. Because of the heterogeneous nature of tumors (discussed earlier) and, because metastases from one tumor may derive from multiple progenitor cells (198), one would expect that tumor cells within different individual metastases would vary in their metastatic potentials, which indeed is the case. (See also the review by Poste [149]). This heterogeneity would occur if the primary tumor were initially heterogeneous. If a tumor had been previously selected for a metastatic phenotype (for example, B16-F10 for lung colonization or B16-BL6 for spontaneous metastases), then the metastatic process would be unlikely to select for cellular subpopulations with an increased metastatic potential (192) and the process of metastasis could not select for a metastatic variant from a homogeneous (clonal) tumor population (158, 159, 193). If the parent tumor population was passaged by trocar transplantation, a technique which tends to limit tumor heterogeneity (48, 205), metastases from such a population would not be expected to exhibit increased metastatic potential, which appears to be true (67, 123).

The conclusion that metastasis is a selective process does not rule out the occurrence of random (chance) events. Subpopulations of tumor cells with metastatic capabilities may be killed during the metastatic process and thus not complete the metastatic "decathalon" to form metastatic foci. During metastasis, tumor cells are exposed to vascular turbulence, the mononuclear phagocytic system, NK cells, and other detrimental conditions that by chance could prevent the fruition of the metastatic process. There is, therefore, some element of chance during metastasis and certainly (fortunately) not all cells with a metastatic phenotype survive to form metastatic foci. However, a tumor cell probably will not form a metastatic focus if it does not express all the attributes needed to metastasize given the constraints imposed by the host.

Stackpole (183) and Weiss and colleagues (222) have also disagreed with the concept of a selective process during metastasis. Stackpole examined the metastatic properties, in both experimental and spontaneous metastases, of an impressibly large number (> 150) of clones and subclones from

B16 melanoma cell lines. In this study, Stackpole reported that the phenotypic diversity with regard to three distinct dissemination-related biological parameters (metastasis, colonization, and cell proliferation rate) was generated so rapidly and with such regularity within B16 melanoma clones that tumor longevity may be inconsequential to the issue of heterogeneity. He also suggested that significant fluctuation in tumor cell subpopulations occurred periodically, affecting both the metastatic and colonizing predilection of a tumor cell line.

This fluctuation in metastatic potential is sufficiently extensive that one should question the reproducibility of any one observation. The early studies of heterogeneity by Fidler and coworkers (53) and Kripke and coworkers (102), based on a variation of the Luria-Delbruck fluctuation analysis, required a control demonstrating that the metastatic phenotype of a tumor line was reproducible. As they stated, the analysis of metastatic phenotype by cloning experiments requires the demonstration that subclones from a recent clone were statistically similar in metastatic potential compared with the metastatic potential of the parent/clone, thereby demonstrating that the heterogeneity observed with the parental tumor was not an artifact of the cloning process. Therefore, the fluctuation observed by Stackpole (183), unsupported by statistical analysis, needs to be supported by the demonstration of an assay reproducible for metastatic predilection.

The concept that metastasis is a nonrandom process involving the selective survival of cellular subpopulations with the phenotypic properties required to complete each step in the metastatic process does not infer that random events do not occur. Tumor cell subpopulations, even those with metastatic properties, are at constant risk during the metastatic process, due to random events. Similarly, metastatic competence to complete any specific step in the metastatic process may be subject to a reversible impairment imposed by its microenvironment. Weiss (222) has suggested that alterations in nutrition or metabolism secondary to cellular proliferation or degenerative events within solid tumors may modulate a number of cellular properties, i.e., site dependent, reversible changes. He suggests that phenotypic modulation could then induce a situation in which metastatic subpopulations may be subject to transitory phenotypic alterations that enhance or restrict metastatic competence (221). It is proposed that cells entering the metastatic process do so from "transient metastatic compartments" and that, after allowance is made for pathophysiologic differences between primary and metastatic lesions, metastases are no more likely to metastasize than their parent primary tumor. Weiss and colleagues (222) report that, in the case of KHT and B16 tumors, when selected primary and secondary groups of animals are compared, cancer cells from the latter gave rise to significantly more metastases than the former. In contrast, cells from selected primary lesions of 3LL and T-24 tumors gave rise to significantly more metastases than cells derived from pulmonary metastases. Therefore, for two tumors, the process of metastasis appeared selective, while with the other two tumors, 3LL and T-241, the process appeared random. However, all the tumor variants were metastatic, and no tumor line established from either primary or metastasis lesions was nonmetastatic. Thus, the cells within the metastatic lesions did express those phenotypic characteristics required for the metastatic process, suggesting that the primary tumor was composed of tumor populations, the majority of which were metastatic. These results are in agreement with the hypothesis that spontaneous metastases arise from preexistent metastatic populations from within the primary tumor, since this does not infer that the metastatic cell populations compose a minor subpopulation within the primary tumor. The studies with homogeneous tumors (clone 40 from UV-2237) or previously selected tumors B16-F10 or B16-BL6 demonstrated that metastases from homogeneous or highly metastatic tumors were similar in metastatic ability to the parental tumor.

DISSIMILARITIES AMONG METASTASES FROM A PRIMARY TUMOR

The observation that a tumor population is heterogeneous, be it either a primary tumor or a metastatic foci, does not suggest that such individual lesions do not, as a population, differ phenotypically from one another. Thus, metastases within one host can exhibit heterogeneity with regard to many characteristics besides metastatic capacity, such as hormone receptors (19, 180); marker enzymes (10, 45), antigenicity or immunogenicity (1, 55, 89, 116, 139, 146, 170, 202), macrophage content (93), metabolic characteristics (10), androgen response (19), karyotypic expression (103, 166), DNA content (164, 184), and response to various chemotherapeutic agents (63, 81, 171, 209).

Evidence that human cancers contain tumor cell subpopulations with divergent phenotypes comes from the comparison of tumor cells from both primary tumors and metastases. Here again one may see divergence in histological type (142). The problem of cellular diversity inherent in some neoplasms is clearly demonstrated by the work of Baylin and co-workers (10). The elevation of serum histaminase, L-dopa decarboxylase, and calcitonin are used as clinical markers for the presence of small-cell lung cancer of humans. However, the simultaneous sampling of primary and metastatic lesions of small-cell lung cancer by Baylin and colleagues demonstrated significant differences in the levels of these markers between the primary tumor and metastases. All primary (chest) lesions produced high levels of these markers. In contrast, either low levels or none of these three products could be detected in four of seven metastases isolated from the livers of several patients. Moreover, immunohistochemical tests for histaminase demonstrated that cells within the primary tumor were heterogeneous in their enzyme content. Therefore, the level of these three markers in a patient's serum may not accurately represent the tumor burden in patients with small-cell lung tumors. Another study reported differences in sensitivity to antineoplastic drugs *in vitro* between cells from primary ovarian carcinomas and their metastases (103, 206). A variable, estrogen receptor content between primary breast cancers and their metastases as well as among multiple metastases in the same patient has been reported (19).

Striking evidence that metastases of primary human tumors may not be uniformly susceptible to control by immunologic manipulation comes from a study performed by McCune and colleagues (116). These investigators used active specific immunotherapy directed against advanced renal carcinoma and its metastases by giving weekly injections of autologous irradiated tumor cells obtained from the primary neoplasm admixed with *Corynebacterium parvum*. They found that not only did the degree of therapeutic efficacy vary from patient to patient but also, in some patients whose overall response was favorable, some metastatic lesions regressed and others simultaneously progressed. This variable responsiveness of metastatic lesions even within the same patient was attributed to the antigenic diversity of the subpopulations of metastatic cells. These observations suggest that antitumor immune responses can be evoked in patients with renal carcinoma but, equally importantly, show that heterogeneity of the metastatic cells with respect to antigenicity is a problem that must be overcome if specific immunotherapy is to be truly effective in eradicating metastatic disease.

In another study, Albino and colleagues (1) examined the antigenic characteristics of six individual metastases from a single patient. These lines showed marked phenotypic diversity, as indicated by characteristic differences in growth rate, morphology, pigmentation, and the expression of surface antigens and glycoproteins. Some lines expressed HLA-DR products, whereas another lacked HLA-DR expression. These lines could also be distinguished on a basis of a profile of radiolabeled glycoproteins. Additional quantitative differences in the surface antigenic phenotype of the three cell lines were revealed by serological tests with a battery of monoclonal and conventional antibodies defining melanoma differentiation antigens. In a study of melanoma-bearing patients by Natali and co-workers (202) examined the antigenic heterogeneity of primary and metastatic lesions surgically removed from nine patients with nodular melanoma. The antigenic expression was investigated using monoclonal antibodies to HLA-A and B antigens to $\beta_2$microglobulin, to Ia antigens, and to melanoma-associated antigens (MAA). The latter included three types of membrane-bound MAA as well as a cytoplasmic MAA. In spite of a homogeneous morphologic appearance, multiple lesions removed from the same patient differed significantly in their reactivity with the panel of monoclonal antibodies when studied using an indirect immunofluorescence test. The extent of antigenic heterogeneity did not correlate with melanin synthesis, site of origin of the primary tumor, site of metastatic foci, or treatment and appeared to be less marked in patients carrying the primary tumor.

Easty and co-workers (39) isolated from a single patient five tumor lines, including primary squamous carcinoma of the tongue, two subsequent local recurrences, and two lymph node metastases. The recurrent line showing the greatest morphological divergence from the primary tumor line also demonstrated the greatest differences at the ultrastructural level, in increased production of plasminogen activator, and in the composition of cell-surface glycoproteins. In another study by Feder and Gilbert (44), cell lines were established from a primary neuroblastoma and, 11 months later, from four different individual metastases. Cells from the primary tumor demonstrated considerable heterogeneity in terms of chromosome number while the cells from four subsequent metastases were all nearly diploid. However, all of the tumor samples contained the same marker chromosome rearrangements, indicating their origin from a common precursor. In addition, each of the cell lines analyzed (including those from the metastases and those from the primary tumor) also contained unique distinguishing chromosomal abnormalities. Feder and Gilbert (44) concluded that the differences in karyotype among these tumor samples and cell lines reflected the different selection pressures at work in each instance. These differences also represent karyotypic variations between the individual metastases.

In a rat mammary adenocarcinoma model, Neri and colleagues (132) studied the phenotypic characteristics of several spontaneous metastases as well as the primary tumor. They examined their cell culture morphologies, histologic structures at the primary site and secondary metastatic sites, and growth characteristics *in vivo* and *in vitro*. In agreement with other studies that we have discussed, there was considerable variation in these phenotypes among the individual metastases (132). In a subsequent study, Welch and co-workers (224) studied the sensitivity of clonal populations from mammary adenocarcinoma metastases and the primary tumor to γ-radiation *in vitro*. This study demonstrated considerable clonal heterogeneity within the tumor and among its metastases with respect to the response to γ-radiation. They found that the inherent sensitivity to radiation could change with time, thereby altering the radiation survival responses.

CLONAL ORIGIN OF METASTASES

As discussed previously in this chapter, metastases in general do not result from the random survival of cells released from the primary tumor but rather from the selected growth of specialized subpopulations of malignant cells that exist as subpopulations within the parent tumor. However, this observation does not address the nature of the emboli released from the primary tumor. The embolus that ultimately develops into a metastatic focus may originate from a single cell or a cellular aggregate comprising both tumor cells and host cells. Such a cell aggregate may be composed of tumor cells from a clonal population due to the zonal nature of neoplasms (48, 205) or a heterogeneous population of tumor cells. In addition, all the secondary tumor foci in a host may originate from a single progenitor cell or from multiple progenitor cells.

We performed a series of experiments (Figure 2) to determine 1) whether individual metastases are clonal or multicellular in origin and 2) whether metastases produced by one tumor originate from a single or different progenitor cells (198). This study was patterned after the classical study by Becker, McCulloch, and Till (11), which demonstrated the pluripotential nature of bone marrow stem cells. In our experiments, cells from a metastatic variant of the K-1735 melanoma (K-1735 met-2) were exposed to 650 rad of x-radiation, which randomly induces chromosomal breaks and rearrangements. A certain number of these breaks and rearrangements (if not lethal) result in the formation of centric fusion chromosomes, and these provided the marker chromosomes for this study. We reasoned that if all the tumor cells populating a single spontaneous metastasis that arose from a primary tumor of x-irradiated tumor cells exhibited the same chromosomal arrangements, the metas-

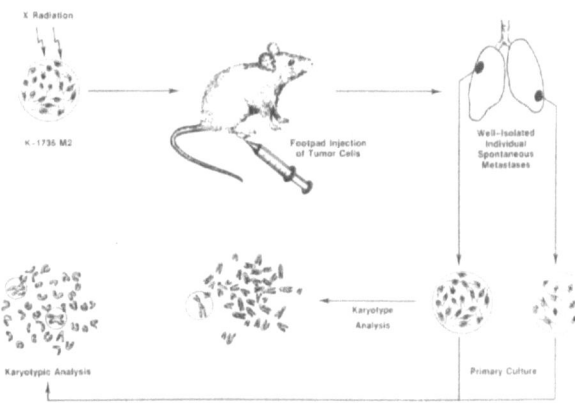

Figure 2. Scheme of experiment used to determine whether metastases are clonal or multicellular in their origin.

tasis would have been derived from one cell. However, if the tumor cells populating an individual spontaneous metastases exhibited multiple chromosomal arrangements, then the metastasis would have arisen from more than one progenitor cell. Obviously, the demonstration of a multiple tumor cell origin of a metastasis would be predicated on the stable expression of the various marker chromosomes.

We chose to induce and use marker chromosomes rather than drug resistance, since a large number of markers would be available. In addition, the frequency of revision to drug resistance is a constant concern in the interpretation of results when drug markers are used. If a metastasis did prove to be clonal in origin, the demonstration of clonality based on two or three parent populations would be far weaker than that associated with a study utilizing a large number of cells with different marker chromosomes.

In these experiments, cells from the metastatic line of the K-1735 melanoma (K-1735, M2) were exposed to 650 rad of x-radiation to induce chromosomal breaks and rearrangements. Cells from the x-irradiated line were implanted into the footpad of syngeneic C3H/HeN mice. When the tumors reached a diameter of 1 cm, the tumor-bearing leg, including popliteal lymph node, was resected at mid femur. Eight to ten weeks after tumor inoculation, spontaneous lung metastases were isolated, grown in culture as individual lines, and karyotyped. In ten of 21 lines, all the chromosomes were telocentric, and, therefore, these metastases were noninformative. In the other 11 lines, single or multiple marker chromosomes (submetacentric, metacentric, minute) were observed. In eight of these lines, unique patterns of chromosome(s) were found in most spreads, suggesting that each metastasis originated from a single progenitor cell. In the remaining three lines, the pattern of markers varied, suggesting a bimodal or multimodal cell origin. However, G-band analysis indicated that these variations probably represented evolution within the individual metastasis. These data show that, although metastasis is a highly selective process, different metastases can originate from different progenitor cells and that most metastases appear to be clonal in origin. This finding of multiple progenitors could account for the biological heterogeneity that exists among various metastases (51). The results suggest that metastases result from either the proliferation of a single viable cell or a single viable cell within a heterogeneous embolus or that a circulating tumor embolus is likely to be homogeneous because it originated from a clonal zone of a primary neoplasm (52).

Previous studies (134) have shown that tumor emboli composed of cellular aggregates, either homotypic (tumor cells) or heterotypic (host cells, generally leukocytes and platelets), are arrested more rapidly in the first capillary bed encountered and have a better rate of survival. In both incidences, this results in a higher frequency of metastasis compared with the circulation of a similar number of single cells. The more rapid rate of arrest is a physical phenomenon associated with the larger embolus size, while the prolonged survival of tumor cell emboli is believed to be due to the "protection" afforded against host effector cells, NK cells, and monocytes as well as the turbulence within the circulation. If larger emboli are better able to metastasize, it would appear logical that metastasis could develop, composed in part of a progenitor cell population, which by itself was unable to complete the metastatic cascade but was able to when associated in an embolus with a metastatic competent cell. We therefore designed experiments to address the following questions: Do tumor emboli that survive the many steps of metastasis consist of single cells or cell aggregates of monoclonal origin? Do metastatic competent cells provide a suitable environment within cellular aggregates whereby metastatic compromised or metastatic incompetent cells could survive and proliferate within the metastatic focus?

In a collaborative study with Fidler, we formed heterotypic cellular aggregates of either a single population of metastatic tumor cells (with a marker chromosome), a mixture of metastatic tumor cell populations, each with a different characteristic marker karyotypes or heterogeneous cellular aggregates composed of metastatic competent tumor cells, and benign tumor cells each with different marker karyotypes. The size and extent of cellular aggregation was monitored by autoradiographic studies using admixed radiolabeled and unlabeled cell populations. In this study, the metastatic variant K-1735 M2-X21 (chromosome mode of 42 and a 3:4 arm length ratio submetacentric chromosome) was admixed with the metastatic parent tumor population, K-1735, M2 (chromosome mode of 44, without any marker chromosomes), or K-1735-cl 26, a nonmetastatic tumor variant (chromosome mode of 54, without any marker chromosomes). These heterotypic (or homotypic) cellular aggregates were injected intravenously into the lateral tail vein of syngeneic mice; 21 to 24 days later, well-isolated metastatic tumor foci were established individually in tissue culture and karyotyped. The karyotypes of the metastases obtained from mice injected with K-1735, M2, or K-1735 M2-X21 (11/11 and 10/10, respectfully) expressed the appropriate characteristics. The mice injected with K-1735 cl 26, a nonmetastatic variant, did not develop metastatic foci. In contrast, all the metastases examined (9/9) from mice injected with cellular aggregates of the metastatic variant K-1735 M2-X21 and the nonmetastatic tumor cell line K-1735 cl 26 expressed the karyotype characteristics of K-1735 M2-X2 in every spread examined (at least 70 per metastasis). The karyotypes of the cells from the metastases of mice injected with cellular aggregates of K-1735, M2, and K-1735 M2-X21, both metastatic variants, were composed of a characteristic spread of one K-1735 M2 [4/12] and K-1735 M2-X21 [8/12] or the other metastatic line. We conclude from this study that, although cellular aggregates are arrested more rapidly and result in an increased metastatic frequency, only a single cell from within the embolus normally survives to form the metastatic focus. Therefore, the metastatic process is clonal in origin and the metastatic foci appears to arise from a single cell that could have been only one of several within the tumor embolus.

Poste and co-workers (155), in a previous study, used tumor cells bearing stable biochemical markers. Syngeneic mice were given intravenous injections of aliquots of wild type B16-F10 cells admixed with equal aliquots of TFT^r and OIua^r B16-F10 variants, and individual lung metastases were established in culture. Clones (5) from each of the 22 metastases obtained from three animals were isolated and tested for resistance to TFT or Oua. Nineteen of 22 lesions were populated by cells with the same drug sensitivity. In addition, two metastases that contained cells with different drug sensitivities were identified, suggesting to the authors a polyclonal origin. One of the metastases expressed cells with either a wild type or a Oua phenotype, while the other was composed of both TFT^r and Oua^r cells. This latter metastasis, discounting the possibility of metastases coalescence, is very probably of a polyclonal origin.. Nonetheless, their study also suggests that a polyclonal event is a very rare occurrence and that most metastases are both clonal in origin and of single cell origin.

Reeve and Twentyman (164), by the flow cytometric analysis of the x-radiation-induced sarcoma RIF-1, have shown that the parent tumor is composed of both diploid and tetraploid subpopulations of cells. They examined both experimental and spontaneous metastases from mice bearing the RIF-1 tumor and observed that, unlike the parent tumor population, they exhibited a single level of ploidy, which was a stable characteristic of cell lines established from metastases. They suggested, based on this observation, that, at least in this tumor system, metastasis is a clonal event. However, a clonal origin denotes a population arising from a single cell, and since only a single ploidy level was observed in the metastases, their observation need not imply a clonal origin but is rather an assessment of the relative distribution of each ploidy level in spontaneous metastases.

Recent studies of human tumors, based on karyotypic analysis, including an ovarian carcinoma (103), neuroblastoma (44), and a neurofibrosarcoma (61), have addressed the clonal versus multicellular origin of metastatic foci. In all these studies, the evidence, while not definitive, supports the observation of a clonal origin for metastases.

THE RAPID GENERATION OF BIOLOGICAL DIVERSITY WITHIN CLONAL METASTASES

The demonstration that spontaneous metastases result from the clonal expansion of highly specialized cells and that cells of metastases demonstrate a high rate of spontaneous mutation (27) compared with nonmetastatic tumorigenic cells suggests that clonal metastases may rapidly become heterogeneous. We were interested, therefore, in investigating whether rapid tumor evolution and progression could occur within a clonal metastasis. If so, this finding would provide a rational explanation for the observed heterogeneity within and among metastases. The demonstration of

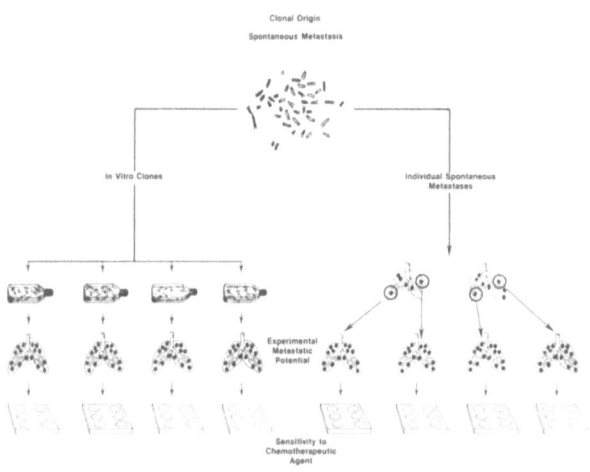

Figure 3. Scheme of experimental design to determine how rapidly metastases of clonal origin develop intralesional heterogeneity with respect to metastatic potential and sensitivity to cytostatic agents

clonal origin metastases (150, 198) provided the experimental basis for this study (Figure 3). The experimental metastatic potential was examined for the cells from the original, demonstrable, clonal origin, X-met-21 line (parent): ten *in vitro* isolated clones: the X-met-21 after growth *in vivo* for 60 days; and seven individual spontaneous lung metastases from the X-met-21 primary tumors. Six of ten clones differed significantly from the parent tumor in their capacity to produce lung tumor colonies, while the metastatic potential of the X-met-21 population did not change after subcutaneous growth for 60 days ($P = 0.45$) compared with X-met-21 cultured line. However, cells from six of seven spontaneous metastases from mice bearing the X-met-21 tumor differed significantly in their metastatic potential from the X-met-21 line growing at a primary site. The cells from the cloned lines and from spontaneous metastases differed greatly in their ability to produce experimental metastases ($P = 0.0001$, Kruskal-Wallis test, Chi square approximation).

In another set of experiments, we used an *in vitro* colony-forming inhibition assay to determine the relative sensitivity of tumor cells from the parent line, tumor cells from the cloned lines, and spontaneous metastases to various chemotherapeutic drugs. The study used the chemotherapeutic drugs amsacrine (AMSA), adriamycin (ADR), bleomycin (BLEO), and vincristine (VCR). Statistical analysis of the differences in drug sensitivity revealed that the following numbers of clones and metastases differed significantly from the parent tumor line: for AMSA, five of ten clones and two of seven metastases; for VCR, one of ten clones and three of seven metastases; for ADR, seven of ten clones and four of seven metastases; and for BLEO, six of ten clones and three of seven metastases. This variability was reproducible and was not caused by artifacts associated with the cloning or selection procedures. This conclusion is based on a study in which five subclones isolated from a benign clone of the K-1735 melanoma were not distinguishable from the parent clone in their response to cytotoxic drugs. In contrast to this diversity in metastatic potential and drug sensitivity, all cells

examined expressed the unique submetacentric chromosome marker, suggesting that its expression was very stable.

In the study of clonal origin by Poste and co-workers (155), the metastatic properties of several tumor cell clones isolated from individual B16 melanoma pulmonary metastases at different stages during the evolution of metastasis were investigated. They found that during the early stages of metastatic growth following intravenous injection of tumor cells, the majority of metastatic lesions contain cells with indistinguishable metastatic phenotypes (intralesional clonal homogeneity). In contrast, the progressive growth of metastatic lesions was accompanied by the emergence of variant tumor cells with altered metastatic properties within clonal homogeneous lesions (intralesional heterogeneity).

In summary, distinct differences in metastatic properties and drug sensitivity were found in most of the *in vitro* and *in vivo* isolated clones. In contrast to the rapid evolution in sensitivity to chemotherapeutic drugs and metastatic potential in our studies as well as the three clinical studies (44, 61, 103), we have observed that marker chromosomes appear to be expressed in an extremely stable manner both *in vitro* and *in vivo*. These intralesion differences could not be attributed to in vivo fusion of tumor cells with each other or normal host cells, since tetraploid karyotypes were only rarely observed. It appears, therefore, that the progressive growth of metastases results in the rapid development of biological intralesional heterogeneity.

CLINICAL IMPLICATIONS

The most feared and devastating aspect of cancer is the propensity of tumor cells to disseminate from their primary site to distant organs and there to develop into metastatic tumor foci. Despite impressive advances in the surgical resection of primary neoplasms and aggressive adjuvant therapies, most cancer deaths are attributable to metastases. There appear to be several reasons for this lack of success in controlling metastatic foci. First, by the time cancer is diagnosed, metastases may already be present in several organs of patient's body, making surgical resection or destruction by radiotherapy or chemotherapy unlikely. Moreover, the metastases may be located in organs that are difficult to treat with effective therapeutic doses without undue toxic effects. Second, in spite of the development of promising anticancer drugs and regimes, their efficiency is hindered by the occurrence of drug-resistant variants within tumors. This tumor cell resistance to conventional therapy is probably the single most important factor responsible for the refractory response of tumor therapy. The emergence of a resistant tumor subpopulation is not limited to chemotherapeutic agents but is also a serious problem when other forms of therapy are used, including hormonal therapy, radiotherapy, hyperthermia, or immunotherapy. This phenotypic diversity, which allows selected variants to develop within the primary tumor, means not only that primary tumors and metastases can differ in their responses to treatment but also that individual tumor cells within a metastasis differ from one another (diagrammatically represented in Figure 4). This diversity can be generated rapidly even when the tumors originate from a single transformed cell. This complication appears to arise because metastatic lesions are

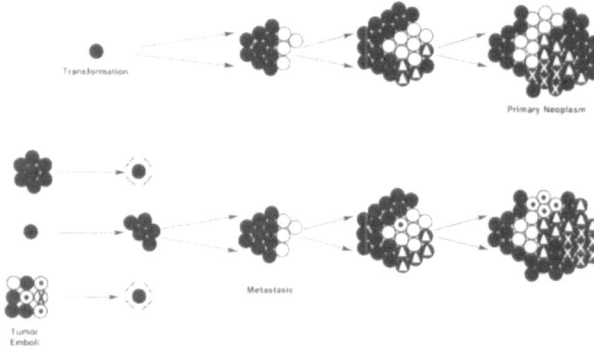

Figure 4. The origin of metastases. Metastases may result from the proliferation of a single cell or multicellular emboli that arrive at secondary sites. Nonetheless, hematogeneous metastases appear to arise from a single surviving cell resulting in a clonal origin of each metastatic foci. Regardless of metastatic origin, the process of tumor progression similar to which occurs in the primary tumor, rapidly results in phenotypic diversity within metastases.

fairly large by the time they are diagnosed. A tumor mass at the lower limit of radiographic detection, for example, 1 cubic centimeter, may contain as many as 10^9 cells; eradication of 99.9% of these cells, a remarkable therapeutic achievement, still leaves 10^6 cells to proliferate, thus providing a large base for the further generation of biological heterogeneity.

The problem of selecting effective therapy for heterogeneous tumors may be further compounded by the existence of interactions between tumor subpopulations, as well as between tumor cells and normal cells, which affect the measured sensitivity of the whole tumor, a concept that has received extensive study by Heppner (82). She and her coworkers have shown that subpopulations of a mouse mammary tumor, which differ in sensitivity to chemotherapeutic agents, can interact in such a way that the apparent sensitivity of one subpopulation is changed in the presence of the other (126). Interactions between cells appear to act through metabolic processes affecting drug metabolism, through factors affecting cell growth, or through immune mechanisms. For example, the well known phenomenon of "metabolic cooperation," a process by which small molecules pass between cells in contact, presumably through gap junctions (113, 189), is one way in which interactions between cells can affect response to therapy. Metabolic cooperation could also result in the rescue of a sensitive cell by molecules from a resistant cell or in the death of a resistant cell due to passage of molecules from a sensitive.

Taken together, the growing body of experimental and clinical evidence suggests that cells within the same cancer exhibit different susceptibilities to the broad range of conventional treatments; therefore, the successful therapy of malignant tumors will require the development of new approaches capable of overcoming this variation and against which resistance is unlikely to develop. Given the extraordinary level of cell diversity apparently present in many tumors, the probability is small that a single anticancer drug, or any other treatment used alone, will be capable of killing all of the cancer cells in a malignant tumor and its metastases. New treatment strategies may be possible that slow the potential of tumor cells that survive initial waves of treatment(s) to generate new variants. To achieve this with existing therapeutic modalities, one has to reduce the time interval between successive administration of different anticancer agents in an attempt to destroy the cancer cell subpopulations that survive each successive treatment before the generation of large numbers of new variants could occur. This conclusion is reflected in the growing trend in cancer medicine to use a combination of anticancer treatments for the patients with malignant tumors.

The heterogeneity of tumors, however it originates, has important implications for the study and treatment of metastases. For example, cells obtained from a primary tumor are not necessarily representative of cancer cells populating metastases or even cells in different regions of the same primary tumor. Thus, experimental efforts must be concentrated on identification of the features that permit malignant cells to metastasize. In addition, the test systems for new therapeutic agents or modalities must address the problem of tumor cell heterogeneity. More effort must be devoted to testing the efficacy of combination therapies with the objective of circumventing the problem of cellular diversity within tumors. The short-term therapeutic goal must be to choose the combination of antitumor agents and to determine the sequence of administration that will be most effective against a particular tumor. The mechanisms by which cancer cells diversify are not fully understood. By limiting the number of different subpopulations of cancer cells within a tumor, we may be able to improve the odds that a combination of anticancer drugs perhaps in conjunction with other adjunct therapeutic modalities will destroy all of the subpopulations of tumor cells. Clearly, the only successful treatment of metastatic disease will be one that circumvents the different phenotypes of tumor cells within individual metastases of a patient and probably will require multiple therapeutic agents and multiple therapeutic modalities.

ACKNOWLEDGMENT

This research was sponsored by the National Cancer Institute, DHHS, under Contract #NO1-CO-23910 with Program Resources, Inc. The contents of the publication do not necessarily reflect the views or policies of the Department of Health and Human Services, nor does mention of trade names, commercial products, or organizations imply endorsement by the U.S. Government.

REFERENCES

1. Albino AP, Lloyd, KO, Houghton, AN, Oettgen HF, Old LJ: Heterogeneity in surface antigen and glycoprotein expression of cell lines derived from different melanoma metastases of the same patient. *J Ex Med* 154:1764–1778, 1981
2. Angello JC, Danielson KG, Anderson LW, Hosick HL: Glycosaminoglycan synthesis by subpopulations of epithelial cells from a mammary adenocarcinoma. *Cancer Res* 42:2207–2210, 1982
3. Ashall F, Bramwell ME, Harris H: A new marker for human cancer cells. I. The Ca antigen and the Ca 1 antibody. *Lancet* ii, 1–6, 1982

4. Aubert C, Rouge F, Galindo JR: Tumorigenicity of human malignant melanocytes in nude mice in relation to their differentiation *in vitro. J Natl Cancer Inst* 64:1029–1040, 1980

5. Barranco SC, Drewinko B, Humphrey RM: Differential response by human melanoma cells to 1,3-bis-(2-chloroethyl)-1-nitrosourea and bleomycin. *Mutation Res* 19:277–280, 1973

6. Barranco SC, Haenelt BR, Gee EL: Differential sensitivities of five rat hepatoma cell lines to anticancer drugs. *Cancer Res* 38:656–660, 1978

7. Barranco SC, Ho DH, Drewinko B, Romsdahl MM, Humphrey RM: Differential sensitivity of human melanoma cells grown *in vitro* to arabinosylcytosine. *Cancer Res* 32:2733–2736, 1972

8. Baylin SB: Clonal selection and heterogeneity of human solid neoplasms. In Fidler IJ, and White RJ (Eds.), *Design of Models for Testing Cancer Therapeutic Agents.* D. Van Nostrand Co., New York. pp. 50–63, 1982

9. Baylin SB, Abeloff MD, Wieman KC, Tomford JW, Ettinger DS. Elevated histaminase (diamine oxidase) activity in small-cell carcinoma of the lung. *N Engl J Med* 293:1286–1290, 1975

10. Baylin SB, Weisburger WR, Eggleston JC, Mendelsohn G, Beaven MA, Abeloff MD, Ettinger DS: Variable content of histaminase, L-dopa decarboxylase and calcitonin in small-cell carcinoma of the lung. Biologic and clinical implications. *N Engl J Med* 299:105–110, 1978

11. Becker AJ, McCulloch EA, Till JE: Cytological demonstration of the clonal nature of spleen colonies derived from transplanted mouse marrow cells. *Nature (London)* 197:452–454, 1963

12. Becker FF, Klein KM, Wolman SR, Asofsky R, Sell S: Characterization of primary hepatocellular carcinomas and initial transplant generations. *Cancer Res* 33:3330–3338, 1973

13. Biorklund A, Hakansson L, Stenstam B, Trope C, Akerman M: On heterogeneity of non-Hodgkin's lymphomas as regards sensitivity to cytostatic drugs. An *in vitro* study. *Eur J Cancer* 16:647–654, 1980

14. Bohm N, Sandritter W: DNA in human tumors: a cytophotometric study. *Curr Top Pathol* 60:152–219, 1975

15. Bosman HB, Winston RA: Synthesis of glycoprotein, glycolipid, protein, and lipid in synchronized L5178Y cells. *J Cell Biol* 45:23–33, 1970

16. Bosslet K, Schirrmacher V: Escape of metastasizing clonal tumor cell variants from tumor-specific cytolytic T lymphocytes. *J Exp Med* 154:557–562, 1981

17. Bosslet K, Schirrmacher V: High-frequency generation of new immunoresistant tumor variants during metastasis of a cloned murine tumor line. *Int J Cancer* 29:195–202, 1982

18. Brattain MG, Fine WD, Khaled FM, Thompson J, Brattain DE: Heterogeneity of malignant cells from a human colonic carcinoma. *Cancer Res* 41:1751–1756, 1981

19. Brennan MJ, Donegan WL, Appleby DE: The variability of estrogen receptors in metastatic breast cancer. *Am J Surg* 137:260–262, 1979

20. Briles EB, Kornfeld S: Isolation and metastatic properties of detachment variants of B16 melanoma cells. *J Natl Cancer Inst* 60:1217–1222, 1978

21. Brock WA, Swartzendruber DE, Grdina DJ: Kinetic heterogeneity in density-separated murine fibrosarcoma subpopulations. *Cancer Res* 42:4999–5003, 1982

22. Brunson KW, Beattie G, Nicolson GL: Selection and altered tumour cell properties of brain-colonising metastatic melanoma. *Nature* 272:543–545, 1978

23. Brunson KW, Nicolson GL: Selection and biologic properties of malignant variants of a murine lymphosarcoma. *J Natl Cancer Inst* 61:1499–1503, 1978

24. Byers VS, Johnston JO: Antigenic differences among osteo-genic sarcoma tumor cells taken from different locations in human tumors. *Cancer Res* 37:3173–3183, 1977

25. Chu MY, Takeuchi T, Yeskey KS, Bogaars H, Calabresi P: Tumor cell heterogeneity in human lung carcinoma LX-1 (Abstract). *Proc Am Assoc Cancer Res* 20:151, 1979

26. Cifone MA, Fidler IJ: Correlation of patterns of anchorage-independent growth with *in vivo* behavior of cells from a murine fibrosarcoma. *Proc Natl Acad Sci USA* 77:1039–1043, 1980

27. Cifone MA, and Fidler IJ: Increasing metastatic potential is associated with increasing genetic instability of clones isolated from murine neoplasms. *Proc Natl Acad Sci USA* 78:6949–6952, 1981

28. Cifone MA, Kripke ML, Fidler IJ: Growth rate and chromosome number of tumor cell lines with different metastatic potential. *J Supramol Struct* 11:467–476, 1979

29. Cikes M, Klein G: Quantitative studies of antigen expression in cultured murine lymphoma cells. I. Cell-surface antigens in 'asynchronous' cultures. *J Natl Cancer Inst* 49:1599–1606, 1972

30. Colcher D, Hand PH, Teramoto YA, Wunderlich D, Schlom J: Use of monoclonal antibodies to define the diversity of mammary tumor viral gene products in virions and mammary tumors of the genus *Mus Cancer Res* 41:1451–1459, 1981

31. Danielson KG, Anderson LW, Hosick HL: Selection and characterization in culture of mammary tumor cells with distinctive growth properties *in vivo. Cancer Res* 40:1812–1819, 1980

32. Dennis JW, Donaghue TP, Kerbel RS: An examination of tumor antigen loss in spontaneous metastases. *Invasion Metastases* 1:111–125, 1981

33. Dethlefsen L: The growth dynamics of murine mammary tumor cells *in situ.* In McGrath CM, Brennan MJ, Rich MA (Eds.), *Cell Biology of Breast Cancer.* Academic Press, New York. pp. 145–160, 1980

34. DeWys WD: Studies correlating the growth rate of a tumor and its metastases and providing evidence for tumor-related systemic growth-retarding factors. *Cancer Res* 32:374–379, 1972

35. Dexter DL, Kowalski HM, Blazar BA, Fligiel Z, Vogel R, Heppner GH: Heterogeneity of tumor cells from a single mouse mammary tumor. *Cancer Res* 38:3174–3181, 1978

36. Dexter DL, Spremulli EN, Fligiel Z, Barbosa JA, Vogel R, Van Voorhees A, Calabresi P: Heterogeneity of cancer cells from a single human colon carcinoma. *Am J Med* 71:949–956, 1981

37. Dominguez OV, Huseby RA: Heterogeneity of induced testicular interstitial cell tumors of mice as evidenced by steroid biosynthetic enzyme activities. *Cancer Res* 28:348–353, 1968

38. Dunn TB: Morphology of mammary tumors in mice. In Homburger F, Fisheman NH (Eds.), *Physiopathology of Cancer.* Karger, New York, pp. 38–84, 1959

39. Easty DM, Easty GC, Carter RL, Monaghan P, Pittam MR, James T: Five human tumour cell lines derived from a primary squamous carcinoma of the tongue, two subsequent local recurrences and two nodal metastases. *Br J Cancer* 44:363–370, 1981

40. Ekman P, Snochowski M, Zetterberg A, Hogberg B, Gustafsson JA: Steroid receptor content in human prostatic carcinoma and response to endocrine therapy. *Cancer (Phila.)* 44:1173–1181, 1979

41. Enders JF, Diamondopoulous GT: A study of variation and progression in oncongenicity in an SV 40-transformed hamster heart cell line and its clones. *Proc Roy Soc Ser B Biol Sci* 171:431–443, 1969

42. Everson LK, Plocinik BA, Rogentine GN Jr: HL-A expression on the G_1, S, and G_2 cell-cycle stages of human

lymphoid cells. *J Natl Cancer Inst* 53:913–920, 1974

43. Ewing SL, Sumner HW, Ophoven JJ, Mayer JE, Humphrey EW: Small cell anaplastic carcinoma with differentiation: a report of 14 cases (abstract). *Lab Invest* 42:115, 1980

44. Feder MK, Gilbert F: Clonal evidence in a human neuroblastoma. *J Natl Cancer Inst* 70:1051–1056, 1983

45. Fialkow PJ: Clonal origin of human tumors. *Biochim Biophys Acta* 458:283–310, 1976

46. Fidler IJ: Selection of successive tumor lines for metastasis. *Nature New Biology* 242:148–149, 1973

47. Fidler IJ, Bucana C: Mechanism of tumor cell resistance to lysis by syngeneic lymphocytes. *Cancer Res* 37:3945–3956, 1977

48. Fidler IJ, Hart IR: Biological and experimental consequences of the zonal composition of solid tumors. *Cancer Res* 41:3266–3267, 1981

49. Fidler IJ, Gruys E, Cifone MA, Barnes Z, Bucana C: Demonstration of multiple phenotypic diversity in a murine melanoma of recent origin. *J Natl Cancer Inst* 67:947–956, 1981

50. Fidler IJ, Hart IR: The origin of metastatic heterogeneity in tumors. *Eur J Cancer* 17:487–494, 1981

51. Fidler IJ, Hart IR: Biological diversity in metastatic neoplasms: origins and implications. *Science* 217:998–1003, 1982

52. Fidler IJ, Hart IR: Biological and experimental consequences of the zonal composition of solid tumors. *Cancer Res* 41:3266–3267, 1981

53. Fidler IJ, Kripke ML: Metastasis results from preexisting variant cells within a malignant tumor. *Science* 197:893–895, 1977

54. Fidler IJ, Nicolson GL: The immunobiology of experimental metastatic melanoma. *Cancer Biol Rev* 2:171–234, 1981

55. Fogel M, Gorelik E, Segal S, Feldman M: Differences in cell surface antigens of tumor metastases and those of the local tumor. *J Natl Cancer Inst* 62:585–588, 1979

56. Foulds L: The histologic analysis of mammary tumors of mice. I. Scope of investigations and general principles of analysis. *J Natl Cancer Inst* 17:701–712, 1956

57. Foulds L: The histologic analysis of mammary tumors of mice. II. The histology of responsiveness and progression. The origins of tumors. *J Natl Cancer Inst* 17:713–754, 1956

58. Foulds L: The histologic analysis of mammary tumors of mice. III. Organoid tumors. *J Natl Cancer Inst* 17:755–782, 1956

59. Foulds L: The histologic analysis of mammary tumors of mice. IV. Secretion. *J Natl Cancer Inst* 17:783–801, 1956

60. Franks LM: Estrogen-treated prostatic cancer. *Cancer* 13:490–501, 1960

61. Friedman JM, Fialkow PJ, Greene CL, Weinberg MN: Probable clonal origin of neurofibrosarcoma in a patient with hereditary neurofibromatosis. *J Natl Cancer Inst* 69:1289–1292, 1982

62. Frost PH, Kerbel RS: Immunoselection *in vitro* of a nonmetastatic variant from a highly metastatic tumor. *Int J Cancer* 27:381–385, 1981

63. Fugmann RA, Anderson JC, Stolfi R, Martin DS: Comparison of adjuvant chemotherapeutic activity against primary and metastatic spontaneous murine tumors. *Cancer Res* 37:496–500, 1972

64. Fuji H, Mihich E: Selection for high immunogenicity in drug-resistant sublines of murine lymphomas demonstrated by plaque assay. *Cancer Res* 35:946–952, 1975

65. Fuji H, Mihich E, Pressman D: Differential tumor immunogenicity of L1210 and its sublines. *J Immunol* 119:983–986, 1977

66. Geier GR, Schwarz JA, Schlag P: Cytologic uniformity of breast cancer from different locations: a pattern analyses study. *Exp Cell Biol* 47:241–249, 1979

67. Giavazzi R, Alessandri G, Spreafico F, Garattini S, Mantovani A: Metastasizing capacity of tumour cells from spontaneous metastases of transplanted murine tumours. *Br J Cancer* 42:462–472, 1980

68. Gorelik E, Feldman M, Segal S: Selection of 3LL tumor subline resistant to natural effector cells concomitantly selected for increased metastatic potency. *Cancer Immunol Immunother* 12:105–109, 1982

69. Gorelik E, Fogel M, Segal S, Feldman M: Tumor-associated antigenic differences between the primary and distant metastatic tumor populations. *J Supramol Struct* 12:385–402, 1979

70. Gray JM, Pierce GB: Relationship between growth rate and differentiation of melanoma *in vivo*. *J Natl Cancer Inst* 32:1201–1211, 1964

71. Hager JC, Fligiel S, Stanley W, Richardson AM, Heppner GH: Characterization of a variant producing tumor cell line from a heterogeneous strain BALB/cfC$_3$H mouse mammary tumor. *Cancer Res* 41:1293–1300, 1981

72. Hager JC, Heppner GH: Heterogeneity of expression and induction of mouse mammary tumor virus antigens in mouse mammary tumors. *Cancer Res* 42:4325–4329, 1982

73. Hakansson L, Trope C: On the presence within tumors of clones that differ in sensitivity to cytostatic drugs. *Acta Pathol Microbiol Scand [A]* 82:35-40, 1974

74. Hakansson L, Trope C: Cell clones with different sensitivity to cytostatic drugs in methylcholanthrene-induced mouse sarcomas. *Acta Pathol Microbiol Scan [A]* 82:41–47, 1974

75. Hanna N, Fidler IJ: Relationship between metastatic potential and resistance to NK cell-mediated cytotoxicity in three murine tumor systems. *J Natl Cancer Inst* 66:1183–1190, 1981

76. Harris JF, Chambers AF, Hill RP, Ling V: Metastatic variants are generated spontaneously at a high rate in mouse KHT tumor. *Proc Natl Acad Sci USA* 79:5547–5551, 1982

77. Hart IR: Selection and characterization of an invasive variant of the B16 melanoma. *Am J Pathol* 97:587–600, 1979

78. Hart IR, Talmadge JE, Fidler IJ: Metastatic behavior of a murine reticulum cell sarcoma exhibiting organ-specific growth. *Cancer Res* 41:1281–1287, 1981

79. Hastings RJ, Franks LM: Cellular heterogeneity in a tissue culture cell line derived from a human bladder carcinoma. *Br J Cancer* 47:233–244, 1983

80. Henderson JS, Rous P: The plating of tumor components on the subcutaneous expanses of young mice. *J Exp Med* 115:1211–1230, 1962

81. Heppner GH, Dexter DL, De Nucci T, Miller FR, Calabresi P: Heterogeneity in drug sensitivity among tumor cell subpopulations of a single mammary tumor. *Cancer Res* 38:3758–3763, 1978

82. Heppner GH, Miller BE: Tumor heterogeneity: biological implications and therapeutic consequences. *Cancer Metastasis Reviews* 2:5–23, 1983

83. Hill HZ, Hill GJ, Miller CF, Kwong F, Purdy J: Radiation and melanoma response of B16 mouse tumor cells and clonal lines to *in vitro* irradiation. *Rad Res* 80:259–276, 1979

84. Isaacs JT, Coffey DS: Adaptation versus selection as the mechanism responsible for the relapse of prostatic cancer to androgen ablation therapy as studied in the Dunning R-3327H adenocarcinoma. *Cancer Res* 41:5070–5075, 1981

85. Isaacs JT, Wake N, Coffey DS, Sandberg AA: Genetic instability coupled to clonal selection as a mechanism for tumor progression in the Dunning R-3327 rat prostatic adenocarcinoma system. *Cancer Res* 42:2353–2361, 1982

86. Ishidate M, Aoshima M, Sakurai Y: Population changes of a rat leukemia by different routes of transplantation. *J Natl Cancer Inst* 53:773–781, 1974

87. Ito E, Moore GE: Characteristic differences in clones isolated from an S37 ascites tumor *in vitro*. *Exp Cell Res* 48:440–447, 1967

88. Kajiji SM, Meitner PA, Bogaars HA, Dexter DL, Cummings FJ, Calabresi P, Turner MD: Establishment of a fast growing variant of human pancreatic cancer (HPC) (Abstract). *Proc AACR* 23:119, 1982

89. Kerbel RS: Implications of immunological heterogeneity of tumors. *Nature* 280:358–360, 1979

90. Kerbel RS: Immunologic studies of membrane mutants of a highly metastatic murine tumor. *Am J Pathol* 97:609–622, 1979a

91. Kerbel RS, Frost P: Heritable alterations induced in tumor cell immunogenicity. *Immunology Today* 3:34–35, 1982

92. Kerbel RS, Twiddy RR, Robertson DM: Induction of a tumor with greatly increased metastatic growth potential by injection of cells from a low-metastatic H-2 heterozygous tumor cell line into an H-2 incompatible parental strain. *Int J Cancer* 22:583–594, 1978

93. Key M, Talmadge JE, Fidler IJ: Lack of correlation between the progressive growth of spontaneous metastases and their content of infiltrating macrophages. *J Reticuloendothelial Soc* 32:387–396, 1982

94. Killion JJ: Immunotherapy with tumor subpopulations. I. Active, specific immunotherapy of L1210 leukemia. *Cancer Immunol Immunother* 4.115-119, 1978

95. Killion JJ, Kollmorgen GM: Isolation of immunogenic tumor cells by cell-affinity chromatography. *Nature* 259:674–676, 1976

96. Kiricuta I, Mustea I, Rogozan I, Simu G: Relations between tumor and metastasis. I. Aspects of the crabtree effect. *Cancer* 18:978–984, 1965

97. Klein E: Gradual transformation of solid into ascites tumors: Permanent differences between the original and the transformed sublines. *Cancer Res* 14:482–485, 1954

98. Klein E: Gradual transformation of solid into ascites tumors: Evidence favoring the mutation-selection theory. *Exp Cell Res* 8:188–212, 1955

99. Kobori O, Oota K: Neuroendocrine cells in serially passaged rat stomach cancers induced by MNNG. *Int J Cancer* 23:536–541, 1979

100. Koch FE: Zur Frage der Metastasenbildung bei Impftumoren. *Z Krebsforsch* 48:495–505, 1939

101. Kripke ML, Fidler IJ: Enhanced experimental metastasis of ultraviolet light-induced fibrosarcomas in ultraviolet light-irradiated syngeneic mice. *Cancer Res* 40:625–629, 1980

102. Kripke ML, Gruys E, Fidler IJ: Metastatic heterogeneity of cells from an ultraviolet light-induced murine fibrosarcoma of recent origin. *Cancer Res* 38:2962–2967, 1978

103. Kusyk CJ, Seski JC, Medlin WV, Edwards CL: Progressive chromosome changes associated with different sites of one ovarian carcinoma. *J Natl Cancer Inst* 66:1021–1025, 1981

104. Larner EH, Rutherford CL: Implementation of micro-methods to resolve problems of human breast tumor heterogeneity in analysis of cyclic 3′:5′ nucleotide phosphodiesterase. *Cancer Res* 42:1661–1668, 1982

105. Law LW: Origin of the resistance of leukaemic cells to folic acid antagonists. *Nature* 169:628–629, 1952

106. Lee SH: Cytochemical study of estrogen receptor in human mammary cancer. *Am J Clin Pathol* 70:197–203, 1978

107. Leith JT, Brenner HJ, DeWyngaert JK, Dexter DL, Calabresi P, Glicksman AS: Selective modification of the X-ray response of two mouse mammary adenocarcinoma sublines by N,N-dimethyl-formamide. *Int J Rad Oncol Biol Phys* 7:943–947, 1981

108. Leith JT, Dexter DL, DeWyngaert JK, Zeman EM, Chu, MY, Calabresi P, Glicksman AS: Differential responses to x-irradiation of subpopulations of two heterogeneous human carcinomas *in vitro. Cancer Res* 42:2556–2561, 1982

109. Leith JT, Gaskins LA, Dexter DL, Calabresi P, Glicksman AS: Alteration of the survival response of two human colon carcinoma subpopulations to X-irradiation by N, N-dimethylformamide. *Cancer Res* 42:30–34, 1982

110. Lerner RA, Oldstone MB, Cooper NR: Cell cycle-dependent immune lysis of Moloney virus-transformed lymphocytes: presence of viral antigen, accessibility to antibody, and complement activation. *Proc Natl Acad Sci USA* 68:2584–2588, 1971

111. Levan A, Hauschka TS: Endomitotic reduplication mechanisms in ascites tumors of the mouse. *J Natl Cancer Inst* 14:1–43, 1953

112. Lippman SM, Mendelsohn G, Trump DL, Wells SA, Baylin SB: The prognostic and biological significance of cellular heterogeneity in medullary thyroid carcinoma: a study of calcitonin, L-Dopa decarboxylase, and histaminase. *J Clin Endocrinol Metab* 54:233–240, 1982

113. Loewenstein WR: Junctional intercellular communication and the control of growth. *Biochim Biophys Acta* 560:1–65, 1979

114. Lotan R: Different susceptibilities of human melanoma and breast carcinoma cell lines to retinoic acid-induced growth inhibition. *Cancer Res* 39:1014–1019, 1979

115. Lotan R, Nicolson GL: Heterogeneity in growth inhibition by B-trans-retinoic acid of metastatic B-16 melanoma clones and *in vivo*-selected cell variant lines *Cancer Res* 39:4767–4771, 1979

116. McCune CS, Schapira DV, Henshaw EC: Specific immunotherapy of advanced renal carcinoma: Evidence for the polyclonality of metastases. *Cancer* 47:1984–1987, 1981

117. McDowell EM, Sorokin SP, Hoyt RF Jr, Trump BF: An unusual bronchial carcinoid tumor: Light and electron microscopy. *Human Pathol* 12:338–348, 1981

118. McGee J O'D, Woods JC, Ashall F, Bramwell ME, Harris H: A new marker for human cancer cells. 2. Immunohistochemical deletion of the Ca antigen in human tissues with the Ca1 antibody. *Lancet* ii:7–10, 1982

119. Macinnes JI, Chan ECM, Percy DH, Morris VL: Mammary tumors from GR mice contain more than one population of mouse mammary tumor virus-infected cells. *Virol* 113:119–129, 1981

120. Mackintosh FR, Louie AC, Evans TL, Amylon MD, Sikic BI: Clonal heterogeneity in a human ovarian adenocarcinoma (Abstract). *Proc AACR* 22:379, 1981

121. MacLean GD, Seehafer J, Shaw ARE, Kieran MW, Longenecker BM: Antigenic heterogeneity of human colorectal cancer cell lines analyzed by a panel of monoclonal antibodies. I. Heterogeneous expression of 1a-like and HLA-like antigenic determinants. *J Natl Cancer Inst* 69:357–364, 1982

122. Makino S: Further evidence favoring the concept of the stem cell in ascites tumors of rats. *Ann NY Acad Sci* 63:818–830, 1956

123. Mantovani A, Giavazzi R, Alessandri G, Spreafico F, Garattini S: Characterization of tumor lines derived from spontaneous metastases of a transplantable murine sarcoma. *Eur J Cancer* 17:71–76, 1981

124. Mathieson BJ, Zatz MM, Sharrow SO, Asofsky R, Logan W, Kanellopoulos-Langevin C: Separation and characterization of two component tumor lines within the AKR lymphoma, AKTB-1, by fluorescence-activated cell sorting and flow microfluorometry analysis. *J Immunol* 128:1832–1838, 1982

125. Michalides R, Wagenaar E, Sluyser M: Mammary tumor virus DNA as a marker for genotypic variance within hormone-responsive GR-mouse mammary tumors. *Cancer Res* 42:1154–1158, 1982

126. Miller BE, Miller FR, Heppner GH: Interactions between tumor subpopulations affecting their sensitivity to the antineoplastic agents cyclophosphamide and methotrexate. *Cancer Res* 41:4378–4381, 1981

127. Miller BE, Miller FR, Leith J, Heppner GH: Growth interaction *in vivo* between tumor subpopulations derived from a single mouse mammary tumor. *Cancer Res* 40:3977–3981,

1980

128. Miller FR: Intratumor immunologic heterogeneity. *Cancer Metastasis Rev* 1:319–334, 1982
129. Miller FR, Heppner GH: Immunologic heterogeneity of tumor cell subpopulations from a single mouse mammary tumor. *J Natl Cancer Inst* 63:1457–1463, 1979
128. Miller FR: Intratumor immunologic heterogeneity. *Cancer Metastasis Rev* 1:319–334, 1982
129. Miller FR, Heppner GH: Immunologic heterogeneity of tumor cell subpopulations from a single mouse mammary tumor. *J Natl Cancer Inst* 63:1457–1463, 1979
130. Mitelman F: The chromosomes of 50 primary Rous rat sarcomas. *Hereditas* 69:155–186, 1971
131. Natali PG, Cavaliere R, Bigotti A, Nicotra MR, Russo C, Ng AK, Giacomini P, Ferrone S: Antigenic heterogeneity of surgically removed primary and autologous metastatic human melanoma lesions. *J Immunol* 130:1462–1466, 1983
132. Neri A, Welch D, Kawaguchi T, Nicolson GL: Development and biologic properties of malignant cell sublines and clones of a spontaneous metastasizing rat mammary adenocarcinoma. *J Natl Cancer Inst* 68:507–517, 1982
133. Nicolin A, Canti G, Marelli O, Veronese F, Goldin A: Chemotherapy and immunotherapy of L1210 leukemic mice with antigenic tumor sublines. *Cancer Res* 41:1358–1362, 1981
134. Nicolson GL, Brunson KW, Fidler IJ: Specificity of arrest, survival, and growth of selected metastatic variant cell lines. *Cancer Res* 38:4104–4111, 1978
135. Nicolson GL, Custead SE: Tumor metastasis is not due to adaptation of cells to a new organ environment. *Science* 215:176–178, 1982
136. Niles RM, Makarski JS: Hormonal activation of adenylate cyclase in mouse melanoma metastatic variants. *J Cell Physiol* 96:355–359, 1978
137. Nowell PC: The clonal evolution of tumor cell populations. *Science* 194:23–28, 1976
138. Ohno S: Genetic implication of karyological instability of malignant somatic cells. *Physiol Rev* 51:496–526, 1971
139. Olsson L, Ebbesen P: Natural polyclonality of spontaneous AKR leukemia and its consequences for so-called specific immunotherapy. *J Natl Cancer Inst* 62:623–627, 1979
140. Olsson L, Kiger N, Kronstrom H: Sensitivity of cloned high and low-metastatic murine Lewis lung tumor cells to lysis by cytotoxic autoreactive cells. *Cancer Res* 41:4706–4709, 1981
141. Panem S, Schauf V: Cell-cycle dependent appearance of murine leukemia-sarcoma virus antigens. *J Virol* 13:1169–1175, 1974
142. Parbhoo SP: Heterogeneity in human mammary cancer. In Stoll BA (Ed.), *Systemic Control of Breast Cancer*. William Heinemann Medical Books, London. pp. 55–77, 1981
143. Pasternak CA, Warmsley AMH, Thomas DB: Structural alterations in the surface membrane during the cell cycle. *J Cell Biol* 50:562–564, 1971
144. Pertschuk LP, Tobin EH, Brigati DJ, Kim DS, Bloom ND, Gaetjens E, Berman PJ, Carter AC, Degenstein GA: Immunofluorescent-detection of estrogen receptors in breast cancer. *Cancer* 41:907–911, 1978
145. Pierce GB: Cellular heterogeneity of cancers. In Pop T, DiPaolo JA (Eds.), *World Symposium on Model Studies in Chemical Carcinogenesis*. Dekker, new York. pp. 463–472, 1974
146. Pimm MV, Baldwin RW: Antigenic heterogeneity of primary and metastatic tumors and its implications for immunotherapy. In Grundmann E (Ed.), *Metastatic Tumor Growth*. Gustav Fischer Verlag, Stuttgart. pp. 305, 1980
147. Pimm MV, Embleton MJ, Baldwin RW: Multiple antigenic specificities within primary 3-methylcholanthrene-induced rat sarcomas and metastases. *Int J Cancer* 25:621–629, 1980
148. Pollack VA, Fidler IJ: Use of young nude mice for selection of subpopulations of cells with increased metastatic potential from nonsyngeneic neoplasms. *J Natl Cancer Inst* 69:137–141, 1982
149. Poste G: Experimental systems for analysis of the malignant phenotype. *Cancer Metastasis Rev* 1:141–199, 1982
150. Poste G, Doll J, Brown AE, Tzeng J, Zeidman I: A comparison of the metastatic properties of B16 melanoma clones isolated from cultured cell lines, subcutaneous tumors and individual lung tumors. *Cancer Res* 42:2770–2778, 1982
151. Poste G, Doll J, Fidler IJ: Interactions between clonal subpopulations affect the stability of the metastatic phenotype in polyclonal populations of B16 melanoma cells. *Proc Natl Acad Sci USA* 78:6226–6230, 1981
152. Poste GH, Doll J, Hart IR, Fidler IJ: *In vitro* selection of murine B16 melanoma variants with enhanced tissue invasive properties. *Cancer Res* 40:1636–1644, 1980
153. Poste, G.: Pathogenesis of metastatic disease; implications for current therapy and for the development of new therapeutic strategies. Cancer Treat Rep 80(1):183–99, 1986
154. Poste G, Fidler IJ: The pathogenesis of cancer metastasis. *Nature* 283:139–146, 1980
155. Poste G, Tzeng J, Doll J, Greig R, Rieman D, Zeidman I: Evolution of tumor cell heterogeneity during progressive growth of individual lung metastases. *Proc Natl Acad Sci USA* 79:6574–6578, 1982
156. Prehn RT: Analysis of antigenic heterogeneity within individual 3-methylcholanthrene-induced mouse sarcomas. *J Natl Cancer Inst* 45:1039–1045, 1970
157. Rabotti G: Ploidy of primary and metastatic human tumours. *Nature* 183:1276–1277, 1959
158. Raz A: Regional emergence of metastatic heterogeneity in a growing tumor. *Cancer Letters* 17:153–160, 1982
159. Raz A, Hanna N, Fidler IJ: *In vivo* isolation of a metastatic tumor cell variant involving selective and nonadaptive processes. *J Natl Cancer Inst* 66:183–189, 1981
160. Raz A, Hart IR: Murine melanoma: A model for intracranial metastasis. *Br J Cancer* 42:331–341, 1980
161. Raz A, McLellan WE, Hart IR, Bucana CD, Hoyer LC, Sela BA, Dragsten P, Fidler IJ: Cell surface properties of B16 melanoma variants with differing metastatic potential. *Cancer Res* 40:1645–1651, 1980
162. Reading CL, Belloni DN, Nicolson GL: Selection and *in vivo* properties of lectin-attachment variants of malignant murine lymphosarcoma cell lines. *J Natl Cancer Inst* 64:1241–1249, 1980
163. Reading CL, Brunson KW, Torriani M, Nicolson GL: Malignancies of metastatic murine lymphosarcoma cell lines and clones correlate with decreased cell surface display of RNA-tumor virus envelope glycoprotein gp70. *Proc Natl Acad Sci USA* 77:5943–5947, 1980
164. Reeve JG, Twentyman PR: Ploidy distribution of tumour cells derived from induced and spontaneously arising metastases of a murine radiation-induced sarcoma, RIF-1. *Eur J Cancer Clin Oncol* 18:1001–1006, 1982
165. Sacchi A, Calabresi F, Greco C, Zupi G: Different metastatic potential of *in vitro* and *in vivo* lines selected from Lewis lung carcinoma: correlation with response to different bleomycin schedulings. *Invasion Metastasis* 1:227–238, 1981
166. Sandberg AA: Chromosome markers and progression in bladder cancer. *Cancer Res* 37:2950–2956, 1977
167. Schirrmacher V, Bosslet K: Tumor metastases and cell-mediated immunity in a model system in DBA/2 mice. X. Immunoselection of tumor variants differing in tumor antigen expression and metastatic capacity. *Int J Cancer* 25:781–788, 1980
168. Schirrmacher V, Bosslet K: Clonal analysis of expression of tumor-associated transplantation antigens and of metastatic capacity. *Cancer Immunol Immunother* 13:62–68, 1982
169. Schirrmacher V, Bosslet K, Shantz G, Clauer K, Hubsch D: Tumor metastases and cell-mediated immunity in a model

system in DBA/2 mice. IV. Antigenic differences between a metastasizing variant, and the parental tumor line revealed by cytotoxic T lymphocytes. *Int J Cancer* 23:245–252, 1979

170. Schirrmacher V, Fogel M, Russmann E, Bosslet K, Altevogt P, Beck L: Antigenic variation in cancer metastasis: Immune escape versus immune control. *Cancer Met Rev* 1:241–275, 1982

171. Schlag P, Schreml W: Heterogeneity in growth pattern and drug sensitivity of primary tumor and metastases in the human tumor colony-forming assay. *Cancer Res* 42:4086–4089, 1982

172. Schmitt M, Daynes RA: Heterogeneity of tumorigenicity phenotype in murine tumors. I. Characterization of regressor and progressor clones isolated from a nonmutagenized ultraviolet regressor tumor. *J Exp Med* 153:1344–1359, 1981

173. Semple TU, Moore GE, Morgan RT, Woods LK, Quinn LA: Multiple cell lines from patients with malignant melanoma: Morphology, karyology and biochemical analysis. *J Natl Cancer Inst* 68:365–380, 1982

174. Shapiro JR, Yung WA, Shapiro WR. Isolation, karyotype and clonal growth of heterogeneous subpopulations of human malignant gliomas. *Cancer Res* 41:2349–2359, 1981

175. Shearman PJ, Longenecker BM: Selection for virulence and organ-specific metastasis of Herpes virus-transformed lymphoma cells. *Int J Cancer* 25:363–369, 1980

176. Shearman PJ, Longenecker BM: Clonal variation and functional correlation of organ-specific metastasis and an organ-specific metastasis-associated antigen. *Int J Cancer* 27:387–395, 1981

177. Shipley WU: Immune cytolysis in relation to the growth cycle of chinese hamster cells. *Cancer Res* 31:925–929, 1971

178. Siracky J: An approach to the problem of heterogeneity of human tumor-cell populations. *Br J Cancer* 39:570–577, 1979

179. Sluyser M, Evers SG, De Goeij CCJ: Sex hormone receptors in mammary tumors of GR mice. *Nature* 263:386–389,1976

180. Sluyser M, Van Nie R: Estrogen receptor content and hormone-responsive growth of mouse mammary tumors. *Cancer Res* 34:3252–3257, 1974

181. Soule HD, Maloney T, McGrath CM: Phenotypic variance among cells isolated from spontaneous mouse mammary tumors in primary suspension culture. *Cancer Res* 41:1154–1164, 1981

182. Stackpole CW: Distinct lung-colonizing and lung-metastasizing cell populations in B16 mouse melanoma. *Nature* 289:798–800, 1981

183. Stackpole CW: Generation of phenotypic diversity in the B16 mouse melanoma relative to spontaneous metastasis. *Cancer Res* 43:3057–3065, 1983

184. Starace G, Badaracco G, Grego C, Sacchi A, Zupi G: DNA content distribution of *in vivo* and *in vitro* lines of Lewis lung carcinoma. *Eur J Cancer Clin Oncol* 18:973–978, 1982

185. Stephens TC, Peacock JH: Clonal variation in the sensitivity of B16 melanoma to m-AMSA. *Br J Cancer* 45:821–829, 1982

186. Stich HF, Florian SF, Emson HE: The DNA content of tumor cells. I. Polyps and adenocarcinomas of the large intestine of man. *J Natl Cancer Inst* 24:471–482, 1960

187. Straus MJ: Growth characteristics of lung cancer. In Straus MJ (Ed.), *Lung Cancer.* Grune and Stratton. New York. pp. 19–32, 1977

188. Strzadala L, Opolski A, Radzikowski C, Mihich E: Differential expression of murine leukemia antigen on L1210 parental and drug-resistant sublines. *Cancer Res* 41:4934–4937, 1981

189. Subak-Sharpe H, Burk RR, Pitts JD: Metabolic co-operation between biochemically marked mammalian cells in tissue culture. *J Cell Sci* 4:353–367, 1969

190. Suzuki N, Withers R, Koehler MW: Heterogeneity and variability of artificial lung colony-forming ability among clones from mouse fibrosarcoma. *Cancer Res* 38:3349–3351,
1978

191. Sweeney FL, Pot-Deprun J, Poupon MF, Chouroulinkov I: Heterogeneity of the growth and metastatic behavior of cloned cell lines derived from a primary rhabdomyosarcoma. *Cancer Res* 42:3776–3782, 1982

192. Talmadge JE, Fidler IJ: Cancer metastasis is selective or random depending on the parent tumour population. *Nature* 297:593–594, 1982

193. Talmadge JE, Fidler IJ: Enhanced metastatic potential of tumor cells harvested from spontaneous metastases of heterogeneous murine tumors. *J Natl Cancer Inst* 69:975–980, 1982

194. Talmadge JE, Key ME, Hart IR: Characterization of a murine ovarian reticulum cell sarcoma of histiocytic origin. *Cancer Res* 41:1271–1280, 1981

195. Talmadge JE, Meyers KM, Prieur DJ, Starkey JR: Role of NK cells in tumour growth and metastasis in beige mice. *Nature* 284:622–624, 1980

196. Talmadge JE, Starkey JR, Davis WC, Cohen AL: Introduction of metastatic heterogeneity by short-term *in vivo* passage of a cloned transformation cell line. *J Supramol Struct* 121:227–243, 1979

197. Talmadge JE, Starkey JR, Stanford DR: *In vitro* characteristics of metastatic variant subclones of restricted genetic origin. *J Supramol Struct Cell Biochem* 15:139–151, 1981

198. Talmadge JE, Wolman SR, Fidler IJ: Evidence for the clonal origin of spontaneous metastases. *Science* 217:361–363, 1982

199. Tan MH, Shimano T, Chu TM: Differential localization of human pancreas cancer-associated antigen and carcino-embryonic antigen in homologous pancreatic tumoral xenograft. *J Natl Cancer Inst* 67:563–569, 1981

200. Tao TW, Burger MM: Non-metastasizing variants selected from metastasizing melanoma cells. *Nature* 270:437–438, 1977

201. Tarin D, Price JE: Metastatic colonization potential of primary tumour cells in mice. *Br J Cancer* 39:740–754, 1979

202. Thistlethwaite P, Davidson DD, Fidler IJ, Roth JA: Syngeneic humoral immune responses to tumor-associated antigens expressed by K-1735 UV-induced melanoma and its metastases. *Cancer Immunol Immunother* 15:11–16, 1983

203. Tilley WD, Keightley DD, Cant EL: Inter-site variation of oestrogen receptors in human breast cancers. *Br J Cancer* 38:544–546, 1978

204. Tropé C: Different sensitivity to cytostatic drugs of primary tumor and metastasis of the Lewis lung carcinoma. *Neoplasma* 22:171–180, 1975

205. Tropé C: Different susceptibilities of tumor cell subpopulations to cytotoxic agents. In Fidler IJ, White RJ (Eds.), *Design of Models for Testing Cancer Chemotherapeutic Agents.* D. Van Nostrand Co., New York. pp. 64–79, 1982

206. Tropé C, Aspergen K, Kullander S, Astredt B: Heterogeneous response of disseminated human ovarian cancers to cytostasis *in vitro*. *Acta Obstet. Gynecol. Scand* 58:543–546, 1979

207. Tropé C, Hakansson L, Dencker H: Heterogeneity of human adenocarcinomas of the colon and the stomach as regards sensitivity to cytostatic drugs. *Neoplasma* 22:423–430, 1975

208. Tseng MT: Ultrastructure of the hormone-dependent N-Nitrosomethylurea-induced mammary carcinoma of the rat. *Cancer Res* 40:3112–3115, 1980

209. Tsuruo T, Fidler IJ: Differences in drug sensitivity among tumor cells from parental tumors, selected variants, and spontaneous metastases. *Cancer Res* 41:3058–3064, 1981

210. Valeriote F, van Putten L: Proliferation dependent cytotoxicity of anticancer agents: A review. *Cancer Res* 35:2619–2630, 1975

211. Varani J, Orr W, Ward PA: A comparison of the migration patterns of normal and malignant cells in two assay systems. *Am J Pathol* 90:159–172, 1978

64   *James E. Talmadge*

212. Vaupel PW, Frinak S, Bicher HI: Heterogeneous oxygen partial pressure and pH distribution in C_3H mouse mammary adeocarcinoma. *Cancer Res* 41:2008–2013, 1981
213. Vindelov LL: Flow microfluorometric analysis of nuclear DNA in cells from solid tumors and cell suspensions. *Virchow Arch [Cell Pathol]* 24:227–242, 1977
214. Vindelov LL, Hansen HH, Christensen IJ, Spang-Thomsen M, Hirsch FR, Hansen M, Nissen NI: Clonal heterogeneity of small-cell anaplastic carcinoma of the lung demonstrated by flow cytometric DNA analysis. *Cancer Res* 40:4295–4300, 1980
215. Vindelov LL, Spang-Thomsen M, Visfeldt J, Povlsen CO, Jensen G, Nissen NI: Clonal evolution demonstrated by flow cytometric DNA analysis of a human colonic carcinoma grown in nude mice. *Exp Cell Biol* 50:216–221, 1982
216. Wagner RK, Schulze RA: Clinical relevance of androgen receptor in human prostate carcinoma. *Acta Endocrinol Suppl* 215:139–140, 1978
217. Walker JR, Rees RC, Teale D, Potter CW. Properties of a Herpes virus-transformed hamster cell line. I. Growth and culture characteristics of sublines of high and low metastatic potential. *Eur J Cancer Clin Oncol* 18:1017–1026, 1982
218. Wang N, Yu SH, Liener IE, Hebbel RP, Eaton JW, McKhann CF: Characterization of high and low metastatic clones derived from a methylcholanthrene-induced murine fibrosarcoma. *Cancer Res* 42:1046–1051, 1982
219. Weiss L: Cancer cells in primary tumors and their metastases. In McGrath CM, Brennan MJ, Rich MA (Eds.), *Cell Biology of Breast Cancer*. Academic Press, New York. pp. 189–205, 1980
220. Weiss L: Vol. 2 Brain Metastasis, Metastasis a monographic series (Workshop on Metastasis to the Brain), Memorial Sloan Kettering Cancer Center, New York, NY, published by Martinus Nijhoff The Hague, pp. 30–49, 1980
221. Weiss L: Differences between cancer cells in primary and secondary tumors. In Ioachim HL (Ed.), *Pathobiology Annual 1980 V* 10. Raven Press, New York. pp. 51–81, 1980
222. Weiss L, Holmes JC, Ward PM: Do metastases arise from pre-existing subpopulations of cancer cells? *Br J Cancer* 47:81–89, 1983
223. Weiss MA, Michael JG, Pesce AJ, DiPersion L: Heterogeneity of B_2-microglobulin in human breast carcinoma. *Lab Invest* 45:46–57, 1981
224. Welch DR, Milas L, Tomasovic SP, Nicolson GL: Heterogeneous response and clonal drift of sensitivities of metastatic 13762NF mammary adenocarcinoma clones to γ-radiation *in vitro. Cancer Res* 43:6–10, 1983
225. Young WW, Jr, Hakomori S: Therapy of mouse lymphoma with monoclonal antibodies to glycolipid: Selection of low antigenic variants *in vivo. Science* 211:487–489, 1981
226. Yung WA, Shapiro JR, Shapiro WR: Heterogeneous chemosensitivities of subpopulations of human glioma cells in culture. *Cancer Res* 42:992–998, 1982
227. Zupi G, Mauro F, Sacchi A: Cloning *in vitro* and *in vivo* of Lewis lung carcinoma: Properties and characteristics. *Br J Cancer* 41:309–310, 1981

NEOPLASTIC HETEROGENEITY AND CLINICAL CHEMOTHERAPY

STEPHEN K. CARTER

Cancer chemotherapy is a modality in transition. In its early days, chemotherapy was viewed with skepticism by many, and its pioneers were forced to emphasize its positives in an aggressively defensive manner. In the early 1970s, chemotherapy appeared poised to possibly become a dominant modality. This was caused by the concept of adjuvant chemotherapy which appeared validated by the early relapse free survival gains reported in the treatment of primary breast cancer. A decade later it is obvious that adjuvant chemotherapy is not a dramatic breakthrough and that the modality itself has plateaued in its ability to cure and palliate malignant disease.

The future of chemotherapy is difficult to precisely predict at this moment in time. Immunotherapy, which was touted as a fourth modality, has proven to be a dismal failure as reflected in the massively negative clinical data base which exists with BCG, C. parvum, MER, levamisole, transfer factor and other new specific approaches. Immunotherapy has been replaced by biologic response modification. The approach of biologic response modification has been developed with such broadness that it fits beneath its umbrella the still large remnants of old immunotherapy as well as growth regulating lymphokines, cytokines, anti-metastatics and redifferentiating agents. Interferon, which has been the most openly publicized cancer treatment development in history, has proven to be far less than a miracle drug. It has demonstrated some activity in a few low incidence tumors, but no activity in the major killers, as well as significant side effects.

The revolution in biotechnology and the exciting ferment in basic science indicates that at some future time, major new approaches to the drug therapy of cancer should be available. It appears unlikely that this will happen in the 1980s and whether it will occur in the 1990s is a matter of conjecture. This conjecture must balance philosophic optimism in the rapid development of scientific progress with the historic reality that conceptual breakthroughs in the laboratory either do not translate into practical clinical reality or take longer to translate than most of enthusiasts are willing to admit. What is often ignored in the pump priming oncopolitical excitement, and publicity generated about new basic science understandings, are the problems and time-frames involved in the targeted processes of developmental therapeutics and drug development.

With this background, it is highly likely that cytotoxic drug treatment will stay a part of the established therapeutic armamentarium for the remainder of the twentieth century. Hopefully, with the discovery of new chemotypes, improved analogs, more specific targeting approaches and increased mechanistic understanding, the therapeutic index of cytotoxics will be significantly improved and its spectrum of activity broadened.

It is the purpose of this review to evaluate the current status of cytotoxic chemotherapy within the framework of our increased understanding about the various aspects of both biologic and therapeutic heterogeneity.

Observational reality

Cancer chemotherapy is a heterogeneous modality with heterogeneous effects against a heterogeneous group of diseases. Cancer is a multitude of different diseases. Cancer of the lung differs from cancer of the breast in terms of clinical presentation, pattern of spread, response to therapeutic modalities and relapse patterns after therapeutic failure. Within a given organ of origin, malignant disease will have histologic heterogeneity as well as biologic heterogeneity. The biologic heterogeneity will relate factors such as invasiveness, metastatic potential, immunogenity and antigenicity. Cytotoxic drug treatment involves a wide range of different chemical compounds each with its own unique spectrum of activity. A given drug will be active against some tumors and inactive against others. For the majority of the drugs, the unresponsive tumors far outweigh the responsive ones. Within a given tumor deemed responsive to a specific drug, response is both heterogeneous and unpredictable. For reasons not completely understood, some patients will respond while others with apparently similar tumor burdens will demonstrate progressive disease while under therapy. A personalized perspective of the role of chemotherapy in various major diseases is given in Table 1.

Why does chemotherapy fail

The cause of cytotoxic chemotherapy's failure to eradicate all the neoplastic cells, in the manifold situations where it fails to do so, is the overgrowth of resistant cells. The concept of resistance is a broad one which encompasses within it a great heterogeneity of mechanistic explanations. Most of these explanations have called forth a range of therapeutic strategies designed to overcome the problem. Some of the newer explanations are still highly investigational and experimental and so no therapeutic strategies have, as yet, been devised. Table 2 outlines the broad mecha-

R. H. Goldfarb (ed.), Fundamental aspects of cancer.
© 1989, Kluwer Academic Publishers, Dordrecht. ISBN 978-94-010-6980-9

Table 1. A personalized perspective of the role of chemotherapy.

Tumor	Clinical role of chemotherapy	Comments
Breast		
	A. Advanced Disease: Palliative treatment with combination chemotherapy in women with aggressive visceral dominant disease or in whom endocrine therapy is no longer reasonable choice	Complete responses seen in 10–20% with overall response in 50–70%
	B. Primary Disease: Adjuvant chemotherapy prolongs disease-free and overall survival in subsets of premenopausal women with positive axillary nodes. No survival benefit in postmenopausal women with positive axillary nodes. Unproven in women with negative axillary nodes	Major impact on overall survival seen in premenopausal women with 1 to 3 nodes. In other subsets, some delay in relapse observed
Lung 1. Small Cell Anaplastic or Oat-Cell	A. Limited Disease: Mainly palliative with some long-term disease-free survival in those who achieve remission either after combination chemotherapy plus irradiation or drug alone	Two-year disease-free survival seen in about 20% of patients. Occasional long-term survival seen
	B. Extensive Disease: Palliative treatment with combination chemotherapy	Complete responses in 20–30% but only a small percentage disease-free at 2 yrs.
2. Squamous Cell, Adeno-carcinoma, and Large Cell	A. Advanced Disease: True palliation not established with chemotherapy despite response rates in the 30% range with combinations	Partial response rates in 30–40% range with combinations.
	B. Primary Disease: No proven value for any adjuvant chemotherapy	–
Gastro-intestinal cancer 1. Colo-Rectal 2. Pancreas 3. Stomach 4. Esophagus	A. Advanced Disease: True palliation not established. No evidence that chemotherapy prolongs survival	Response rates in bowel and pancreas in 10–25% range with no survival gain. Response rates higher in gastric cancer
	B. Primary Disease: Several positive studies for methyl CCNU plus 5-Fu combination	Rectal cancer studies appear to be more positive
Ovarian cancer	A. Advanced Disease: Mainly palliation but some long-term disease-free survival in patients achieving pathologic complete remission after combination chemotherapy	Pathologic CR seen in about 30% of women treated with minimal residual disease. Some will have long-term survival
	B. Primary Disease: No proven value for adjuvant chemotherapy	–
Gynecologic cancer 1. Uterine Cervix 2. Endometrium	A. Advanced Disease: While responses occasionally seen, true palliation not established	Response rates in 20–30% range but complete responses rare
	B. Primary Disease: No proven value for adjuvant chemotherapy	–
Testicular cancer	A. Advanced Disease: High curative potential with achievement of complete remission	Complete responses in about 70%. Surgery in those with PR can convert some to CR

Table 1. cont..

Tumor	Clinical role of chemotherapy	Comments
	B. Primary Disease: Overall survival advantage for adjuvant chemotherapy versus using treatment at time of relapse not established	Major U.S. national study should soon resolve issue
Genitourinary cancer 1. Prostate 2. Bladder 3. Kidney	A. Advanced Disease: While responses occasionally seen, true palliation not established B. Primary Disease: No proven value for adjuvant chemotherapy	In prostate cancer, objective responses uncommon but also difficult to evaluate. If stability accepted, response rates are in 50% range but no survival impact shown
Head and neck cancer	A. Advanced Disease: While responses occasionally seen, true palliation not established B. Primary Disease: No proven value for adjuvant chemotherapy. Preliminary encouraging evidence for induction, or neo-adjuvant drug treatment but role not yet established	Response rate in 30% range but CR uncommon High response rates now reported for induction drug treatment. Data not available on long-term survival from randomized studies
Malignant melanomas	A. Advanced Disease: No palliation established B. Primary Disease: No proven value for adjuvant chemotherapy	Partial responses in 20% range –
Soft tissue and bone sarcomas	A. Advanced Disease: Some slight palliation achieved in those who obtain complete remission B. Primary Disease: No proven value for adjuvant chemotherapy	Response rates in 40–50% range with occasional CR Both positive and negative studies currently exist
Osteogenic sarcoma	A. Advanced Disease: Some palliation achieved for those who obtain complete remission B. Primary Disease 1) Induction, or preoperative drug treatment allows limb salvage 2) Role of adjuvant chemotherapy controversial	Significant benefit observed when surgical removal of pulmonary metastases is combined with chemotherapy Limb salvage approaches with pre- and postoperative drug appear to achieve excellent local control. Whether adjuvant chemotherapy has increased, the long-term cure rate is still open to controversy

Table 1. cont..

Tumor	Clinical role of chemotherapy	Comments
Hodgkin's disease	A. Stage 3 and 4 Disease 1) High curative potential 2) Occasional salvage potential and palliation for second line treatment	There now exist several curative combinations which are not cross-resistant. The sequential use of these combinations may give even higher initial cure rates. Whether this compromises secondary salvage, and what impact this has on overall cure, has not been fully determined
	B. Stage 1 and 2 Disease Adjuvant chemotherapy after radiation does not give a higher overall survival than salvage chemotherapy in those relapsing after radiation alone	More aggressive chemotherapy in classic adjuvant approach is unlikely to be successful
Non-Hodgkin's lymphoma	A. Stages 3 and 4 Disease 1) High curative potential for diffuse lymphomas 2) Palliation achieved for nodular lymphomas	Diffuse lymphoma literature dominated by uncontrolled highly aggressive combination regimens from major cancer centers with increasing long-term disease-free survival rates. In nodular lymphomas, more aggressive approaches do not appear to be successful
	B. Stage 1 – 2: Adjuvant chemotherapy of no proven value	
Acute lymphocytic leukemia	A. Primary Treatment: High curative potential in children	Drug treatment so successful that major focus is on isolating prognostic subsets for poorer survival who can be treated more aggressively
	B. Secondary Treatment: Occasional salvage obtained but mainly palliation	
Acute myelogenous leukemia	A. Primary treatment: Occasional cure obtained but mainly palliation in those achieving complete remission	High dose chemotherapy plus total body irradiation supported by bone marrow transplantation for patients in drug induced remission appears to give a reasonable cure potential. The proof of this in randomized trials has been difficult to demonstrate so far
	B. Secondary Treatment: Only palliation for those achieving complete remission	

Table 1. cont..

Tumor	Clinical role of chemotherapy	Comments
Chronic leukemias 1. CML 2. CLL	A. Palliation achieved for those who respond	Whether highly aggressive treatments can meaningfully perturb the natural history of those initially indolent diseases remains to be determined
Multiple myeloma	A. Palliation achieved for those who respond	Plateau in what highly aggressive drug treatment can achieve
Childhood solid tumors 1. Rhabdomyo-sarcoma 2. Ewing's sarcoma 3. Wilms' tumor	A. Advanced Disease: Palliation for those responding B. Primary Disease: Increased cure rate with adjuvant chemotherapy	Currently in a plateau phase awaiting the discovery of new active drugs

Table 2. Concepts of resistance and clinical strategies designed to overcome them.

Concept of resistance	Strategies designed to combat	Comment
Kinetic – Postulates that drugs not actively moving within the cell cycle (Go Cell) are the most resistant	1. Cytoreduction – Small residual tumor cell masses will be kinetically more sensitive	1. Positive uncontrolled data exist to support approach in ovarian cancer
	2. Adjuvant chemotherapy – Microscopic metastatic disease after removal of primary local and regional disease will be kinetically more sensitive	2. Generally a disappointment to date. Positive data only in some pediatric solid tumors and possibly in premenopausal breast cancer and large bowel cancer
	3. Sequential combination chemotherapy – Cytoreduction achieved with drug active against Go cells (alkylating agent or nitrosourea) and then followed by cell cycle specific anti-metabolite (ARA-C, hydroxyurea, methotrexate)	3. No successful example ever demonstrated
	4. Synchronization – Pile tumor cells up in a sensitive phase of cell cycle	4. Never shown to work
Pharmacologic – Assumes that a critical concentration over time of the active moiety of drug is not achieved at the tumor cell level 1. Pharmacologic sanctuaries	(A) Sanctuary therapy with drugs placed directly into the sanctuary, e.g., intrathecal drug administration	1A) Intrathecal methotrexate and ARA-C have proven successful in both the treatment and prophylaxis of CNS leukemia
2. Inadequate blood supply to tumor cells (*hypoxia*)	B) Drugs designed to penetrate the sanctuary, e.g., nitrosoureas for blood-brain barrier	B) Nitrosoureas are most active drugs in brain tumors but are still only weakly active. No drugs effective against solid tumor brain metastases

Table 2. Cont.

Concept of resistance	Strategies designed to combat	Comment
	2A) Regional drug delivery to achieve higher concentration – Intra-arterial or intraperitoneal delivery	2A) Case selection bias was high in pilot studies. Never demonstrated effective in randomized studies with drugs utilized to date
	B) Drugs designed to passively diffuse into hypoxic areas and become activated	B) Still investigational
3. Transport resistance – Resistance is caused by rapid efflux of drug out of the tumor cell as seen with anthracyclines and vinca alkaloids in some *in vitro* systems	3. Modulation of efflux through the use of drugs such as the calcium channel blocker verapamil	3. Clinical trials underway but preliminary data with adriamycin + verapamil not encouraging
Biochemical – Assumes that a specific biochemical target is the critical mechanism of action and that some change in target, or drug access to target, is cause of resistance	1. "Rational" drug design to more specifically attack the target	1A) While 5-fluorouracil was a rationally designed drug, analogs with greater rational support have failed to improve the therapeutic index
		B) More rationally designed thiopurines and anti-foles have failed to improve upon parent structures despite elegant experimental rationales
	2. Sequential combination use of anti-metabolites	2. Has never been shown to be superior to empiric drug combinations
	3. Biochemical modulation – Use of a noncytotoxic modulator of an anti-metabolite to increase its effectiveness (example: 5-Fu + thymidine)	3. Has never been shown to be superior to single agent alone in a controlled trial
Genetic – 1. Hypothesis that tumor cells spontaneously mutate to become resistant (by whatever mechanism) to drugs they have never been exposed to (Goldie-Coldman)	1A) Neo-adjuvant or induction therapy which involves giving drugs prior to surgery to improve local control and attack tumor cells earlier	1A) Preliminary data in head and neck cancer encouraging but not proven in controlled trials. In osteosarcoma can achieve local control with limb salvage but impact on cure rate not proven
	B) Sequential use of non crossresistant combinations	B) Data in Hodgkin's Disease with MOPPABVD is positive. Data in breast cancer and small cell lung cancer negative so far

Table 2. Cont.

Concept of resistance	Strategies designed to combat	Comment
2. Pleiotropic drug resistance occurs because of gene amplification or other genetic changes	2. None as yet	2. Still in basic science stage

Table 3. Potential approaches to overcome plateau of cancer chemotherapy.

Short term approach	Strategy
Discovery of new chemotypes	1. Utilize a mixture of human tumor cells *in vitro* and heterotransplantation systems *in vivo* to achieve superior prediction
	2. Switch clincial trial emphasis to phase 2 studies in major solid tumors where combination chemotherapy has achieved minimal to no success in improving survival
Discover improved analogs of existing chemotypes	1. Improve screening techniques as mentioned above
	2. Utilize cell culture systems designed to overcome different mechanisms of resistance
Improve drug delivery to achieve greater specificity	1. Link drugs with monoclonal antibodies to tumor related antigens

Long term approach	Strategy
Selective treatment to overcome resistance	*1. Test individual patients for specific mechanisms of resistance and tailor therapy to award or overcome the problem*
	2. Specific treatments to block or overcome resistance
Ancillary biologic therapy	*1. Utilization of adjuvant therapies to improve efficacy or diminish side effects*
	2. Therapies designed to optimize cell kill potential

nisms of postulated resistance and some of the strategies devised to combat them.

A major problem with most of these concepts and strategies is that we are unable to routinely measure or evaluate what is happening at the tumor cell level in deep seated metastatic lesions. Therefore, it is not possible to know what the kinetics of the tumor cells are, what concentration of the drug active moiety is being achieved or what type of biochemical heterogeneity may exist. Because of this, most of therapeutic strategies can only be empirically extrapolated from the experimental *in vitro* and *in vivo* studies which support their rationale.

Reality is probably some amalgamation of the various concepts of resistance outlined in Table 2. Almost surely, for any given malignancy in an individual patient, there are combined factors of pharmacologic inability to deliver optimal amounts of drug, kinetic, biochemical and transport factors, which lead to some, or most, tumor cells not being killed. The strategies designed to overcome resistance all seem to naively view the problem as a unifactorial one, ignoring all the other aspects. When this bypassing of probable multifactorial reality is combined with the empiricism required by our inability to routinely study deep-seated human malignancy, then the failure of the approaches undertaken so far are easier to comprehend.

How can we get off the plateau on which cancer chemotherapy is currently sitting? In the short term, this can be accomplished in several ways (Table 3). The first is by discovering new active chemotypes. With the discovery of each new active chemotype in the past, the therapeutic index of one or more tumor types has been improved. The current plateau exists mainly because of the failure to find new active chemotypes in recent years. It is unreasonable to assume that all the active cytotoxic chemotypes have already been discovered. It is more likely that the currently used predictive systems are finding compounds which cannot overcome the more difficult hurdles of today's clinical testing realities. In the past, a new drug could be tested in fresh cases of the most responsive tumor types. Today, a new drug can be evaluated in the lymphomas, leukemias, or testicular cancer only after extensive prior aggressive combination chemotherapy. Only the classically insensitive solid tumors remain to be utilized for phase 2 studies without prior exposure to some "standard" cytotoxic regimen. What will be required is the utilization of predictive systems which are closer to the human tumor reality than rodent transplantable ascitic leukemias used previously. Current approaches include the use of panels of human tumor cells grown in culture combined with *in vivo* testing of the same cell lines in heterotransplantation systems in order to achieve some semblance of pharmacologic reality in the prediction process.

Targeting drugs more specifically utilizing the drug delivery system of monoclonal antibodies is a highly attractive hypothesis which will be technically demanding in its application. The major conceptual hurdle to overcome will be the inability, to date, of finding any tumor specific antigens. Utilizing tumor associated antigens requires a strategy which will assume that some tumor cells will be "immunologically resistant" to targeting. It also assumes that some normal cells will be hit as well. This is one reason that favors established cytotoxic moieties for targeting which have some demonstrated selectivity over non-selective potent poisons.

A second hurdle will involve the number of cytotoxic molecules which can be linked to an antibody and a third hurdle involves the development of linkage which will be stable until the tumor cell is reached but then allow cell killing to occur. This could occur either through release at the tumor cell or incorporation of the complex into the cell through the mechanism of antigenic modulation.

In summary, the biologic heterogeneity of neoplastic disease is reflected in the heterogeneity of cancer chemotherapy's effectiveness. Within given diseases, cytotoxic drugs can cure, palliate or have no effect in varying proportions of patients. The major problem is the outgrowth of resistant cells with the mechanisms of resistance also reflecting biologic heterogeneity. While cancer chemotherapy is currently in a plateau, there is still reason for optimism about its future in improving the care of cancer patients.

REFERENCES

1. Carter SK, Bakowski M, Hellmann K: Chemotherapy of Cancer, 2nd edition. John Wiley and Sons, NY, 1981
2. Carter SK, Livingston RG, Glatstein E: *Principles of Cancer Treatment.* McGraw-Hill, NY, 1982
3. De Vita VT, Hellman S, Rosenberg SA: *Cancer Principles and Practice of Oncology*, 2nd edition. J.B. Lippincott Co., Philadelphia, 1985
4. Carter SK: Some Thoughts on Resistance to Cancer Chemotherapy *Cancer Treatment Reviews* 11:3–7, 1984
5. Skipper HE, Simpson-Herren L: Relationship between Tumor Stem Cell Heterogeneity and Resistance to Chemotherapy. In: De Vita VT, Hellman S, Rosenberg SA: *Important Advances in Oncology*, 1985. J.B. Lippincott, Philadelphia, pp. 63–78 1985
6. Chabner BA, Fine RL, Allegra CJ et al: Cancer Chemotherapy Progress and Expectations, 1984. *Cancer* 54:2599–2608, 1984
7. Fidler IJ: Recent Concepts of Cancer Metastasis and Their Implications for Therapy. *Cancer Treat Rep* 68:193–198, 1984
8. McGuire WL (Moderator), Goldie JH, Salmon SE, Ling V: Strategies to Identify or Prevent Drug Resistance in Cancer – A Panel Discussion. *Breast Cancer Res and Treatment* 5:257–268, 1985

THE ATTRACTION OF WANDERING METASTATIC CELLS

JAMES VARANI, J. PHILIP McCOY and PETER A. WARD

INTRODUCTION

The cascade of events leading to the formation of metastases from primary tumors is a complex and incompletely understood phenomenon. The current concept envisions the initial invasion of local tissue and separation of individual cells or small groups of cells from the primary tumor. The invading cells gain access to the blood vascular and/or lymphatic circulatory systems and are distributed throughout the body. Most of the cells which enter the circulation, however, are rapidly killed. Only a few go on to establish themselves at secondary sites and carry on the processes that lead to the formation of metastatic growths. These processes include attachment to the appropriate structures (i.e., either the vascular endothelial cells or the sub-endothelial basement membranes), invasion of these structures and ultimately, proliferation. The process of tumor cell invasion through the endothelial layer and the sub-endothelial cell basement membrane most likely involves both active cell motility and substrate degradation.

While each of the steps in the metastatic cascade is critical, one of the most intriguing is the manner in which the localization of circulating tumor cells at secondary sites occurs. Although we have known for decades that factors such as adherence, motility and the release of hydrolytic enzymes are involved in secondary localization, much of our current understanding of this process is the result of the classic study by Fidler (13) showing that the B16 murine melanoma is composed of heterogeneous subpopulations. As a result of this study and subsequent work by a large number of investigators, it has become apparent that most tumors are heterogeneous and that subpopulations of cells within these tumors differ in many of the features that are critical to the process of metastasis. Thus, it is possible to isolate from a parent tumor, subpopulations which differ in specific characteristics and then to compare these populations with regard to metastatic capability. In this chapter, we will focus on one property (i.e., adhesiveness) which we feel is central to the entire process of secondary localization. Evidence will be presented which suggests that differences in adhesiveness among populations of tumor cells correlates directly with differences in secondary localization. The possible mechanisms of adhesiveness will be examined along with events which may occur as a consequence of adhesion of tumor cells. Finally, evidence will be presented which suggests that the adhesiveness of tumor cells is not an intrinsic and unalterable property but rather is subject to modulation.

Secondary localization

Mechanical entrapment. Tumor cells travel to sites of secondary localization suspended in the fluid environment of the hematogenous or lymphatic circulation. The exact mechanism by which these cells arrest and establish secondary growths remains unclear although numerous theories exist to explain this phenomenon. Perhaps the simplest concept to explain arrest of circulating tumor cells is the mechanist or hemodynamic theory of metastasis, in which the simple mechanical lodging of tumor cells in the microcirculation determines the site of secondary tumor formation. While not conclusive, there does exist considerable evidence to suggest that mechanical entrapment plays a role in secondary localization. The main arguments favoring this hypothesis come from studies using animal models in which tumor cells were injected intravenously and found to lodge in the first organ bed encountered (54, 8). Additionally, Sugarbaker and coworkers (64) have observed that, in general, the most frequent metastases occur in the first organ which would be encountered by cells shed from the primary tumor.

If, in fact, mechanic entrapment does play a role in the secondary localization process, there must be some physical features which allow certain tumor cells to be "selected" to form secondary tumors. There are at least two characteristics which could easily be envisioned as playing a role in this process; cell size and rigidity. Although there is no direct evidence indicating a relationship between increased cell size and enhanced metastatic capability, studies have indicated an association between the presence of cell clumps and the formation of metastases (82, 13, 37). It is unclear, however, if size *per se* is the dominant factor in enhancing metastasis or if other factors, such as protective effects of clumping, are dominant. Increased cell rigidity, on the other hand, has been shown to correlate with increased colonization of the first organ through which the cells circulated (57), although this may actually result in decreased secondary metastases. Similarly, disruption of the cytoskeleton of tumor cells with agents such as cytochalasin B, which makes the cells less rigid, inhibits the localization of the cells in the first organ bed encountered and leads to a more disseminated pattern of metastasis (24, 22). In spite of the evidence supporting it, the majority of studies suggest that the mechanistic theory is, by itself, insufficient to explain the various patterns of metastasis observed. Included among these are the study of Weiss et al. (84) dealing with hemodynamic considerations of human material and those by several other groups which

R. H. Goldfarb (ed.), Fundamental aspects of cancer.

show organ-specific metastasis in animal models regardless of the route of inoculation of tumor cells (3). Furthermore, experimental models have shown that, while tumor cells may lodge in the first organ bed encoutered, they do not necessarily remain there (14). It is likely therefore that mechanical lodging by itself does not determine the pattern of metastasis, but this does not exclude mechanical entrapment from being one of a number of factors involved in secondary localization.

Coagulation factors. Evidence has accumulated over the past several decades suggesting a role for coagulation factors in the development of metastases. Of particular interest is the data implying that blood platelets may play a role in the secondary localization of hematogenously spread tumor cells. The data supporting a role for platelet involvement in the localization of circulating tumor cells include the fact that tumor cells induce aggregation of platelets both *in vitro* and *in vivo* (17, 30, 33, 80), the fact that the process of tumor metastasis is accompanied by the induction of thrombocytopenia (17) and the fact that anti-coagulant therapy and anti-platelet aggregation therapy have a profound effect on the development of metastasis – at least in experimental animals (18, 29). In a simplified context, one could postulate that tumor cells form secondary loci as a result of becoming entrapped due to platelet aggregation around the circulating cells. The lodged cells could then attach to the vessel wall and subsequently invade surrounding tissue. This concept is supported by the histological findings of tumor cells surrounded by activated platelets in lung capillaries shortly after intravenous injection of the lung metastasizing tumor cells (28).

The possibility that platelet-tumor cell aggregates are involved in the arrest of circulating tumor cells raises several interesting questions. Among these is the nature of the tumor cell-platelet interaction. It could be argued that with regard to the tumor cells, the process is entirely passive. That is, that the tumor cells serve only as an appropriate foreign surface and that the very active aggregation mechanism in platelets is solely responsible for the formation of the platelet-tumor cell clumps. The ability of agents which inhibit platelet aggregation to also block the formation of tumor metastases is at least consistent with this hypothesis (29). However, as will be described below, there is evidence that these same treatments which have a direct, anti-aggregatory effect on platelets may also be inhibitory to active tumor cell adherence mechanisms as well. Thus it cannot be ruled out that the tumor cells themselves are active participants in the aggregation process. In fact, there is evidence that tumor cells may be active participants. Hara et al. (23) have described a membrane-bound factor on murine tumor cells that induces aggregation of platelets with the tumor cells. Whether a similar mechanism exists in other types of tumor cells activating platelets remains to be determined. In any event, this is one example of a direct active involvement of the tumor cells in a process which leads to the attachment of the tumor cells to elements of the host. Indeed, whether the host target is a circulating cell such as the platelet or whether the appropriate host target is a structure of the vascular bed such as the endothelial cells or exposed basement membrane, there is now considerable evidence to suggest that the attachment of the circulating tumor cell to the structures is

an active process and that the interaction is mediated by specific adherence molecules. Some of this evidence is described in the following section.

Attachment factors. One aspect of metastasis research which has been vigorously studied in recent years is the role that specific attachment factors may play in tumor cell arrest. Whether the circulating cells attach initially to the vascular endothelium and cause retraction of these cells of whether they attach directly to exposed basement membrane, they ultimately must come into contact with and traverse the matrix material of the basement membranes in order to enter the extravascular space (35). It is known that attachment of cells (both normal and neoplastic) is mediated through specific attachment factors. Fibronectin is one of the best known and several good reviews have been written on this subject (see, for example (51)). However, this is not the only known factor which can specifically mediate cell attachment. Other factors which have been described include laminin, chondronectin and the heparan sulfate proteoglycan (34). Among these recently described factors, laminin may be the most interesting with regard to tumor metastasis. This is a high molecular weight glycoprotein which was originally purified from the EHS sarcoma (69). Some of the characterisitics of laminin are summarized in Table 1. Laminin is a normal component of basement membranes and has a high affinity for Type IV collagen (2, 16). Studies by Terranova et al. (66) have shown that laminin is involved in the attachment of epithelial cells to their basement membranes. Recent studies by Murray et al. (43) showed that tumor cells, as well, could attach to Type IV collagen. What makes this interesting is the fact that there

Table 1. Properties of murine laminin.

Structural characteristics:
    MW = 850, 000 – 1, 000, 000 D (11, 68)
    subunits: α – 3 per molecule, MW = 200, 000 D (55)
    β – 1 per molecule, MW = 400, 000 D (55)
    joined by disulfide bonds (69) cross-shaped configuration with globular end regions (11)

Biochemical characteristics:
    Contains terminal α-d-galactopyranosyl groups (55)
    Removal of globular end regions destroys attachment function (55)
    lacks 3- and 4-hydroxyproline (69, 68).
    β subunit digested by alpha thrombin (55)

Binding substrates:
    Type IV collagen (66)
    entactin (5)

Distribution:
    Basement membranes (69)
    Low concentrations ($< 1\mu g/ml$) in serum (34)
    Surface of high metastatic fibrosarcoma cells (75)
    Surface of rat kidney (26)

Biological function:
    Attachment of various cell types to basement membranes (65, 66, 75)
    Contributes to structural integrity of basement membranes (69)

was a good correlation between the metastatic level of a given cell population and the ability of the cells to attach to Type IV collagen. Subsequent studies provided strong evidence that, like the epithelial cells, tumor cell attachment to the type IV collagen was also mediated by laminin (65). This evidence includes the fact that exogenous laminin stimulated attachment to the collagen substrate and that antibodies to laminin inhibited attachment. Furthermore the same treatment that reduced cell attachment to the Type IV collagen substrate also reduced metastasis formation by the high metastatic tumor cells. Based on these results it could be postulated that circulating tumor cells become localized at secondary sites *in vivo* as a result of their ability to bind to the collagenous material of the basement membranes. This binding is mediated (at least in part) by laminin, and tumor cells which utilize laminin may have a selective advantage in forming metastasis.

Recent studies in our own laboratory (75) have extended this interesting theory. Our studies involved a number of high and low malignant fibrosarcoma cell lines which had previously been isolated in our laboratory and characterized with regard to several properties (76, 77, 73). Following the observations of Murray et al. (43) we compared the high and low malignant fibrosarcoma cells for attachment to type IV collagen. As would be expected, the high malignant cells attached to the type IV collagen substrate faster and to a greater extent than the low malignant cells. When the collagen was pretreated with laminin, the attachment of the low malignant cells was increased. In contrast, however, the addition of exogenous laminin had no dramatic effects on the attachment of the high malignant cells. Although the results were quite variable from experiment to experiment, we observed that in some cases, the addition of exogenous laminin actually inhibited the attachment of the high malignant cells.

In experiments conducted simultaneously with the collagen-binding studies (and thought at the time to be unrelated) we observed that the high malignant cells bound fluorescein-labeled *Griffonia simplicifolia* isolectin B_4 (GS I-B_4) while the low malignant cells did not. This lectin is specific for terminal α-d-galactopyranosyl groups (42) and the difference in lectin binding between the high and low malignant fibrosarcoma cells demonstrates a dissimilarity in their surface carbohydrate pattern. That this difference in carbohydrate pattern could be related to differences between the cells in their expression of laminin was suggested by the finding that murine laminin contains terminal α-d-galactopyranosyl groups as part of its carbohydrate structure (58). In light of these findings immunochemical studies were carried out to determine if, in fact, there were a dissimilarity between the high and low malignant cells in their expression of laminin. These studies showed that the high malignant fibrosarcoma cells, but not the low malignant cells, express a moiety on their surface (75, 41) which immunologically cross reacts with murine laminin. It has yet to be conclusively determined whether this factor is whole intact laminin, a fragment of laminin, or a closely related molecule. Regardless, the results of these studies show that the high malignant fibrosarcoma cells express a factor which has immunochemical and biochemical similarities with laminin. The low malignant cells do not. The factor expressed by the high malignant cells may function in a manner similar to laminin since

the cells possessing it attach readily to type IV collagen in the absence of exogenous laminin. The cells not expressing this substance, on the other hand, do not readily attach to type IV collagen in the absence of exogenous laminin but do attach if exogenous laminin is added. To extend the theory originally put forward as a result of the work by Terranova et al. (65), it is possible that in addition to utilizing exogenous laminin, the expression of endogenous laminin (or substance with laminin-like characteristics) may facilitate tumor cell attachment to type IV collagen and ultimately, the secondary localization process.

The difference in laminin expression by the high and low malignant cells is interesting in light of the methods originally used to select these populations. The high malignant cells were originally selected from metastases which developed in the lungs of mice from primary subcutaneous tumors (77). The low malignant cells were selected by adapting the unselected parent cells for survival and growth in medium containing pooled normal human serum (76). Human blood group B antigen is defined by its carbohydrate structure which contains terminal α-d-galactopyranosyl groups (83) and since the blood group specific antibodies are directed toward the carbohydrate part of the molecule (32) it seemed reasonable to postulate that the anti-blood group B antibodies in the pooled human serum eliminated (by complement-dependent killing) those cells with α-d-galactopyranosyl end groups on their surface. To test this, we obtained commercially-prepared hyperimmune blood typing sera and compared them for cytotoxicity against the high and low malignant cells in the presence of complement (41). A summary of the results obtained in this study are seen in Figure 1. It can be seen that the low malignant cells were resistant to the cytotoxic activity of all of the sera. On the other hand, the high malignant cells (i.e., those cells expressing terminal α-d-galactopyranosyl groups as determined by lectin binding) were sensitive to sera with anti-B or anti-A, B activity but were not sensitive to the anti-A sera. These results strongly suggest that the elimination of those cells expressing the α-d-galactopyranosyl groups gave rise to the population of cells with reduced capacity for tumorigenicity and metastasis formation. If, as we suspect, it was the elimination of those cells expressing laminin which was effected by the human serum, then it implies that the original population was a mixture of laminin-positive and negative cells and that it was those cells expressing laminin which were the most malignant within the population. Whether these findings are unique to this particular tumor model or are, in fact, of general significance remains to be determined. It is reasonable to suspect that not all tumors (indeed even all methylcholanthrene-induced murine tumors) will use the same mechanisms of attachment. Rather, we will probably find a number of attachment factors and mechanisms used by circulating tumor cells to attach to the capillary wall. What is likely is that in all cases we will find that the cells intrinsically better able to accomplish this task will be more malignant than the cells less able.

EVENTS SUBSEQUENT TO ATTACHMENT

The attachment of circulating tumor cells to the vessel wall is essential to allow them to be removed from the general

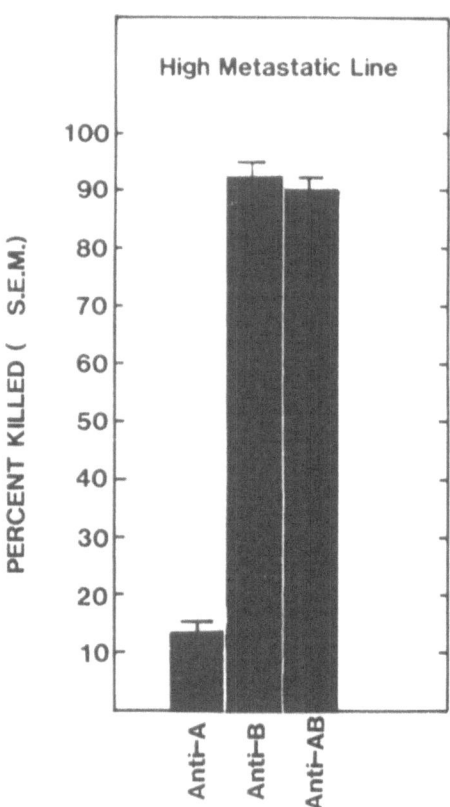

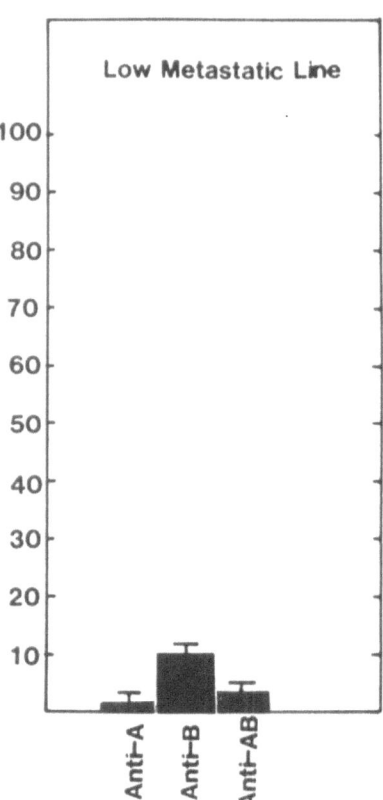

Figure 1. Cytotoxicity of hyperimmune human anti-A, anti-B and anti-A, B sera to high and low metastatic murine fibrosarcoma cells. The cells were incubated with the hyperimmune serum in the presence of rabbit complement. The cells surviving treatment for one hour were enumerated. See: McCoy et al., (41) for complete details.

circulation. Failure to accomplish this will almost certainly result in cell death. Once this occurs and the cells are removed from the circulation, then other processes ensue that lead to the formation of tumors at the secondary site. These processes, which include both invasion and cell proliferation probably require prior cellular attachment for them to occur. First consider invasion. It is generally accepted that both active cell motility (62, 35) and tissue destruction (38, 52) are involved in the invasion process. The mechanisms by which these events occur are attachment-dependent. Cell motility in higher organisms is a continuous process of making and breaking contacts with the substratum as the cell "pulls" itself over the surface (9, 61). Our intention is not to review the molecular basis of this process; rather it is to underscore the fact that motility of cells (both normal and neoplastic) in higher organisms is intrinsically associated with adherence. Numerous experimental studies have validated this relationship (1, 79, 6, 44, 53, 71).

Substrate attachment is also necessary for effective hydrolysis. This may be because the reorganization of the cell as it undergoes attachment allows for enzyme exocytosis (or perhaps activation of latent surface enzymes). On the other hand, hydrolytic enzymes may be released by tumor cells in suspension but under these conditions be quickly swept away and diluted in the fluid milieu or be inactivated by soluble plasma enzyme inhibitors. There is evidence to suggest that both of these mechanisms may be operating. In polymorphonuclear leukocytes, which may be considered the prototypic cell capable of degrading biological substrates, a rapid release of lysozomal enzymes occurs upon stimulation with various factors if the cells are first allowed to adhere to a substratum (27). Enzyme release, however, by the same cells is very inefficient if the cells are stimulated and maintained in suspension. It is primarily for this reason that cytochalasin B is routinely added to leukocyte cultures when chemotactic factor-induced enzyme release in suspension is being monitored (59). In contrast, when macromolecular substances such as zymosan particles and precipitated immune complexes are used as the stimulating agents rather than soluble chemotactic factors, active release of enzymes by cells in suspension occurs (31).

Even if tumor cell proteases are released from cells in suspension, it is likely that they would quickly be diluted and inactivated by the plasma inhibitors which include α_1-antitrypsin, α_2-macroglobulin and a specific plasmin inhibitor, as well as several others. In order to study protein hydrolysis by cells in the presence of inhibitors, a model system has been developed in our laboratory in which radio-labeled protein substrates absorbed onto the surface of a microtiter cell culture dish were used as the substrates (72, 31). In this system, the addition of proteolytic enzymes in solution induced protein hydrolysis with the release of labeled fragments into the supernatant fluids. The simultaneous addition of proteolytic enzyme inhibitors prevented this. When viable leukocytes or tumor cells were added to the microtiter wells, they rapidly attached to the surface and hydrolyzed the protein substrate. However, with the cells in direct contact with substrate, the addition of enzyme inhibitors to the supernatant was much less efficient at inhibiting hydrolysis. To effectively inhibit the cell-induced hydrolysis, the specific inhibitors had to be absorbed onto the surface along with the protein substrate. This suggests that exclusion of the protease inhibitors from the site of hydrolysis by the direct contact of cells and substrate could explain, at least in part, how protein hydrolysis could occur in the presence of high levels of protease inhibitors. Although our studies focused on the proteases, recent studies by Campbell et al., (4) suggested that a similar mechanisms may operate to prevent the inactivation of cell-derived oxygen radicals by their specific inhibitors. Thus, whether or not the attachment of cells to the substrate is necessary for triggering the activation and/or release of hydrolytic enzymes (and other degradative substances), the absence of direct contact would make the process much less efficient.

Finally, cell proliferation must occur in order for the tumor cells which have survived passage through the circulation to actually become clinically evident metastases. That cell proliferation will occur at the colonized site is not a foregone conclusion as evidence by both the clinical and experimental observations regarding the tumor dormant state (15, 63, 10, 74). Is the signal for proliferation related to substrate attachment? It might seem that proliferation is one aspect of behavior not influenced by attachment since the ability to grow in suspension (at least in culture) is one of the properties associated with the transformed state (85). However, even with transformed cells, growth in suspension is often limited to several generations. Among experimental tumor lines arising from solid tumors, the lines which grow as ascites tumors are exceptions. Likewise, during the natural course of malignancy, the development of ascites occurs very late. Thus, it seems reasonable to speculate that *in vivo* proliferation of the tumor cells at secondary site follows from the successful attachment of the cells to an appropriate substratum.

ACTIVATION OF TUMOR CELLS BY CHEMOTACTIC FACTORS

In the preceding sections of this chapter, we focused on the interaction of circulating tumor cells with elements of the hosts vascular system. With the possible exception of purely mechanical entrapment, the adhesive properties of the tumor cells are likely to be critical determinants of this interaction. In this section we will describe findings which suggest that the adhesive properties of tumor cells are not constant, but rather are capable of being modulated by soluble facors. These factors are refered to as chemotactic factors-having been originally defined by their ability to stimulate directional motility in the Boyden chamber assay. Although the concept of chemotaxis implies motility, it should be remembered that these same factors induce other physiological responses in susceptible cells and that the effects on motility may be secondary to some of these.

Early studies by Hayashi and his colleagues (25, 86) and by Romualdez and Ward (56) identified chemotactic respon-

ses in a number of different types of tumor cells. The chemotactic response in these cells was similar to that of the well-characterized polymorphonuclear leukocytes. Because of the apparent similarities, subsequent studies to characterize the chemotactic response in tumor cells have borrowed heavily from the approaches taken by others with leukocytes. A recent, good review of the chemotactic response in leukocytes is available (60). Studies in tumor cell chemotaxis have also been recently reviewed (70). In the present work, we will limit our discussion to the effects of chemotactic factors on the adherence of tumor cells and the implications of this for secondary tumor cell localization.

Effects of Chemotactic Factors on Tumor Cell Adhesiveness. Using a nylon fiber assay described previously by Mac-Gregor, Spagnuolo and Lentnek (39) we demonstrated that chemotactic stimulation of the Walker 256 carcinosarcoma cells would lead to a rapid, transient hyperadherence response (74). In this study two chemotactic factors, i.e., the factors derived from the fifth complement component and the synthetic tripeptide, N-formyl-methionyl leucyl phenyl-alanine, were used. Subsequent studies showed that the tumor promoter, 12-0-tetradecanoyl phorbol acetate would induce a similar response (71). It was also shown that the response could be observed on a variety of substrates which include serum-coated plastic culture dishes and monolayers of bovine corneal endothelial cells. The hyperadherence response in the Walker tumor cells occurred rapidly following stimulation (within 5–15 minutes) and was transient. By two hours after stimulation, the response was over and, in fact, the cells had entered a desensitization phase. Restimulation produced no response during this period. Responsiveness returned gradually over the course of 48–72 hours if the cells were allowed to proliferate during this period (21).

This hyperadherence response observed with the Walker cells is not unique to these cells. We have been able to show that a chemotactically-responsive line of murine fibrosarcoma cells also demonstrates a response in the adherence assay following stimulation (71). In contrast, a line of murine fibrosarcoma cells which were not chemotactically responsive as well as the non-chemotactic normal fibroblasts do not become hyperadherent when stimulated under the same conditions. Recent studies by Magro and his colleagues (40) also suggest that chemotactic factors induce a hyperadherence response. Working with the previously described chemotactic factor obtained during bone breakdown (48, 49), they found a correlation between the amount of chemotactic factor released in organ culture and the number of tumor cells that would adhere to the bone tissue. What makes this finding of interest is the fact that the bone tissue is a highly complex, natural substrate which often is invaded by metastasizing tumor cells.

It should be noted that our emphasis on the adherence response is not meant to imply that other biological responses to chemotactic stimulation are not important. Once cells have become localized, their ability to migrate directionally toward an increasing concentration of a chemoattractant could facilitate their passage through the endothelial cell layer and subendothelial basement membrane into the extravascular space. This has, in fact, been demonstrated nicely in an experimental model by Thorgeirsson et al. (67).

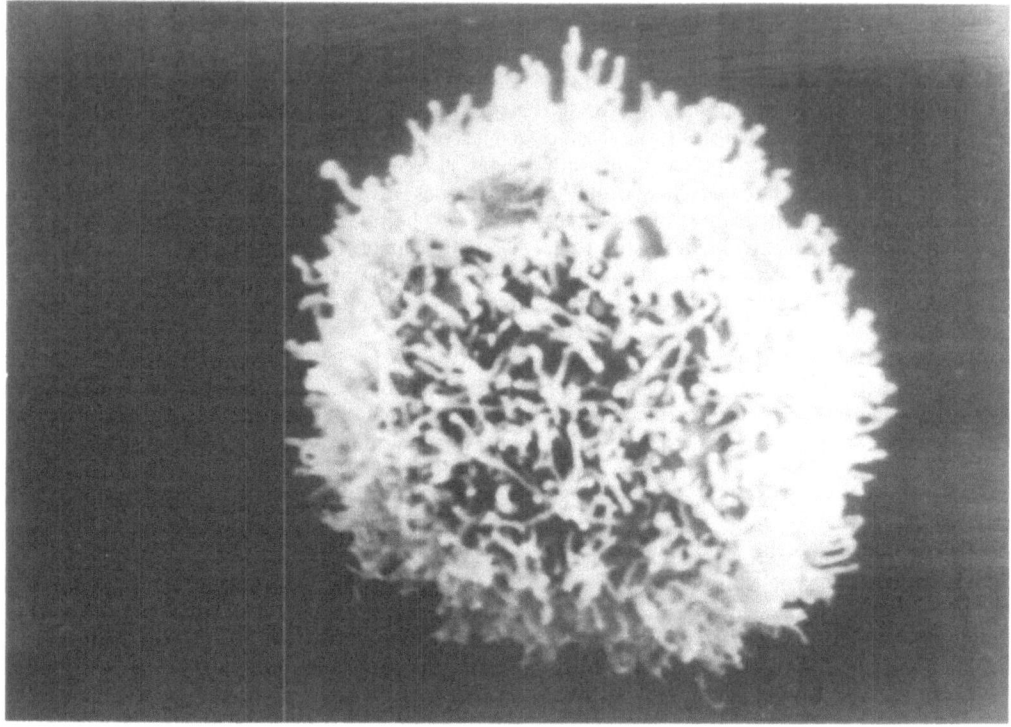

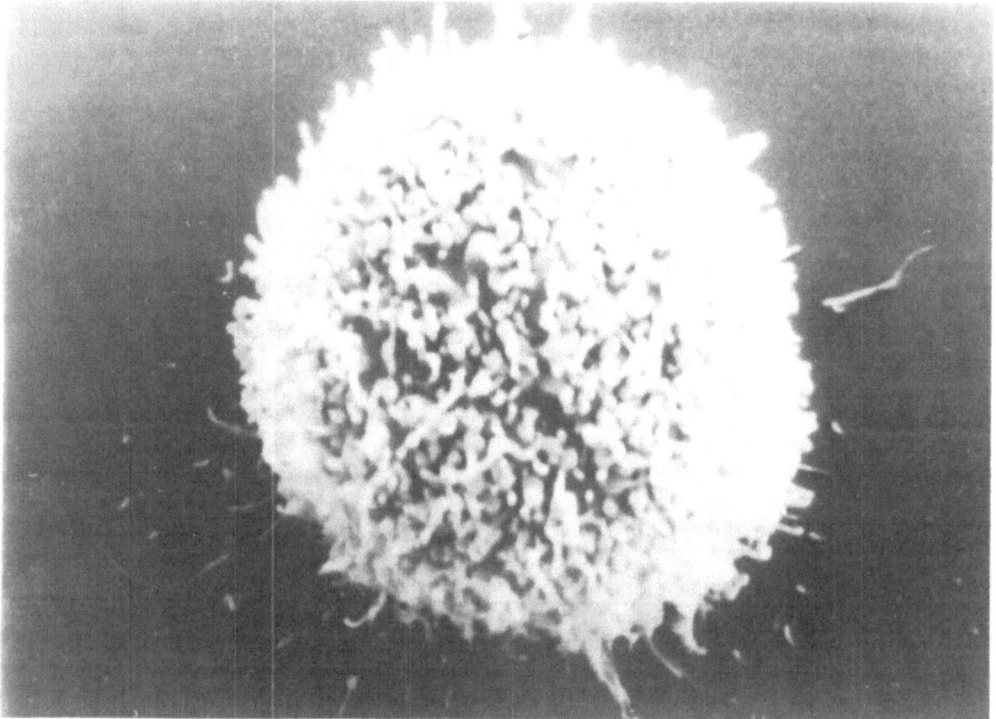

Figure 2. Morphological changes accompanying the stimulated adherence responses in Walker 256 carcinosarcoma cells. The cells in suspension were treated with 12-O-tetradecanoyl phorbol acetate as described earlier (71) and then examined by scanning electron microscopy. a) In suspension the cells are round and covered with a large number of short microvilli. ($\times$ 9800). b) Shortly after stimulation, the cells begin to attach to the substratum which in this case is serum-coated glass through long, slender filopodia ($\times$ 9800). c) The cells

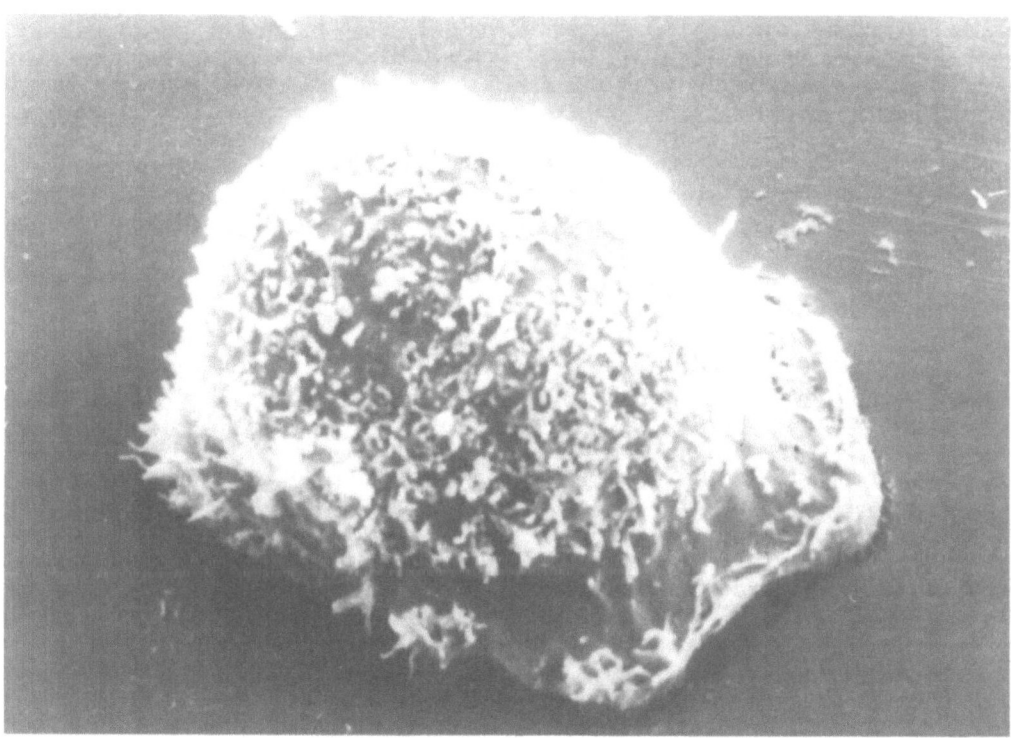

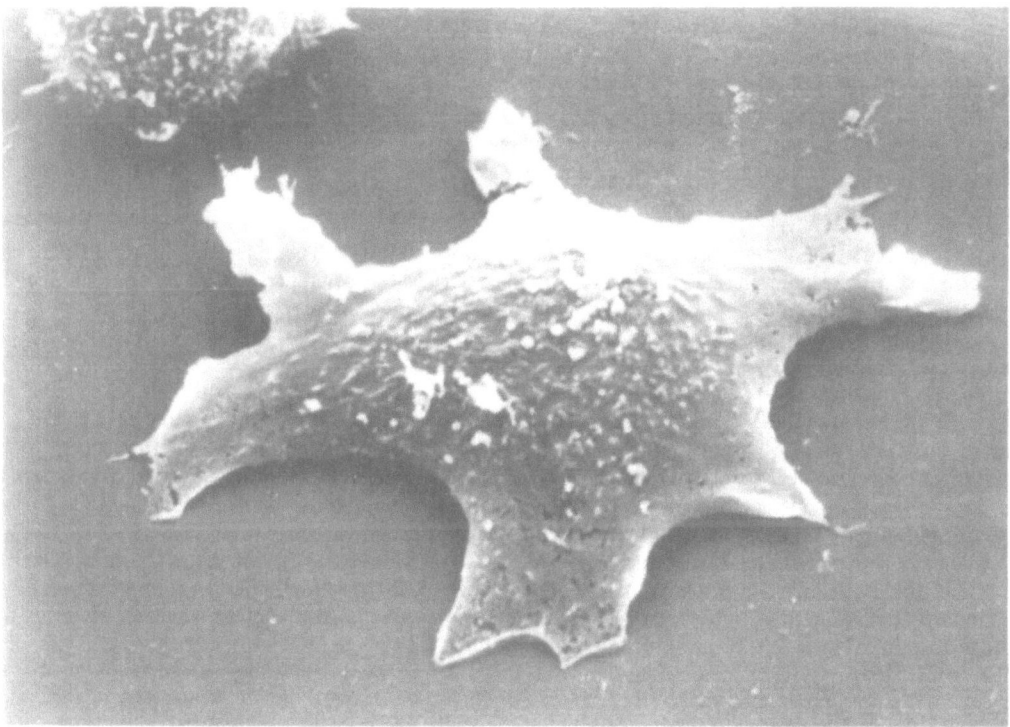

undergo a morphological transformation. The cells become flattened and the microvilli disappear (× 7350). d) The cells are completely flattened at this stage which is approximately 30 minutes after treatment (× 5200). Following this, the cells begin to round up and eventually detach from the substratum. By two hours after stimulation, nearly all of the cells are again in suspension.

They showed that a chemotactically-responsive line of reticulum sarcoma cells would invade through the collagenous stroma prepared from human amnion when placed on the stromal surface. Although invasion occurred in the absence of chemotactic stimulation, invasion was greatly increased when a chemotactic factor was added to the distal side of the membrane.

Since invasion involves tissue breakdown as well as cell migration, it would be very worthwhile to determine if stimulated tumor cells produce and/or release hydrolytic enzymes which facilitate the tissue breakdown. There is no conclusive evidence to support this, however. Studies in our laboratory with the Walker carcinosarcoma cells demonstrated only a very slight increase in the release of hemoglobin-hydrolyzing enzymes into the supernatant fluid following stimulation (47). Likewise, Thorgeirsson et al. (67) observed no change in the secretion of collagenolytic enzyme from reticulm sarcoma cells by stimulation with a chemotactic factor. Although only a limited amount of data is available, these results suggest that unlike polymorphonuclear leukocytes, enzyme release is not one of the major consequences of chemotactic stimulation in tumor cells. Perhaps there are other types of stimuli for release of these substances. On the other hand, their release may occur continually or, as suggested above, occur as a consequence of direct interaction between the cells and substratum.

Biological Basis of Stimulated Adherence. The sequence of events which occurs during tumor cell stimulation with chemotactic factors is only partially understood. However, studies carried out in the past few years allow us to suggest that the activation process in these cells is in many ways similar to what occurs in leukocytes. It is not our intention to review the voluminous leukocyte literature, but a brief synopsis of the major findings is warranted. A recent review on the molecular and cellular mechanisms of leukocyte chemotaxis is available (60). Briefly, leukocyte chemotaxis is initiated by the binding of chemoattractants to specific plasma membrane receptors. Following binding, rapid alterations in membrane potential, cyclic mucleotide levels and ion fluxes are observed. Membrane protein and phospholipid alterations occur. Arachidonic acid is released from the membrane phospholipids and is subsequently metabolized through both the cychlooxygenase and lipoxygenase pathways to produce bioactive intermediates. Within minutes, microtubule structures and microfilaments undergo reorganization. Some, or all, of these changes are, no doubt, responsible for the morphological changes undergone by stimulated cells and for the subsequent movement of the cells toward the source of the attractant.

Studies carried out in our laboratory using the Walker 256 carcinosarcoma have shown that these cells have specific binding sites for the synthetic N-formylated tripeptides (Marasco and Varani, submitted for publication). Peptide binding is dose and time dependent, saturatable and partially reversible. Scatchard analysis of the binding data indicates a single class of non-interacting binding site (approximately 7000/cells). While this appears to be a very small number of sites per cell, it must be remembered that this is a very heterogeneous tumor and that only 10–15% of the cells demonstrate responsiveness in the most sensitive assay of responsiveness (adherence). Specific binding sites on

tumor cells for chemotactic factors other than the formulated peptides have not been conclusively demonstrated, but there is no reason to believe that these are unique. It has been shown by Chiang et al. (7) that normal fibroblasts have specific bindings sites for the chemotactic collagen peptides. Based on these limited studies, it appears that the chemotactic response in non-leukocytic cells, as in leukocytes, follows from the binding of the chemotactic factor at specific sites on the cell surface. Following the binding of the chemotactic factor, a series of events are initiated which lead to the biological responses.

Using the adherence response as an indicator of biological activity, some of the cellular requirements for responsiveness have been examined in our laboratory (71, 70). The synthesis of new protein is probably not involved. In addition to the fact that the response is very rapid (within 5 min after stimulation), it will occur in the presence of high concentrations of cychlohexamide. Previous studies in our laboratory have also demonstrated similar findings using the cell swelling assay (8). In contrast, Gauss-Müller et al. (19) reported that migration in the Boyden chamber assay was inhibited by cyclohexamide. This may be a secondary consequence of the inhibition of other basic cellular functions. The response to chemotactic factors is an energy-dependent process as shown by the ability of agents such as iodacetate and 2-deoxyglucose to completely abrogate it (71).

Adherence also demonstrates a requirement for an intact cytoskeleton (78, 71). In the presence of high concentrations of either colchicine or cytochalasin B, the adherence response is blocked. Furthermore, we have been able to show by scanning electron microscopy a dramatic alteration in cell shape accompanying the stimulated adherence of the cells to the substratum. The cells, which in the unstimulated state are round and covered with numerous microvilli, attach to the foreign surface through long slender filopodia and rapidly undergo spreading. These kinds of changes, which are illustrated in Figure 2a–d, have been shown in other cell types to be dependent on the reorganization of cytoskeletal elements.

Cellular response to chemotactic factors require both Ca^{2+} and Mg^{2+}. The requirements for divalent cations exist regardless of whether the stimulus is a classic chemotactic peptide or a non-specific agent such as the phorbol esters (21). In the tumor cells there is a rapid exchange of Ca^{2+} between the cells and the extracellular environment and factors which prevent the cells from responding to the stimulating agents inhibit Ca^{2+} uptake (21).

The biological response of the tumor cells to stimulation can be blocked by several agents which interfere with phospholipid metabolism or with the metabolism of arachidonic acid through the lipoxygenase pathway (71,70). These results are compatible with the suggestion that, as with leukocytes (20), chemotactic activation induces phospholipid turnover with the resultant release of arachidonic acid. Presumably, the arachidonic acid is then available for metabolism through the lipoxygenase pathway. In preliminary studies we have found that there is, in fact, a very rapid turnover of phosphatidyl inositol in the stimulated cells. We have also found that at least one lipoxygenase product of arachidonic acid (i.e., leukotriene B_4) stimulates the hyperadherence response in the Walker cells in much the same way as the chemotactic factors. If these initial observations can be confirmed they will provide a strong basis for the assumption of a biochemical similarity between leukocytes and tumor cells in their response to chemotactic factors.

In contrast to the effects of the lipoxygenase metabolites, we observed that cyclooxygenase products of arachidonic acid (i.e., the anti-aggregatory prostaglandins) blocked the ability of the cells to respond to stimulation. Inhibition was associated with an elevation of the intracellular cAMP levels in the treated cells. The inhibitory effect on the tumor cells could be duplicated by the addition of exogenous dibutyryl cAMP or by agents which are known to raise cAMP levels (12).

In summary these studies, though far from complete, provide an insight into the biological events associated with the hyperadherence phenomenon induced in the Walker cells by chemotactic factors. In many respects the process in these cells appear similar to the process which occurs in stimulated leukocytes.

In Vivo Effects. What evidence is there to suggest that the ability of tumor cells to respond to chemotactic factors affects their *in vivo* behavior? Studies carried out with the tissue-derived chemotactic factors (25, 50) and studies carried out with the complement-derived factor (36, 45) suggest that the localization of circulating tumor can be influenced by chemotactic factors. In Hayashi's experiments, the chemotactic factors were injected intradermally and tumor cell localization monitored by histological examination of the injected sites. Within 24 hours after injection, tumor cells could be identified at the injection sites. The histological sections revealed the apparent sticking of the tumor cells to the endothelium with evidence that some of the cells were emigrating into the exravascular space. The response was specific for the chemotactic factors since control buffers, leukocyte-specific chemotactic factors and vasodilating agents did not have this effect. At periods longer than 24 hours, there were large numbers of extravascular tumor cells and there was widespread invasion of the underlying tissue.

In our studies with the complement-derived chemotactic factor, animals were injected intravenously with the Walker cells and intraperitoneally with the chemotactic factor or with a variety of control substances. An increased number of tumors developed in the peritoneal mesenteries of the chemotactic factor-treated animals (36). When radiolabeled tumor cells were used, it was shown that an increased number of tumor cells localized in the mesenteries of the treated animals (45). In contrast, the chemotactic factor had no effect on proliferation of the tumor cells. Subsequent studies (46) showed that the same pattern of metastasis was observed in animals injected intraperitoneally with glycogen to activate endogenous complement-derived chemotactic activity. These studies strongly support the concept that the localization of circulating tumor cells can be influenced by the presence of chemotactic factors. This could account, at least in part, for the dissimilar patterns of metastasis formation observed with different tumor types.

Summary and Conclusions

There is now a large body of evidence which indicates that the localization of circulating tumor cells is a non-random event and that the adhesive properties of the cells are of critical importance in this process. Several questions remain to be answered. The relevant substrata to which the circulating tumor cells attach to initially must be clearly defined. In some cases this may be the endothelial cell layer while in other cases, the tumor cells may attach directly to exposed areas of basement membranes. There is evidence that in some cases the tumor cells attach to circulating platelets and that this facilitates their subsequent localization. There is no reason to suspect that all tumors behave identically. In addition to defining the relevant substrates, the molecular basis for the adherence of tumor cells to these substrates must be clearly defined. It is obvious, however, that there are multiple mechanisms depending on the cell type and the substrate. Once we understand the mechanisms which circulating tumors cells use in their attachment processes, we may be able to interfere with it and this may ultimately have a real impact on the outcome of the disease.

ACKNOWLEDGMENTS

These studies were supported in part by grants CA29550 and CA29551 from the USPHS.

REFERENCES

1. Abercrombie M: Contact inhibition in tissue culture. *In Vitro* 6:128–142, 1970
2. Bender BL, Jaffe R, Carlin B, Chung AE: Immunolocalization of entactin, a sulfated basement membrane component, in rodent tissues, and comparison with GP-2 (laminin). *Am J Path* 103:419–426, 1981
3. Brunson KW, Nicolson GL: Selection of malignant melanoma variant cell lines for ovary colonization. *J Supramol Struct* 11:517–528, 1979
4. Campbell EJ, Senior RM, McDonald JA, Cox DL: Proteolysis by neutrophils: Relative importance of cell-substrate contact and oxidative interaction of protease inhibitors *in vitro. J Clin Invest* 70:845–852, 1982
5. Carlin B, Jaffe R, Bender B, Chung AE: Entactin, a novel basal lamina-associated sulfated glycoprotein. *J Biol Chem* 256:5209–5214, 1981
6. Carter SB: Principles of cell motility: The direction of cell movement and cancer invasion. *Nature* 206:1183–1187, 1965
7. Chiang TM, Postlethwaite AE, Beachey EH, Seyer JM, Kang AH: Binding of chemotactic collagen-derived peptides to fibroblasts: The relationship to fibroblast chemotaxis. *J Clin Invest* 62:916–922, 1978
8. Coman DR, deLong RP, McCutcheon M: Studies on the mechanisms of metastasis. The distribution of tumors in various organs in relation to the distribution of arterial emboli. *Cancer Res.* 11:648–651, 1951
9. Dunn GA: Mechanisms of fibroblast locomotion. In: ASG Curtis and JD Pitts (eds.) *Cell Adhesion and Motility.* Cambridge University Press. New York. p. 409–424, 1980
10. Eccles SA, Alexander P: Immunologically-mediated restraints of latent tumor metastases. *Nature* 257:52–53, 1975
11. Engel J, Odermatt E, Engel A, Madri JA, Furthmayr H, Rohde H, Timpl R: Shapes, domain organizations and flexibility of laminin and fibronectin, two multifunctional proteins of the extracellular matrix. *J Mol Biol* 150:97–120, 1981
12. Fantone J, Kunkel SL, Varani J: Inhibition of tumor cell

adherence by prostaglandins. In: *Prostaglandins and Cancer: First International Conference*. Alan R. Liss, Inc. New York, pp. 673–677, 1982

13. Fidler IJ: Selection of successive tumor lines for metastases: *Nature New Biol* 242:148–149, 1973
14. Fidler IJ, Nicolson GL: Organ selectivity for implantation survival and growth of B16 melanoma variant tumor lines *J Natl Cancer Inst* 57:1199–1202, 1976
15. Fisher B, Fisher ER: Experimental evidence in support of the dormant tumor cell. *Science* 130:918–919, 1959
16. Foidart J.M, Bere EW, Yaar M, Rennard SI, Gullino M, Martin GR, Katz SI: Distribution and immunoelectron microscopic localization of laminin, a noncollagenous basement membrane glycoprotein. *Lab Invest* 42:336–342, 1980
17. Gasic G, Gasic T, Galanti N, Johnson T, Murphy S: Platelet-Tumor cell interactions in mice. The role of platelets in the spread of malignant disease. *Int J Cancer* 11:704–718, 1973
18. Gastpar H, Ambrus JL, Ambrus CM: Platelet cancer cell interaction in metastasis formation. Platelet aggregation inhibitors: a possible approach to metastasis prevention. In: *Interaction of platelets and tumor cells* (Jamieson GA, ed) Alan R. Liss, Inc., New York, pp. 63–82, 1982
19. Gauss-Müller V, Kleinman HK, Martin GR, Schiffman E: Role of attachment factors and attractants in fibroblast chemotaxis. *J Lab Clin Med* 96:1071–1080, 1980
20. Goetzl EJ: A role for endogenous mono-hydroxi-eicosatetraenoic acids (HETEs) in the regulation of human neutrophil migration. *Immunology* 40:709–726, 1980
21. Grimstad IA, Wass J, Spirnak J, Fantone JC, Varani J: Chemotactic factor and tumor promoter-induced adherence of tumor cells: Involvement of Ca^{2+} and Mg^{2+}. *Invasion Metastasis* Vol 2:274–288, 1982
22. Hagmar B, Ryd W: Tumor cell locomotion-a factor in metastasis formation? Influence of cytochalasin B on a tumor dissemination pattern. *Int J Cancer* 19:576–580, 1977
23. Hara Y, Steiner M, Baldini MG: Characterization of the platelet-aggregating activity of tumor cells. *Cancer Res* 40:1217–1222, 1980
24. Hart IR, Raz A, Fidler IJ: Effect of cytoskeleton-disrupting agents on the metastatic behavior of melanoma cells. *J Natl Cancer Inst* 64:891–900, 1980
25. Hayashi H, Yoshida K, Ozaki T, Ushijima K: Chemotactic factor associated with invasion of cancer cells. *Nature* 226:174–175, 1970
26. Hayman EG, Engvall E, Ruoslahti E: Concomitant loss of cell surface fibronectin and laminin from transformed rat kidney cells. *J Cell Biol* 88:352–357, 1981
27. Henson PM: Interaction of cells with immune complexes. Adherence, release of constituents and tissue injury. *J Exp Med* 134:1145–1154, 1971
28. Hilgard P: The role of blood platelets in experimental metastases. *Br J Cancer* 28:429–435, 1973
29. Honn KV, Cicone B, Jkoff A: Prostacyclin: A potent antimetastatic agent. *Science* 212:1270–1272, 1981
30. Jamieson GA, Bastida E, Ordinas, A: Mechanisms of platelet aggregation by human tumor cell lines. In: *Interaction of Platelets and Tumor Cells* (Jamieson GA, ed) Alan R. Liss, Inc., New York, pp. 405–413, 1982
31. Johnson, KJ, Varani, J: Substrate hydrolysis by immune complex-activated neutrophils: Effect of physical presentation of complexes and protease inhibitors. *J Immunol* 127:1875–1879, 1981
32. Kabat, E, Leskowitz, S: Immunochemical studies on blood groups. XVII. Structural units involved in blood groups A and B specificity. *J Am Chem Soc* 77:5159–5164, 1955
33. Karpatkin S, Pearlstein E, Salk PL, Yogeeswaran G: Role of platelets in tumor cell metastases. *Ann N Y Acad Sci*: 370:101–118, 1981
34. Kleinman, HK: Role of cell attachment proteins in defining

cell-matrix interactions. In: *Tumor Invasion and Metastasis* (Liotta L, Hart IR, eds). *Dev Oncol* 7:291–308, 1982
35. Kramer R, Nicolson GL: Interactions of tumor cells with vascular endothelial cell monolayers: A model for metastatic invasion. *Proc Nat Acad Sci USA*. 76:5704–5708, 1979
36. Lam WC, Delikatny EJ, Orr FW, Wass J, Varani J, Ward PA: The chemotactic response of tumor cells: A model for cancer metastasis. *Am J Path* 104:69–76, 1981
37. Liotta LA, Kleinerman J, Saidel GM: The significance of hematogenous tumor cell clumps in the metastatic process. *Cancer Res* 36:889–894, 1976
38. Liotta LA, Tryggvason K, Garbisa S, Hart I, Foltz CM Shafie S: Metastatic potential correlates with enzymatic degradation of basement membrane collagen. *Nature* 284:67–68, 1980
39. MacGregor R, Spagnuolo P, Lentnek A: Inhibition of granulocyte adherence by ethanol, prednisone and aspirin measured with an assay system. *New Eng J Med* 291:642–646, 1974
40. Magro C, Orr, FW, Manishen WJ, Sivananthan K, Mokashi SS: Adhesion, chemotaxis, and Walker carcinosarcoma cells in response to products of resorbing bone. *JNCI* 74(4):829–836 1985
41. McCoy JP, Schrier D, Lovett EJ, Judd WJ, Varani J: Hyperimmune human ABO blood-typing sera: Reactivity with murine laminin and cytotoxicity for metastatic murine tumor cells. *J Cell Sci* 59, 245–256, 1983
42. Murphy LA, Goldstein IJ: Five α-d-galactopyranosyl-binding isolectins from *Bandeiraea simplicifolia* seeds. *J Biol Chem* 252:4739–4742, 1977
43. Murray JC, Liotta L, Rennard SI, Martin GR: Adhesion characteristics of murine metastatic and nonmetastatic tumor cells *in vitro*. *Cancer Res* 40:347–351, 1980
44. O'Flaherty JT, Kreutzer DL, Ward PA: The influence of chemotactic factors on neutrophil adhesiveness. *Inflammation* 3:37–48, 1978
45. Orr FW, Lam WC, Delikatny EJ, Mokashi S, Varani J: Localization of 125-I-iododeoxyuridine-labeled tumor cells at tissue sites injected with chemotactic stimuli. *Invasion Metastasis* 1:239–247, 1981
46. Orr FW, Mokashi S, Delikatny J: Generation of a complement-derived chemotactic factor for tumor cells in experimentally-induced peritoneal exudates and its effect on the local metastasis of circulating tumor cells. *Am J Path* 108:112, 1982
47. Orr FW, Varani, J: Chemotactic mechanisms and cancer. *Path Annual* 17:307–330, 1982
48. Orr W, Varani J, Gondek MD, Ward PA, Mundy GR: Chemotactic responses of tumor cells to products of resorbing bone. *Science* 203:176–179, 1979
49. Orr FW, Varani J, Gondek MD, Ward PA, Mundy GR: Partial characterization of a bone-derived chemotactic factor for tumor cells. *Am J Path* 99:43–52, 1980
50. Ozaki T, Yoshida K, Ushijima K, Hayashi, H: Studies on the mechanisms of invasion in cancer. II: *In vivo* effects of a factor chemotactic for cancer cells. *Int J Cancer* 7:93–100, 1971
51. Pearlstein E, Gold LI, Garcia-Pardo, A: Fibronectin: A review of its structure and biological activity. *Molecular and Cellular Biochemistry* 29:103–128, 1980
52. Poole AR, Tiltman KJ, Recklies AD, Stober, TAM: Differences in secretion of proteinase cathepsin B at the edges of human breast carcinomas and fibroadenomas. *Nature* 273:545–547, 1978
53. Postlethwaite AE, Keski-Oja J, Balian G, Kang AH: Induction of fibroblast chemotaxis by fibronectin: Localization of the chemotactic region to a 140, 000 molecular weight nongelatin-binding fragment. *J Exp Med* 153:494–499, 1980
54. Proctor JW: Rat sarcoma model supports both 'soil seed' and 'mechanical' theories of metastatic spread. *Br J Cancer* 34:651–654, 1976
55. Rao CN, Margulies IMK, Tralka TS, Terranova VP, Madri

JA, Liotta LA: Isolation of a subunit of laminin and its role in molecular structure and tumor cell attachment. *J Biol Chem* 257:9740–9744, 1982

56. Romualdez AG, Ward PA: A unique, complement-derived chemotactic factor for tumor cells. *Proc Natl Acad Sci USA* 72:4128–4132, 1975
57. Sato H, Suzuki M: Deformability and viability of tumor cells by transcapillary passage, with reference to organ affinity of metastasis in cancer. In: *Fundamental Aspects of Metastasis* (Weiss L. ed.) North Holland Publ. Co., New York, pp. 311–17, 1976
58. Shibata S, Peters BP, Roberts DD, Goldstein IJ, Liotta LA: Isolation of laminin by affinity chromatography on immobilized *Griffonia simplicifolia* I lectin. *FEBS Lett.* 142:194–198, 1982
59. Showell HJ, Freen RJ, Zigmond SH, Schiffman E, Aswanikumar S, Carcoran B, Becker EL: The structure activity relations of synthetic peptides as chemotactic factors and inducers of lysozomal enzyme secretion for neutrophils. *J Exp Med* 143:154–168, 1976
60. Snyderman R, Goetzl EJ: Molecular and cellular mechanisms of leukocyte chemotaxis. *Science* 213:830–836, 1981
61. Stossel TP: The mechanism of leukocyte locomotion. *Leukocyte Chemotaxis: Methods, Physiology and Clinical Implications.* Gallin JI, Quie PG, (eds.) Raven Press, New York, pp. 143–157, 1978
62. Strauli P, Weiss L: Cell locomotion and tumor penetration. *Euro J Cancer* 13:1–12, 1977
63. Sugarbaker EV, Ketcham AS, Cohen AM: Studies on dormant tumor cells. *Cancer* 28:545–552, 1971
64. Sugarbaker EV, Weingrad DN, Roseman JM: Observations on cancer metastasis in man. *Develop Oncology* 7:427–465, 1982
65. Terranova VP, Liotta LA Russo RG, Martin GR: Role of laminin in the attachment and metastasis of murine tumor cells. *Cancer Res* 42:2265–2269, 1982
66. Terranova VP, Rohrbach DH, Martin GR: Role of laminin in the attachment of PAM 12 (epithelial) cells to basement membrane collagen. *Cell* 22:719–726, 1980
67. Thorgeirsson UP, Kalebic T, Russo RG Liotta LA: Effects of chemotactic agents and protease inhibitors on tumor cell invasion of native human connective tissue barriers *in vitro.* *Fed Proc* 41:334, 1982
68. Timpl R, Rohde H, Ott-Ulbricht U, Risteli L, Bachinger HP: Chemical characterization of laminin, a major glycoprotein of basement membranes. In: *Glycoconjugates* (Shaver et al., eds.), Georg Thieme, Stuttgart, pp. 145–146, 1979b
69. Timpl R, Rohde H, Robey PG, Rennard SI, Foidart JM, Martin GR: Laminin-a glycoprotein from basement membranes. *J Biol Chem* 254:9933–9937, 1979a

70. Varani J: Chemotaxis of metastatic tumor cells. *Cancer Metastasis Reviews* 1:17–28, 1982
71. Varani J, Fantone JC: Phorbol myristate acetate-induced adherence of Walker 256 carcinosarcoma cells. *Cancer Res* 42:190–197, 1982
72. Varani J, Johnson KJ, Kaplan J: Development of a solid phase assay for measurement of proteolytic enzyme activity. *Analyt Biochem* 107:377–384, 1980
73. Varani J, Lovett EJ, Elgebaly S, Lundy J, Ward PA: *In vitro* and *in vivo* adherence of tumor cell variants correlated with tumor formation. *Am J Path* 101:345–352, 1980
74. Varani J, Lovett EJ, Lundy J: A model of tumor dormancy: Effects of anesthesia and surgery. *J Surg Oncol* 17:9–14, 1981
75. Varani J, Lovett EJ, McCoy JP, Shibata S, Maddox DE, Goldstein IJ, Wicha M: Differential expression of a laminin-like substance by high and low metastatic tumor cells. *Am J Path* 111:27–34, 1983
76. Varani J, Orr W, Ward PA: Comparison of subpopulations of tumor cells with altered migratory activity, attachment characteristics, enzyme levels and *in vivo* behavior. *Euro J Cancer* 15:585–592, 1979a
77. Varani J, Orr W, Ward PA: Hydrolytic enzyme activities, migratory activity and *in vivo* growth and metastatic potential of recent tumor isolates. *Cancer Res* 39:2376–2380, 1979b
78. Varani J, Wass J, Piontek G, Ward PA: Chemotactic factor-induced adherence of tumor cells. *Cell Biol. International Reports* 5:525–530, 1981
79. Vasiliev JM, Gelfand IM: Morphogenetic reactions and locomotory behavior of transformed cells in culture. In: *Fundamental Aspects of Metastasis.* North Holland Publishing Co., Inc. Weiss L, (ed.) New York, pp. 71–98, 1976
80. Warren BA: Environment of the blood-borne tumor embolus adherent to vessel wall. *J Med* 4:150–177, 1973
81. Wass JA, Varani J, Piontek GE, Goff D, Ward PA: Characteristics of the chemotactic factor-mediated cell swelling response in tumor cells. *J Nat Cancer Inst* 66:927–933, 1981
82. Watanabae S: The metastasizing ability of tumor cells. *Cancer* 7:215–223, 1954
83. Watkins WM: Blood-group substances. *Science* 152:172–181, 1966
84. Weiss L, Haydock K, Pickren JW, Lane WW: Organ vascularity and metastatic frequency. *Am J Path* 101:101–113, 1980
85. Wright TC, Ukena TE, Campbell R, Karnovsky MJ: Rates of aggregation, loss of anchorage dependence and tumorigenicity of cultured cells. *Proc Nat Acad Sci USA* 74:258–262, 1977
86. Yoshida K, Ozaki T, Ushijima K, Hayashi H: Studies on the mechanism of invasion in cancer. I. Isolation and purification of a factor chemotactic for cancer cells. *Int J Cancer* 6:123–132, 1970

11

TUMOR-CELL INTERACTIONS WITH BLOOD VESSELS DURING CANCER METASTASIS

PETER A. NETLAND and BRUCE R. ZETTER

INTRODUCTION

The metastatic process can be subdivided into a series of discrete steps that must be completed before a metastatic tumor colony can flourish in a new environment. After passing into a vessel, a metastatic cell must survive in the bloodstream, come to rest in a vessel in the new organ, and pass out of that vessel into the new organ site. Further, the growth of a new tumor cell colony can be sustained only after a blood supply is recruited from the host vasculature. While it is obvious that the vascular circulation transports tumor cells to distant organ sites, it is sometimes overlooked that the vasculature has a crucial role in nearly all steps of metastasis.

In this chapter, we will outline the steps during which metastatic tumor cells must interact with the vasculature and we describe the nature of those interactions. The processes to be considered include:
1. Cell shedding and tumor vascularity
2. Tumor blood vessels as an impaired barrier to tumor cell release
3. Vascular permeability and metastasis
4. Intravasation of tumor cells
5. Transport of tumor cells in the bloodstream
6. Initial arrest of tumor cells
7. Adherence of tumor cells to vascular components
8. Extravasation of tumor cells
9. Tumor cell motility
10. Degradation of vascular basement membrane
11. Secondary tumor growth and angiogenesis

ENTRY OF TUMOR CELLS INTO THE CIRCULATION

Cell shedding and tumor vascularity

One of the earliest host responses to a solid tumor is angiogenesis, the growth of new capillaries toward a growing tumor. Since proximity to blood vessels should facilitate entry of tumor cells into the circulation, the number of tumor cells released into the circulation would be expected to correlate with the density of blood vessels in the primary tumor. In support of this prediction, Liotta *et al.* (112) found tumor cells in the effluent of a mouse fibrosarcoma implanted in the thigh of C57BL/6 mice coincident with the appearance of new blood vessels in the tumor. The number of cells shed from the primary tumor correlated with the

density of tumor blood vessels and with the number of lung metastases observed six days later. These results indicate that increased tumor vascularity can facilitate cell shedding into the circulation and thereby increase the number of blood-borne metastatic cells.

Clinical observations also demonstrate the importance of tumor vascularization for the escape of tumor cells into the circulation. The *in situ* phase of carcinoma of the cervix, breast, colon, bladder, or skin is characteristically avascular and metastasis-free. Only after blood vessels penetrate the basement membrane and invade the tumor does the *in situ* phase end and metastases become apparent (50).

It should be noted that tumor angiogenesis may have other roles in the spread of tumors. When aggregates of a squamous cell carcinoma of the bladder were cultured with microvascular networks in a plasma clot, the pattern of neoplastic growth changed abruptly after vessels contacted the tumor aggregates (148). The tumor cells accumulated along a periendothelial route even though there was no blood flow through these *in vitro* capillaries. These results suggest that vessels may promote the local spread of tumors, perhaps by enzymatically carving a path of least resistance or by providing an adhesive substrate for the migration of tumor cells.

Tumor blood vessels as an impaired barrier to tumor cell release

Although endothelial cells for the tumor vasculature are recruited from host tissues, there are differences between normal and tumor blood vessels. The proliferation rate of vascular endothelial cells is 20–2000 times faster in tumor endothelium compared with normal tissue endothelium (88). Structural defects found in tumor vessels include the absence of a basal lamina and the presence of large gaps between adjacent endothelial cells (122 and Figure 1, 216). Such defects are common in newly-formed capillaries. However, new capillaries in healing wounds and other tissues eventually form a mature vascular network of arterioles, capillaries, and venules. In contrast, tumor capillaries persist as tubes of endothelium that lack sheaths of smooth muscle or pericytes (2). Tumor-induced capillaries regress completely after the tumor is removed (4); this suggests that the maintenance of these immature vessels requires the continued presence of a tumor-derived factor. It has been suggested that these morphological abnormalities in the tumor vasculature may facilitate the entry of tumor cells into the circulation (179).

R. H. Goldfarb (ed.), Fundamental aspects of cancer.
© 1989, Kluwer Academic Publishers, Dordrecht. ISBN 978-94-010-6980-9

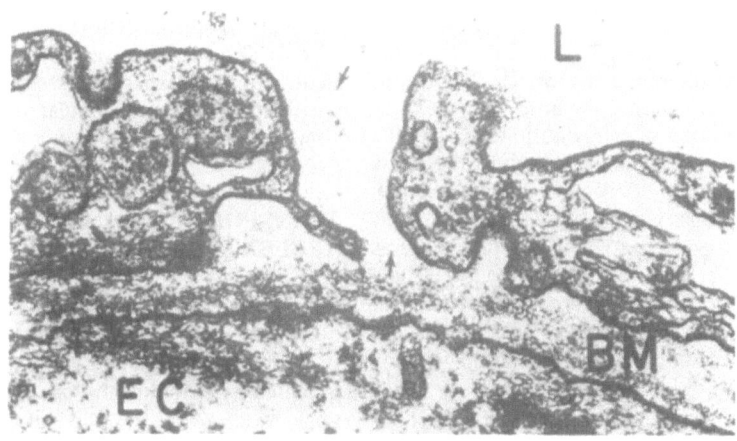

Figure 1. Demonstration of an intercellular gap between endothelial cells in a human metastatic brain tumor (× 57,000 magnification). The lumen of the vessel (*L*) is in direct communication with extracellular space (*EC*) and basement membrane (*BM*). Such gaps along with abnormalities of the basal lamina are characteristic of tumor-induced blood vessels. [Reprinted from D.M. Long. J. Neurosurg. 51:53–8, 1979.]

Vascular permeability and metastasis

It has long been noted that the vessels in and around growing tumors are abnormally "leaky" for both fluid and solutes in the blood stream. Abnormal accumulation of fluid commonly accompanies the growth of solid and especially ascites tumors. In the brain, malignant tumors are characterized by a breakdown of the blood-brain barrier to protein as well as a great propensity for the production of brain edema (122).

There are several possible mechanisms for the increased permeability of tumor blood vessels. Tumor cells themselves may produce a vascular permeability factor. One such factor has been purified to near homogeneity from tumor-conditioned media and from native tumor ascites fluid (35, 186, and Figure 2). This factor appears to be a $M_r 38,000$ protein that is released both *in vitro* and *in vivo* from a variety of tumors and species, and its activity can be specifically inhibited with antibody. A second type of permeability factor has been identified in the ascites fluid of several different tumor strains (70, 97). Another possibility is that lymphocyte products may increase vascular permeability (125). Presumably, the action of a lymphocyte-derived factor on vascular permeability would require an immune reaction at the tumor site. However, the increased permeability of tumor vessels can precede and therefore be independent of an immune response (35).

The increased permeability of tumor blood vessels could facilitate the process of metastasis in several different ways. Because high levels of procoagulant are present in tissues, increased vascular permeability may result in extravascular coagulation and deposition of fibrin (36), which in turn could depress the immune response, influence angiogenesis, or otherwise alter metastasis. In addition, tumor cell motility may be increased by exposure to serum chemotactic factors such as the fifth component of complement (171, 172). Such increased tumor cell motility might potentiate the passage of tumor cells into the circulation. Alternatively, the morphological changes in the vascular endothelium and basal lamina that lead to increased permeability may coincidentally provide a less effective barrier to the transvascular passage of tumor cells. Whatever the mechanism, the processes that lead to increased vascular permeability at tumor sites should increase the probability of tumor cells entering the circulation and consequently forming metastases.

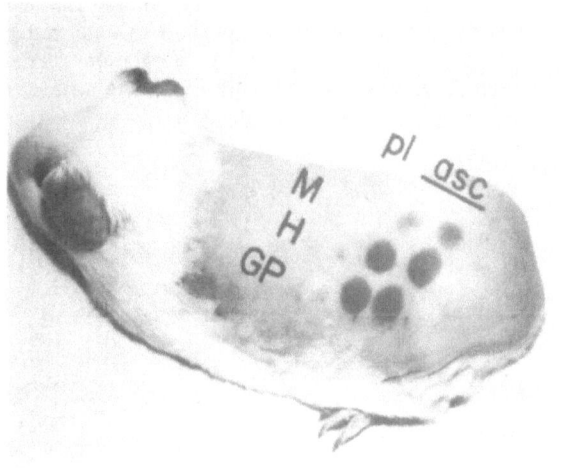

Figure 2. Demonstration of the action of a vascular permeability factor in plasma and ascites fluid from tumor bearing animals. In the Miles assay, depilated guinea pigs were injected i.v. with 0.5% Evans Blue dye. Samples tested for permeability-increasing activity were injected intradermally in a volume of 0.1 ml isotonic buffer at neutral pH. Abbreviations: *pl*, control plasma; *asc*, ascites fluid; *M*, mouse TA3-St tumor; *H*, hamster HSV-NIL8 tumor; and *GP*, guinea pig line 10 tumor. Factors that increase vascular permeability may be responsible for the accumulation of fluid that commonly accompanies the growth of solid or ascites tumors. [Reprinted by permission of Science (D.R. Senger *et al.*, 219:983–5, 1983), copyright 1983 by the American Association for the Advancement of Science.]

Intravasation of tumor cells

An essential early event in metastasis is intravasation, the entry of tumor cells into the blood stream. This important event has been the subject of relatively little study in comparison with the later process of extravasation whereby the tumor cells exit the blood stream and pass into the tissue space. Both intravasation and extravasation occur in small capillaries rather than in larger vessels with thicker vascular walls. Although the two processes may have some features in common, it would probably be a mistake to consider them identical events simply occurring in reverse. As pointed out earlier, for example, the vessels through which tumor cells intravasate may be easier to penetrate than normal capillaries.

Recently, a model for intravasation was developed in which B16 and K-1735 melanoma cell lines were incubated with intact brain capillaries (170). In this model, metastatic tumor cells adhered to the surface of capillaries in greater numbers and at a faster rate than normal cells. These results suggest that attachment to vascular components may play a role during the initial contact between tumor cells and blood vessels. It would be of interest to examine additional mechanisms such as enzymatic degradation of the basement membrane or tumor cell motility in order to identify the factors that enable metastatic cells to traverse from outside the blood vessel to the vascular lumen.

Passage of tumor cells through an endothelial layer can take place in two distinct ways. The tumor cells can either pass through the junctions *between* adjacent endothelial cells (intercellular passage) or pass directly *through* the cytoplasm of an intact endothelial cell (transcellular passage). DeBruyn and Cho (1982) found that rat W/Fu AML cells as well as mouse B16 melanoma cells could pass from the outside to the inside of capillaries by direct penetration through individual endothelial cells (Figure 3). This transcellular passage was non-destructive and the migration pore was transient. Further experiments are necessary to determine whether this form of vascular transmural passage is more common in intravasation than in extravasation.

TRANSPORT IN THE BLOODSTREAM AND ARREST AT DISTANT SITES

Large numbers of tumor cells are released into the blood during the metastatic process. Liotta *et al.* (112) found that the number of cells released from an implanted MTW9 mammary carcinoma increased as the vascularized tumor grew, with 1.4×10^3 cells shed per 24 hours on day 5, 3.0×10^4 cells on day 10, and 1.5×10^5 cells on day 15. Butler and Gullino (17) quantitated cell shedding into the efferent blood of a rat mammary adenocarcinoma and found $3-4 \times 10^6$ cells/24 hr/gram tumor, or $1.6-2.0 \times 10^4$ cells/ml of blood. Recently, Glaves (64) showed that Lewis lung carcinoma cells and B16 melanoma cells were detectable in the circulation after one to three days of primary tumor growth. Glaves also showed that the median number of cells shed throughout tumor growth was 1×10^8 for Lewis lung carcinoma cells and 2.4×10^6 for B16 melanoma cells, whereas the number of spontaneous pulmonary metastases was orders of magnitude less. In human malignancies, circulating tumor cells have been identified in the venous blood (61, 67, 73, 104, 177). Although the transport of tumor cells in the blood sream is an essential component of the metastatic process, it is important to note that the mere presence of tumor cells in the circulation *does not* insure that those cells will eventually give rise to metastases.

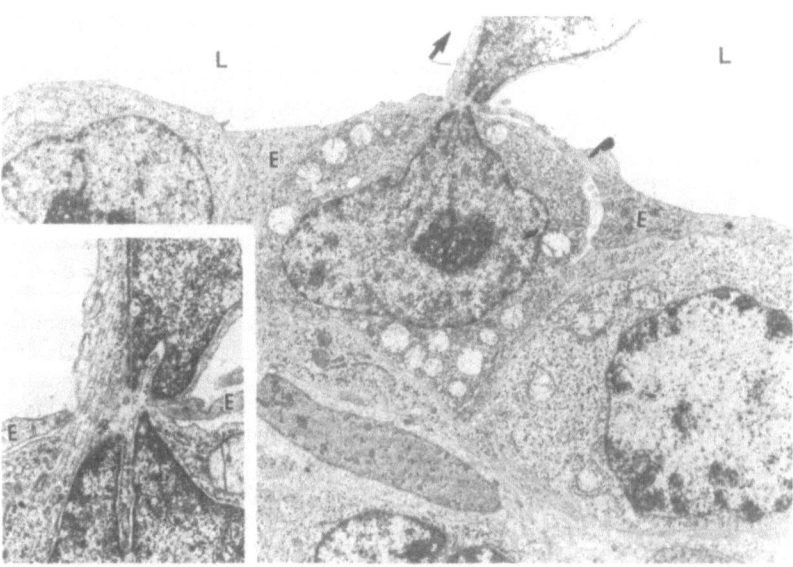

Figure 3. Tumor cell intravasation. A rat W/Fu AML tumor cell is seen entering into a vessel lumen in a syngeneic Wistar-Furth rat (× 2900 magnification). Inset shows an enlargement of the temporary migration pore (× 12,600 magnification). *E*, endothelial cell: *L*, lumen. Arrow shows the direction of tumor cell movement. [Reprinted by permission from P.P.H. DeBruyn & Y. Cho. J. Ultrastruct. Res. 81:189–201, 1982 (copyright© 1982 by Academic Press Inc.).]

Transport of tumor cells in the bloodstream

While in the blood, tumor cells may interact with themselves as well as other blood components. Homotypic aggregation of tumor cells can influence implantation in the microcirculation and have a positive effect on the frequency of successful metastasis (39, 113, 123, 230). Similarly, heterotypic interactions with platelets (55, 60, 157, 218), lymphocytes (40, 42), and polymorphonuclear leukocytes (195) can increase the frequency of metastasis. In addition, the release of platelet-derived factors that increase vascular permeability or stimulate tumor cell growth and/or motility could enhance the metastatic process (80, 100, 135). In support of this hypothesis various treatments that interfere with tumor cell-platelet interactions have been shown to decrease metastatic frequency (56–59, 89–91).

Circulating tumor cells are thromboplastic and can elicit fibrin formation in the blood stream. Tumor cell-associated procoagulant activities (PCAs) include: an activity similar to tissue factor (25, 149), procoagulants capable of activating factor X (26, 68, 69, 161), and procoagulant activity associated with plasma membrane vesicles that acts at the level of prothrombinase generation (34, 35). The large literature that describes the effects of anticoagulant (e.g. warfarin and heparin) or fibrinolytic agents on tumor progression is complicated because such agents may alter immunologic mechanisms or may directly inhibit tumor cell motility and growth. Nonetheless, pharmacologic and histologic data suggest a role for fibrin deposition in the metastatic process. This view has been supported by a correlation between procoagulant activity and metastatic capacity of B16 melanoma variants (62). On the other hand, only small amounts of fibrin are found around certain tumor cell types or fibrin formation may be transient, and in many cases fibrin formation is not required for the circulatory arrest or metastatic spread of tumor cells (219). Although the exact role of fibrin formation around tumor cells remains uncertain, fibrin deposited around tumor cells could serve as a physical barrier or "cocoon" that interferes with the host's immune response (33) or could facilitate the arrest of tumor cells in the microvasculature (21, 225).

Despite such favorable interactions, the blood compartment is a hostile environment for tumor cells. Injecting radiolabeled murine B16 melanoma cells into the venous circulation, Fidler (38) found that most cells were destroyed within 24 hours, and that after 3 days less than 0.1% remained viable. Similar observations have been reported using other experimental models (86, 103, 114, 167, 223). The rapid destruction of tumor cells has been ascribed to a variety of mechanisms, including natural killer cells (77–79, 85), macrophages (45, 96, 101), polymorphonuclear leukocytes (65), antibodies (54, 205, 224) or mechanical trauma (180). Such cytotoxic mechanisms could operate while tumor cells circulate or after they lodge in the microcirculation.

Initial arrest of tumor cells

Studies of circulating radiolabeled tumor cells have demonstrated that the vast majority of tumor cells are arrested in the first capillary bed they encounter, probably due to nonspecific trapping. With the possible exception of lymphoid tumors (93, 176), circulating tumor cells are rapidly cleared from the blood (38, 75, 173). After injection into the tail vein, radiolabeled cells from a variety of tumors are trapped in the first encountered capillary bed in the lung (15, 38, 46). Similarly, radiolabeled tumor cells injected into the rat portal vein are initially arrested in the liver. Certain tumor cell lines that produce pulmonary metastases after tail vein injection may produce hepatic metastases when injected into the portal vein (72, 167). Based on such observations, a "mechanical" hypothesis has been proposed. According to this hypothesis, the largest number of metastases should appear in the organ that had initially trapped the most tumor cells. *Frequently, however, there is no correlation between the initial arrest of circulating tumor cells and the subsequent pattern of metastatic growth.*

Divergence of metastatic distribution and initial arrest pattern has been documented using a variety of experimental systems (43, 46, 81, 168). Two murine tumor cell lines that exhibit widely divergent metastatic patterns *in vivo* are the B16 melanoma and the reticulum cell sarcoma (M5076). As shown in Table 1, B16-F10 melanoma selectively colonized the lung after tail vein injection, whereas reticulum cell sarcoma grew preferentially in the liver and rarely metastasized to the lung. In contrast, the initial arrest patterns of the two cell types were nearly identical (Figure 4). It is clear, therefore, that the initial pulmonary arrest pattern for most of the reticulum cell sarcoma cells is in marked contrast to their later preferential formation of hepatic metastases. These findings agree with previous reports that the initial arrest pattern does not correlate with the subsequent metastatic distribution for these cell lines (82, 83, 155).

The lack of correlation between initial arrest pattern and subsequent tumor development is not surprising. Metastasis is a selective process and specific properties of select tumor cell subpopulations influence their metastatic potential (44,

Table 1. Experimental metastases found after intravenous injection of B16-F10 melanoma cells and murine reticulum cell sarcoma cells.*

Cell line	Pulmonary metastases		Hepatic metastases		All other sites[†]	
	% mice	mean ± SD	% mice	mean ± SD	% mice	mean ± SD
B16-F10 melanoma	100	112 ± 25	13	0.2 ± 0.7	25	0.4 ± 0.7
Reticulum cell sarcoma	25	0.4 ± 0.5	100	58 ± 16	75	1.2 ± 0.9

*Metastases were counted 25 days after tail vein injection of 3×10^5 trypsinized viable cells into groups of 8 C57BL/6 mice each.
[†]"All other sites" refers to metastases found in organs other than lung and liver, which included mesentery, lymph node, and adrenal for B16-F10 melanoma cells as well as spleen and kidney for reticulum cell sarcoma cells.

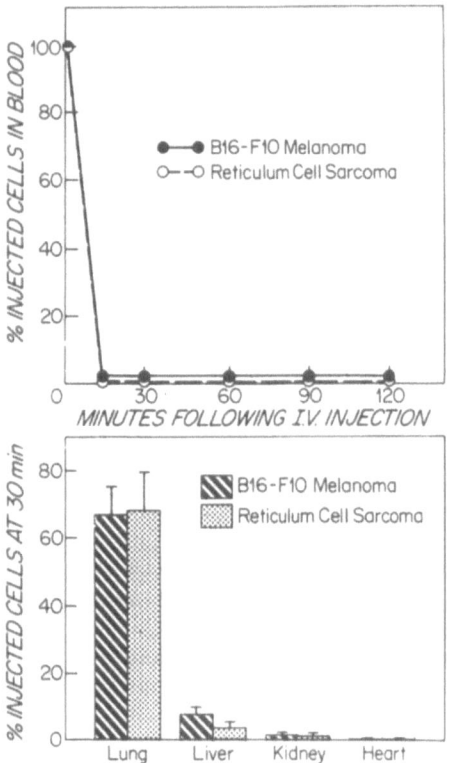

Figure 4. Clearance from the blood and initial arrest pattern of B16-F10 melanoma cells and reticulum cell sarcoma cells. B16-F10 melanoma cells and reticulum cell sarcoma cells were labeled with [51]chromate then trypsinized and injected into groups of four C57BL/6 mice each. Blood samples were removed at various times following injection, organs were removed at necropsy, and radioactivity was measured in a gamma counter. The blood volume was determined by measuring the dilution of [51]chromate-labeled homologous erythrocytes. The percent injected cells in the blood (top) and in organs after 30 minutes (bottom) are shown. The values shown are means ± S.D. Where error bars are not shown, the S.D. was within the range of the datum point. The initial arrest patterns are very similar for these two cells and do not correlate with their very different *in vivo* metastatic distributions. The initial arrest of tumor cells is probably due to mechanical trapping in the first capillary bed encountered. Most nonspecifically trapped tumor cells are rapidly destroyed. [P.A. Netland & B.R. Zetter, unpublished data.]

144, 165, 198). Most tumor cells are destroyed at the site of their initial arrest (38, 86, 103, 114, 167, 223). Surviving cells can be released and recirculated to other organs (41, 81, 221). Furthermore, a small proportion of injected tumor cells are distributed to organs ubiquitously (15, 38, 71, 82, 155, 160). Thus, the formation of metastases distant from the initial arrest site may result from the arrest of only a small and probably select subpopulation of tumor cells. Not all arrested cells, however, produce metastases. Tumor cells must undergo subsequent steps to develop into a metastasis.

Adherence of tumor cells to vascular components

Clinical and experimental observations have demonstrated

the preferential metastasis of certain tumors to one or more select organs (144, 165, 184, 197). To explain this organ-selectivity, Greene and Harvey (71) postulated that a "tumor cell-endothelial bond" promotes subsequent development of tumor cells into gross metastases. Because different organs exhibit varying susceptibility to metastasis by cells of the same tumor, they predicted organ-specific differences in "receptivity" to the binding of tumor cells.

Organ-specific adhesive interactions have correlated with metastatic patterns in a variety of experimental systems. Nicolson and Winkelhake (142) found that heterotypic aggregation of tumor cells with lung cells correlated with lung-colonizing potential of B16 melanoma variants. Aggregation of tumor cells with cells from other organs was less extensive and did not vary with lung-colonizing potential. Similarly, liver-colonizing lymphoma variants formed rosettes with hepatocytes according to their metastatic potential (18), and spleen-colonizing leukemia cells preferentially bound to suspended cells from their target organ (159). Lymphoid tumor cells that metastasize to liver bound selectively to isolated liver endothelial cells (175) and a Lewis lung carcinoma variant that metastasizes to liver adhered preferentially to mouse hepatocytes (Pnina Brodt, personal communication). Moreover, several investigators have observed specific adherence of tumor cells to monolayers of cells from organs that are selectively colonized by those tumor cells *in vivo* (1, 76, 98, 145). Use of syngeneic tissue has provided convincing evidence for organ-selective adhesion. Schirrmacher *et al.* (181) and Nicolson *et al.* (147) found that the metastatic distribution of mouse tumor cells *in vivo* was correlated with the selectivity of their binding to specific organ tissue fragments *in vitro*.

By use of a cryostat section assay, evidence has been obtained for specific binding of tumor cells to the tissues that they selectively colonize *in vivo* (102, 139, 140). As shown in Figure 5, B16-F10 melanoma cells that metastasize preferentially to lung *in vivo* bound preferentially to cryostat sections of mouse lung in comparison with other organs. Similarly, liver-colonizing reticulum cell sarcoma cells bound preferentially to cryostat sections of mouse liver *in vitro* with significantly less binding to other tissues. In similar studies with an avian system, Kieran and Longnecker (102) found that chick AL-2 cells that metastasize preferentially to the liver bind preferentially to cryostat sections of chick liver tissue. Together these results present strong evidence for a specific adhesive interaction between tumor cells and the cells of the tissues that they preferentially colonize. Recently, it has been demonstrated that B16 melanoma variant cell lines can be selected for altered adhesion to cryostat sections of specific tissues (141). Cell lines selected for increased adhesion to lung cryostat sections showed increased lung colonization *in vivo*, which indicates that adhesive interactions between metastatic tumor cells and specific host tissues can influence the frequency of metastasis in those tissues *in vivo* (141). The absence of such specific cellular adhesions may in part explain the failure of some tumor cells to colonize a given organ.

The biochemical mechanisms that mediate organ-specific adhesion of tumor cells to host tissues are currently under investigation. Elegant work by Nicolson and co-workers has implicated cell surface molecules in tumor cell implantation (144). Incubation of B16 melanoma cells with tunicamycin

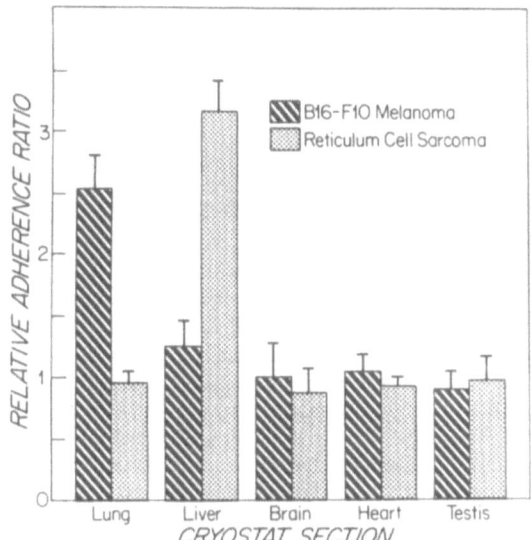

Figure 5. Organ-specific binding of murine B16-F10 melanoma cells and reticulum cell sarcoma cells *in vitro*. A cryostat section assay (Stamper & Woodruff, 1976: Butcher *et al.*, 1980) was modified as described (Netland & Zetter, 1983, 1984). Briefly, tumor cells were labeled with ^{51}chromate and incubated with gentle agitation for 40 minutes at 5–7°C on fresh cryostat sections prepared from various host organs. After gentle washing to remove nonadherent cells, the radioactivity associated with individual sections was counted to determine the number of adherent cells per section. The relative adherence ratio was determined from the ratio of the number of adherent tumor cells to the number of control mouse Balb/c 3T3 cells that bound to duplicate sections. The values shown are the means ± S.D. for at least 5 samples. Murine B16-F10 melanoma cells and reticulum cell sarcoma cells demonstrate a specificity in their binding to syngeneic organ sections *in vitro* that reflects the selectivity of their metastatic homing *in vivo*. [Reprinted by permission of Science (P.A. Netland & B.R. Zetter, 224:1113–5, 1984), copyright 1984 by the American Association for the Advancement of Science.]

decreased cell surface sialogalactoproteins, reduced adhesion of tumor cells to endothelial cell monolayers, and inhibited lung colony formation *in vivo* (94, 95). Other glycoconjugates (12, 29, 30, 74, 193, 227) or tumor cell surface lectins (169, 185) may also have a role in adhesive interactions.

Development of antibodies against tumor cell surface antigens provides another promising approach for the study of adhesion and metastatic events (146, 182, 187). Indeed, monoclonal antibodies can inhibit the adhesion of B16 melanoma cells to plastic and inhibit lung metastasis *in vivo* (213). These antibodies react with two antigenic sites on the B16 melanoma cell surface that have apparent molecular weights of 40,000 and 50,000 (214) and inhibit tumor cell adhesion to the adhesive glycoprotein laminin (215).

Because tumor cells rapidly adhere to exposed endothelial cell extracellular matrix or basal lamina (107, 145, 166, 183), they may bind *in vivo* to regions of damaged endothelium or interendothelial cell junctions. Using anti-fibronectin antibodies, Nicolson *et al.* (143) reported that host fibronectin plays only a minor role in the adhesion of B16 melanoma cells to endothelial cells or basal lamina. Metastatic cells may, however, attach selectively to type IV collagen (134) or

to laminin via a specific cell-surface receptor (126, 203). Antibodies to laminin have been reported to decrease metastatic frequency in mouse lungs *in vivo* as well as to inhibit the attachment of tumor cells to a laminin-coated plastic substratum *in vitro* (202). Furthermore, alterations in laminin or laminin receptors on the cell surface of certain tumor cells can influence metastatic frequency (8, 127, 204). Although these results indicate that adhesion of certain tumor cells via laminin is an important step in the metastasis of those cells, it should be emphasized that other adhesive molecules in specific tissues or on different tumor cells may mediate adhesive interactions during metastasis.

Since tumor cells are rapidly destroyed in the bloodstream, specific adhesive interactions between tumor cells and vascular components that promote the removal of tumor cells from the circulation would likely promote subsequent metastasis formation. Such specific interactions could enhance extravasation of tumor cells by providing a necessary adhesive substrate for cell motility or by facilitating enzymatic degradation of the vascular basement membrane. There are probably several biochemical determinants that mediate adhesive interactions between tumor cells and host vascular components. Further elucidation of such adhesive interactions will permit better understanding of the relative contributions to the metastatic process of specific tumor cell adherence and other factors such as organ-modulation of tumor cell proliferation.

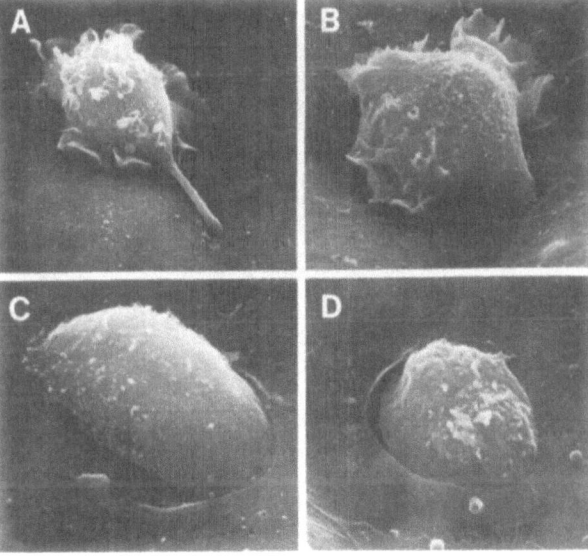

Figure 6. Model system for tumor cell extravasation. Murine ESb lymphoma cells are seen penetrating into a confluent monolayer of cultured bovine aortic endothelial cells. The tumor cells penetrate at intercellular junctions between adjacent endothelial cells. 6 hours (A), 18 hours (B, C), and 24 hours (D) after seeding, the cultures were washed, fixed, and processed for scanning electron microscopy (magnification: A × 3350, B × 6200: C × 6900: D × 9200). [Scanning electron micrographs provided by Israel Vlodavsky, Hadassah University Hospital, Israel.]

EXTRAVASATION OF TUMOR CELLS

After arrest in host organs, tumor cells may extravasate through the vascular endothelium and subsequently form metastases. To penetrate the layer of endothelium, tumor cells may pass between endothelial cells *in vivo* (37, 124, 189, 217). Such intercellular passage has also been observed *in vitro* (106, 145, 183, 210 and Fig. 6). However, tumor cells may extend protrusions or pseudopodia into endothelial cells and penetrate the endothelium by a transcellular route (31, 174). In addition, tumor cell entry into the organ parenchyma can be facilitated by destruction of the vascular wall (10, 19, 20, 121).

Tumor cell motility

Extravasation of metastatic cells may involve active tumor cell motility (196). This motility could be chemokinetic (non-directional) or chemotactic (directional) and would require adhesion to a component of the host vasculature. When tumor cells were assayed for their ability to move across gold coated coverslips in a quantitative phagokinetic assay, highly metastatic melanoma cell lines displayed significantly increased chemokinetic motility in comparison with low-metastatic melanoma cell lines (141, 212). Factors chemotactic for tumor cells have been reported (206). Such factors were first identified in tumor tissue (84, 228). However, tumor-derived factors probably have little involvement in the movement of tumor cells into tumor-free tissues. Other chemoattractants for tumor cells that have been identified include the complement component C5 (171), a bone resorption factor (150), low molecular weight peptides (220), collagen fragments (133), and a factor in inflammatory exudates (152). Recently, it was shown that extracts of specific organs stimulated the chemotactic migration of tumor cells that metastasize to those organs *in vivo* (92). Although

additional studies are needed, the current evidence does suggest a functional role for tumor cell motility during metastasis (151, 154). Because tumor cell motility may have a role in metastasis, inhibition of tumor cell migration by the host may have a protective function against metastasis. In support of this notion, lymphokine-containing supernatants obtained from cultures of activated lymphocytes were found to inhibit the migration of tumor cells *in vitro* (23, 24).

In addition to chemotaxis, the directed motility of tumor cells could be due to haptotaxis, which involves migration across a substratum-bound gradient of adhesive or attractant factors. Using a Schwann cell tumor line, tumor cells migrated by haptotaxis in response to substratum-bound laminin (128). B16 melanoma cells also demonstrated haptotactic migration in response to gradients of fibronectin or laminin (109, 129). Serum spreading factor promoted the haptotactic migration of murine and human tumor cells (9). Furthermore, highly metastatic murine fibrosarcoma cells migrated by haptotaxis in response to both laminin and fibronectin, whereas weakly metastatic cells did not demonstrate a haptotactic response (207). These results are of great interest and could help explain the migration of invading tumor cells across the extracellular matrix and the vascular basement membrane.

Degradation of the vascular basement membrane

The extravasation of metastatic cells is not complete until the tumor cells penetrate the vascular basement membrane. This step involves focal lysis of the basement membrane at points of contact with tumor cells followed by penetration of tumor cell pseudopodia through the basement membrane (6, 208). Experimental evidence indicates that degradative enzymes facilitate the penetration of metastatic tumor cells through the basement membrane (for reviews see 11, 66, 119, 120, 144, 156, 192, 226).

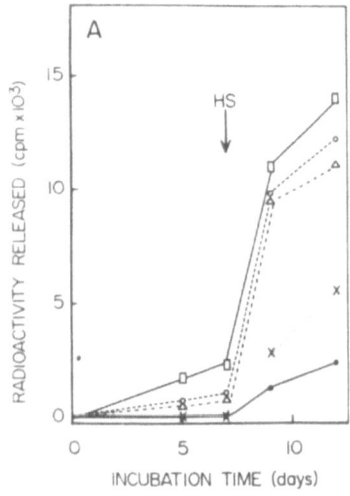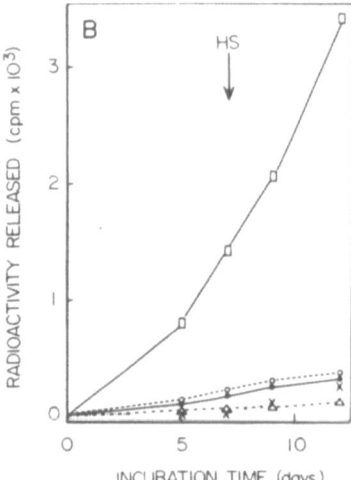

Figure 7. Digestion of complete (A) or glycoprotein-depleted (B) extracellular matrices by human tumor cells or fibroblasts. Matrices were labelled with [³H]fucose (A) or [³H]proline (B). Degradation of glycoprotein-depleted matrices represents tumor cell mediated collagen degradation. Enzymatic degradation of basement membrane components, such as collagen, may facilitate tumor cell penetration of the vascular wall. □, human fibrosarcoma; ○, human rhabdomyosarcoma; △, human neuroblastoma; ×, human osteogenic sarcoma; ●, normal human fibroblasts. [Reprinted from W.E. Laug *et al*. Cancer Res. 43:1827–34, 1983.]

Several enzymes have been implicated as mediators of tumor cell invasion of the vascular wall. Plasminogen activator, a serine protease, can activate latent collagenase and cause conversion of plasminogen to plasmin, which in turn can degrade basement membrane components (117, 131, 222). Antibodies to plasminogen activator were found to inhibit metastasis but not primary tumor growth in the chick embryo, which suggests that plasminogen activator is involved during tumor dissemination (153). In a recent study, a strong correlation between plasminogen activator activity and metastatic potential was found in comparison of clonal tumor cell populations isolated from a rat mammary adenocarcinoma (18). However, plasminogen activator levels have not correlated well with metastatic potential in all studies, perhaps because these studies compared different tumors or heterogeneous tumor sublines. Also, the variable results may be due to tumor release of inhibitors of plasminogen activator (87, 136) or diffusible factors that may induce adjacent normal cells to produce plasminogen activator (27). Other proteases, such as lysosomal cathepsin B, may have some role in the degradation of the basement membrane (105, 130, 164, 190, 191).

Because collagen is a major component of vascular basement membranes, it seems likely that collagenases could have a role in tumor cell invasion. Indeed, complete degradation of endothelial cell matrix was achieved by incubation of the matrix with tumor cells (11 and Figure 7). Tumor cells produce variable amounts of types I, IV, and V collagenases (118), which may be related to the predominant collagen types found in the different organs that metastatic cells colonize *in vivo*. In particular, type IV collagen is a major structural protein of basement membrane and type IV collagen-degrading activity has been correlated with metastatic potential (116). A neutral protease activity preferential for type IV collagen was isolated from metastatic tumor cells (115), then further purified and characterized (178).

Endo- and exoglycosidases may also have a role in degradation of the vascular basal lamina. Tumor cells can solubilize subendothelial glycoproteins and proteoglycans (108 and Figure 8; 209). Because heparan sulfate is a major scaffolding proteoglycan of the subendothelial basal lamina, it is especially interesting that heparan sulfate endoglycosidase activity correlated with metastatic capabilities of murine B16 melanoma variants (137) and murine T-lymphoma variants (211). The enzyme responsible for the degradation of heparan sulfate by B16 melanoma cells is heparanase, a heparan sulfate-specific endoglucuronidase (138). The relative contributions of endoglycosidases and other degradative enzymes to tumor cell extravasation and colonization of host organs remains to be determined.

demonstrated that an avascular tumor spheroid will reach a diameter of only 1–2 mm (approximately 10^6 cells) before the loss of cells due to death at the center of the sphere equals the rate of expansion due to cell proliferation at the periphery (49, 63). When this equilibrium point has been reached, the tumor can remain constant at this size *in situ* for over 20 years (158).

It is now apparent that a 1 mm tumor may commence rapid growth after the appearance of new host capillary blood vessels. The signal for the growth of these new capillaries is complex as it involves the production of not only angiogenic factors from the tumor itself (3, 47) but also products from accessory cells such as mast cells (5), lymphocytes (188) and macrophages (162, 163) at the tumor site. Virtually all angiogenic factors studied to date have been shown to stimulate capillary endothelial cell migration (184, 231) and most, but not all (7) can stimulate capillary endothelial cell proliferation *in vitro* (99, 232). The ubiquity of angiogenic factors in solid tumors has prompted their use as markers of neoplastic and preneoplastic tumor growth in

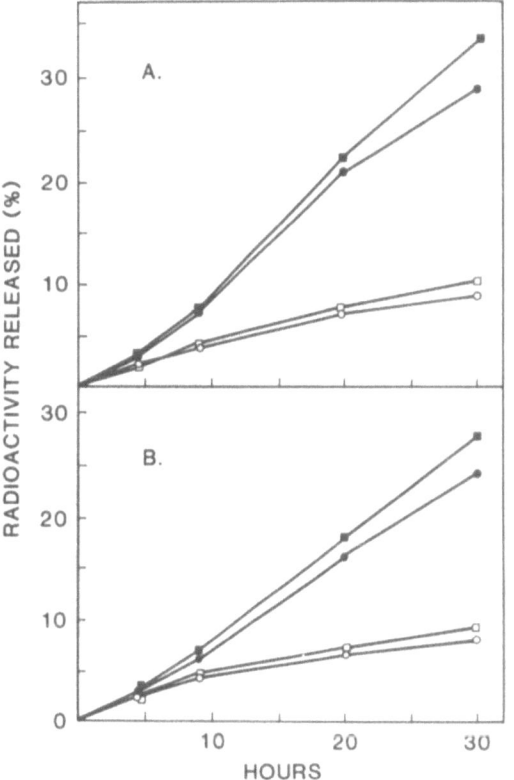

Figure 8. Solubilization of subendothelial matrix components by murine B16 melanoma cells. Matrix components were prelabeled with [^{35}S]Na$_2$SO$_4$ (A) or [^{3}H] leucine (B). Intact endothelial cell monolayers (■, □) or matrix (●, ○) were incubated with (■, ●) or without (□, ○) tumor cells at 37°C. As discussed in text, Nicolson and co-workers have subsequently demonstrated that the enzyme responsible for the degradation of ^{35}S-labeled proteoglycans is a heparanase and that the heparan sulfate endoglycosidase activity correlates with metastatic capabilities of B16 melanoma variants. [Reprinted from R.H. Kramer, K.G. Vogel, G.L. Nicolson. J. Biol. Chem. 257:2678–86, 1982.]

SECONDARY TUMOR GROWTH AND ANGIOGENESIS

The growth of a solid tumor in a new organ site depends primarily on two factors: the suitability of the microenvironment in supporting proliferation of those tumor cells and the ability of the growing tumor to elicit new blood vessels (48, 52, 53). The new vascular network is needed not only to provide nutrients to the growing tumor but also to carry away organic acids and other waste products. It has been

Table 2. Inhibition of metastasis formation with heparin plus cortisone.* Male C57BL/6 mice were treated with heparin (Abbott Panheparin; 200 U/ml delivered orally in the drinking water), hydrocortisone (Sigma; 250 mg/day administered subcutaneously), or both drugs as described by Folkman et al. (51). Inhibition of angiogenesis by heparin administered with cortisone prevented metastasis.

	Cell line	
Treatment	B16-F2 melanoma (lung metastases/mouse)	Reticulum cell sarcoma (liver metastases/mouse)
Water	38	129
Heparin	18	303
Cortisone	38	156
Heparin + cortisone	1	0

*Unpublished data, kindly provided by Judah Folkman.

sites including the human breast (14), eye (199, 200) and bladder (22).

Perhaps the most compelling evidence for the role of neovascularization in tumor growth is from anti-angiogenesis studies. Local and regional administration of cartilage or a cartilage extract inhibited angiogenesis and restricted tumor growth (13, 110). Taylor and Folkman (201) demonstrated that the heparin antagonist protamine could inhibit angiogenesis in two *in vivo* assay systems, the chick chorioallantoic membrane and the rabbit cornea. In addition, these investigators showed that protamine administered locally or systemically could inhibit primary *and* secondary solid tumor growth in mice, rats and rabbits. More recently, Folkman and co-workers (51) have shown that the combination of cortisone with heparin or a heparin fragment could inhibit angiogenesis, cause regression of large tumor masses, and prevent metastases of four murine tumors (Table 2). These dramatic results suggest that it is possible not only to inhibit growth but also to eradicate solid tumors by the use of agents whose primary action is to inhibit tumor-induced vascularization.

Once a metastatic tumor has established a proper vascular supply, its growth may be limited by the presence of inhibitors (chalones), by a suboptimal growth environment in the new organ, or by a cytotoxic response by the host. If such events fail to stop the growth of the metastases, they can easily saturate an entire organ. Furthermore, the new vessels that have grown in response to the tumor can serve as a conduit for the passage of further cells into the circulation to start the metastatic process anew.

ACKNOWLEDGEMENTS

PAN is a recipient of NIH Fellowship 5 T32 GM 07258. BRZ is a Glick-Franzheim Cancer Research Scholar and holds a Faculty Research Award (# 263) from the American Cancer Society. We are grateful to Mrs. P. Breen for manuscript preparation. We thank Ms. Catherine L. Hill and Drs. Patricia A. D'Amore, Julie Glowacki, and John C. Voyta for critical review of the manuscript.

REFERENCES

1. Alby L, Auerbach R: Differential adhesion of tumor cells to capillary endothelial cells *in vitro. Proc Natl Acad Sci USA* 81:5739–43, 1984
2. Algire GH, Chalkley HW: Vascular reactions of normal and maglinant tissues *in vivo*. I. Vascular reactions of mice to wounds and to normal and neoplastic transplants. *J Natl Cancer Inst* 6:73–85, 1945
3. Auerbach R: Angiogenesis-inducing factors: a review. *Lymphokines* 4:69–88, 1981
4. Ausprunk DH, Falterman K, Folkman J: The sequence of events in the regression of corneal capillaries. *Lab Invest* 38:284–94, 1978
5. Azizkhan RG, Azizkhan JC, Zetter BR, Folkman J: Mast cell heparin stimulates migration of capillary endothelial cells in vitro. *J Exp Med* 152:931–44, 1980
6. Babai F: Étude ultrastructural sur la pathogénie de l'invasion du muscle strié par des tumeurs transplantables. *J Ultrastr Res* 56:287–303, 1976
7. Banda MJ, Knighton DR, Hunt TK, Werb Z: Isolation of a nonmitogenic angiogenesis factor from wound fluid. *Proc Natl Acad Sci USA* 79:7773–77, 1982
8. Barsky SH, Rao CN, Williams JE, Liotta LA: Laminin molecular domains which alter metastasis in a murine model. *J Clin Invest* 74:843–8, 1984
9. Basara ML, McCarthy JB, Barnes DW, Furcht LT: Stimulation of haptotaxis and migration of tumor cells by serum spreading factor. *Cancer Res* 45:2487–94, 1985
10. Baserga R, Saffiotti U: Experimental studies on histogenesis of blood-borne metastases. *AMA Arch Pathol* 59:26–34, 1955
11. Bernacki RJ, Niedbala MJ, Korytnyk W: Glycosidases in cancer and invasion. *Cancer Metas Rev* 4:81–102, 1985
12. Brackenbury R, Greenberg ME, Edelman GM: Phenotypic changes and loss of N-CAM-mediated adhesion in transformed embryonic chicken retinal cells. *J Cell Biol* 99:1944–54, 1984
13. Brem H, Folkman J: Inhibition of tumor angiogenesis mediated by cartilage. *J Exp Med* 141:427–39, 1975
14. Brem SS, Jensen HM, Gullino PM: Angiogenesis as a marker of preneoplastic lesions of the human breast. *Cancer* 41:239–44, 1978
15. Brown JM: A study of the mechanism by which anticoagulation with warfarin inhibits blood-borne metastasis. *Cancer Res* 33:1217–24, 1973
16. Butcher EC, Scollay RG, Weissman IL: Organ specificity of lymphocyte migration mediation by highly selective lymphocyte interaction with organ-specific determinants on high endothelial venules. *Eur J Immunol* 10:556–61, 1980
17. Butler TP, Gullino PM: Quantitation of cell shedding into efferent blood of mammary adenocarcinoma. *Cancer Res* 35:512–16, 1975
18. Carlsen SA, Ramshaw IA, Warrington RC: Involvement of plasminogen activator production with tumor metastasis in a rat model. *Cancer Res* 44:3012–6, 1984
19. Carr I, McGinty F, Norris P: The fine structure of neoplastic invasion: invasion of liver, skeletal muscle and lymphatic vessels by the Rd/3 tumor. *J Pathol* 118:91–99, 1976
20. Chew EC, Josephson RL, Wallace AC: Morphologic aspects

of the arrest of circulating cancer cells. In: *Fundamental Aspects of Metastasis*, Weiss L, (ed). Amsterdam: North-Holland, pp 121–50, 1976

21. Chew EC, Wallace AC: Demonstration of fibrin in early stages of experimental metastases. *Cancer Res* 36:1904–9, 1976

22. Chodak GW, Scheiner C, Zetter BR: Urine from patients with transitional-cell carcinoma stimulates migration of capillary endothelial cells. *N Engl J Med* 305:869–874, 1981

23. Cohen MC, Goss A, Yoshida T, Cohen S: Inhibition of tumor cells *in vitro* by lymphokine-containing supernatants. *J Immunol* 121:840–3, 1978

24. Cohen MC, Forouhar F, Donskoy M, Cohen S: *In vitro* migration of tumor cells from human neoplasms: inhibition by lymphokines. *Clin Immunol Immunopath* 34:94–9, 1985

25. Colucci M, Giavazzi R, Allesandri G, Semeraro N, Mantovani A, Donati MB: Procoagulant activity of sarcoma sublines with different metastatic potential. *Blood* 57:733–5, 1981

26. Curatolo L, Colucci M, Cambini AL, Poggi A, Morasca L, Donati MB, Semeraro N: Evidence that cells from experimental tumours can activate coagulation factor X. *Br J Cancer* 40:228–33, 1979

27. Davies RL, Rifkin DB, Tepper R, Miller A, Kucherlapati R: A polypeptide secreted by transformed cells that modulates human plasminogen activator production. *Science* 221:171–3, 1983

28. De Bruyn PPH, Cho Y: Vascular endothelial invasion via transcellular passage by malignant cells in the primary stage of metastasis formation. *J Ultrastr Res* 81:189–201, 1982

29. Dennis J, Waller C, Timpl R, Schirrmacher V: Surface sialic acid reduces attachment of metastatic tumor cells to collagen type IV and fibronectin. *Nature* 300:274–6, 1982

30. Dennis JW, Carver JP, Schachter H: Asparagine-linked oligosaccharides in murine tumor cells: comparison of WGA-resistant (WGA^r) nonmetastatic mutant and a related WGA-sensitive (WGA^s) metastatic line. *J Cell Biol* 99:1034–44, 1984

31. Dingemans KP: Invasion of liver tissue by blood-borne mammary carcinoma cells. *J Natl Cancer Inst* 53:1813–24, 1974

32. Donati MB, Poggi A: Malignancy and haemostasis. *Br J Haem* 44:173–82, 1980

33. Dvorak HF, Dvorak AM, Manseau EJ, Wiberg L, Churchill WH: Fibrin-gel investment associated with line 1 and line 10 solid tumor growth, angiogenesis, and fibroplasia in guinea pigs. Role of cellular immunity, myofibroblasts, microvascular damage, and infarction in line 1 tumor regression. *J Natl Cancer Inst* 62:1459–72, 1979

34. Dvorak HF, Quay SC, Orenstein NS, Dvorak AM, Hahn P, Bitzer AM, Carvalho AC: Tumor shedding and coagulation. *Science* 212:923–4, 1981

35. Dvorak HF, Senger DR, Dvorak AM: Fibrin as a component of the tumor stroma: origins and biological significance. *Cancer Metas Rev* 2:41–73, 1983

36. Dvorak HF, Senger DR, Dvorak AM, Harvey VS, McDonagh J: Regulation of extravascular coagulation by microvascular permeability. *Science* 227:1059–61, 1985

37. Fasske E, Fetting R, Rühland D, Schubert T, Themann H: Colonization of the mouse liver by transplanted virogenic leukemia cells. Electron microscopic investigations. *Z Krebsforsch* 84:257–69, 1975

38. Fidler IJ: Metastasis: quantitative analysis of distribution and fate of tumor emboli labeled with ^{125}I-5-iodo-2′-deoxyuridine. *J Natl Cancer Inst* 45:773–82, 1970

39. Fidler IJ: The relationship of embolic homogeneity, number, size, and viability to the incidence of experimental metastasis. *Eur J Cancer* 9:223–7, 1973

40. Fidler IJ: Biological behavior of malignant melanoma cells

correlated to their survival in vivo. *Cancer Res* 35:218–24, 1975

41. Fidler IJ, Nicholson GL: Organ-selectivity for implantation, survival, and growth of B16 melanoma variant tumor lines. *J Natl Cancer Inst* 57:1199–202, 1976

42. Fidler IJ, Bucana C: Mechanism of tumor cell resistance to lysis by syngeneic lymphocytes. *Cancer Res* 37:3945–56, 1977

43. Fidler IJ, Gersten DM, Riggs CW: Relationship of host immune status to tumor cell arrest, distribution, and survival in experimental metastasis. *Cancer* 40:46–55, 1977

44. Fidler IJ, Hart IR: Biological diversity in metastatic neoplasms: origins and implications. *Science* 217:998–1003, 1982

45. Fidler IJ: Eradication of metastases by tumoricidal macrophages: therapeutic implications. In: *Tumor Invasion and Metastasis*, Liotta LA, Hart IR (eds). Boston: Martinus Nijhoff, pp 15–27, 1982

46. Fisher B, Fisher ER: The organ distribution of disseminated ^{51}Cr-labeled tumor cells. *Cancer Res* 27:412–20, 1967

47. Folkman J, Merler E, Abernathy C, Williams G: Isolation of a tumor factor responsible for angiogenesis. *J Exp Med* 133:275–88, 1971

48. Folkman J, Cotran R: Relation of vascular proliferation to tumor growth. *Int Rev Exp Pathol* 16:207–48, 1976

49. Folkman J, Hochberg M: Self-regulation of growth in three dimensions. *J Exp Med* 138:745–53, 1973

50. Folkman J, Tyler K: Tumor angiogenesis: its possible role in metastasis and invasion. In: *Cancer Invasion and Metastasis: Biologic Mechanisms and Therapy*. Day SB *et al.* (eds). New York: Raven Press, pp 95–103, 1977

51. Folkman J, Langer R, Linhardt RJ, Haudenschild C, Taylor S: Angiogenesis inhibition and tumor regression caused by heparin or a heparin fragment in the presence of cortisone. *Science* 221:719–25, 1983

52. Folkman J: Angiogenesis. In: *The Biology of Endothelial Cells*, Jaffe E (ed). Boston: Martinus Nijhoff, pp 412–28, 1984

53. Folkman J: Tumor angiogenesis. *Adv Cancer Res* 43:175–203, 1985

54. Galtin JE, Xue B, Hochwald GM, Thorbecke GJ: Derivation of transplantable, dimethylbenzanthracene-induced chicken fibrosarcoma lines with differences in metastasizing properties and organ specificity. *J Natl Cancer Inst* 69:535–41, 1982

55. Gasic GJ, Gasic TB, Stewart CC: Antimetastatic effects associated with platelet reduction. *Proc Natl Acad Sci USA* 61:46–52, 1968

56. Gasic GJ, Gasic TB, Murphy S: Anti-metastatic effect of aspirin. *Lancet* 2:932–3, 1972

57. Gasic GJ, Gasic TB, Galanti N, Johnson T, Murphy S: Platelet-tumor cell interactions in mice. The role of platelets in the spread of malignant disease. *Int J Cancer* 11:704–18, 1973

58. Gasic GJ, Koch PA, Hsu B, Gasic TB, Niewiarowski S: Thrombogenic activity of mouse and human tumors: effects on platelets, coagulation, and fibrinolysis, and possible significance for metastasis. *Z Krebsforsch* 86:263–77, 1976

59. Gasic GJ, Gasic TB, Jiminez SA: Effects of trypsin on the platelet-aggregating activity of mouse tumor cells. *Thromb Res* 10:33–45, 1977

60. Gasic GJ: Role of plasma, platelets, and endothelial cells in tumor metastasis. *Cancer Metas Rev* 3:99–116, 1984

61. Gerson JM, Schlesinger HR, Sereni P, Moorhead PS, Hummeler K: Isolation and characterization of a neuroblastoma cell line from peripheral blood in a patient with disseminated disease. *Cancer* 39:2508–12, 1977

62. Gilbert LC, Gordon SG: Relationship between cellular procoagulant activity and metastatic capacity of B16 mouse melanoma variants. *Cancer Res* 43:536–40, 1983

63. Gimbrone MA Jr, Leapman SB, Cotran RS, Folkman J: Tumor dormancy in vivo by prevention of neovascularization. *J Exp Med* 136:261–76, 1972

64. Glaves D: Correlation between circulating cancer cells and incidence of metastases. *Br J Cancer* 48:665–73, 1983a

65. Glaves D: Role of polymorphonuclear leukocytes in the pulmonary clearance of arrested cancer cells. *Inv Metas* 3:160–73, 1983b

66. Goldfarb RH: Proteases in tumor invasion and metastasis. In: *Tumor Invasion and Metastasis*, Liotta LA, Hart IR (eds). Boston: Martinus Nijhoff, pp 375–90, 1982

67. Golinger RC, Gregorio RM, Fisher ER: Tumor cells in venous blood draining mammary carcinomas. *Arch Surg* 112:707–8, 1977

68. Gordon SG, Franks JJ, Lewis B: Cancer Procoagulant A: a factor X activating procoagulant from malignant tissue, *Thromb Res* 6:127–37, 1975

69. Gordon SG, Cross BA: A factor X-activating cysteine protease from malignant tissue. *J Clin Invest* 67:1665–71, 1981

70. Greenbaum LM: Pepstatin, an inhibitor of acid kininogenases and ascites retardant in neoplastic disease. *Fed Proc* 38:2788–91, 1979

71. Greene HSN, Harvey EK: The relationship between the dissemination of tumor cells and the distribution of metastases. *Cancer Res* 24:799–811, 1964

72. Griffiths JD, Salsbury AJ: The fate of circulating Walker 256 tumour cells injected intravenously into rat. *Br J Cancer* 17:546–57, 1963

73. Griffiths JD, McKinna JA, Rowbotham HD, Tsolakidis P, Salsbury AJ: Carcinoma of the colon and rectum: circulating malignant cells and five-year survival. *Cancer* 31:226–36, 1973

74. Grimstad IA, Varani J, McCoy JP Jr: Contribution of α-D-galactopyranosyl end groups to attachment of highly and low metastatic murine fibrosarcoma cells to various substrates. *Exp Cell Res* 155:345–58, 1984

75. Guaitani A, Květina J, Garattini S: Isolated perfused liver: a model for studies on cancer-cell dissemination. *Eur J Cancer* 8:79–84, 1972

76. Guy D, Latner AL, Sherbet GV, Turner GA: Surface properties of cells isolated from non-metastasizing and metastasizing hamster lymphosarcomas. *Br J Cancer* 42:915–21, 1980

77. Hanna N: Expression of metastatic potential of tumor cells in young nude mice is correlated with low levels of NK cell-mediated cytotoxicity. *Int J Cancer* 26:675–80, 1980

78. Hanna N: Inhibition of experimental tumor metastasis by selective activation of natural killer cells. *Cancer Res* 42:1337–42, 1982

79. Hanna N, Fidler IJ: Role of natural killer cells in the destruction of circulating tumor emboli. *J Natl Cancer Inst* 65:800–12, 1980

80. Hara Y, Steiner M, Baldoni MG: Platelets as a source of growth-promoting factor(s) for tumor cells. *Cancer Res* 40:1212–6, 1980

81. Hart IR, Fidler IR: Role of organ selectivity in the determination of metastatic patterns of B16 melanoma. *Cancer Res* 40:2281–7, 1980

82. Hart IR, Talmadge JE, Fidler IJ: Metastatic behavior of a murine reticulum cell sarcoma exhibiting organ-specific growth. *Cancer Res* 41:2181–87, 1981

83. Hart IR: 'Seed and soil' revisited: mechanisms of site-specific metastasis. *Cancer Metas Rev* 1:5–16, 1982

84. Hayashi H, Yoshida K, Ozaki T, Ushijima K: Chemotactic factor associated with invasion of cancer cells. *Nature (London)* 226:174–5, 1970

85. Herberman RB, Holden HT: Natural cell-mediated immunity. *Adv Cancer Res* 27:305–77, 1978

86. Hewitt HB, Blake A: Quantitative studies of tranlymphonodal passage of tumor cells naturally disseminated from a non-immunogenic murine squamous carcinoma. *Br J Cancer* 31:25–35, 1975

87. Hisazumi H, Naito K, Misaki T, Kosaka S: Urokinase in-

88. hibitor in patients with bladder cancer. *Urol Res* 2:137–42, 1974

89. Hobson B, Denekamp J: Endothelial proliferation in tumours and normal tissues: continuous labelling studies. *Br J Cancer* 49:405–13, 1984

89. Honn KV, Cicone B, Skoff A: Prostacyclin: a potent antimetastatic agent. *Science* 212:1270–2, 1981

90. Honn KV, Meyer J, Neagos G, Henderson T, Westley C, Ratanatharathorn V: Control of tumor growth and metastasis with prostacyclin and thromboxane synthetase inhibitors: evidence for a new antitumor and antimetastatic agent (BAY g 6575). *Progr Clin Biol Res* 89:295–331, 1982

91. Honn KV, Onoda JM, Pampalona K, Battaglia M, Neagos G, Taylor JD, Diglio CA, Sloane BF: Inhibition by dihydropyridine class calcium channel blockers of tumor cell-platelet-endothelial cell interactions *in vitro* and metastasis *in vivo*. *Biochem Pharmacol* 34:235–41, 1985

92. Hujanen ES, Terranova VP: Migration of tumor cells to organ-derived chemoattractants: *Cancer Res* 45:3517–21, 1985

93. Ioachim HL, Pearse A, Keller SE: Role of immune mechanisms in metastatic patterns of hemopoietic tumors in rats. *Cancer Res* 36:2854–62, 1976

94. Irimura T, Nicolson GL: The role of glycoconjugates in metastatic melanoma blood-borne arrest and cell surface properties. *J Supramol Struct Cell Biochem* 17:325–36, 1981

95. Irimura T, Gonzales R, Nicolson GL: Effects of tunicamycin on B16 metastatic melanoma cell surface glycoproteins and blood-borne arrest and survival properties. *Cancer Res* 41:3411–18, 1981

96. James K, McBride B, Stuart A: *The Macrophage and Cancer*. Edinburgh: Econoprint, 1977

97. Johnston MM, Greenbaum LM: Leukokinin-forming system in the ascitic fluid of a murine mastocytoma. *Biochem Pharmacol* 22:1386–9, 1973

98. Kahan B: Ovarian localization by embryonal teratocarcinoma cells derived from female germ cells. *Somatic Cell Genet* 5:763–80, 1979

99. Keegan A, Hill C, Kumar S, Phillips P, Schor A, Weiss J: Purified tumor angiogenesis factor enhances proliferation of capillary but not aortic endothelial cells *in vitro*. *J Cell Sci* 55:261–276, 1982

100. Kepner N, Lipton A: A mitogenic factor for transformed fibroblasts from human platelets. *Cancer Res* 41:430–2, 1981

101. Key ME: Macrophages in cancer metastasis and their relevance to metastatic growth. *Cancer Metas Rev* 2:75–88, 1983

102. Kieran MW, Longnecker BM: Organ specific metastasis with special reference to avian systems. *Cancer Metas Rev* 2:165–82, 1983

103. Kodama M, Kodama T: Enhancing effect of hydrocortisone on hematogenous metastasis of Ehrlich ascites tumor in mice. *Cancer Res* 35:1015–21, 1975

104. Koo J, Fung K, Siu KF, Lee NW, Lett Z, Ho J, Wong J, Ong GB: Recovery of malignant tumor cells from the right atrium during hepatic resection for hepatocellular carcinoma. *Cancer* 52:1952–6, 1983

105. Kramer MD, Robinson P, Vlodavsky I, Barz D, Friberger P, Schirrmacher V: Characterization of an extracellular matrix-degrading protease derived from a highly metastatic tumor cell line. *Eur J Cancer Clin Oncol* 21:307–16, 1985

106. Kramer RH, Nicolson GL: Interactions of tumor cells with vascular endothelial cell monolayers: a model for metastatic invasion. *Proc Natl Acad Sci USA* 76:5704–8, 1979

107. Kramer RH, Gonzalez R, Nicolson GL: Metastatic tumor cells adhere preferentially to the extracellular matrix underlying vascular endothelial cells. *Int J Cancer* 26:639–45, 1980

108. Kramer RH, Vogel KG, Nicolson GL: Solubilization and degradation of subendothelial matrix glycoproteins and pro-

teoglycans by metastatic tumor cells. *J Biol Chem* 257:2678–86, 1982

109. Lacovara J, Cramer EB, Quigley JP: Fibronectin enhancement of directed migration of B16 melanoma cells. *Cancer Res* 44:1657–63, 1984

110. Langer R, Conn H, Vacanti J, Haudenschild C, Folkman J: Control of tumor growth in animals by infusion of an angiogenesis inhibitor. *Proc Natl Acad Sci USA* 77:4331–5, 1980

111. Laug WE, DeClerck YA, Jones PA: Degradation of subendothelial matrix by tumor cells. *Cancer Res* 43:1827–34, 1983

112. Liotta LA, Kleinerman J, Saidel GM: Quantitative relationships of intravascular tumor cells, tumor vessels, and pulmonary metastasis following tumor implantation. *Cancer Res* 34:997–1004, 1974

113. Liotta AL, Kleinerman J, Saidel GM: The significance of hematogenous tumor cell clumps and the metastatic process. *Cancer Res* 36:889–94, 1976

114. Liotta LA, DeLisi C: Method for quantitating tumor cell removal and tumor cell-invasive capacity in experimental metastases. *Cancer Res* 37:4003–8, 1977

115. Liotta LA, Abe S, Gehron-Robey P, Martin GR: Preferential digestion of basement membrane collagen by an enzyme derived from a metastatic murine tumor. *Proc Natl Acad Sci USA* 76:2268–72, 1979

116. Liotta LA, Tryggvason K, Garbisa S, Hart I, Foltz CM, Shafie S: Metastatic potential correlates with enzymatic degradation of basement membrane collagen. *Nature (London)* 284:67–8, 1980

117. Liotta LA, Goldfarb RH, Brundage R, Siegal GP, Terranova SV, Garbisa S. Effect of plasminogen activator (urokinase), plasmin, and thrombin on glycoprotein and collagenous components of basement membrane. *Cancer Res* 41:4629–36, 1981a

118. Liotta LA, Lanzer WL, Garbisa S: Identification of a type V collagenolytic enzyme. *Biochem Biophys Res Commun* 98:184–90, 1981b

119. Liotta LA, Garbisa S, Tryggvason K: Biochemical mechanisms involved in tumor cell penetration of the basement membrane. In: *Tumor Invasion and Metastasis*, Liotta LA, Hart IR (eds). Boston: Martinus Nijhoff, pp 319–33, 1982

120. Liotta LA, Rao CN, Barsky SH: Tumor invasion and the extracellular matrix. *Lab Invest* 49:636–49, 1983

121. Locker J, Goldblatt PJ, Leighton J: Ultrastructural features of invasion in chick embryo liver metastasis of Hoshida ascites hepatoma. *Cancer Res* 30:1632–44, 1970

122. Long DM: Capillary ultrastructure in human metastatic brain tumors. *J Neurosurg* 51:53–8, 1979

123. Lotan R, Raz A: Low colony formation *in vivo* and in culture as exhibited by metastatic melanoma cells selected for reduced homotypic aggregation. *Cancer Res* 43:2088–93, 1983

124. Ludatscher RM, Luse SA, Suntzeff V: An electron microscopic study of pulmonary tumor emboli from transplanted Morris hepatoma 5123. *Cancer Res* 27:1939–52, 1967

125. Maillard JL, Pick E, Turk JL: Interaction between 'sensitized lymphocytes' and antigen in vitro. V. Vascular permeability induced by skin reactive factor. *Int Arch Allergy* 42:50–68, 1972

126. Malinoff HL, Wicha MS: Isolation of a cell surface receptor protein for laminin from murine fibrosarcoma cells. *J Cell Biol* 96:1475–9, 1983

127. Malinoff HL, McCoy JP Jr, Varani J, Wicha MS: Metastatic potential of murine fibrosarcoma cells is influenced by cell surface laminin. *Int J Cancer* 33:651–5, 1984

128. McCarthy JB, Palm SL, Furcht LT: Migration by haptotaxis of a Schwann cell tumor line to the basement membrane glycoprotein laminin. *J Cell Biol* 97:772–7, 1983

129. McCarthy JB, Furcht LT: Laminin and fibronectin promote the haptotactic migration of B16 mouse melanoma cells in

130. Mort JS, Recklies AD, Poole AR: Characterization of a thiol proteinase secreted by malignant human breast tumours. *Biochim Biophys Acta* 614:134–43, 1980

131. Mullins DE, Rohrlich ST: The role of proteinases in cellular invasiveness. *Biochim Biophys Acta* 695:177–214, 1983

132. Mullins DE, Rifkin DB: Stimulation of motility in cultured bovine capillary endothelial cells by angiogenic preparations. *J Cell Physiol* 119:247–54, 1984

133. Mundy GR, DeMartino S, Rowe DW: Collagen and collagen-derived fragments are chemotactic for tumor cells. *J Clin Invest* 68:1102–5, 1981

134. Murray JC, Liotta L, Rennard SI, Martin GR: Adhesion characteristics of murine metastatic and nonmetastatic tumor cells *in vitro*. *Cancer Res* 40:347–51, 1980

135. Nachman RL: The platelet as an inflammatory cell. In: *Platelets: A Multidisciplinary Approach*, deGaetano G, Gerattini S (eds). New York: Raven Press, pp 199–203, 1978

136. Naito S, Kinjo M, Nanno S, Kohga S, Oka K, Tanaka K: Fibrinolysis-inhibitory activity of cultured human cancer cell lines. *Gann* 72:1–7, 1981

137. Nakajima M, Irimura T, DiFerrante D, DiFerrante N, Nicolson GL: Heparan sulfate degradation: relation to tumor invasive and metastatic properties of mouse B16 melanoma sublines. *Science* 220:611–3, 1983

138. Nakajima M, Irimura T, DiFerrante N, Nicolson GL: Metastatic melanoma cell heparanase. Characterization of heparan sulfate degradation fragments produced by B16 melanoma endoglucuronidase. *J Biol Chem* 259:2283–90, 1984

139. Netland PA, Zetter BR: Organ-specific binding of tumor cells *in vitro*. *J Cell Biol* 97:90a, 1983

140. Netland PA, Zetter BR: Organ-specific adhesion of metastatic tumor cells *in vitro*. *Science* 224:1113–5, 1984

141. Netland PA, Zetter BR: Metastatic potential of B16 melanoma cells after *in vitro* selection for organ-specific adherence. *J Cell Biol*, 101(3):720–24, 1985

142. Nicolson GL, Winkelhake JL: Organ specificity of blood-borne tumour metastasis determined by cell adhesion? *Nature (London)* 255:230–2, 1975

143. Nicolson GL, Irimura T, Gonzalez R, Ruoslahti E: The role of fibronectin in adhesion of metastatic melanoma cells to endothelial cells and their basal lamina. *Exp Cell Res* 135:461–5, 1981

144. Nicolson GL: Cancer metastasis: organ colonization and the cell-surface properties of malignant cells. *Biochim Biophys Acta* 695:113–76, 1982a

145. Nicolson GL: Metastatic tumor cell attachment and invasion assay utilizing vascular endothelial cell monolayers. *J Histochem Cytochem* 30:214–20, 1982b

146. Nicolson GL, Mascali JJ, McGuire EJ: Metastatic RAW117 lymphosarcoma as a model for malignant-normal cell interactions: possible roles for cell surface antigens in determining the quantity and location of secondary tumors. *Oncodev Biol Med* 4:149–59, 1982

147. Nicolson GL, Dulski K, Basson C, Welch DR: Preferential organ attachment and invasion *in vitro* by B16 melanoma cells selected for differing metastatic colonization and invasive properties. *Invasion Metas* 5:144–58, 1985

148. Nicosia RF, Tchao R, Leighton J: Angiogenesis-dependent tumor spread in reinforced fibrin clot culture. *Cancer Res* 43:2159–66, 1983

149. O'Meara RAQ: Coagulative properties of cancer. *Irish J Med Sci* 6:474–9, 1958

150. Orr W, Varani J, Gondek MD, Ward PA, Mundy GR: Chemotactic responses of tumor cells to products of resorbing bone. *Science* 203:176–9, 1979

151. Orr FW, Mokashi S, Delikatny J: Generation of a complement-derived chemotactic factor for tumor cells in experi-

mentally induced peritoneal exudates and its effects on the local metastasis of circulating tumor cells. *Am J Pathol* 108:112–8, 1982

152. Orr FW, Adamson IYR, Young L: Pulmonary inflammation generates chemotactic activity for tumor cells and promotes lung metastasis. *Am Rev Respir Dis* 131:607–11, 1985

153. Ossowski L, Reich E: Antibodies to plasminogen activator inhibit human tumor metastasis. *Cell* 35:611–9, 1983

154. Ozaki T, Yoshida K, Ushijima K, Hayashi H: Studies on the mechanism of invasion in cancer. II. *In vivo* effects of a factor chemotactic for cancer cells. *Int J Cancer* 7:93–100, 1971

155. Parks RC: Organ-specific metastasis of a transplantable reticulum cell sarcoma. *J Natl Cancer Inst* 52:971–3, 1974

156. Pauli BU, Schwartz DE, Thonar EJ-M, Kuettner KE: Tumor invasion and host extracellular matrix. *Cancer Metas Rev* 2:129–52, 1983

157. Pearlstein E, Salk PL, Yogeeswaran G, Karpatkin S: Correlation between spontaneous metastatic potential, platelet-aggregating activity of cell surface extracts, and cell surface sialylation in 10 metastatic-variant derivatives of rat renal sarcoma cell line. *Proc Natl Acad Sci USA* 77:4336–9, 1980

158. Petersen O: Spontaneous course of cervical precancerous lesions. *Am J Obstet Gynecol* 72:1063–71, 1956

159. Phondke GP, Madyastha KR, Madyastha PR, Barth RF: Relationship between concanavalin A-induced agglutinability of murine leukemia cells and their propensity to form heterotypic aggregates with syngeneic lymphoid cells. *J Natl Cancer Inst* 66:643–7, 1981

160. Pilgrim HI: The metastatic behavior of a spleen-tropic reticulum cell sarcoma in splenectomized mice. *Proc Soc Exp Biol Med* 138:178–80, 1971

161. Pineo GF, Rogoeczi E, Hatton MWC, Brian MC: The activation of coagulation of extracts of mucus: a possible pathway of intravascular coagulation accompanying adenocarcinomas. *J Lab Clin Med* 82:255–64, 1973

162. Polverini PJ, Cotran RS, Gimbrone MA, Unanue E: Activated macrophages induce vascular proliferation. *Nature (London)* 269:804–6, 1977

163. Polverini PJ, Leibovich SJ: Induction of neovascularization *in vivo* and endothelial proliferation *in vitro* by tumor-associated macrophages. *Lab Invest* 51:635–42, 1984

164. Poole AR, Tiltman KJ, Recklies AD, Stoker TAM: Differences in secretion of the proteinase cathepsin B at the edges of human breast carcinomas and fibroadenomas. *Nature (London)* 273:545–7, 1978

165. Poste G, Fidler IJ: The pathogenesis of cancer metastasis. *Nature (London)* 283:139–46, 1980

166. Poste G, Doll J, Hart IR, Fidler IJ: *In vitro* selection of murine B16 melanoma variants with enhanced tissue-invasive properties. *Cancer Res* 40:1636–44, 1980

167. Proctor JW: Rat sarcoma model supports both "soil seed" and "mechanical" theories of metastatic spread. *Br J Cancer* 34:651–4, 1976

168. Raz A, Hart IR: Murine melanoma: a model for intracranial metastasis. *Br J Cancer* 42:331–41, 1980

169. Raz A, Lotan R: Lectin-like activities associated with human and murine neoplastic cells. *Cancer Res* 41:3642–7, 1981

170. Repesh LA, Fitzgerald TJ: Interactions of tumor cells with intact capillaries: a model for intravasation. *Clin Expl Metastasis* 2:139–50, 1984

171. Romualdez AG, Ward PA: A unique complement-derived chemotactic factor for tumor cells. *Proc Natl Acad Sci USA* 72:4128–32, 1975

172. Romualdez AG, Ward PA, Torikata T: Relationship between the C5 peptides chemotactic for leukocytes and tumor cells. *J Immunol* 117:1762–6, 1975

173. Roos E, Dingemans KP, Van de Pavert IV, Van den Bergh-Weerman M: Invasion of lymphosarcoma cells into the perfused mouse liver. *J Natl Cancer Inst* 58:399–407, 1977

174. Roos E, Dingemans KP: Mechanisms of metastasis. *Biochim Biophys Acta* 560:135–66, 1979

175. Roos E, Tulp A, Middelkoop OP, Van de Pavert IV: Interactions between lymphoid tumor cells and isolated liver endothelial cells. *J Natl Cancer Inst* 72:1173–80, 1984

176. Sadler TE, Alexander P: Trapping and destruction of blood-borne syngeneic leukaemia cells in lung, liver, and spleen of normal and leukaemic rats. *Br J Cancer* 33:512–20, 1976

177. Sako K, Marchetta FC: Radioautography of *in vitro* labeled tumor cells in postoperative wound drainage. *Cancer* 19:735–7, 1966

178. Salo T, Liotta LA, Tryggvason K: Purification and characterization of a murine basement membrane collagen-degrading enzyme secreted by metastatic tumor cells. *J Biol Chem* 258:3058–63, 1983

179. Salsbury AJ, Burrage K, Hellmann K: Histological analysis of the anti-metastatic effect of ($\pm$)-1,2-bis (3,5-dioxopiperazin-1-yl)-propane. *Cancer Res* 34:843–9, 1974

180. Sato H, Suzuki M: Deformability and viability of tumor cells by transcapillary passage, with reference to organ affinity in metastasis in cancer. In: *Fundamental Aspects of Metastasis*, Weiss L (ed). Amsterdam: North-Holland, pp 311–7, 1976

181. Schirrmacher V, Shantz G, Clouer K, Komitowski D, Zimmerman H-P, Lohman-Matthes M-L: Tumor metastases and cell-mediated immunity in a model system in DBA/2 mice. I. Tumor invasiveness *in vitro* and metastasis formation *in vivo*. *Int J Cancer* 23:233–44, 1979

182. Schirrmacher V, Cheingsong-Popov R, Arnheiter H: Hepatocyte-tumor cell interaction *in vitro*; I. Conditions for rosette formation and inhibition by anti-H-2 antibody. *J Exp Med* 151:984–9, 1980

183. Schirrmacher V, Vlodavsky I: *In vitro* interactions of aortic endothelial cell monolayers with tumor cell lines of different invasive and metastatic capacity. *Prog Appl Microcirc* 1:103–13, 1983

184. Schirrmacher V: Cancer metastasis: experimental approaches, theoretical concepts, and impacts for treatment strategies. *Adv Cancer Res* 43:1–73, 1985

185. Schlepper-Schäfer J, Friedrich E, Kolb H: Galactosyl specific receptor on liver cells: binding site for tumor cells. *Eur J Cell Biol* 25:95–102, 1981

186. Senger DR, Galli SJ, Dvorak AM, Perruzzi CA, Harvey VS, Dvorak HF: Tumor cells secrete a vascular permeability factor that promotes accumulation of ascites fluid. *Science* 219:983–5, 1983

187. Shearman PJ, Gallatin WM, Longenecker BM: Detection of a cell-surface antigen correlated with organ-specific metastasis. *Nature (London)* 286:267–9, 1980

188. Sidky YA, Auerbach R:Lymphocyte-induced angiogenesis: a quantitative and sensitive assay of the graft-vs.-host reaction. *J Exp Med* 141:1084–100, 1975

189. Sindelar WF, Tralka TS, Ketcham AS: Electron microscopic observation on formation of pulmonary metastasis. *J Surg Res* 18:137–61, 1975

190. Sloane BF, Dunn JR, Honn KV: Lysosomal cathepsin B: correlation with metastatic potential. *Science* 212:1151–3, 1981

191. Sloane BF, Honn KV, Sadler JG, Turner WA, Kimpson JJ, Taylor JD: Cathepsin B activity in B16 melanoma cells: a possible marker for metastatic potential. *Cancer Res* 42:980–6, 1982

192. Sloane BF, Honn KV: Cysteine proteinases and metastasis. *Cancer Metas Rev* 3:249–63, 1984

193. Springer GF, Cheingsong-Popov R, Schirrmacher V, Desai PR, Tegtmeyer H: Proposed molecular basis of murine tumor cell-hepatocyte interaction. *J Biol Chem* 258:5702–6, 1983

194. Stamper HB Jr, Woodruff JJ: Lymphocyte homing into lymph nodes: *in vitro* demonstration of the selective affinity

of recirculating lymphocytes for high endothelial venules. *J Exp Med* 144:828–33, 1976

195. Starkey JR, Liggitt HD, Hosick HL: Influence of migratory blood cells on the attachment of tumor cells to vascular endothelium. *Int J Cancer* 34:535–43, 1984
196. Sträuli P, Weiss L: Cell locomotion and tumor penetration. *Eur J Cancer* 13:1–12, 1977
197. Sugarbaker EV: Patterns of metastasis in human malignancies. *Cancer Biol Rev* 2:235–78, 1981
198. Talmadge JE: The selective nature of metastasis. *Cancer Metas Rev* 2:25–40, 1983
199. Tapper D, Langer R, Bellows AR, Folkman J: Angiogenesis capacity as a diagnostic marker for human eye tumors. *Surgery* 86:36–40, 1979
200. Tapper D, Albert DM, Robinson NL, Zetter BR: Capillary endothelial cell migration: stimulating activity of aqueous humor from patients with ocular cancers. *J Natl Cancer Inst* 71:501–5, 1983
201. Taylor S, Folkman J: Protamine is an inhibitor of angiogenesis. *Nature (London)* 297:307–12, 1982
202. Terranova VP, Liotta LA, Russo RG, Martin GR: Role of laminin in the attachment and metastasis of murine tumor cells. *Cancer Res* 42:2265–9, 1982
203. Terranova VP, Rao CN, Kalebic T, Margulies IM, Liotta LA: Laminin receptor on breast carcinoma cells. *Proc Natl Acad Sci USA* 80:444–8, 1983
204. Terranova VP, Williams JE, Liotta LA, Martin GR: Modulation of the metastatic activity of melanoma cells by laminin and fibronectin. *Science* 226:982–5, 1984
205. Vaage J: *In vivo* and *in vitro* lysis of mouse cancer cells by anti-metastatic effectors in normal plasma. *Cancer Immunol Immunother* 4:257–61, 1978
206. Varani J, Ward PA: Tumor cell chemotaxis. In: *Tumor Invasion and Metastasis*, Liotta LA, Hart IR (eds). Boston: Martinus Nijhoff, pp 99–112, 1982
207. Varani J, Fligiel SEG, Perone P: Directional motility in strongly malignant murine tumor cells. *Int J Cancer* 35:559–64, 1985
208. Vlaeminck MN, Adenis L, Mouton Y, Demaille A: Étude expérimentale de la diffusion métastatique chez l'oeuf de poule embryonné. Répartition, microscopie et ultrastructure des foyers tumouraux. *Int J Cancer* 10:619–31, 1972
209. Vlodavsky I, Ariav Y, Atzmon R, Fuks Z: Tumor cell attachment to the vascular endothelium and subsequent degradation of the subendothelial extracellular matrix. *Exp Cell Res* 140:149–59, 1982
210. Vlodavsky I, Fuks Z, Schirrmacher V: In vitro studies on tumor cell interaction with the vascular endothelium and the subendothelial basal lamina: relationship to tumor cell metastasis. In: *The Endothelial Cell – A Pluripotent Control Cell of the Vessel Wall*, Thilo-Körner DGS, Freshney RI (eds). Basel: S. Karger, pp 126–57, 1983a
211. Vlodavsky I, Fuks Z, Bar-Ner M, Ariav Y, Schirrmacher V: Lymphoma cell mediated degradation of sulfated proteoglycans in the subendothelial extracellular matrix: relationship to tumor cell metastasis. *Cancer Res* 43:2704–11, 1983b
212. Volk T, Geiger B, Raz A: Motility and adhesive properties of high- and low-metastatic murine neoplastic cells. *Cancer Res* 44:811–24, 1984
213. Vollmers HP, Birchmeier W: Monoclonal antibodies inhibit

the adhesion of mouse B16 melanoma cells *in vitro* and block lung metastasis *in vivo*. *Proc Natl Acad Sci USA* 80:3729–33, 1983a
214. Vollmers HP, Birchmeier W: Monoclonal antibodies that prevent adhesion of B16 melanoma cells and reduce metastasis in mice: Crossreaction with human tumor cells. *Proc Natl Acad Sci USA* 80:6863–7, 1983b
215. Vollmers HP, Imhof BA, Braun S, Waller CA, Schirrmacher V, Birchmeier W: Monoclonal antibodies which prevent experimental lung metastases: interference with the adhesion of tumour cells to laminin. *FEBS Lett* 172:17–20, 1984
216. Warren BA: The ultrastructure of capillary sprouts induced by melanoma transplants in the golden hamster. *J Roy Micr Soc* 86:177–87, 1966
217. Warren BA, Vales O: The adhesion of thromboplastic tumour emboli to vessel walls *in vivo*. *Br J Exp Pathol* 53:301–13, 1972
218. Warren BA: Environment of the blood-borne tumor embolus adherent to vessel wall. *J Med* 4:150–77, 1973
219. Warren BA: Origin and fate of blood-borne tumor emboli. *Cancer Biol Rev* 2:95–169, 1981
220. Wass JA, Varani J, Ward PA: Size increase induced in Walker ascites cells by chemotactic factors. *Cancer Lett* 9:913–8, 1980
221. Weiss L: Cancer cell traffic from the lungs to the liver: an example of metastatic inefficiency. *Int J Cancer* 25:385–92, 1980
222. Werb Z, Mainardi CL, Vater CA, Harris ED Jr: Endogenous activation of latent collagenase by rheumatoid synovial cells: evidence of a role of plasminogen activator. *N Engl J Med* 296:1017–23, 1977
223. Weston BJ, Carter RL, Easty GC, Connell DI, Davies AJC: The growth and metastasis of an allografted lymphoma in normal, deprived, and reconstituted mice. *Int J Cancer* 14:176–85, 1974
224. Wolosin LB, Greenberg AH: Murine natural anti-tumor antibodies. I. Rapid *in vivo* binding of natural antibody by tumor cells in syngeneic mice. *Int J Cancer* 23:519–27, 1979
225. Wood S Jr: Experimental studies of the intravascular dissemination of ascitic V2 carcinoma cells in the rabbit with special reference to fibrinogen and fibrinolytic agents. *Bull Swiss Acad Med Sci* 20:92–121, 1964
226. Woolley DE: Collagenolytic mechanisms in tumor cell invasion. *Cancer Metas Rev* 3:361–72, 1984
227. Yogeeswaran G, Salk PL: Metastatic potential is positively correlated with cell surface sialylation of cultured murine tumor cells. *Science* 212:1514–6, 1981
228. Yoshida K, Ozaki T, Ushijima K, Hayashi H: Studies on the mechanism of invasion in cancer. I. Isolation and purification of a factor chemotactic for cancer cells. *Int J Cancer* 6:123–32, 1970
229. Zacharski LR: The biological basis for anticoagulant treatment of cancer. *Progr Clin Biol Res* 89:113–29, 1982
230. Zeidman I, Buss JM: Transpulmonary passage of tumor cell emboli. *Cancer Res* 12:731–3, 1952
231. Zetter BR: Migration of capillary endothelial cells is stimulated by tumor derived factors. *Nature* 285:41–3, 1980
232. Zetter BR: The endothelial cells of large and small blood vessels. *Diabetes* 30:Sup 2; 24–8, 1981

COMPARATIVE IMPORTANCE OF THE LYMPHATIC SYSTEM DURING NEOPLASTIC PROGRESSION: LYMPHOHEMATOGENOUS SPREADING

H.E. KAISER

with a contribution of D. Berens von Rautenfeld and C. Hunneshagen

INTRODUCTION. COMPARATIVE ASPECTS: MAMMALS EXHIBIT THE HIGHEST TYPE OF LYMPHATIC STRUCTURES

The phylogenetic development of body fluids and related structures spans from lowest eumetazoans to man (74, 127–129).

Phyla without-open- and closed circulatory systems can be distinguished. The earliest lymphatic systems appear in the jawless vertebrates, such as the lowest fishes (see Chapter 17/V). The comparative aspects have to be considered as evidence that lymphatic metastasis is phylogenetically a younger phenomenon than hematogenous metastases, which are already known, although only superficially, from highly developed molluscs and arthropods.

On the basis of its development, neoplastic growth reaches its most specialized state in the mammal, because it shows the highest development of the lymphatic system, especially the pronounced multiplicity of its most advanced organs, the lymph nodes. The transformation of malignant cells, especially those of true tissues, can occur in each tissue with the exception of the cell invariable (neurons and, perhaps, the cardiac musculature) or nonliving tissue, as in certain tissues of the vascular plants, such as the sclerenchyma.

Man with his action and behavior, including the environmental changes produced by him (see Chapter 7/IX) contributed to his own neoplastic diseases. The fact that we know our own tumor histology best, makes our body the central point of neoplastic development, not only ethically but realistically; it also explains why primary neoplasms also occur in invertebrates and lower vertebrates and that metastasis and secondary spreading is less common there, whereas metastasis as such is unknown in vascular plants due to the rigid cell wall (cellulose) and the lack of floating cells in the body fluid.

The lymphatic system as part of the circulatory system is involved in both primary tumorigenesis in the tumors of the lymphoid tissues and secondary tumor spreading as in mammary cancers, head and neck cancers and lung-infiltration of lymphatic vessels and deposits in lymph nodes. The high rate of development in the lymphatic system shows a remarkable diversification to the spreading of metastatic cells. Theoretically, four comparative types of metastatic spreading can be distinguished in the organisms:

1. Malignant neoplasms without metastatic spreading; the crown gall disease of vascular plants, and the majority of generally non-metastasizing cancers such as the basal cell cancer in man.

2. Hematogenous spreading of neoplasms by free cells such as certain tumors in the fruit fly, *Drosophila* sp.

3. Hematogenic and lymphatic spreading in lower vertebrates, changing gradually to type four. Lymph nodes are generally not present.

4. The mammalian stage of tumor spreading, with extensive lymphatic involvement, including also the other types (see Chapters 1, 3, 4/VII and 22/VIII).

In addition, the mammalian lymph nodes are affected by diseases such as acute leukemias and others.

Comparative aspects of the various types of lymphatic structures are not well known, therefore it is not surprising that it is not generally understood why the mammal exhibits the highest type of the lymphatic system development. But mammals range in body size from a few grams and a few centimeters to organisms weighing many tons and reaching a body length of more than 30 m (see Chapter 5/I). Accordingly, the life span also shows a wide range, and there are more than 4000 species of living mammals which show many environmental adaptations. The most important peculiarity in the lymphatic system is the lymph node as a separate structure. Figure 1 (after Feneis, (74)) shows the lymph nodes in the trunk of man. Observing the other classes of vertebrates we find that only in mammals the lymph nodes are widely distributed. From a species-specific standpoint several types can be distinguished: the lymph node as such; the hemal node typical for ruminant species; and the hemal lymph node, known from the rat and, perhaps, appearing in man. Lymph nodes are located in the path of the extensive lymph vessels, sometimes more than one in a row, filtering the lymph before it is returned to the blood stream.

Lymph nodes in birds are known only from the mesentery of a few species such as the ostrich and in ducks; in reptiles, they occur only in the mesentery of crocodiles but they are missing in amphibians and fishes. Nevertheless, lymph hearts or comparable structures appear in amphibians with the other structures of body fluids and defense; these splinter groups are discussed at the end of the chapter.

In the leopard frog (*Rana pipiens*), the effect of temperature on metastasis is applied directly on the neoplastic cells and/or the endogenous environment of the animal (123).

Here, I will outline the involvement of the lymphatic system of man and other mammals in tumorigenesis of

R. H. Goldfarb (ed.), Fundamental aspects of cancer.

Table 1. Review of maligant neoplasms of the human lymphatic system.

I. Malignant lymphomas	Condition of lymph nodes

A. Non-Hodgkin's malignant lymphomas
    1. Nodular (follicular) lymphomas
        lymphocytic, poorly differentiated, mixed lymphocytic "histiocytic",
        "histiocytic"
    2. Diffuse lymphomas
        well-differentiated lymphocytic type lymphocytic, intermediate
        differentiation type poorly differentiated lymphocytic type mixed,
        lymphocytic "histiocytic" type large cell lymphomas – "histiocytic" and
        undifferentiated pleomorphic (non-Burkitt's type) types
        lymphoblastic lymphoma
    3. Less common lymphoreticular malignancies
        mycosis fungoides
        Sezary's syndrome
        malignant histiocytosis (histiocytic medullary reticulosis)
	Partial retention of sinus pattern, infiltration with large histiocyte-like cells with atypia and frequent mitosis

hairy cell leukemia (leukemic reticuloendotheliosis)
        heavy chain disease
        Burkitt's lymphoma
	Diffuse infiltration of sinuses and medullary cords
	Especially mediastinal and abdominal nodes are involved

B. Hodgkin's malignant lymphomas
    Hodgkin's disease
        nodular sclerosis
        lymphocytic predominance
        mixed cellularity
        lymphocytic depletion
	Lymph nodes are often enlarged, discrete and hard. The structure and consistency varies during the course of the disease. The tissue appears gray-white when cut; in more pronounced lesions stripes of dense fibrous tissue appear. The stages of the disease shows therefore variable structure.

II. Disease with additional involvement of lymph nodes(?)

Acute leukemia
Myeloid leukemia
Myelomatosis
–
Kaposi's sarcoma
Plasma cell tumor
Glomus tumor

III. Primary neoplasms of diffuse lymphatic tissue

IV. Primary tumors of lymphatic organs

Tonsil
    Lymphoepithelioma

Thymus
    Thymolipomas
    Thymoma
    Thymus involvement in a primary sense occurs in other neoplasms

Spleen
    Hemangio-endotheliomatous structure in spleen
    Extraosseous multiple myelomatosis

Bone marrow
    Lymphoma
    Leukaemic nodules (rarely present as primary malignant tumors of bone)
    Myeloma and myelomatosis

V. Places of embryonal development of the lymphatic system

    e.g.,
Mesenchyme
Tissue spaces
Capillary loops
Esophagus
Liver

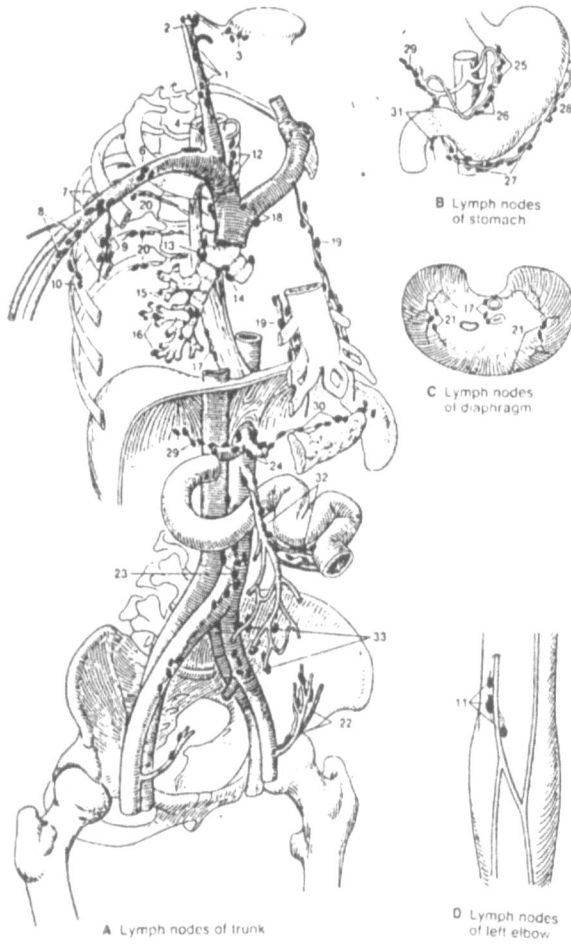

Figure 1. A Lymph nodes of trunk, B Lymph nodes of stomach, C Lymph nodes of diaphragm, D Lymph nodes of left elbow (After Feneis (74)) with permission of Thieme Publisher.

Review of the lymph nodes in man. Occipital nodes. Retroauricular nodes. Parotid nodes. Retropharyngeal nodes. Submandibular nodes. Buccal nodes. Submental nodes. Mandibular nodes. Superficial cervical nodes. Deep cervical nodes (1), Jugulodigastric nodes (2), Lingual nodes (3), Jugulo-omohyoid node (4), Axillary nodes (5), Apical nodes (6), Central nodes (7), Lateral nodes (8), Pectoral nodes (9), Subscapular nodes (10), Cubital nodes (11), Tracheal nodes (12), Superior tracheobronchial nodes (13), Inferior tracheobronchial nodes (14), Bronchopulmonary nodes (15), Pulmonary nodes (16), Posterior mediastinal nodes (17), Anterior mediastinal nodes (18), Parasternal nodes (19), Intercostal nodes (20), Phrenic nodes (21), Epigastric nodes (22), Lumbar nodes (23), Celiac nodes (24), Left gastric nodes (25), Right gastric nodes (26), Right gastric epiploic nodes (27), Left gastroepiploic nodes (28), Hepatic nodes (29), Pancreaticosplenic nodes (30), Pyloric nodes (31), Superior mesenteric nodes (32), Ileocolic nodes, Right colic node, Middle colic nodes, Inferior mesenteric nodes, Left colic nodes, Common iliac nodes, Internal iliac nodes, External iliac nodes, Sacral nodes, Superficial inguinal nodes, Deep inguinal nodes, Popliteal nodes, Anterior tibial node.

malian lymph nodes, and, finally, the tumorigenesis of the lymphatic system *per se*.

Lymphatic and hematogenic metastasis

Primary neoplasms are easily eradicated by surgery, radiotherapy or other methods. The problems of neoplastic diseases are caused by the dispersal of secondary neoplasms, generally via the hematogenic and lymphatic systems. Neoplasms vary in accordance with the manner in which they spread, the subject of this chapter.

The mammalian lymph nodes are the most highly organized of all the lymphatic organs. Of all lymphatic organs they are the only ones which have afferent and efferent lymph vessels and sinuses (Figure 2: Schematic drawing of the lymph node after Dellman and Brown, 1981. With permission of Lea & Febiger Publishers.)

The most diversified artificial tumor progression is found in man and the most diversified tumor progression, in the mammal.

The human body is not only the one for which we have the most extensively knowledge of neoplastic progression, but it is also the one most widely exposed to the most extensive therapeutic treatments which produce the greatest variation in tumor modification. There is variable involvement of the lymphatic system and especially, lymph nodes, in metastatic spreading of various neoplasms.

Neoplastic diseases with lymph node involvement, other than metastatic spreading as, for example, the Brill-Symmers disease and lymphosarcomas, have been dealt with in Chapter 10/VII. Of interest here is only the role of the lymph nodes in the spreading of selected neoplasms, as listed in Table 2.

Relative stimulation or suppression as changes of nodal activity are in correlation with the distance of the lymph node from the nearest primary or metastatic melanoma (48). Also, Hoon and coworkers (111) found in the study of histology and immunohistology of tumor-draining lymph nodes that nodes closer to the tumor showed reduced paracortical activity responses than nodes located further away. The early establishment of metastases may be facilitated by early immunosuppression of nodes in closest vicinity to a tumor.

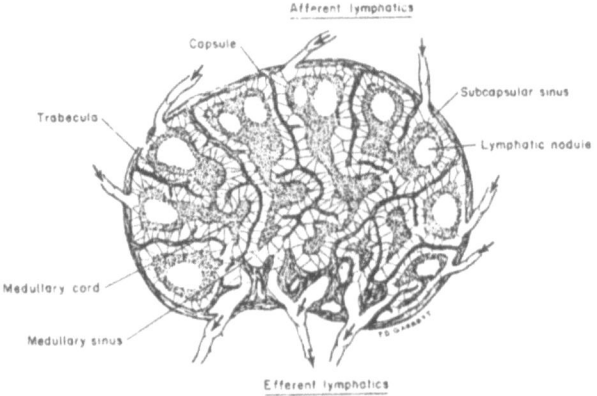

Figure 2.

nonlymphatic and lymphatic tumors, Table 1, the role of the lymphatic system in tumor dissemination from the mam-

Table 2. The lymphatic system and secondary tumorigenesis of nonlymphatic neoplasms (adapted after Manual for Staging of Cancer (2nd edition), Beahrs OH, Myers MH (eds.) American Joint Committee on Cancer. Philadelphia: JB Lippincott, 1983)

Species	Topographic region organ	Main histologic tumor type	Location of primary tumor	Primary regional lymph nodes	Secondary regional lymph nodes	Distant site
Man	Lip and oral cavity	squamous cell cancer	Lip and oral cavity	Jugulodigastric, jugulo-omohyoid, upper deep cervical, lower deep cervical, sub-maxillary and submental lymph nodes. Sometimes bilateral affected	Parotid lymph nodes (juxtaposition nodes).	Lung (common), also skeleton & liver, mediastinal lymph nodes
	Pharynx	Squamous cell cancer	Pharynx epithelium	Jugulodigastric, jugulo-omohyoid, upper deep cervical, lower deep cervical, sub-maxillary & submental, (retropharyngeal & parapharyngeal). Sometimes, bilateral affected	Parotid lymph nodes.	Lung (common), other sites, mediastinal nodes
	Larynx	Squamous cell cancer	Larynx epithelium	Jugulodigastric, jugulo-omohyoid, paratracheal and deep cervical nodes	—	Lung (common), skeleton, other sites, mediastinal nodes.
	Paranasal sinuses	Squamous cell cancer	Larynx epithelium	Submaxillary, parotid, jugulo-digastric, retropharyngeal and deep cervical nodes	—	Lung (common), occasionally bone & distant lymph nodes
	Major salivary glands	Acinic cell ca, adenoid cystic ca, adenoca, squamous cell ca. ca in pleomorphic adenoma, mucoepidermoid ca	Parotid, submaxillary, submental and deep cervical lymph nodes.			
	Thyroid gland	Papillary ca, follicular ca, medullary ca, undifferentiated ca, unclassified malignant neoplasm		Tracheoesophageal nodes bilaterally, upper anterior mediastinal nodes, delphian node, bilaterally to nodes of jugular chain, retropharyngeal nodes		Lung, bone & others by haematogenous or lymphatic route
	Esophagus	Squamous cell carcinoma (98%), Adenocarcinoma (2%)		Cervical, supraclavicular and adjacent lymph nodes		Liver, lungs, adrenals
	Stomach	Adenocarcinoma		Lesser curvature, left gastro-pancreatic, juxtacardiac, gastro-duodenal, gastropyloric, supra-pyloric, pancreatoduodenal, celiac, splenic, hepatic lymph nodes.	Para-aortic nodes	Liver, bone, supraclavicular lymph nodes, lung and widespread visceral involvement
	Colon & rectum	Adenocarcinoma	Cecum, ascending colon, hepatic flexure, transverse colon, splenic flexure, descending colon, sigmoid colon, rectosigmoid, rectum.	Anterior cecal; posterior cecal, ileocolic nodes for cecum ileo-, right and middle colic for ascending colon; right and middle colic for hepatic flexure; middle colic for transverse colon; left colic, inferior mesenteric for	?	Peritoneum, liver, lung and bones.

Table 2. cont.

Species	Topographic region organ	Main histologic tumor type	Location of primary tumor	Primary regional lymph nodes	Secondary regional lymph nodes	Distant site
				splenic flexure, descending and sigmoid colon; perirectal, left colic, sigmoid mesenteric, inferior mesenteric for rectosigmoid; perirectal, left colic, sigmoid & inferior mesenteric, internal iliac, lateral sacral, common iliac, sacral promontory nodes for rectum.	Para-aortic nodes	
	Liver and bilary tract	Hepatocellular ca, cholangio-carcinoma, mixed hepatocellular cholangioca, bile duct cystadenoca, hepatoblastoma, undifferenciated ca,	Liver and biliary tract	Regional hilar nodes, those along the common bile duct and subsequently the para-aortic lymph nodes.		Liver & lung, less frequent bone, brain and other regions.
	Gallbladder	Adenocarcinoma, squamous cell ca, adenosquamous ca, oat cell ca, others.	gall bladder			
	Extrahepatic bile ducts (without ampulla & intra-pancreatic duct	Adenoca, squamous cell ca, adenosquamous ca, oat cell ca, others	Extrahepatic bile ducts			
	Exocrine pancreas	Duct cell adenoca, giant cell ca, giant cell ca with osteoid, adenosquamous ca, microadenoca, mucinos ca, cystadenoca, acinar cell adenoca, pancreatoblastoma, papillary cystic tumor, mixed type, unclassified	Pancreas	Celiac, splenic, suprapancreatic, left gastropancreatic, hepatic artery, inferior pancreatic, juxta-aortic, anterior pancreatic duodenal, posterior pancreatic duodenal, inferior paraaortic, mediastinal and mesenteric nodes.		
	Lung	Squamous cell (epidermoid) ca, adenoca, undifferentiated large-cell ca, undifferentiated small-cell ca.	bronchial mucosa	Intrapulmonary, peribronchial and hilar nodes.	Mediastinal, para-esophageal, subcarinal, paratracheal, aortic, pre- or retrotracheal nodes.	Scalene, supra-clavicular, & other cervical & contralateral hilar nodes. Any site, mainly liver, brain, bones, adrenals, kidneys, and contralateral lung
	Breast (Mammary glands)	Ductal, lobular ca	Glandular tissue and ductal linings	Axillary, axillary apex, infra-clavicular, internal mammary, inter-pectoral, subclavicular, & supra-clavicular.		Bone, lung, brain & liver, but also to all other remote sites
	Cervix uteri	Carcinoma of cervix	Vaginal portion or canal portion of cervix	Parametrial, hypogastric (obturator), external iliac, presacral and common iliac nodes.	Para-aortic nodes	Lung & skeleton
	Corpus uteri	Adenoca predominates	Endometrium	Hypogastric, external iliac, common iliac, presacral, and para-aortic nodes.	Para-aortic nodes	Vagina & lung

Organ	Histological type	Site of origin	Regional lymph nodes	Other nodes	Metastases
Testis	Seminomatous and non-seminomatous (teratoma, embryonal cell carcinoma, teratocarcinoma, yolk sac and choriocarcinoma	Testis	Paracaval, para-aortic and nodes of renal hilus; external iliac and inguinal nodes.	All other nodes	Lung, bone and liver
Bladder	Transitional cell ca	Mucosa of bladder	Nodes of true pelvis	All other nodes	Bone, liver, lung & brain
Kidney	Adenocarcinoma (clear-cell and granular cell ca)	Kidney	Para-aortic lymph nodes & lateral caval node at right, and a hilar-located renal vein node on the left.		Hematogenic, lymphatic and direct spreading
Eyelids	Basal cell & squamous cell ca Sebaceous ca Adnexal carcinomas	Epidermis, Meibomian and other glands and other adnexal structures	Preauricular, submandibular, and cervical lymph nodes		
Conjunctiva	Mucoepidermoid and squamous cell carcinoma	Conjunctiva	Preauricular, submandibular, and cervical nodes		Lung, bone, liver, brain, lymph nodes, bone marrow pleura, skin.
Conjunctiva	Melanoma	Conjunctiva	Preauricular, submandibular, and cervical nodes		
Lacrimal gland	Carcinoma in pleomorphic adenoma, adenoid cystic ca arising de novo, adenoca, mucoepidermoid & squamous cell carcinoma	Lacrimal gland	Preauricular, submandibular, and cervical nodes		Lung, bone, and remote viscera
Kidney	Nephroblastoma	Kidney	Hilar nodes, para-aortic nodes, and the paracaval nodes between diaphragm and bifurcation of the aorta.		
Soft tissues: Orbit Head & neck Limbs	Soft tissue sarcomas	Soft tissue: Orbit Head & neck Limbs	Cervical and supraclavicular lymph nodes for head & neck. Sub-diaphragmatic, intra-abdominal and ilio-inguinal lymph nodes for	In case of unilateral tumors all contra-lateral lymph nodes which are involved.	
Ovary	Serous tumors, mucinous tumors, endometriod tumors, clear cell (mesonephroid) tumors, undifferentiated and unclassified tumors.	Ovary	External iliac, common iliac, hypogastric, lateral sacral, para-aortic nodes, (rarely) inguinal nodes		Peritoneum with omentum, pelvic, abdominal viscera, diaphragma, liver (common); lungs and pleura
Vulva			Inguinal, external iliac and hypogatric nodes.		
Prostate	Nearly always adenocarcinoma	Prostate, multifocal in true parenchyma	Nodes of true pelvis	All others	Bones, lung & liver most common.

Table 2. cont.

Species	Topographic region organ	Main histologic tumor type	Location of primary tumor	Primary regional lymph nodes	Secondary regional lymph nodes	Distant site
	Pelvis Abdomen Thorax Other			Abdominal & pelvic location. Homolateral epitrochlear and axillary lymph nodes for upper limbs. Homolateral popliteal & inguinal lymph nodes for lower limbs.		
	Various locations	Alveolar soft-part sarcoma angiosarcoma, epithelioid sarcoma, extraskeletal chondrosarcoma, extraskeletal osteosarcoma, fibrosarcoma, leiomyosarcoma, liposarcoma, malignant fibrous histiocytoma, malignant hemangiopericytoma, malignant mesenchymoma, malignant schwannoma, rhabdomyosarcoma, synovial sarcoma, unclassified and other sarcomas.	Dependable	Regions related to location of primary tumor		Most common the lung but nearly any other viscera and site
	Various locations	Melanoma of skin (lentigo maligna type, with radial growth phase of the radial spreading type, nodular type, acral lentiginous type, unclassified).	Variable	Preauricular and cervical nodes for head & face; anterior and posterior cervical, supraclavicular & axillary for neck & upper chest wall; anterior & posterior chest wall & upper arm axillary nodes; hands & upper extremities epitrochlear or axillary nodes; abdominal wall & thigh femoral inguinal nodes; for feet and leg up to the knees popliteal or femoral inguinal nodes.		Wide metastasis, to skin, subcutaneous tissues, M1 and lymph nodes, liver, bone, lung, brain and v. cera (M2).
	Skin of face, ears, hands, scalp, much less protected regions of body & extremities	Squamous and basal cell carcinoma	Variable	Face: Parotide, submaxillary and cervical nodal areas; hands to epitrochlear axillary and supraclavicular nodal aeras.	Nodes after first regional ones.	Lung

Bone	Osteosarcoma and juxtacortical osteosarcoma are boneforming; Chondrosarcoma, juxta-cortical and mesenchymal chondrosarcoma are cartilage-forming; malignant giant cell tumor; Ewing's sarcoma, and myeloma are tumors of the marrow; hemangioendothelioma, hemangiopericytoma, and angiosarcoma are vascular tumors, fibrosarcoma liposarcoma, malignant mesenchymoma, and undifferentiated sarcoma are connective tissue tumors; chordoma and adamantinoma of long bones are rare	Skeleton
Lymph nodes, minor accumulations of lymphatic tissue, thymus, spleen	Hodgkin's disease, Nodular or diffuse Non-Hodgkin's lymphomas	
Different regions	Neuroblastoma	Different regions	Cervical and supraclavicular nodes for the cervical region; intrathoracic and supraclavicular nodes for the thoracic region; subdiaphragmatic, intra-abdominal and pelvic nodes with external iliac nodes for abdominal and pelvic regions; appropriate lymph nodes in other regions.

THE ADDITION OF THE HIGHEST ORGANISMIC DEVELOPMENT OF THE LYMPHATIC SYSTEM TO THE HEMATOPOIETIC SYSTEM IN THE MAMMAL AS THE REASON FOR THE MOST ADVANCED METASTASIS

Neoplastic progression depends not only on histologic characteristics but, to a great deal, on the possible ways of distribution which the metastatic cells can use. Absence and presence, as well as the magnitude of development of the lymphatic system is an excellent example of this. Immunologically active phagocytic or lymphocytic cells appear in many invertebrates, but a lymphatic system is missing. The correlated circulatory system is missing in small and certain parasitic groups, but appears in the open, mixed or closed condition in others. In vertebrates, the lymphatic system develops as mesenchymal structure, but reaches its highest state in the lymph nodes in the mammals. Here, the lymphatic system is in its highest development as a supplement to the closed circulatory system which includes the remnant of an open circulatory system in the spleen, again a lymphatic organ. The combination of both systems makes possible the widest general distribution and dissemination of the neoplastic diseases in the mammal. Other ways of secondary neoplastic distribution, such as the direct spread of neoplasms, implantation on epithelial surfaces, or coelomic distribution, are of subordinate importance (see Chapters 1, 3, 4/VII, 22/VIII).

Connections of lymphatic and hematogenous system

The lymphatic system is intimately connected with the circulatory system, one reason why hematogenous and lymphatic metastasis cannot be separated meaningfully. The connections between both systems are given in Table 3.

The most important connections, besides those of tissue spaces and from surfaces as the peritoneum, are the lymph nodes, where interchange of neoplastic cells between blood and lymph may take place, especially if we think of the enzymatic capabilities of neoplastic cells.

Hematogenic and lymphatic dissemination of mammalian, especially human, neoplasms, cannot be meaningfully separated. They act together. Not much is known of metastases in invertebrate neoplasms or of those of lower chordates. Also, in fishes only very few metastases are

Table 3. Connections between the hematogenic and lymphatic systems.

1. Hilus of lymph nodes: entrance and outlet of blood vessels to the lymph node. Through the number of lymph nodes they are quite important.
2. The thoracic duct enters the venous system at the angulus venosus.
3. The jugular trunk runs also to the angulus venosus.
4. The subclavian trunk opens at right into the lymphatic duct; on the left in an angle between internal jugular and subclavian vein.
5. The bronchiomediastinal trunk opens into the thoracic duct or the brachiocephalic vein.
6. The right lymphatic duct arises from the junction of the jugular trunk, the subclavian trunk, and the brachiomediastinal trunk.
7. Spleen: vessels enter and leave at the hilum.

Table 4. Review of the combined conditions of the systems of body fluids in the organisms with true tissues, excluding plants.

Small and parasitic forms of invertebrates without a circulatory system, but with lymphocytic and phagocytic cells (e.g., tardigrads and acanthocephalans)

Phyla with an open circulatory system, including such highly developed groups as the insects with an open circulatory system, abundant cells of body fluids, with lymphatic and phagocytic cells, immunologic reaction and endocrinologic structures (glands).

Pulmonate snails and decapod cephalopods with a mixed circulatory system, lymphatic and phagocytic cells, immunologic reactions, and endocrine structures (glands).

Phyla with closed circulatory systems, but without lymphatic channels, often abundant lymphocytic cells and phagocytes, endocrine structures and immune reactions, such as nemertine or annelid worms.

Vertebrates with a closed circulatory system and a system of lymphatic channels, as in fishes, amphibians, the majority of reptiles and birds. Immunologic and endocrine structures.

Mammals with closed circulatory system, highest development of the lymphatic system with abundant lymph nodes, a highly developed immunology and highly developed endocrine organs (a few species of reptiles and also birds).

known (see Chapters 8/V and 11/V). This lack of knowledge is not due to few observed cases but because this condition is caused by the combination of the hematogenic and lymphatic systems, which are missing in invertebrates, lower chordates, and, of course, plants. (In the latter, this is due to the lack of floating cells in the body fluids, in the phloem and the xylem and the rigid cell wall composed of cellulose.)

The combination of the lymphatic system as an addition to the circulatory or hematogenic system, and the advanced development of both systems, are the most important preconditions for mammalian neoplastic dissemination and distribution. It is interesting that solid tumors appear generally in a restricted location, whereas the hematogenic or lymphatic neoplasms occur in a systematic manner. The normal makeup of the hematogenic and lymphatic systems provides one of the most important preconditions for the extensive development of neoplastic metastasis in mammals.

DEVELOPMENT OF THE LYMPHATIC SYSTEM AND THE INTERRELATION BETWEEN LYMPHOID HEMATOPOIETIC SYSTEMS

Growth of the lymphatic system

The ontogenetically normal development is as follows: The mesenchyme, a mesodermal tissue, gives rise to the lymph nodes, lymph vessels and spleen, the myocardium, the musculature of the blood vessels, the endocardium and endothelium of blood vessels, as well as the different varieties of blood cells. The parenchyma of the thymus derives from the embryonic endoderm. The lymphatic system, as well as the hematopoietic system, return the fluid from the tissues and both are closely related. This is true also with regard to the process of metastasis in general and neoplastic metastasis in particular.

Two views exist which explain the ontogenetic origin of the lymphatic system: The first states that all lymphatic channels develop as saccular outgrowths of venous endothelium. The main sacs are the jugular lymph sacs, the iliac lymph sacs, the retroperitoneal or mesentery sac, and the cisterna chyli. Continuous elongation and branching lead to the penetration into the various body regions. How the connection with the veins is established is not yet clearly understood.

The second opinion states that the lymphatic system develops from perivenous spaces of the mesenchyme which later are transferred to continuous vessels, finally opening into the venous system. In early stages the spaces are lined with mesenchyme and the cells change later to the flattened lining of the endothelium of the lymphatic vessels. During ontogeny, the beginning of the lymphatic system appears first in the jugular region of embryos 10 to 11 mm C.R. long. The cranial part of the thoracic duct appears next. In the second month of fetal life, the valves appear in the region of the jugular lymph sacs. The valves attain near completion at the beginning of the fifth month of fetal life. The valves of the veins appear a month later than those of the lymphatics.

CONNECTION OF DIRECT AND METASTATIC SPREADING

Spreading of a malignant tumor can begin and proceed via the direct way and via metastatic spreading. Both processes are related as shown by the sequence of steps occurring during both types of spreading. The main variation between both is the way of detachment of the metastatic cells. But this may also occur during the direct spreading of large neoplasms if the inner part of the tumor becomes necrotic in certain areas.

It is only natural that direct and metastatic spreading may establish an interchangeable sequence of steps as shown in Table 5.

The sequence of lymphatic neoplastic spreading can be seen as follows: The lymphatic system, in contrast to the circulatory system, is a one-way system, extending from the tissue spaces via the lymph capillaries, larger lymph vessels and passing through at least one lymph node and larger collecting ducts (of which the most prominent one is the thoracic duct), to the venous portion of the circulatory system. This structure of the lymphatic system, to be given

in more detail later, explains why neoplastic metastasis, at a later stage, will proceed by hematogenic and lymphatic ways in the same time frame established by the connection between the hematogenic and lymphatic systems.

(1) Departure of single cells or clusters of neoplastic cells from the primary tumor into the tissue spaces, destruction of metastatic clusters.

(2) Penetration of single, neoplastic cells into the lymph capillaries and small lymphatic vessels, transport to regional lymph nodes.

(3) Destruction or growth in regional lymph nodes and/or possible passage to collecting duct and thoracic duct and from there into the blood stream.

(4) General dissemination:

Neoplastic cells, simultaneously may or may not enter the circulatory system at each portion of the way through the lymphatic vessels. As the lymphatic system is involved not only in the building but also in the destruction of leukocytes, lymphocytes and erythrocytes, cells, like killer cells, will not only eliminate neoplastic cells traveling in the lymphatic system, but the killer cells themselves will later be destroyed as used cells. The components of the neoplastic cells secreted into a possibly existing, larger accumulation of neoplastic cells, will finally overextend the protective capacity of the lymphatic defense system. This means spreading will pass through the regional lymph nodes and the next higher hierarchic group of lymph nodes, if present, and general dissemination will occur via additional steps of metastasis.

THE COMPONENTS OF THE MAMMALIAN SYSTEM OF BODY FLUIDS AND THEIR ACTION ON NEOPLASTIC SPREADING

Because of the lymphatic-circulatory systems link neoplastic spreading of certain tumors occurs more often via one or the other route. In reality, a combined distribution via both

Table 6. The components of the lymphatic system and their connections with the circulatory system.

The connection of the lymphatic system with the circulatory system
a. Lymph vessels
    (a) Lymph capillaries
    (b) Small and medium-sized lymph vessels
    (c) Large lymph vessels and conducting ducts
    (d) The thoracic duct
b. Lymph nodes
    (a) Lymph nodes *per se*
    (b) Hemal nodes
    (c) Hemal lymph nodes
c. Diffuse lymphatic tissue
    (a) Scattered tissue
    (b) Isolated nodules
d. Lymph organs
    (a) Tonsils
    (b) Thymus
    (c) Spleen
e. Involvement in building and destruction of leukocytes, lymphoocytes and erythrocytes
f. The bone marrow
g. Places of embryonal lymphatic development during embryogenesis in the mammal comparable to similar structures in other vertebrate classes

Table 5. Interchanging of direct and indirect (metastatic) neoplastic spread.

Start of direct spreading	Metastatic start
1. Expanding growth from primary tumor following path of least resistance	1. Detachment (see Chapter XX)
2. Penetration	2. Penetration
3. Direct growth, e.g. in a vein	3. Swimming of neoplastic emboli in lymph or blood vessel
4. Seeding in vein	4. Settling in venule of target organ
5. Continuation also as metastatic spread	5. Direct spread also from metastasis

ways may occur. In one case the lymphatic distribution involves carcinomas and in the other the hematogenic distribution sarcomas.

The following sections review the structures and their connections involved in neoplastic spreading.

Lymph vessels

Lymph vessels are of great importance for the transport and harboring of metastatic cells. Not only do they form an extensive system, but the walls of these vessels are easily penetrated like those of veins and arteries. Their transport speed and fluid pressure also vary, especially in lymph vessels and veins, on one hand, and the arteries, on the other (see Chapter 1/VII). Additional renal factors are multifocality and small vessel infiltration. These conclusions are drawn from studies by Fossa et al (1985) regarding bladder cancer. As found in 56 cases of renal cell carcinoma, lymphadenectomy is useful in treating lymph node metastasis (170).

(a) Lymph capillaries

The anastomosing lymph capillaries are the starting points of the lymph vessels; they drain from the tissue spaces, particularly those of the connective tissues (especially the collagen, one of the basic substances which contains large amounts of hyaluronic acid). They are lined by endothelium, whose cells are joined by intimate interdigitations, simple overlapping or zonulae adherents. Gaps of variable size between these cells occur frequently. In general, lymph capillaries are larger than blood capillaries. A basal lamina is usually absent or, if present, discontinuous.

(b) Small- and medium-sized lymph vessels

Depending on location, the vessels exhibit a great species-specificity and a great variation. The diameter of the post capillary lymph vessels is larger than that of the lymph capillaries; a complete basement membrane is present. Connective tissue and, after further enlargement, smooth musculature and elastic fibers occur in the wall.

(c) Large lymph vessels and collecting ducts

The walls of these structures are composed of three layers: tunica intima (endothelium, basement membrane and collagenic and elastic fibers, and, at times, an internal elastic lamina); tunica media (smooth) muscle cells, elastic and collagenic fibers); and tunica externa (collagenic and elastic fibers, and, sometimes, smooth muscle cells). Valves characterize all larger lymph vessels, but they can also be found in some capillaries, and, occasionally, in lymph capillaries. They are mainly endothelial folds with some connective tissue support.

(d) The thoracic duct

This portion is characterized by the presence of musculature. The thoracic duct's intima exhibits an endothelium, its thin intermediate layer containing fibroelastic tissue and especially longitudinally arranged musculature and an internal elastic membrane.

The tunica media shows abundant longitudinal and circular musculature. The muscle bundles are separated from each other by collagenous fibers of the richly developed connective tissue. Separate elastic fibrils occur. The poorly developed tunica externa is composed of coarse longitudinally oriented collagenous fibers, elastic tissue, and some longitudinally oriented muscle fibers. The fibrils in the inner layer are more coarse than in the outer layer, where they blend into the connective tissue.

Lymph nodes

Some researchers consider lymph nodes as a protection against metastatic spreading, others as a sanctuary for progressing neoplastic cells. The question is still unresolved, but the reality may point at variations as to how neoplasms deriving from different tissues proceed. The following cases are a selection of recent reports on the subject.

The second landmark of tumor progression after the primary tumor are the regional lymph nodes or adjacent anatomic structures (102). The tumor doubling time of high-grade or poorly differentiated malignant tumors is shorter. They are less cohesive, exhibit often irregular borders and invade by small aggregates and individual cells. The pattern of invasion offers considerable information on neoplastic aggressiveness (51).

Regional lymph nodes may be considered as indicators but not as governors of survival in cancer. It is also shown that many lymphatic and lymphatico-circulatory shunts exist that bypass regional lymph nodes and permit combined dissemination on the basis of hematogenic and lymphatic interaction. In many cases, the traditional regional lymph node filter function appears therefore doubtful, based on information obtained from the clinical and animal experimental aspects in certain tumors (41). The lymph nodes are bean-shaped organs with a slight indentation, the hilus, surrounded by a capsule and composed of stroma and trabeculae, sinuses and lymphatic parenchyma. The functional morphology is reflected in the structure of the organ. Filtration and phagocytosis make the lymph nodes so important for tumor spreading. When the lymph percolates through the coarse mesh it comes into contact with lymphocytes, reticular cells and macrophages. Particulate matter is filtered out and antigenic material is made available to macrophages and lymphocytes (59). In addition to filtration and phagocytosis, lymphopoiesis and immunologic resections are the other important functions of the lymph nodes. Foreign particles, such as infectious agents, like bacteria, etc., and neoplastic cells, stimulate cell formation in the lymphatic tissue. It must be assumed that by overextension this capability will break down, making the lymph node ineffective. If a second filter station, in the form of a second lymph node, follows, then immediate metastasis by infection or formation of a neoplasm may still be prevented. Otherwise, total dissemination of infectious agents or neoplastic cells may occur. It is still questionable whether the breakdown of the antigen response occurs in one or several steps.

Lymph nodes produce a remarkable amount of lymphocytes only second to the bone marrow, the main site of lymphopoiesis. The different types of lymphocytes are bound to special locations. Antigenic experience stimulates the lymphoproliferative response. T-lymphocytes (thymus-dependent lymphocytes) are found in the subcapsular and mantle zone of the lymph node and surround the lymphatic nodules. Their function is cell-mediated immunity; they influence the cooperation of other cell types, control B-cell functions, and are able to act as cytotoxic cells or as killer cells. Some B-lymphocytes develop surface markers. They need maturation in the peripheral lymphatic organs. B-lymphocytes in the germinal centers and medullary cords produce humoral antibodies. The recirculating, long-lived lymphocytes are of both the B- and T-form. There are plenty of active macrophages and plasma cells, with macrophages exhibiting antigens on their cell surfaces. Immunologic is-lands are composed of a central macrophage surrounded by B- or T-lymphocytes. B-lymphocytes change into plasma-blasts as a result of the interaction, described earlier, which takes place primarily in the medullary cords. T-lymphocytes exhibit activation and differentiation in several subtypes with various antigenic functions. Recirculation is important because these long-lived lymphocytes are involved in cellular immune responses. B-lymphocytes are short-lived, T-lymphocytes are long-lived (month to year).

Augmented generation of cytotoxic lymphocytes may be ascribed to local effects of PSK in the lymph nodes, since this is mediated by Lyt-1+2+ cells. Local administration of PSK increased the threshold number of metastatic tumors eliminated by hosts (280). The importance of puncture cy-tology also in regard to unknown primary tumors must be stressed (136). Thin-needle aspirates from palpable lymph nodes were investigated with antibodies to intermediate filament proteins. Metastatic adenocarcinoma cells from breast, ovary, endometrium, cervix, colon, and stomach, as well as from squamous cell carcinoma or mesothelioma stained especially with antibodies to keratin. Mesenchymal originated tumor cells, such as lymphomas from fibrosarco-mas and neurosarcoma as well as those of melanoma were only positive for vimentin. In lymph nodes, keratin staining of the cells aspirated was a direct indication of metastatic carcinoma (220). In the therapy of murine Lewis lung car-cinoma, monoclonal antibodies were effective against the T-cell differentiation antigen Lyt-1. The potentiation of Lyt-1+ cell activity by passively administered anti Lyt-1 antibodies produces tumor rejection (107). Movement by metastatic cells through the lymph nodes seems to be vari-able in different neoplasms as, shown by Carr and cowor-kers (44). The lining of the lymph node sinusoid by active cell movement is invaded by the Walker rat carcinoma, whereas the 13762 mammary carcinoma of the rat does not do this. In the mouse, severe combined immune deficiency is uniformly characterized by lymphopenia, a rudimentary thymic medulla without cortex, relatively empty splenic follicles and lymph nodes, and undeveloped bronchial and gastrointestinal lymphocytic foci (53).

Stratified squamous epithelium
Transcapsular spread of metastatic squamous cell car-cinoma of the head and neck from cervical lymph nodes can be either macroscopic or microscopic. Macroscopic trans-capular spread derives most frequently from large nodal masses with a diameter measuring more than 3 cm, but occurs also in specimens from smaller lymph nodes. Macro scopic spreading invades mainly skeletal muscle, the adven-titia of the internal jugular vein. These metastatic tumors coincide with a high incidence of 44% of recurrency in the ipsilateral neck, mainly in the first 12 months. Microscopic transcapsular growth has a smaller incidence (45). Extracap-sular spread is associated with a statistically significant re-duction of survival (121).

Recurrence in 140 cases of intrathoracic esophageal car-cinoma was 40% in lymph nodes and organs as well. Local recurrence appeared frequently in cervical and mediastinal lymph nodes and regarding the organs in lung, liver and bone. The survival after recurrence in lymph nodes was 8 months and 4 months in other organs. Peritoneal recurrence

showed only a survival of 2 months (119). Computed tomo-graphy is important in the determination of tumor extent in more advanced carcinoma of the cervix (290). Two-hundred-three patients of squamous cell carcinoma of head and neck exhibited 137 positive specimens of transcapsular spread, of which 74 were macroscopic and 63 were micro-scopic. Macroscopic spread occurred mainly with large nodal masses. Macroscopic infiltration exhibited a high in-cidence of recurrent tumor spread in the ipsilateral neck. Microscopic transcapsular spread showed a lower incidence of recurrent tumor which did not reach statistical signifi-cance (45).

Simple cuboidal epithelium
The tumor, nodes and metastasis system clearly document that the survival of patients with renal cell carcinoma de-pends on the local extent of the primary tumor, determined at the time of surgical exploration (17).

Simple columnar epithelium
Fifty-four cases of colonic and rectal carcinoma showing no absolute noncurative resection were evaluated according to the noncurative factors (liver metastasis, peritoneal dissem-ination, lymph node metastasis, and distant metastasis). Longer survival would be expected if the primary tumor could be resected (243).

Pseudostratified columnar epithelium
In 248 patients with squamous cell carcinoma of the supra-glottic larynx, no correlation could be seen between the histologic grade of the primary tumor and initial lymph node status (295); see also (15).

Mammary gland
Histologic grade and number of involved lymph nodes are two important prognostic factors in the development of breast cancer (147). The location of breast tumors does not influence the prognosis, and irradiation of internal mam-mary nodes in patients with inner quadrant lesions does not improve survival (77). Among patients with positive nodes, 97.9% of women treated with radiation and 63.8% of those receiving no radiation remained tumor-free, although both groups received chemotherapy (77). The presence of epider-mal growth factor receptors is associated with metastatic potential (234). Individual risk of breast cancer progression depends on tumor size, tumor fixation and nodal fixation (8). Maximum diameter of the primary tumor affects signifi-cantly the survival of patients with axillary and internal mammary nodes (289). Histopathologic features of the pri-mary tumor and axillary lymph nodes from 97 breast cancer patients from Japan were compared with those from 164 English patients. There appeared statistically significant dif-ferences regarding the primary tumor. In axillary lymph nodes, Japanese women had much more sinus histiocytosis and British women exhibited a diminished frequency of axillary lymph node metastases. Germinal centers were more common in the lymph nodes of Japanese women and were again related with diminished frequency of metastases (80). Three patients with breast carcinoma presented in-clusions of benign-appearing nevus cells in an axillary lymph node. The lesions were exclusively limited to the lymph node capsule (83). Treatment with antimetastatic doses of maleic

anhydride-divinyl ether in rats bearing mammary adenocarcinoma showed significant reduction in size and/or incidence of lymph node metastasis, but no effect on the primary tumor (139).

Only ultrasound or CT are able to diagnose directly tumors of the mesentery and greater omentum resulting, in general, from lymph node metastasis from abdominal carcinoma, or involvement of lymph nodes in cases of general lymphatic malignancy (100).

Testis
Vascular invasion of neoplastic cells leads to an additionally increased metastatic risk, as experienced in the development of non-seminoma testicular neoplasms (285).

Reticular connective tissue
The host macrophage-tumor relationship seems to differ from neoplasm to neoplasm (117). Homing receptors serve as functional markers in investigations of leukemias and lymphomas (131). Adult T-cell leukemia is a disease first described in Japan and different from convoluted T-cell acute lymphocytic leukemia. The lymph nodes are diffuse, infiltrated by medium-sized lymphoblasts with irregular nucleid. Bone marrow and lymph node of one European patient showed lymphoblasts with the helper/inducer phenotype, whereas this phenomenon was only seen in the lymph node of the other patient (276).

Fibrous connective tissue
A relationship between neoplastic diseases and the coagulation system was assumed by Trousseau more than 100 years ago. The role of fibrin in today's scientific investigation is based on the evidence that fibrin appears in tumors. The mechanism of deposit ion in the neoplasm and the importance of fibrin deposition and degradation are discussed by Dvorak, (66). Coagulation may play a role in immune responses, angiogenesis, desmoplasia and metastasis.

Melanogenic system
Lymphoscintigraphy, together with gallium-67, is a useful combination in order to decide treatment, particularly in patients with melanoma of the trunk. Forty-one patients were investigated with gallium-67 for the detection of regional lymph node spread or distant metastases. The latter were demonstrated in brain, lung, bone and liver (232).

Bone
Bone biopsy is not without risk because particles in the size of neoplastic cells, freed by bone biopsy can move fast via the venous system to the lung. The lymphatic system seems not to participate, but may perhaps do so in chronic processes (223).

Lymphatic circulation and the role of lymph nodes in immunological surveillance are important for the role of lymph nodes in tumor spreading (197). CT scanning is useful for diagnosing abdominal lymph node metastasis (270). See also Takeda et al. (263) for metastatic foci of a mature testicular teratoma.

Veins
Veins are much involved in tumor spreading. Their walls are more easily penetrated by disseminating malignant cells than those of arteries because of the absence of elastic fibers. Movement of venous blood is slower than that of arterial blood but there are some exceptions; and the blood pressure is diminished. Neoplastic tissues extend easily into the veins (see Chapter 1/VII) and tumors also grow along larger veins in the so-called "arteries-veins-nerves-avenue" (Arterien-Venen-Nervenstrasse). The importance of the veins for metastatic dissemination can be seen in the general use of veins for centripetal metastasis.

The grade of involvement of the vena cava by a neoplastic thrombus has prognostic significance in renal cell carcinoma. A review of 24 patients showed a two-year-survival of 45.8% and a mean survival of 38.9 months. The extension of the tumor thrombus in the inferior caval vein was paralleled by a worsening of prognosis (253); 5 to 10% of patients with renal cell carcinoma experience an extension of the tumor into the vena cava, 14 to 39% of these patients have a tumor extension into the right atrium. No other evidence of metastasis may be present (143). Operative management in form of cardiopulmonary bypass, hyperthermia and total circulatory arrest are the surgical methods of choice in patients with renal cancer extending into the inferior vena cava and right atrium because the tumor extension into the right atrium poses an immediate risk to life by acute obstruction of the tricuspid valve or pulmonary emboli (152). After application of an intravenous contrast bolus, CT scans of 62 patients with hepatocellular carcinomas showed that the proximal portal vein was involved in 40% of patients and the distal portal vein in 16%. The CT signs of portal vein involvement consisted of hypodensity and enlargement, periportal arterial hypervascularization, inability to visualize the lobar portal vein, arterioportal shunting, and differences in lobar attenuation (171).

A benign leiomyoma arose in the uterus, passed through both ovarian veins, the inferior vena cava, the right atrium and ventricle, and the pulmonary trunk, and extended to both pulmonary arteries (1).

A 35-year-old patient with a tumor of the urinary bladder exhibited massive tumor embolism which showed multiple small tumor emboli within small pulmonary arteries at autopsy (133).

Capillaries, Arterioles
The capillaries are a very important place for the trapping of metastatic cell clusters or single cells (76). The transit of cancer cells through the microvasculature as an interaction of the surfaces of the blood vessels and those of the cancer cells separated by a thin liquid film, is discontinuous, interrupted by adhesions of the two surfaces (298).

Arteries
The arteries, especially the elastic ones, are harder to penetrate by metastatic cells, a condition seen from cases in which undamaged arteries run through a tissue penetrated totally by neoplastic growth. According to Weiss (298), the soil effect divides the target organs into the two major groups; however, within these groups the incidence of tumors is explicable in terms of the "mechanical" hypothesis. Local ischemia decreases grafting of tumors, the growth rate and formation of regional distant metastases and the quantity of tumor cells in the peripheral blood (44). The endovasal transcatheteral blockage of arteries which

supply tumors is a palliative measure and can be used before operation to reduce bleeding and spread of neoplastic cells. Blood exposed to *in vitro* effect of anodic direct current acts like an endogenic thrombogenic substance. Monoclonal antibodies and immunohistochemistry are useful for the differentiation of lymphocyte subpopulations in thymoma (145, 277). No clear correlation could be established between the level of glucocorticoid receptor and the tissue (109).

Diagnosis and staging of neoplasms in the mediastinum were dramatically improved by computed tomography (184, 245). Resistance to metastases after treatment with immunomodulators developed by cyclic nucleotides is topographically variable (287). Regarding fundamentals of the fight against metastasis by the oxygen multistep immunostimulation process see Chapters 16/IX and 17/IX (291). It is difficult to estimate specific cytotoxicity from phytohemagglutinin-lymphogenesis (308). Thymoma is uncommon in dogs (7).

Tonsils (16, 154)

The characteristic neoplasms are the carcinoma and the lymphosarcoma, as well as the association with the lymphomas of the bowel. The first tumor is also known as squamous cell carcinoma, transitional epithelioma or lymphoepithelioma and occurs generally in elderly males. Metastasis involves regional lymph nodes and dissemination to lung, liver, and bones. Lymphocytic lymphoma (lymphosarcoma) is a malignant lymphoid tissue tumor, metastasizing to regional lymph nodes and distant organs.

Bone marrow

Bone is a characteristic of vertebrates but bone marrow is more restricted. Fishes have no bone marrow; the hematopoietic function is performed by the pronephros (see Chapter 11/V). Amphibians and reptiles exhibit bone marrow but its greatest importance is found in birds and mammals. The majority of neoplasms in birds are not epithelial but mesenchymal (see Chapter 12/V). Bone marrow plays a significant role in the development of leukemia and lymphoma, especially in the form of the systemic dissemination of the diseases mentioned earlier. This role must be viewed in connection with those of spleen, thymus and tonsils.

Studies in 26 patients with neoplastic bone marrow involvement in the peripheral blood of granulocyte-macrophage clusters and colony-forming cells showed that the concentration of colony-forming cells in normal persons and in cancer patients without bone marrow invasion ranged from 0–99 ml, while 9 patients with invasion exhibited an increase of colony-forming cells in the blood of 100 to 21 000/ml (9 patients) and 41 to 9000/ml (5 patients). Bone marrow involvement by neoplastic cells may cause spatial redistribution of the granulocyte-macrophage progenitor cells (58).

Blood

Killer cells, suppressor cells, monocytes and platelets will be singled out for review.

Autologous and allogenic tumors were lysed by the same effector cells and multiple metastases from the same patient were similarly lysed by these allo-activated killer cells. Ac-

tivated T-cells represent a population of non-natural killer cells with broad lytic specificity for fresh tumor cells which may be important in the adaptive immunotherapy of human solid tumors (176, 222) – see also Chapter 14/I. The incidence of metastasis from human tumor cell lines grown in the nude mouse seems to be dependent primarily on the biologic characteristics of the individual tumor cell line (149). The percentage of large granular lymphocytes in the peripheral blood of patients with less advanced tumors exhibited an average of 2.15 +/− 1.3, whereas it was 3.8 +/− 1.5 in patients with more progressive cases and with metastases (146, 222). Antigen may induce specific activation of helper lymphocytes, while cyclophosphamide inhibits the activation of suppressor cells (199). Blood T-lymphocyte populations and functions are not altered at time of diagnosis (exception: elderly patients with disseminated disease), but a reduced cellular immune response is well known from patients with advanced breast cancer (166). Cellular interactions following treatment with a biological response modifier regulate natural killer cell-mediated cytotoxicity and antimetastatic activity (99); see Chapters I/8 and 2/X). Operative stress facilitates tumor metastasis (264); see Chapter 2/II).

In 120 patients with gastrointestinal tract, lung and breast cancer, melanoma, and lymphomas, antibody-dependent cellular cytotoxicity, mediated by peripheral blood monocytes, showed a significant decrease in maximal cytotoxicity for patients with gastrointestinal tract cancer and melanoma, but not for the other groups (62). Superoxide-generating activity of blood monocytes, the precursors of macrophages, from patients with advanced cancer seems to indicate that monocytes of cancer patients are defective in secreting 0_2- but the activity may be stimulated by infection (190); see Chapter 19/VII. A week-long or month-long consistency of platelet morphology occurs in whole blood (231).

The blood platelets as part of the coagulation-fibrinolysis system play an important part in the lodgement of circulating tumor cells (268, 269). Platelets form aggregates with tumor cells in circulation and adhere to vascular endothelium. The aggregates of platelets with neoplastic cells and their sequestration in end-organs may result in thrombocytopenia. Tumor metastasis may be inhibited through lack of platelet factors, as seen in thrombocytopenic animals (180). Some tumors are able to activate platelets and the coagulation mechanism *in vivo* (3, 84, 196). The underlying extracellular matrix, contrast to blocking microcirculation and main artery of an organs results in parenchyma loss (242).

Spleen

The only important single tumor of the spleen is the hemangioma (168). The spleen is an organ which has influence on the metastatic process, most clearly known from the effect of T-lymphocytes as killer cells. Some recent aspects of the connection of the spleen and metastatic development of various tissues are discussed in this section.

Local administration of PSK increased the generation of cytotoxic lymphocytes and the induction of opposition against metastatic neoplasms (280). Puncture cytology to detect metastases of known and unknown primary tumors is significant (136).

Simple/stratified squamous epithelium

Non-invasive tests for preoperative staging of esophageal carcinoma comprise the CT (computed tomographic) scan of the thorax and the radionuclide bone scan. These methods were compared to conventional full-lung linear tomography, radionuclide liver plus spleen and bone scans, and thoracic and abdominal CT (116). A 67-year-old male exhibited an advanced inoperable gastric cancer with tissue and peripheral eosinophilia and metastases to pancreas, bone marrow, ileum, lungs, and lymph nodes. In this case of scirrhous cancer, increased numbers of eosinophils occurred in the signet ring cells of the primary tumor and its metastases. It is possible that the signet ring cells produced a factor which mobilized the eosinophils in this patient (281). Carcinoembryonic antigen (CEA) gave the most sensitive test for the detection of occult metastases in 57% of a high-risk patient population with colon and rectal cancer. Computerized tomograms of the abdomen; including the spleen and the other organs complemented well the method cited above (87).

Animals

Natural killer cells of male C57BL/6 mice at the single cell level showed that estramustine phosphate did not change the number of natural killer cells but their lytic activity, therefore reducing their actual killer capacity. Spleen cells from diethylstilbestrol-treated mice had a proximal equal activity as control animals, but this compound reduced the number of lymphocytes with the ability to recognize target cells, and the natural killer cells showed an increased lytic activity and recycling capacity. The changes that these two compounds effected on the natural killer cell activity were reversible in one week (130). Plasma cell membranes or the products which they release play an important role in dormant metastatic growth. But the presence of the spleen is prerequisite (144). No direct correlation between granulocytosis-splenomegaly and the number of lung metastases was observed using the murine TS/A cell line (193). Mice bearing the immunosuppressive plasmacytoma TEPC-183 exhibit a marked splenic hyperplasia. Cyclophosphamide treatment resulted in an expansion of the splenic T-lymphocyte population. The immune response directed against primary TEPC-183 tumor cells was not inhibitory to metastatic tumor cells (244). Natural killer cells are most effective in the early phase of melanoma metastasis (309). Winn's assay using splenocytes revealed a postoperative enhanced suppressor activity in the cases undergoing laparatomy stress (264). The role of cyclic nucleotides in the development of resistance to metastases after treatment with immunomodulators shows on the one hand a close negative correlation between the increase in the cAMP/cGMP coefficient in thymus and spleen, and on the other, an inhibition of metastatic spreading in the lungs under the influence of levamisol and zymosan (289). Properties derived from normal T-cells when fused into non-invasive T-lymphoma cells cause invasive and metastatic hybrids (229). Small numbers of micrometastases in the spleen are detected only by the agarose cloning technique (158). Hybrids by fusion of T-lymphoma cells with normal lymphoid cells to study separation of tumorigenicity and metastatic potential showed no correlation between initial DNA content and tumorigenicity. Complete hybrids always exhibited reduction in the ploidy levels in the cells of primary and metastatic tumors (159). The appearance of potent antitumor immune potential in tumor-bearer splenic cells containing metastatic tumor cells was induced by a low concentration of L-phenylalanine mustard (melphalan) (29). The liver colony assay is useful in the determination of the number of viable tumor cells in a suspension (125). Using the MC-2 fibrosarcoma of the mouse, T-cell-mediated anti-tumor immunity was seen in the murine spleens with small tumors of the host but disappeared during increased tumor growth. The antitumor immune response by the suppressor cells seems to be connected with metastasis in this model. In the lymph nodes of the region, the late appearance of suppressor and metastatic cells may be due to similar processes, as in the spleen (61). Isolated lung metastasis exhibited significantly lower blood supply than the surrounding tissue in two murine models. In an experimental study in dogs pulmonary emboli were localized by using chest radiographs made in multiple projections (260).

Thymus (56, 294)

Types of neoplasms connected with more than 20 parathymic syndromes (most important: myasthenia gravis, pure red cell aplasia, and hypogammaglobulinemia) affected around 40% of patients afflicted with thymoma; 35% of thymomas are malignant (104, 140, 161, 187, 230). The apical surface of vascular endothelium lacks adhesive glycoproteins. Blood platelets may participate in the steps of blood vessel invasion by neoplastic cells, such as adhesion of blood-borne cells to the luminal surface of the vascular endothelium, penetration through the endothelial cell layer and local dissolution of the subendothelial basement membrane (306). Adherence of circulating neoplastic cells in the microvasculature must be considered a key event in metastasis formation (106, 250). Certain drug effects on vascular endothelium are accessible with the vascular endothelial cell monolayer model (194).

An acid-sensitive protein able to support the expression of the transformed phenotype of human melanoma seems to be contained in human platelets (246). Nimodipine, a dihydropyridine calcium channel blocker, is able to inhibit neoplastic cell-platelet-endothelial cell interactions (110). The platelet aggregation inhibitor RA233 is able under certain circumstances to inhibit metastases and prolong survival in experimental animals (162). Protamine and persantine were the most effective metastasis inhibitors in the rat prostate adenocarcinoma model (64).

Lymph

See section on B- and T-lymphocytes.

HEMATOGENIC METASTASES

Frequency of specific neoplasms (epithelial and mesenchymal)

The progression and distribution of malignant neoplasms exhibits a tumor-specific pattern, not only in regard to the soil where metastatic cells may settle or the topography of the organs, but also with regard to the way neoplastic cells are going to travel. The epithelial tumors prefer more the route through the lymphatic system, whereas the mesenchymal tumors, such as sarcomas or leukemias, prefer the

Table 7. Lymphatic hematogenic dissemination.

Neoplasm	Lymphatic	Hematogenic
Endometrial carcinoma	+	+
Carcinoma of gall-bladder	+	
Carcinoma of liver		+
Carcinoma of exocrine pancreas	+ may simulate carcinoma of lung (bronchus)	
Mammary carcinoma	+	+
Melanoma	+	+
Osteosarcoma	(+)	+

hematogenous way. Of course, as pointed out above, the connections between the hematogenic and the lymphatic portion of the system of body fluids prevents a total separation of these two types of secondary tumor distribution. In reality, phases of hematogenous and lymphatic tumor spreading may interchange. The following table provides a few selected cases of neoplasms and their dissemination via the system of body fluids.

Development of lymph nodes
The lymph nodes appear after the development of the lymph sacs by the aggregation of lymphoblasts in the mesenchyme around the plexuses of lymphatics developing from the primary lymphatic sacs. These lymphoblast aggregations occur in 30 mm embryos, but the first real lymph nodes cannot be recognized before 50 mm C.R. length of the embryo. They are first found in the axillary and iliac regions. The complete histological differentiation of the lymph nodes with cortex and medulla does not occur before birth. Lymph nodes produce erythrocytes in their early phase comparable to the hemolymph nodes, as, for example, in ruminants. This activity ceases after full development and only lymphopoiesis remains.

Histogenesis of the spleen
The spleen appears as a concentration of the mesenchyme in the mesogastrium dorsale (10 mm embryos) and extends

into the abdominal cavity in embryos with a length of 15 mm. The ability to produce spleen tissue shows a wide distribution in the subperitoneal mesenchyme. The simultaneous development of parasplenic structures is common. The mesenchyme of the spleen produces lymphocytes and reticulocytes and during the middle of gestation develop erythroblastic and myeloic cell clusters. The ability to produce myeloic cells ceases soon, whereas the production of erythrocytes continues until after birth. In emergencies, the spleen regains its erythroblastic capacity (256).

Most metastases in patients occur by hematogenous metastasis (278). This assumption may be clouded with doubt. It is more likely that human metastasis occurs in reality by a mixture of hematogenous and lymphatic steps, and even a combination with direct spreading. Ultrastructural findings regarding the interaction of neoplastic cells and blood vessels during hematogenous development of metastasis in animal models such as Yoshido sarcoma and others indicated two different ways of intravasation and extravasation: (1) tumor cells produced pores in the vascular walls and migrated through those; (2) the cytoplasm of endothelial cells enclosed neoplastic cells which moved the tumor cells intra- or extravascularly. Metastatic lesions involved tumor nodules accompanying neovasculature, spreading of tumor cells along the perivascular tissue of an organ, and diffuse infiltration of tumor cells in an organ (135). Hemorrhages (72.4%) were much more common than ischemic infarcts in patients with leukemia. The incidence of cerebral bleeding was lower (36.3%) in lymphoma patients. Cerebral infarctions (54.1%) were more frequent than hemorrhages in patients with carcinoma (94), see also Chapter 17/III. Four times more Lewis carcinoma cells than B16 melanoma cells were shed in the circulation. The numbers of cells shed from each neoplasm were orders of magnitude more than the numbers of spontaneous pulmonary metastases developing (92). In this regard the seeding by single cells and thrombi or emboli of different size should not be underestimated.

The metastatic pathways of malignant solid tumors, especially mammary carcinomas, could be seen as hematogenous, lymphogenous, or hematogenous-lymphogenous combined, depending on the capacity of the tumor cells to

Table 8. Characteristic features of the circulatory system.

Structures	Components	Histology
Heart	Endocardium	endothelium
	cardiac valves	endothelium, connective tissue
	Myocardium	cardiac musculature
	impulse conducting system cardiac skeleton	
	Epicardium (and pericardium, continuation)	endothelium
	Cardiac blood and lymph vessels and nerves	
Arteries	External tunic	Endothelium and subendothelial connective tissue
elastic type	Middle tunic	Smooth muscle and/or elastic connective tissue
Arterioles, metarterioles	Internal tunic	Elastic and collagen fibers and connective tissue
Capillaries	One layer of cells composing wall	Endothelial cells with tight junctions
Sinusoids	Present in liver	Larger than capillaries, with variable diameter
Sinusoidal capillaries	Present in endocrine organs	

intravasate the lymphatic and/or vascular channel and traverse the pulmonary artery. This metastatic pattern can be reproduced with cells of any of the organs involved, indicating that it is inherent in all cells of a given tumor, rather than being determined by the organs they colonize (142). Hematogenous metastasis of bronchial carcinoma depends on tumor size and presence of lymph node metastases (155).

Free metastatic cells
These cells have been discovered in the blood stream and lymph and were derived from several types of tumors. (For details see Chapter 14/IV.)

Tumor emboli
In Stedman (257), p. 455), a "tumor embolus" is defined as an embolus, comprised of neoplastic tissue, which is transported and lodged in a blood or lymphatic vessel and which may grow as a metastasis. One of the especially important steps is the arrest of circulating emboli in capillary beds with the formation of a thrombus. Billroth in 1878 was the first to describe thrombus formation in the process of metastasis of human cancer (278). A carcinoma begins as an epithelial lesion which penetrates the basement membrane and compresses or destroys surrounding normal cells. From this invading neoplasm detach small numbers of neoplastic cells and float as tumor emboli in the interstitial space. These neoplastic emboli are able to travel a remarkable distance and may stay dormant for long periods of time until circumstances such as the ingrowth of blood vessels enables them to grow and divide. From the interstitial fluid some neoplastic emboli will enter small lymphatic capillaries, travel in the lymph stream to regional lymph nodes or the vascular system. The neoplastic cells may pass through lymphatic venous anastomoses, disseminate without passing through lymph nodes, and may return through arterial capillaries to the interstitial spaces (236). Surface active phospholipids may act as surfactants opposing adhesion of neoplastic emboli (105). Faster growing neoplasms release more metastatic cells (177). Thrombocytopenia reduces lodgement of metastatic cells (247, 248). Mobility as well as release of degradative enzymes are characteristic of neoplastic cells (43). The shedding of viable cells parallels the linear, not the volumetric dimensions of the neoplasm (97). Subacute pulmonary hypertension may be due to carcinomatous microembolism (221), and embolism of the CNS due to carcinoma of the seminal vesicle (148).

(1) Entry of tumor emboli into the vessels
For this process details have been given above (135). But many specifics of the relevant processes are still unknown.

(2) Structure and size of tumor emboli
The size of tumor emboli as well as their structural components vary from two points of view; the processes can be considered tumor-specific. The first variability is given by the cell content of the thrombus, depending on the parent tissue of the primary metastasizing tumor; the second variability is given by the types of cellular blood or lymph components added. All these cells united in the neoplastic embolus are able to secrete different compounds and to interfere in the metastatic process. The size of the embolus is variable and depends on the number of cells involved.

(3) Arrest of tumor emboli

The main problem of arrest is adhesion which takes place mainly in the microvasculature. The firmness of adhesion is positively correlated with the metastatic potential of the neoplastic cells (265). The lodgement process is influenced by activated platelets and the release of bioactive substances (249). Immunocytochemical stains and antibodies to type IV collagen increase the rate of detection in histological examination (27). In the microcirculation in rat liver studied with microscopy and electron microscopy it was found that the neoplastic cells mainly became arrested by mechanical trapping in narrow liver sinusoids (13). Peritoneovenous shunting provides a unique opportunity for collecting data on the spread of tumors in man (271). The intravenous propagation of a clear cell renal tumor was preoperatively diagnosed by gallium imaging and computed tomography scanning (302). Radiolabelled B16 and Walker 256 cancer cells when injected into the portal vein of mice or rats showed that all of the cells were temporarily arrested in the liver and the majority later slowly released (299).

Complete intrinsic occlusion of the inferior caval vein was seen by renal cell carcinoma (164), and iliac arterial embolism after lung cancer resection (297). Surgical block dissection of inguinal lymph nodes is characterized by serious complications, especially those of wound healing (292).

Paranodal embolism, retrograde venous embolism, transpulmonary passage, uninterrupted passage through capillaries

The types of neoplastic progression mentioned here are not usual and depart somewhat from the general path of metastatic progression. Paranodal embolism appears when the lymph node is only partially involved or totally circumscribed in the path of the neoplastic metastatic cells. Retrograde venous embolism, also a sideline of spreading, was observed many times and is characterized by embolic distribution in the reverse direction of venous flow and leading to the arrest of tumor cells. The death of the majority of circulating neoplastic cells in the first organ, such as the liver, leads to a strong limitation of continued spread. Metastasis from the first organ encountered after the primary tumor, as to the lung may be a metastasis from metastasis (299) or may even pass through the lungs and seed in a third organ. Uninterrupted passage through capillaries is not the usual way but it occurs.

Fate of arrested tumor emboli

Neoplastic metastasis is an inefficient process. Many more neoplastic cells circulating in the body fluids and with a chance of being metastatic are destroyed than those which survive. The destruction of arrested circulating cells continues in the place of settlement. In this regard, the participation of non-neoplastic cells, such as thrombocytes and other components of the body fluid, play a significant role. An additional precondition to the fate of arrested tumor emboli is the heterogeneity of the different cell clones departing from the primary tumor. Another point to be considered is the topographic situation which directs the path of the

tumor emboli and, therefore, the spot in which they are arrested.

The tumor-characteristic hemostasis of malignant disease and clotting initiation as well as fibrin deposition of solid tumors growing outside the blood vasculature may result in protection from host inflammatory cells, change of the immune response and induction of angiogenesis (67).

Superimposed metastatic cells

Metastatic cycles are present when metastasis develops from metastasis (see Chapter 15/I), when metastasis and direct spreading are combined in sequence or when a combination of other types which are not as usual as metastasis on coelomic surface occurs (see Chapter 3/VII). Especially underestimated is the fact of parallel metastasis as it appears in two ways: (a) a consecutive one and (b) a simultaneously parallel one. In the consecutive case, a primary tumor will, for example, seed to the liver, which seeds again to the lung, etc. But the liver itself does not seed only into the lung but also to the other organs, and the lung, somewhat later, also starts to seed to other organs. The result is general dissemination via various organs involved in secondary spreading. The second way is given when a primary tumor seeds simultaneously into different organs, such as lymph nodes and they begin to seed again at the same time. This process also results in general dissemination.

The most important predictors for metastasis and general relapse in the prognosis of patients with Wilms' tumor lacking metastasis are anaplastic histology and microscopically confirmed involvement of the lymph nodes. Tumor thrombi in the renal vein or inferior caval vein increased the risk of metastasis; intrarenal vascular invasion was combined with a general relapse (38).

THE ROLE OF THE LYMPHATIC SYSTEM IN MAMMALIAN TUMORIGENESIS: LYMPHATIC METASTASIS

Neoplastic lymphatic metastasis varies according to the application of the intra- and interspecies comparison.

The lymphatic system and secondary tumorigenesis of nonlymphatic tumors:

Intraspecies comparative aspects of metastasis of nonlymphatic tumors are discussed in the following sections.

Lymphatic neoplastic metastasis involves in a large percentage of cases, participation in secondary tumor spreading of nonlymphatic tumors, such as colon cancer and other solid neoplasms. Similar to nonlymphatic tumors, lymphatic metastasis of sarcomas is also of lesser magnitude.

Nonhematopoietic cancers are able to produce marked effects on leucocytes, platelets and blood coagulation. Virtually every cancer can metastasize to the marrow but, in general, such reactions have been reported in cases of metastatic melanoma and breast adenocarcinoma. In bone marrow biopsies and aspirations cells of breast, prostate and lung tumors are found most common (2, 120).

Comparison of lymphatic metastasis in carcinomas and sarcomas

Carcinomas have the tendency to metastasize at a relatively early developmental stage to local and regional lymph nodes and they do so much earlier than sarcomas. Hematogenic-lymphatic neoplasms are not included in this comparison because they, such as leukemias, originate in a systemic way.

Lymph nodes, as other metastatic sites, may have been reached by blood-borne metastasis and by afferent lymph vessels as well. They must be retained there but the metastatic spread of the blood-borne cells may continue from the lymph nodes. Blood-borne metastatic cells may have been there after passing through the lymph nodes, but they may have left prior to the diagnostic investigation (20 and 27).

The role of lymph nodes in the staging system of neoplastic diseases

The participation of the lymph nodes in the neoplastic process is of great importance because it is of prognostic value for the planning of therapy and the outlook for survival ((18); and Chapter 5/IX).

Retention of cancer cells within lymph nodes and especially dormancy of residual cells and, finally, metastasis from lymph node metastasis can in their importance not be overestimated.

(1) Regional lymph nodes

It is not decided yet whether the lymph nodes when involved with a tumor in a particular region increase or decrease the risk of the patient. It has to be assumed that this may be different for the individual tumors. A review of the involvement of the regional lymph nodes according to the neoplasms of the body region is given in Table 3. The involvement of regional lymph nodes characterizes the second step of neoplastic development.

(2) General dissemination

This is the third and most dangerous step in neoplastic development, connected to or followed by cachexia. In general dissemination, a parallel involvement of lymph nodes and other structures and a continuous involvement of several lymph nodes and other structures as a chain reaction can be distinguished.

The activated human *ras* oncogene may confer metastatic potential onto lymphoid tumor cells (49). Tumor-associated macrophage content of murine solid tumors is accompanied by tumor cell proliferation and is a factor in radiation response of tumors (182).

Frequency of specific neoplasms (epithelial and mesenchymal)

The frequency of lymphatic metastases of epithelial and mesenchymal neoplasms invites an intraspecies and interspecies comparison regarding the various neoplasms involved. Selected examples have been given in Table 2. Our knowledge concerning non-human species is incomplete. Some variations are known from zoo, domestic and laboratory animals.

Lymph gland metastases as deposits for further metastases

The deposits in lymph nodes serve as deposits for further metastasis in uncounted cases. Lymph nodes can be seen as switching places for other types of metastasis or for tumor spreading other than lymphatic metastases.

Lymph gland deposits secondary to metastatic tumors in viscera

In switching from one type of neoplastic distribution to

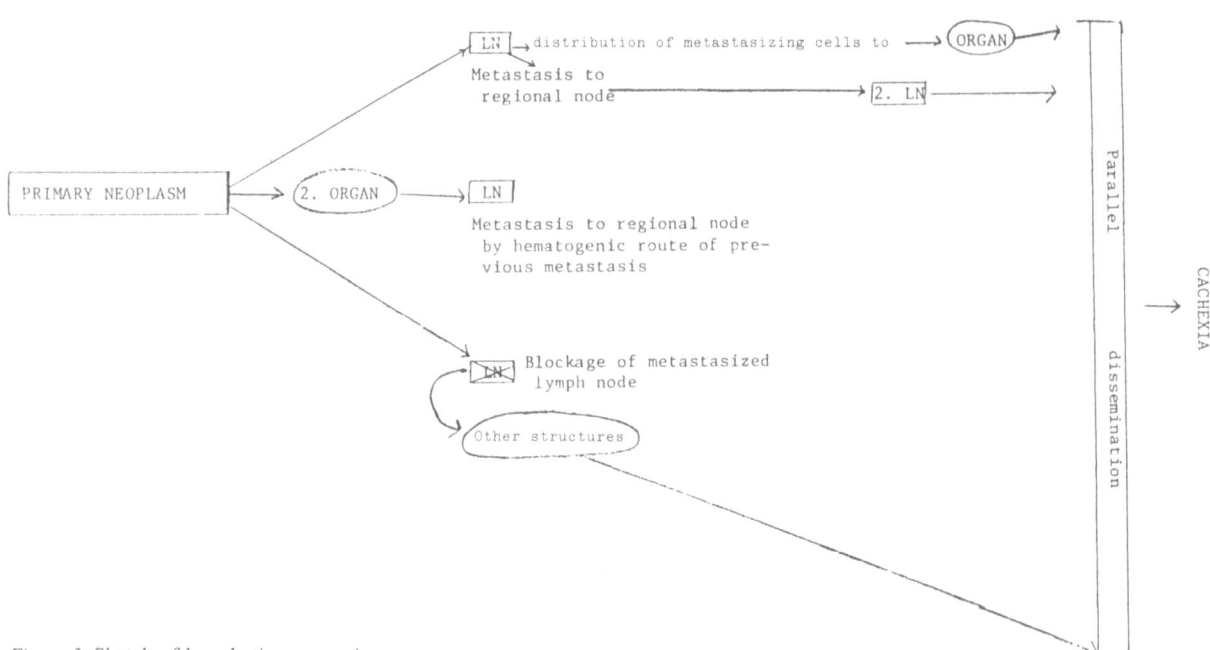

Figure 3. Sketch of lymphatic metastasis.

another, the involvement of lymph nodes may be secondary to metastases in the viscera, if the metastatic spread from a special organ, such as the liver (secondary involved), includes the regional lymph nodes of this organ.

The cancerous thoracic duct and thoracic duct lesions in further neoplastic spreading

The neoplastic lesions of the thoracic duct are a source of embolic dissemination comparable to lesions of large veins. The neoplastic occlusion of the thoracic duct is the most common cause of chylous ascites, but this phenomenon is not common but rare (Willis, RA: The Spread of Tumours in the Human Body. 3rd ed., 1973 – London: Butterworth, pp. 34/35).

THE ROLE OF ENZYMES SUCH AS ANGIOTONIN AND OTHER COMPOUNDS

Variations of serum enzymes in patients with malignancies relate to heavy tumor involvement or metastases (258).

The development of new blood vessels is an essential feature of the growth of solid tumors. This process is known as angiogenesis and induced by factors secreted by neoplastic cells (283). The prediction of the amino acid sequence of human angiogenin from the gene sequence corresponded with that determined by amino acid sequence analysis (156). Angiogenin is the first tumor angiogenesis factor to be isolated in pure form from human sources with proper amino acid sequence (261). Only 3.5 pmol is required to induce extensive blood vessel growth in the rabbit cornea (75).

In case of well-differentiated carcinoma of the thyroid,

patients with vascular invasion incline to show lymph node metastasis and/or extraglandular extension (112).

BIOPHYSICAL ASPECTS

The hemodynamic destruction of circulating neoplastic cells seems to be an important underlying cause of metastatic inefficiency. Large numbers of circulating neoplastic cells seem to be killed in the microvasculature. If we would understand these processes, better therapies against tumor spreading would be possible. The circulating neoplastic cells may be killed by friction or adhesion between cancer cells and capillary wall which result in an increase of tension in the cancer cell peripheries above a critical level due to (blood) pressure differentials between their free end. The increase of tension at the peripheries of neoplastic cells which pass through the myocardial capillaries will exceed the critical levels for rupture. Analysis of autopsy data for solid tumors reveals a low (less than 3%) incidence of myocardial metastases in the absence of lung metastases and a higher (15%) incidence in their presence. Relatively few neoplastic cells enter the coronary arteries from primary tumors with systemic venous drainage when lung metastases are absent, because many are retained or destroyed passing through the pulmonary vasculature. Most of these neoplastic cells delivered to the myocardium suffer hemodynamic destruction. When pulmonary metastases are present, large numbers of neoplastic cells liberated enter the pulmonary venules direct and are delivered to the myocardium without exposure to the arterial site of microcirculation. Increased delivery and protective effects of those arrested cells preceding them are responsible for a higher incidence of myocardial metastases (300).

Peritumoral vessel invasion in patients with breast cancer showing axillary lymph node metastasis seems to be a sign of increased systemic disease burden. Studies of 1510 women showed that the presence of vessel invasion was significantly associated with increasing numbers of positive axillary lymph nodes, rising tumor grade, nonstellate tumor border, growth pattern, and higher steroid hormone receptor content of the primary tumor. Depending on the subpopulation, patients with vessel invasion had a 41% to 54% greater risk of treatment failure than those without vessel invasion and a 29% to 64% greater risk of death (55). Oxygen tensions in tumors were substantially lower than in surrounding tissues (85). Invasion to the adjacent organs and limited lymphatic spread of gastric cancer can be controlled by wide combined resection of adjacent organs, and extended lymphadenectomy (95, 198). For kinetics of 13N-ammonia incorporation in human tumors, see Schelstraete (238). Recombinant interferon-gamma administered by short i.v. infusion can induce biological activities and causes less toxicity than when given by prolonged i.v. infusion (282).

COMPARATIVE TUMORIGENESIS

This is reflected in an inter- and intraspecies comparison. To understand the point here, comparative aspects are provided below.

Variations are: (1) the differences of circulation and lymphatics in the phyla. Due to free cells in body fluids of invertebrates and immunologic capabilities in these animals, these organisms may not be excluded from our comparison. (2) Selected species of the classes of vertebrates can be seen as phylogenetic steps in the arrangement of the lymphatic system. (3) The variations are composed of a complicated morphologic and functional mosaic of facts. (4) These host factors interact with factors of the neoplasms themselves.

a. Interaction of morphologic factors, producing a variability in the presence of tumors.

(1) primary tumors of vessel walls
(2) primary tumors of free cells
(3) primary tumors of lymphoreticular organs

b. Seeding to and implantation of secondary tumors in (1), (2), (3).

c. Variability of intraspecies and interspecies tumor types.

Variable involvement of the lymphatic system, especially of lymph nodes

The class of mammals with its high state of lymph node development represents, with the class of birds, the two warm-blooded taxonomic units.

As stated in other chapters such as 12/V birds are characterized by the predominance of mesenchymal neoplasms, with the exception of those of the ovary; mammals show a predominance of epithelial neoplasms. The species of birds exhibit a unique body plan, that cannot be said of the so diversified body plan of mammals (bat, whale, horse). In comparative oncology, it is possible to speak of metastasis in molluscs, arthropods, birds, and mammals, for example;

but metastasis is only relevant when it is seen as neoplastic cell distribution, occurring in body fluids and in settlement. It is misleading to equalize or simplify the various mechanisms involved.

The topography of avian and mammalian lymph nodes exhibits differences which are of remarkable value for the comparative study of neoplastic and, also infectious metastasis. In lower vertebrates with the "beginning" of lymph node development, patches of lymphatic tissue appear in the vessel walls. These structures are still present in birds, where the further developed lymph nodes, the avian lymph nodes, also appear.

Avian lymph nodes exhibit a thin capsule, thin lymphoreticular cords and no trabeculae. The distinction of cortex, paracortex and medulla is impossible. In the Pekin duck two cervicothoracic lymph nodes, 3 cm long and 2 lumber lymph nodes occur close to the synsacrum. Afferent lymphatic vessels continue from cranial into the node efferent vessels exit caudally. No hilus occurs. More avian germinal centers appear in avian lymph nodes of free ranging domesticated birds than in housed domestic birds. In birds, the phallus is erected by lymph and not by blood.

The phylogeny of the lymphatic system indicates that in invertebrates only hematogenic neoplastic and infectious metastasis may occur; but phagocytic and lymphocyte-like cells may participate. In the vertebrate, lymphatic metastasis develops as an offspring from hematogenous metastasis with the appearance of lymphatic vessels in the Dipnoi. The lymph nodes from mere tissue patches in cold-blooded tetrapod vertebrates to mammalian lymph nodes complicate this process more and more. Lymphatic metastasis exhibits therefore the step by step background of the development of the lymphatic system.

In the mammal, the lymph nodes are interspersed in the lymphatic system in a regional pattern. If a woman has breast cancer at the lateral side of the organ, other lymph nodes will be primarily involved in contrast to a tumor of the medial side. As mentioned above, the development of the lymphatic system led from fishes to amphibians, to reptiles, and from there to birds and mammals. It should not be forgotten that the mammals appeared earlier in the Triassic period than the birds which came later in the Jurassic of the Earth's history. Thus, this development of both vertebrate classes, at least in the advanced stages, continued in parallel manner. The avian lymph nodes, to a certain degree comparable to mammalian lymph nodes, occur only in certain species of birds. In contrast to the mammal with the regional lymph node distribution (Figure 1) the four main lymph nodes are interspersed in main vessels such as the thoracic duct. This means that they have less influence on a specific distribution of neoplastic or infectious metastasis, but, of course, are able to prevent or, perhaps, to promote general dissemination of neoplastic cells. The condition in the birds with avian lymph nodes is more comparable with lower organisms where hematogenic metastasis dominates or is solely present. The birds stand therefore on the level of a lower type of neoplastic metastasis. These theoretical questions are of utmost importance when neoplastic metastasis or infectious metastasis are compared in various classes and phyla of animals. Metastasis in the one and metastasis in another may be similar, but they must not be necessarily so in different species.

Table 9. Comparison of lymph node like structures and lymph nodes of vertebrates in regard to neoplastic metastasis.

Amphibians, reptiles, birds	Birds	Mammals
Patch-like structures in vessel wall	Avian lymph nodes	Mammalian lymph nodes
In different vessels	Only in largest lymph vessels	Regional arrangement
	No cortex, paracortex and medulla	Hilus, capsule, cortex, medulla
	Due to lymph node topography no regional, tumor-specific metastasis to be expected	Regional lymphatic metastasis as seen in table 2

Comparison of lymphatic and hematogenic spreading of neoplastic diseases

In our species, the frequency of hematogenic and lymphatic spreading of selected tumors differs, but varies also in different body regions by the histologic same tumor type. We have elaborated on this topic throughout this chapter.

Angiotensin I–II increased the blood flow of human tumors, in agreement with the findings in animal tumors (134). In radiation or tumor treatment, lymphostasis development was determined by injury to the lymphatic collectors only, or their combination with injury to the major veins (138). Intravascular and intralymphatic therapy of neoplastic diseases are aimed at the prevention or cure of lymphatic metastases. Chemotherapeutica and other agents should be brought closer and more directly to the tumor (225).

Extramedullary disease in Philadelphia chromosome-positive chronic myelogenous leukemia supports a poor prognosis (273).

Computed tomography of the chest is valuable in determining at three levels lymphangitic spread of neoplasms in the lung (259). Resection of subaortic lymph nodes in patients with bronchogenic carcinoma should be undertaken for a full investigation (212).

THE SIGNIFICANT ROLE OF THE LYMPHATIC SYSTEM IN TUMOR DISSEMINATION FROM THE MAMMALIAN LYMPH NODES

Sonographic examinations permit differentiation between inflammatory involvement of lymph nodes and primary lymphoma or lymph nodes involved in metastasis. Another possibility is the detection of the ability of lymphomas to respond to antibiotic, cytostatic and radiation treatment (39). For *in vivo* disposition of adriamycin in human tumors with different responses to the drug, see Cummings (52), and for gamma scintigraphy of lymphatic nodes with metastasis (179). Early metastasis to liver, lung, cerebellum and ovary occurred postoperatively by hematogenous spreading after tumor resection of pancreatic cancer (173).

I. C. PRIMARY NEOPLASMS OF LYMPH NODES

In the primary malignant disease of lymphoid tissue the proliferation of tumorous cells, either in the form of follicle-like structures or in a diffuse, sheath-like manner, upsets the normal architecture of the node – the true follicles disappear

and the lymph cords and the sinuses are obliterated (9). The lymph nodes can be involved, either as the source of the primary tumor on the one hand or as an additional involvement on the other. Fluorine-18-2-fluorodeoxyglucose is a more sensitive radiopharmaceutical for non-Hodgkin's lymphoma than gallium-67 citrate (213). Media from target organ tissues and other factors (organ-specific adhesion mechanisms) stimulate murine RAW117-P large cell lymphoma for blood-borne metastatic organ colonization (195).

DEFENSE, THE MAIN PURPOSE OF THE LYMPHATIC SYSTEM

The defense capabilities of the lymphatic system can be grouped in the following way: (1) collecting of unnecessary fluid from tissue spaces and its return to the circulatory system; (2) cellular defense by so-called killer cells and other cells of the lymphatic system (see Chapter 14/I); (3) humoral defense (see Chapter 17/IV); and (4) improvement of circulation.

A trial of adoptive immunotherapy showed that long-term cultured tumor-derived T-cells may be transferred safely into humans and enhance immune responses and tumor reduction (150). Studies by Matsuzaki and coworkers (175) showed that transnodal administration of emulsionized bleomycin in the rat is an effective and safe treatment for metastatic lymph nodes.

COMPARATIVE STRUCTURES IN NONMAMMALIAN DEFENSE SYSTEMS

The characteristic cells: B- and T-lymphocytes in mammals

B- and T-lymphocytes are the characteristic cells in mammals and can be compared to typical cells with similar functions in other vertebrates and even invertebrates.

(1) Comparable cells in invertebrates

B- and T-lymphocytes are concepts based on structural and organic entities of mammals; both cells derive from either the bone marrow or thymus. A comparison with respective cells in invertebrates can only be made randomly based on such characteristics as phagocytosis (126). In the description of the lymphocytic and hematogenous cells in vertebrates the outline given by Andrew & Hickman (5) is followed.

The lymphatic system is typical for vertebrates, reaching its highest point of development in the mammal. The beginning of lymphatic development can already be visualized in such protozoans as the amoebae, which in their life style show one of the important characteristics, namely, phagocytosis. Therefore, these animals can be seen as the starting point of the principle which will later develop into the lymphatic system. Ranging from the protozoans to the mammals, we find four stages in the development of lymphatic functions: (1) the premetazoan stage, from protozoans to porifera; (2) the stage of lymphatic cells or the prestage of the lymphatic system (according to Mislin*), eumetazoan invertebrates; (3) the lymphatic system, primarily without lymph nodes, from fishes to birds. (4) the complete lymphatic system with lymph nodes: crocodiles, certain birds, such as the ostrich, and especially, the mammals.

(1) The situation as found in the protozoans has been already mentioned. In the placozoa, amoeboid activity of fiber cells may exist. The totipotent archeocytes serve the function of phagocytosis. Immunologic aspects have been described for the cells of these animals (126).

(2) In this, the second group of lymphatic development through phylogeny, no separate lymphatic vessels have been developed in addition to the circulatory systems found in the majority of phyla, which may be either open or closed. Lower phyla, and very small ones, have no circulatory systems but also phagocytic cells and other cells attributable to the range of the lymphatic activity. Pulmonate snails and cephalopods develop a partially closed circulatory system through the development of vessels, but not in all portions of the body. This condition I have called "a mixed" circulatory system. Table 10 gives a review of the circulatory systems, because transport and action of free cells with lymphatic capacity depend on these conditions. In the following section, a brief review is given of selected examples of cells with lymphatic capacities for the invertebrate phyla, but it should not be considered exhaustive beyond the scope of this chapter.

B-Lymphocytes
Immunological effects were correlated with clinical in thymostimulin therapy in melanoma patients. The survival rate of patients on DTIC plus TS did not differ significantly from that of DTIC alone (25). Metastatic competence of cloned tumor cell populations may be controlled by immunogenetics (69). The immune response to oncofetal antigens may be inhibiting tumor growth and metastases in mice bearing a malignant fibrosarcoma (86).

T-lymphocytes (10, 93, 137, 141, 214, 266, 291, 303, 316).
It appears to be difficult to estimate specific cytotoxicity from phytohemagglutinin-blastogenesis (308). Melanoma patients with normal T-Ea, T-Et, and total lymphocyte values showed a significant, prolonged survival when compared to those with lower values (25). The metastasis of B16 melanoma cells differed significantly in obese and lean female mice of strain C57BL/6J. The primary tumor grew more slowly in obese than in lean littermates (275). Thymosin fraction 5 acted successfully as an adjuvant to irradiated tumor cells (266). A patient with invasive thymoma treated with radiotherapy, steroids, cis-platinum, and dox-

orubicin later developed a chronic lymphocytic leukemia (274). T-cell-mediated immunity is mainly important for protection against tumors induced by oncogenic viruses and not for many other types of spontaneous or chemical carcinogen-induced tumors (103). In the thymus are only two predominant cell types but nearly 15 histologically different neoplasms (230). A teratoma group tumor of the testicle exhibited mature teratoma in the metastatic foci (263). The acquisition of metastatic properties following somatic cell fusion with normal lymphoreticular cells may represent a mechanism of tumor progression *in vivo* (57) – see Chapter 12/III.

The lymphatic system in the different classes of vertebrates in relation to neoplastic spreading
Mammals have a very extensively developed lymphatic system characterized by the presence of lymph nodes. Therefore, the metastatic spreading of mammalian neoplasms encounters a special situation, uncommon in all other organisms. The other vertebrates, especially birds and fishes, in which a great number of neoplasms have been observed, show a characteristic variation of metastatic spreading whenever the lymphatic system is involved. This sharp contrast does not occur when we observe the hematogenic spreading of tumors in different vertebrate classes. The variability must be due to the lymph nodes, because other lymphatic organs, such as the spleen, are also present in the other vertebrate classes besides mammals. Birds exhibit lymph nodes only in the mesentery of some species such as the ostrich. In reptiles, they are known only from the mesentery of crocodiles. In amphibians, lymph nodes are not known but their lymphatic system is very active. Therefore, in experimental oncology it was difficult to apply chemical carcinogens to frogs (personal communication I. Berenblum). Fish, have neither lymph nodes nor bone marrow.

New aspects to the phylogenesis of the lymphovascular system
Electronmicroscopic investigations indicate that in the kingdom animalia the Dipnoi exhibit for the first time lymph vessels (personal communication by Vogel). In more primitive vertebrates than the Dipnoi, according to Casley-Smith (46), a special opening-apparatus in the wall of peripheral blood vessels enables the transport of larger molecules and particles from the interstitial connective tissue into the lumen of the vessel. Amphibians (160), reptiles (113), birds (24), and mammals (23) possess specialized lymph vessels with comparable structural and systemic make-up. Lymph hearts are present in the form of modified portions of lymph vessels, and in regulating stations between the lymphatic and hematogenic systems in some fishes, and in amphibians (239). The genesis of these mural lymphoreticular formations (MLF) ensues in the bird postembryonally and is antigen-dependent (20). Regular lymph nodes occur only in some bird species (duck, goose, swan) (22) and in the mammal. A possible analogy of the MLF and ALN, but also of the mammalian lymph nodes, is indicated by the presence of lymphoreticular cords with B- and T-lymphocytes and the macrophage and lymphocyte transfer through the endothelial coat of the lymph sinus and the post-capillary venules as well (20). The synthesis of the avian lymph nodes

---

* Ztschr Lymphologie 5(1):3–12, 1981.

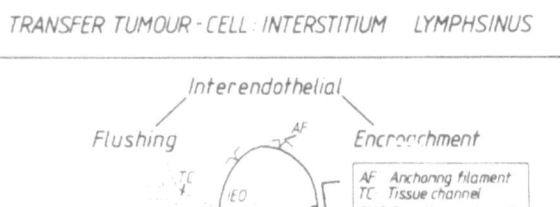

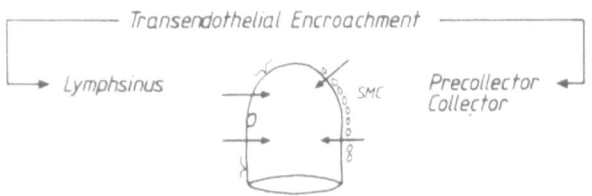

Figure 4. Representation of the tumor-cell-transfer into the initial lymphsinus lumen.

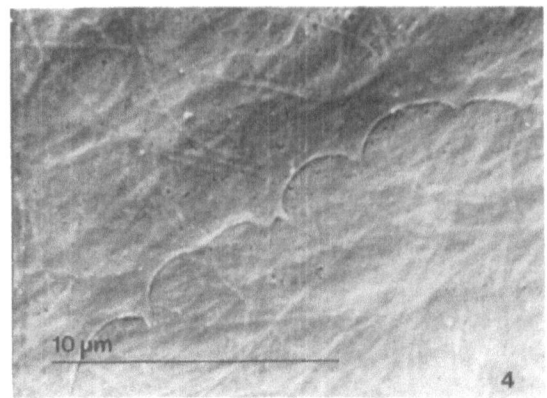

Figure 6. Luminal aspect lymph capillary of interendothelial openings of testis (*Pseudemys scripta elegans*). SEM-situation after indirect application of glutaraldehyde. Courtesy of C. Hunneshagen.

(ALN) shows common structural characteristics with the lymph nodes of primitive mammals (*Echidna*). A possible homology of the regular lymph nodes in birds and mammals is given by the identical ontogenesis.

3. Review of systems in the invertebrate phyla and their importance for comparative oncology

Invertebrates also exhibit metastatic spreading of tumors as described by Cooper (Chapter 6/V) for molluscs, and by Gateff and others for the fruit fly *Drosophila* sp. A metastatic process takes place in these organisms and mammals but we must not underestimate the big differences between these groups. In the invertebrates, we often find catastrophic development, as in the holometabolic insects. Larvae, as roundabouts of development, live longer than the imago and, therefore, should be able to produce larval neoplasms, which can be lethal, as known from *Drosophila*. During

development an animal may change from aquatic to terrestrial life; this, consequently, brings about a change in the respiratory organs with histolytic processes and, more or less well known, variations in the system of body fluids, including the hematogenic and lymphatic portions. Sometimes it can be very difficult to distinguish between the two. In the following a brief review of the lymphatic systems in the main invertebrate phyla is given (Table 4).

The control of cancer metastases is crucial for therapy. The grading system of many neoplastic diseases, such as different types of breast cancer, prostatic cancers or soft tissue tumors, takes into account how the lymph nodes are involved is, when the diagnosis is confirmed. HM Maurer and coworkers established four groups for the development of the rhabdomyosarcoma. Group 1 is localized and exhibits no involvement of regional lymph nodes; group 2 is regional, completely resectable with or without lymph node involvement; group 3 exhibits residual disease and is incompletely resectable; whereas group 4 is characterized by distant metastases at diagnosis. (70).

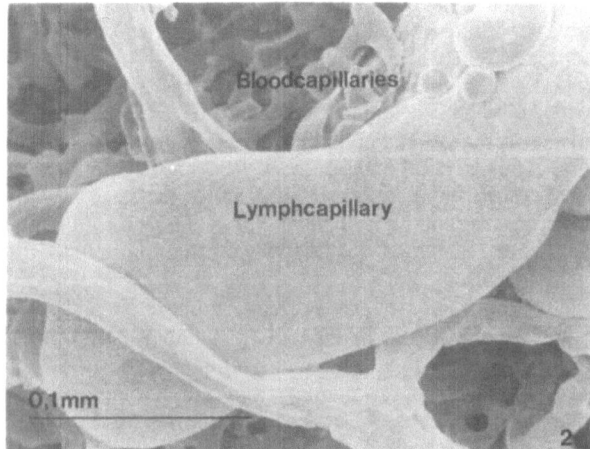

Figure 5. SEM-demonstration of a lymph capillary and blood capillaries in the stomach (submucosa) of a turtle (*Pseudemys scripta elegans*) after indirect application of MERCOX[R]. Courtesy of C. Hunneshagen.

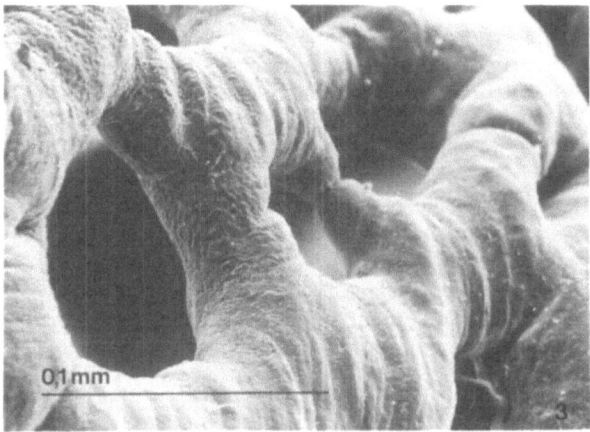

Figure 7. Net of lymphatic capillaries in the small intestine (mucosa) of a turtle (*Pseudemys scripta elegans*). SEM-situation after indirect application of MERCOX[R]. Courtesy of C. Hunneshagen.

The following topics should be briefly considered:

1. The role of the lymphatic system, including lymph nodes in the mammal

(a) Neoplasms of the lymphatic system *per se*

(b) Variable involvement of the lymphatic system and especially lymph nodes in metastatic spreading of various neoplasms

2. Review of the lymphatic system of the different classes of vertebrates in relation to neoplastic spreading

3. Review of lymphatic systems in the invertebrate phyla and their importance for comparative oncology

4. Comparison of lymphatic and hematogenic tumor spreading in man and mammals according to selected tumor types

5. Brief review of the hematogenic system in non-mammalian animals:

The role of the lymphatic system, including lymph nodes in the mammal. Functionally, the lymphatic system can be divided into the channels which a) collect fluid interspersed between tissues and transport it to regional lymph nodes and b) return it from there through the thoracic duct. Therefore, two units, the channels and the lymph nodes, can be distinguished in the mammalian body. For other animal species the situation is described later. Table 3 gives a short review of make-up and variation of lymphatic channels of different size and variable function. This is of importance for the classification of the classical lymphangioma. Figure 2 gives a review of the lymph nodes of the trunk in man (after Feneis, (74)).

(a) Neoplasms of the lymphatic system *per se*

Five disease groups can be considered as neoplastic diseases of the lymphatic system *per se*. In the first group, the lymphangiomas, it is not always easy to state whether such a disease is a true neoplasm, a hamartoma or a lymphangiectasis. Lymphangiomatosis is an extremely rare disease. The third unit, lymphangiosarcoma, generally cannot be separated from the angiosarcoma. In the case of the two last diseases, lymphangiomyoma and lymphangiomyomatosis, as the name implies, these diseases develop from the muscular coat. The tumors of the lymphatic system *per se* are grouped together according to the site of this appearance, not according to the tissue distribution as such. Therefore, they may be mentioned again in other chapters of the book.

Phagocytic wandering cells occur in the Cnidaria. The collenchyme in the Ctenophora exhibits amebocytes. The blood corpuscles of nemertini which have, phylogenetically, the first closed circulatory system, are nucleated cells. Gnathostomulida exhibit a rare connective tissue with cells for which a lymphatic function is not known. The Entoprocta also have a mesenchyme but the situation may be the same as in Acanthocephala where no wandering cells or amebocytes occur. In the Rotifera, wandering amebocytes or fixed phagocytes seem to be present. In the phylum Gastrotricha no wandering amebocytes are present in the pseudocoelomic spaces, as may apply to Kinorhyncha and Nematoda. In the first class of Nematomorpha, the Gordioidea, a mesenchyme is found. In the phylum Priapulida, coelomocytes are seen in the body cavity which are either erythrocytes or leukocytes. The leukocytes of *Priapulus caudatum* (174) are ameboid mobile cells with a cytoplasm containing numerous organelles, of which oval particles, possibly developmental stages of lysosomes, are especially

impressive. The histological picture, although complicated, shows some resemblance to the lymphoepithelial tissues of vertebrates (174). The blood of molluscs contains different types of amebocytes. The gastropod, *Biomphalaria glabrata*, exhibits hemocytes containing five monoclonal antibodies (mass) against antisurface antigens connected with hemoglobin-depleted ultracentrifuged fractions of snail hemolymph. Circulating *B. glabrata* hemocytes consist of a single predominant population of adherent cells which is composed of several distinct antigenic subpopulations (310).

Amebocytes of the pond snail, *Lymnea stagnalis* synthesize agglutinin opsonin and carry it on their surfaces as receptors for foreign material (284). The coelom of Sipunculida contains free or fixed ciliated corpuscles and amebocytes. The knowledge of the condition of the body fluid of Echiurida is insufficient as to draw any conclusions. The annelid worms exhibit different types of coelomocytes. The body fluid of the polychaete, *Flabelliderma commensalis* shows a blood pigment with the absorption characteristics of a chlorocruorin with maxima at 438, 558, and 606 nm (254). Application of scanning and transmission electron microscope low-dose and digital image processing techniques (203) to the annelid extracellular hemoglobin of *Lumbricus terrestris* have shown the existence of a central substructure. A coelomic fluid is present in onychophora and the large coelom of Pentastomida contains floating cells; the free cells of the body fluids of the largest phylum, Arthropoda, are complicated and the studies for a comparison of these cells with lymphatic characteristics, in my opinion, are still not conclusive. The difficulties are shown in the variation in the respiratory structures connected with the systems of body fluids. In the majority of adult insects (imago) of the phylum Arthropoda, the body fluids have nothing to do with respiration because that function is assumed by the tracheids, working with infusion. Other animals like the Meristomata and the crustaceans exhibit gills and body appendages. Book lungs occur in spiders. Aquatic insect larvae breathe through gills and use hemoglobin or other blood pigments. From these differences we can conclude that the unifying factor among the various phagocytes, coelomocytes or ameboid cells is the immunologic activity. The blood cells of insects have been reviewed by Jones (122) and Storch and Welsch (301). Studies by Smith and Soderhall (251) led to the conclusion that the attaching proteins of the prophenoloxidase cascade are strong nonself signals for the hemocytes in the freshwater crayfish *Astacus astacus*, causing them to degranulate and release previously cell-bound recognition factors into the hemolymph, where they are free to trigger activation of adjacent hemocytes. Five proteins of the prophenoloxidase-activating system in the hemocytes were attached to foreign surfaces (including the blastospores) after activation and it was suggested that these attaching proteins (one being phenoloxidase) are responsible for the opsonic function of the hemocyte lysate on crayfish blood cells (252). Reciprocal functional and structural adaptations in the circulatory and ventilatory systems in adult insects show adaptation to an economic and efficient use of a small hemolymph quantity for hydraulic functions in light-weight flight adapted insects (296). Proteins of the hemolymph of bees and hemolysin of rabbits were compared after separation by Sephadex G-200 (88). Glutaminic acid, aspartic acid and prolin have been found in the hemolymph of the honey bee, *Apis mellifera* L. (89).

Hemocytes of *Drosophila melanogaster* and *Drosophila yakuba* larvae have been defined by Brehelin (37) in terms of their ultrastructure and functions in "coagulation", wound healing, encapsulation, phenoloxidase activity, and phagocytosis. The position of these cells among the classical hemocyte types of insects was determined. Brehelin distinguished two plasmatocyte types (macrophage-plasmatocytes and lamellocytes) which do not seem to belong to the same lineage, and oenocytoids, which are crystal cells of the literature.

The red blood corpuscles in species of the Phoronida contain hemoglobin as respiratory pigment; brown bodies are found in the Ectoprocta, comparable to those in the Sipunculida. Coelomocytes occur in the phylum of Brachiopoda.

Three types of systems of body fluids, the hemal system, the water vascular system and the coelom appear in Echinoderms. The situation therefore is complicated. In the axial complex of the sea urchin, *Sphaerechinus granularis* (Lam.), intense phagocytotic activity was encountered by Bachmann (11). The phagocytes ingest morula cells and other phagocytes; a lysosomal digestion is assumed.

In Chaetognatha, the immunology remains to be investigated. The Pogonophora, such as *Siboglinum fiorticum*, exhibit a well-developed circulatory system; new studies of the cells with lymphocytic function would be necessary. Immunology of cells in Hemichordata with an open circulatory system are unknown. The open circulatory system of Urochordata contains a large number of cells with different pigments (183). Heart capillaries and respiratory pigments are missing in the blood of Cephalochordata, in which the coelom also is very restricted exhibiting therefore a unique situation. Moller and Philpott (183) suggested that the endothelial cells of *amphioxus*, like the endothelial cells in capillaries of higher chordates, most likely play a role in the physiology of the circulatory system by removing residues of filtration from the basal lamina, thereby facilitating an exchange of materials to and from the surrounding tissues.

3. The lymphatic system of vertebrates mainly without lymph nodes: fishes to birds

This group of animals is composed of the pisces or fishes; the amphibians; the majority of reptiles (with exception of crocodiles), and the birds (aves) with exception of the ostrich and a few other species.

I(1) Pisces, fishes: Agnatha

Centrifugation of the blood from the arctic lamprey, *Lampetra japonica*, by Fujii (82) yielded a uniform population of leukocytes containing about 90% of polymorphonuclear leukocytes (PMNs). Observations by both SEM and TEM revealed the formation of prominent pseudopodia, lamellipodia and phagosomes by the PMN during the process of engulfing erythrocytes.

Chondrichthyes

The lymphatic system is poor, often not distinct from the venous system but efficient in collecting fluid from the tissue spaces. Lymphatic valves or lymph nodes are lacking. In the spleen, true lymphoid tissue first occurs phylogenetically. The well-developed spleen is very similar to that of the mammal.

Osteichthyes

A well-developed lymphatic system with subcutaneous, intramuscular vessels, including those in the walls of viscera and glants, is found. In some species, pulsating lymph hearts occur near the opening into the vein. Lymph nodules without germinal centers have been observed. A spleen is present. Unique eosinophils, each of which contained only one eosinophilic granule, have been found in the peripheral blood of the loach (*Misgurnus anguillic caudatus*). Eosinophils are produced mainly in the spleen and to a small extent in the kidney, but not in other organs. The crystal line cores are almost pure protein (118).

The number of circulating erythrocytes in sexually mature male brown trout, (*Salmo trutta* L.) increases during October–December and a lymphocytopenia in both sexes from October–March (215). The increase in susceptibility to disease (furunculosis, *Saprolegnia* infection and fin-rot), was not accompanied by a reduction in the number of circulating lymphocytes. Chronically elevated cortisol levels may be better indicators of reduced disease resistance than changes in blood cell count (216).

Amphibia

Large lymph spaces, lymph capillaries and larger vessels are present; the lymphatic vessels are poorly developed. Four lymph hearts occur in the frog. Valves in vessels are lacking but are exhibited in some lymph hearts.

Lymph nodes are lacking in amphibians. Lymph nodules (dense clusters of lymphoid tissue, without germinal center) are common. In the frog, the spleen is the largest hemolymphatic organ.

Studies by Obara (201) suggested that in *Xenopus laevis* thymus-dependent lymphocytes preferentially localize in the splenic white pulp, and thymus-derived lymphocytes possibly in the red pulp. In contrast to its mammalian counterpart, the splenic white pulp of this anuran, the African clawed toad, *Xenopus laevis*, is the site where thymus-independent lymphocytes commence blast formation and transformation into plasma cells.

Birds, Aves

In contrast to findings in mammals, follicular dendritic cells in chicken spleen exhibit apparent acid-phosphatase activity and possess considerable numbers of primary lysosomes (68).

4. The complete lymphatic system with lymph nodes: crocodiles; certain birds, as the ostrich; and especially the mammals

In newborn rats, the marrow cavity of tail vertebrae is hemopoietic and contains no adipose tissue (272). The kinetics and the route of migration in the spleen and lymph nodes in the pig are comparable to data for other species, despite the peculiar structures of pig lymph nodes and the paucity of lymphocytes in efferent lymphatics in pigs (205). Not only splenic tissue seems to be an important factor in the protective function of the spleen (208). In normal young pigs, the bone marrow is an integral part of the migratory route of lymphocytes (209). There was no obvious redistribution between organ compartments with time after autoradiographical labeling of the spleen, using an extracorporal perfusion circuit. The spleen produces large numbers of lymphocytes which show typical organ distribution and homing to areas in lymphoid and nonlymphoid organs

Table 10. Selected aspects of cell structures and respiratory pigments in body fluids from nemertini to chordates.

Groups	Cells	Pigments

Nemertini	red cells
	white cells: hyaline amebocytes
	             amebocytes – eosinophil
	                       basophil
		hemoglobin, intracellular

Nemathel- minthes	spindle-shaped cells	diluted pigments. Ascaricruorin: *Ascaris* sp.
Priapulida	–	hemerythrin

Mollusca	lymphocytes
	macrophages
	eosinophil granular leukocytes
		diluted pigments:
		hemoglobin: *Planorbis cornuus*
		                   Planorbis umbilicatus
		Pulmonata:
		    Buccinum undatum
		    Helix pomatia
		    Littorina littorea
		    and others
		Cephalopoda:
		    Eledone moschata
		    Octopus vulgaris
		    Sepia officinalis
		    and others
		pigments in cells:
		hemoglobin: Pulmonata
		                Arca sp.

Sipunculida	blood cells, see annelida	hemerythrin in cells of body
		cavity: *Aspidosiphon* sp.
		           Phascolion sp.
		           Phascolosoma sp.
		           Physcosoma sp.
		           Sipunculus sp.

Annelida	eleocytes e.g.
	leukocytes: lymphoblasts earth-
	             eosinophils worm
	             neutrophils
	             basophils
		diluted pigments: hemoglobin
		(*Lumbricus terrestris* – this
		member of the Oligochaeta has
		been
		placed in this unusual systemic
		position in regard to the follow-
		ing forms because the author
		intends to show the blood cells
		of this very common form at the
		beginning)

Polychaeta		*Arenicola marina* *Eumenia crassa* *Nereis virens* and others
Hirudinea		*Hirudo medicinalis* *Haemopsis sanguisuga* chlorocruorin: *Spirographis spallanzanii* pigments in cells: hemoglobin Polychaeta *Glycera goesi* *Notomastus latericius*
Onycho- phora		blood has almost no respiratory function because of the tracheids
Tardi- grada	swimming cells in myxocoel	
Lingua- tulida	no circulatory organs	
Arthro- poda	hemocytes, clotting hemocytes granular oenocytes, ultrastructure oenocytes, histochemistry hemocytes hemocytes hemocytes hemocytes	*Limulus polyphemus* *Leucophaea maderae* Pterygota *Gryllus bimaculatus* *Periplaneta americana* *Galleria mellonella* *Calpodes ethlius* *Calliphora erythrocephala*

Table 10. cont.

Groups	Cells	Pigments
		The body fluid of *Limulus* contains blood pigments which the imagines of insects lack, because they respirate by tracheids (Dumont, Hagopian, Romer, Baerwald, Neuwirth, Lai-Fook, Zachary, Kaiser)
Tenta-culata (Lopho-phorata) Phoronida		changing of direction of contraction of blood stream
Bryozoa	ameboid cells in coelomic fluid, no circulatory systems as such	
Brachio-poda	amebocytes granulocytes, etc.	one subtype of the granulocytes contains hemerythrin (compared to the coelomic circulation of sipunculids and certain poly-chaetes)
Branchio-tremata Entero-pneusta	few floating cells in the well-developed circulatory system	
Ptero-branchia	similar to Enteropneusta	serum without color
Echino-dermata	red blood cells ameboid phagocytic leukocytes leukocytes spherule cells or trophocytes (big class variation)	cells of the body fluids of echinida contain, with other body parts echinochrom. This compound is not responsible for oxygen transport. The oxygen need shall be increased by this compound as it is the case with the eggs of *Halla parthenopeia* by the compound hallachrom, a red color
Pogo-nophora	new studies on the closed circulatory system of these animals are needed	
Chaetog-natha	the animals lack a circulatory system	
Chordata	all blood pigments are contained in the blood cells of chordates (in contrast to arthropods)	
Tunicata	hemoblastic cells, macrophages, vacuolated cells and special types	hemovanadin (shall not transport oxygen) *Phallusia mammillata*
Primitive fishes, hagfish	the principal types of cells of vertebrates occur in general: erythrocytes spindle cells (lymphocytic) monocytes thrombocytes granulocytes	hemoglobin remains the respiratory pigment in all following groups
fishes amphibians reptiles birds	the cells show in general a decrease in size and changes in the topographical center of development	
mammals	a characteristicum is the anucleated erythrocyte as typical red blood corpuscle of this class	

Table 11.

Coelomocytes in Echinoderms	Size	Function	Class*
Lymphocytes	4–6 μ	stem cells	1, 2
Phagocytes		phagocytose	1, 2, 3, 5?
Morula cells (colorless)	8–20 μ	ameboid behavior	1, 2, 3, 4, 5
Morula cells (colored)		ameboid behavior	1, 2, 4
Fusiform cells	6–12 μ	?	1, 2, 4, 5
Hemocytes	8–11 μ	colonization	1, 5?
Crystal cells		?	1
Vibratile cells		movement by flagellum	1
Eleocytes		metabolic, contain glycogen	2
Large spherical cells		?	2
Explosive cells	9–14 μ	removal of tissue debris	2
Red cells	8–18 μ (1)	red pigment	2
Reniform cells	39–46 μ (1)	?	2, 5
Osmiphil cells	10–12 μ	?	2
Small pigment cells	4–8 μ	?	3, 5
Hyaline plasma cells	17–32 μ	?	3
Phagocytes with short pseudopods	11 μ	phagocytic	4
Cells with rods and granules		?	4

* 1 = holothuroids, 2 = echinoids, 3 = asteroids, 4 = crinoids, 5 = ophiurids.

Source: The Coelomocytes and Coelomic Fluid, by Rob Endean in "Physiology of Echinodermata". ed. by R.A. Boolootian, Interscience 1966.

(206). The spleen also produces large numbers of lymphocytes during the secondary immune response with sheep red blood cells, many of which migrated to different organs, probably as memory cells, while others were found in the bone marrow as effector cells from the immune response (207). The bone marrow of pigs is an integral part of the migratory route of lymphocytes (209). Abundant connections between arterial capillaries and venous sinuses (i.e. closed circulation) exist in dog spleen. An "open" circulation also exists, inasmuch as the majority of all capillaries end in the marginal zone around lymphatic nodules (240). A crypto-lymphatic unit was observed at the left lateral aspect of the uvula of a mature female monkey, Macaca fascicularis. Three other monkeys of the same species failed to reveal similar structures at the same time site (189).

In the heterophil granulocytes of the guinea pig and rat, three morphologically identifiable granules are formed successively in early promyelocytes, azurophil granules in late promyelocytes, and specific granules in myelocytes. All three types of granule remain present during the maturation of the cells and can be found in the mature heterophils (34). Three types of granule originate in consecutive stages of heterophil maturation. Three cell stages were observed in mitosis: the early promyelocyte, the late promyelocyte and the myelocyte. In mature cells, roughly 14% nucleated granules, 10% azurophil granules, and 76% specific granules occur (35). In a study on the effect of pinealectomy of the rat by McMillan et al. (178) on thyroid cell numbers, 8 animals out of 66 were found to have thymic tissue in close association with the thyroid.

The development of the granule population of rat heterophil promyelocytes is identical to that of the granules in guinea pig heterophils. Both have in mature cells a gra-nule population composed of three types of granule, i.e., nucleated, azurophil, and specific (33). Since the formation of nucleated granules and azurophil granules in the guinea pig is restricted to promyelocytes, both can be considered to be primary granules. The moderately dense specific granules (secondary granules) appear later during granulopoiesis and are first present in the myelocyte (32). Bone marrow from hematologically healthy adults contained four main cell stages of neutrophil granulocytes: early promyelocyte, late promyelocyte, myelocyte, and mature neutrophil granulocyte. The existence of three successively formed and morphologically distinguishable types of granule in heterophil (neutrophil) granulocytes has been demonstrated for three mammalian species: guinea pig, rat, and man (36).

Lymphocytes in the palatine tonsils of normal young pigs were selectively labelled by minute, multiple injections of fluorescein isothiocyanate into the tonsils. One day later, considerably more lymphocytes were determined in cervical, bronchial and mesenteric lymph nodes; spleen; Peyer's patches; thymus; bone marrow, and blood. Relatively more lymphocytes were found in lymph nodes than in the spleen, but very few in the thymus, Peyer's patches, and bone marrow. This organ distribution differed from the results of selectively labelling lymphocytes in lymph nodes, spleen and bone marrow (208).

Monolayer cultures of endothelial cells of human dermal microvascular origin formed junctional complexes seen in uncontracted microvessels and specialized attachment sites at their basal cell membrane contained a complex network of bundled micro- and intermediate filaments and numerous Weibel-Palade bodies and accumulated electron-opaque deposits between the cells and the culture dish surface (19).

Electron microscopic studies of lymphoid tissues from bovine fetuses and from calves disclosed a non-lymphoid cell type in the thymus-dependent zones of secondary lymphoid tissues and in the thymus, distinguishable from reticulum cells, epithelial and endothelial cells, and macrophages. These interdigitating cells originate from monocytoid cells which undergo differentiation in the thymus-dependent zones during an immune response (28). The location and temporal appearance of the different classes of lymphocytes were investigated by Dijkstra and Döpp (63) in the developing white pulp of the rat spleen. It was shown that (1) already at birth, strong Ia-positive cells are present in the T-cell area; (2) the marginal zone develops as a distinct compartment, independent of the PALS and follicles; and (3) follicles are recognizable at day 14, the capacity to trap immune complexes on follicular dendritic cells occurs one week later.

SUMMARY AND CONCLUSION

The importance of the lymphatic system with regard to neoplastic progression is due to the following factors:

(1) The lymphatic system reaches its highest stage of structural and functional development in the mammals, including man. It influences neoplastic progression in man decisively.

(2) In its most diversified structure, the lymphatic system resembles a filter-station for body fluids, including metastatic cells, and an immunologic factory at the same time.

(3) The cells, vessels, diffuse aggregations and organs of the lymphatic system give rise to characteristic neoplasms, such as leukemias, lymphomas, lymphangiomas, and lymphosarcomas. Lymph nodes are frequently involved in the growth of primary lymphomas.

(4) Lymph nodes are breeding grounds for secondary metastatic neoplasms: those starting from primary neoplasms; those from metastatic neoplasms; or tumors from lymph nodes located closer to primary neoplasms.

(5) Carcinomas are more prone to lymphatic spreading than sarcomas. Several tumors can vary if compared with one another in this respect.

(6) Lymph nodes appear phylogenetically first in crocodiles, are rarely found in birds, such as the ostrich or the duck, and occur abundantly in the mammals.

(7) Primary and secondary neoplasms of the lymphatic system metastasize in a neoplasm-specific way.

(8) The stages of tumor spreading via the lymphatic system decide the survival or death of the patient. The lymphatic system is one of the central points of neoplastic progression for many neoplasms. Therefore, they are of important prognostic value.

(9) The lymphatic system is connected to the circulatory system not only morphologically and functionally but also as regards neoplastic progression.

(10) Metastasis from metastasized lymph nodes appears to be a general phenomenon of secondary or tertiary metastasis in the progression of many neoplasms, especially cancers.

(11) The question whether the lymph node in the cancer patient is supporting the patient or the tumor is not clear to date. There are divided opinions about the question whether metastatic cells in the lymph node are weakened or strengthened. Is the process of metastasis, after passing the regional lymph nodes, stronger or weaker as compared to metastatic progression bypassing the regional lymph nodes? It seems doubtful that this applies to all cancers.

(12) Lymph nodes are a barrier against foreign matter such as microbes and others. Neoplastic cells can be regarded as "foreign" matter because they do not obey the regulatory control of the body. More research efforts should be undertaken to enhance the role of lymph nodes as a barrier to cancer-spreading in man and more efforts should be made to clarify the immunologic and filter action of lymph nodes with respect to particular neoplasms.

(13) When the first set of regional lymph nodes is passed, a secondary set of lymph nodes may be present in certain body regions; when these are passed also, general dissemination most often occurs.

(14) In contrast to cancer, the invasion of lymphoma cells into lymph nodes can lead to dissemination and the disease may change from a lymphoma to a leukemia of the lymphatic type.

(15) In a broad comparative sense, as indicated above, the progression of malignant neoplasms is generally similar to the action of lymph nodes.

REFERENCES

1. Akatsuka N, Tokunaga K, Isshiki T, et al: Intravenous leiomyomatosis of the uterus with continuous extension into the pulmonary artery. *Jpn Heart J* 25(4):651–9, 1984

2. Alfrey CP Jr, White MR, Zelnick PW: Abnormalities of white blood cells, platelets, and hemostasis. In: *Medical Complications of Malignancy*, Smith FE, Lane M (eds). New York: Wiley and Sons, pp. 207–17, 1984

3. Al-Mandhiry H: Tumor interaction with hemostasis: the rationale for the use of platelet inhibitors and anticoagulants in the treatment of cancer. *Am J Hematol* 16(2):193–202, 1984

4. Almagro UA: Argyrophilic prostatic carcinoma. Case report with literature review on prostatic carcinoid and "carcinoid-like" prostatic carcinoma. *Cancer* 55(3):608–14, 1985

5. Andrew W, Hickman P: *Histology of the Vertebrates*. St. Louis, Mo.: CV Mosby, 1974

6. Ariyama J, Shimaguchi S, Suyama M, Shirakabe H: Intraarterial digital subtraction angiography in the diagnosis and treatment of gastrointestinal disorders. *Gastrointest Radiol* 11(2):177–82, 1986

7. Aronsohn M: Canine thymoma. *Vet Clin North Am* (Small Anim Pract) 15(4):457–67, 1985

8. Arriagada R, Mouriesse H, Sarrazin D, et al: Radiotherapy alone in breast cancer. I. Analysis of tumor parameters, tumor dose and local control: the experience of the Gustave-Roussy Institute and the Princess Margaret Hospital. *Int J Radiat Oncol Biol Phys* 11(10):1751–7, 1985

9. Ashley DJB: Evans' Histological Appearances of Tumours. vol. 1 (3rd edition). Edinburgh–London–New York: Churchill Livingstone, 1978

10. Ba DN: Cancer metastasis and immunology. *Chung Hum Chung Liu Tsa Chih* 6(2):154–6, 1984

11. Bachmann S, Phin H, Goldschmid A: Phagocytes in the axial complex of the sea urchin, *Sphaerechinus granularis* (Lam.). *Cell Tiss Res* 213:100–8; Bachmann S, Pohla SH, Goldschmidt A pp. 109–20, 1980

12. Baerwald RJ, Mallory Boush G: Fine structure of the hemocytes of *Periplaneta americana* (Orthoptera: Blattidae)

with particular reference to marginal bundles. *J Ultrastr Res* 31:151–61, 1970

13. Bagge U, Skolnik G, Ericson LE: The arrest of circulating tumor cells in the liver microcirculation. A vital fluorescence microscopic, electron microscopic and isotope study in the rat. *J Cancer Res Clin Oncol* 105(2):134–40, 1983

14. Bagshaw MA: Radiotherapy of prostatic cancer: Stanford University experience. *Prog Clin Biol Res* 153:493–512, 1984

15. Barberis M, Valagussa E, Pieri Nerli F, et al: Carcinoid tumors of the lung. Report of 66 cases. *Pathologica* 75(1040):803–11, 1983

16. Barnes L, Johnson, JT: Pathological and clinical considerations in the evaluation of major head and neck specimens resected for cancer. Parts I and II. Pathol Annu 21:173–250, 83–110, 1986

17. Bassil B, Dosoretz DE, Prout GR, Jr: Validation of the tumor, nodes and metastasis classification of renal cell carcinoma. *J Urol* 134(3):430–4, 1985

18. Beahrs OH: Surgery of the head and neck, 1896–1982. *Surg Gynecol Obstet* 157(2):1804, 1983

19. Bensch KG, Davison PM, Karaser MA: Factors controlling the *in vitro* growth pattern of human microvascular endothelial cells. *J Ultrastr Res* 82:76–89, 1983

20. Berens v. Rautenfeld D: Comparative aspects on the avian lymph system. In: Duncker/Fleischer (eds.) *Vertebrate Morphology*, Fortschr. der Zoologie, Bd. 30, 411–414, G. Fischer, Stuttgart/New York, 1985

21. Berens v. Rautenfeld D, Budras K-D: TEM and SEM investigations of lymph hearts in birds. Lymphology 14:186–190, 1981

22. Berens v. Rautenfeld D, Budras K-D: Topography, ultrastructure and phagozytic capacity of avian lymph nodes. *Cell Tissue Res.* 228:389–403, 1983

23. Berens v. Rautenfeld D, Lubach D, Wenzel-Hora B, Klanke J, Hunneshagen C: New techniques of demonstrating lymph vessels in skin biopsies and intact skin with the scanning electron microscope. *Archives of Dermatological Research*, in press

24. Berens v. Rautenfeld AD, Wenzel-Hora BI, Hickel EM, Henschel E: The system of lymphatic vessels and lymphography in the bird (2). *Tieraerztl Prax* 12:21–32, 1984

25. Bernengo MG, Fra P, Lisa F, et al: Thymostimulin therapy in melanoma patients: correlation of immunologic effects with clinical course. *Clin Immunol Immunopathol* 28(3):311–24, 1983

26. Bernengo MG, Lisa F, Meregalli M, et al: The prognostic value of T-lymphocyte levels in malignant melanoma. A five-year follow-up. *Cancer* 52(10):1841–8, 1983a

27. Bettelheim R, Mitchell D, Gusterson BA: Immunocytochemistry in the identification of vascular invasion in breast cancer. *J Clin Pathol* 37(4):364–6, 1984

28. Bielefeldt Ohmann H, Basse A: Interdigitating cells in the lymphoid tissues of bovine fetuses and calves. *Cell Tiss Res* 235:153–8, 1984

29. Bocian RC, Dray S, Ben-Efraim S, Mokyr MB: Melphalan-induced enhancement of tumor cell immunostimulatory capacity as a mechanism for the appearance of potent antitumor immunity in the spleen of mice bearing a large metastatic MOPC-315 tumor. *Cancer Immunol Immunother* 20(1):61–8, 1985

30. Bockus D, Remington F, Friedman S, Hammar S: Electron microscopy what izzits. *Ultrastruct Pathol* 9(1–2):1–30, 1985

31. Boon ME, Veldhuizen RW, Ruingard C, et al: Qualitative distinctive differences between the vacuoles of mesothelioma cells and of cells from metastatic carcinoma exfoliated in pleural fluid. *Acta Cytol* (Baltimore) 28(4):443–9, 1984

32. Brederoo P, Daems WTh: A new type of primary granule in guinea pig heterophil granulocytes. *Cell Biol Internatl Rep* 1(4):363–8, 1977

33. Brederoo P, van der Meulen J: Granule formation in rat heterophil promyelocytes. In: *Electron Microscopy* 1980, edited by Brederoo P and W. de Priester, vol. 2. Biology. Proc 7th Eur Congr on Electron Microscopy, The Hague, Aug 24–29, 1980, pp. 64–65, 1980

34. Brederoo P, van der Meulen J: Three types of granule formed in guinea pig and rat heterophil granulocytes. In: *Biochemistry and Function of Phagocytes*, Rossi F, Patriarca P (eds). Plenum Publishing Corp., pp. 1–7, 1982

35. Brederoo P, van der Meulen J: Development of the granule population in heterophil granulocytes from rat bone marrow. *Cell Tissue Res* 118:433–49, 1983

36. Brederoo P, van der Meulen J, Mommaas-Kienhuis AM: Development of the granule population in neutrophil granulocytes from human bone marrow. *Cell Tiss Res* 234:469–96, 1983

37. Brehelin M: Comparative study of structure and function of blood cells from two *Drosophila* species. *Cell Tiss Res* 221:607–15, 1982

38. Breslow N, Churchill G, Beckwith JB, et al: Prognosis for Wilms' tumor patients with nonmetastatic disease at diagnosis – results of the second National Wilms' Tumor Study. *J Clin Oncol* 3(4):521–31, 1985

39. Brockmann WP, Maas R, Voigt H, et al: Changes in the lymph nodes seen by ultrasonics. *Ultraschall Med* 6(3):164–9, 1985

40. Brodt P: Tumor immunology – three decades in review. *Annu Rev Microbiol* 37:447–76, 1983

41. Cady B: Lymph node metastases. Indicators, but not governors of survival. *Arch Surg* 119(9):1067–72, 1984

42. Carcangiu ML, Steeper T, Zampi G, Rosai J: Anaplastic thyroid carcinoma. A study of 70 cases. *Am J Clin Pathol* 83(2):135–56, 1985

43. Carr I, Orr FW: Invasion and metastasis. *Can Med Assoc J* 128(10):1164–7, 1983

44. Carr I, Levy M, Orr K, Bruni J: Lymph node metastasis and cell movement: ultrastructural studies on the rat 13762 mammary carcinoma and Walker carcinoma. *Clin Exp Metastasis* 3(2):125–39, 1985

45. Carter RL, Barr LC, O'Brien CJ, et al: Transcapsular spread of metastatic squamous cell carcinoma from cervical lymph nodes. *Am J Surg* 150(4):495–9, 1985

46. Casley-Smith JR: The Phylogeny of Lymphatic System. In: Földi/Casley-Smith (Eds.) *Lymphangiology*, 1–25, F.K. Schattauer, Stuttgart/New York, 1983

47. Chissov VI, Rusakov KG, Shchitkov KG, et al: Experimental study of the need for the dearterialization of tumors. *Eksp Onkol* 6(4):66–70, 1984

48. Cochran AJ, Pihl E, Wen D-R, et al: Zone immune suppression of lymph nodes draining malignant melanoma: histologic and immunohistologic studies. *JNCL* 78(3):399–405, 1987

49. Collard JG, Schijwen JF, Roos E: Invasive and metastatic potential induced by ras-transfection into mouse BW5147 T-lymphoma cells. *Cancer Res* 47(3):754–9, 1987

50. Craighead JE, Juliano EB: Asbestos-associated disease: can the issue be resolved in the courtroom? *Monogr Pathol* (26):211–21, 1985

51. Crissman JD: Tumor-host interactions as prognostic factors in the histologic assessment of carcinomas. *Pathol Annu* 21 Pt 1:29–52, 1986

52. Cummings J, McArdle CS: Studies on the *in vivo* disposition of adriamycin in human tumours which exhibit different responses to the drug. *Br J Cancer* 53(6):835–8, 1986

53. Custer RP, Bosma GC, Bosma MJ: Severe combined immunodeficiency (SCID) in the mouse. Pathology, reconstitution, neoplasms. *Am J Pathol* 120(3):464–77, 1985

54. Dalal BI, Slinger RP: Formaldehyde-induced fluorescence in melanomas and other lesions. *Arch Pathol Lab Med* 109(6):551–4, 1985

55. Davis BW, Gelber R, Goldhirsch A, et al: Prognostic significance of peritumoral vessel invasion in clinical trials of adjuvant therapy for breast cancer with axillary lymph node metastasis. *Hum Pathol* 16(12):1212–8, 1985

56. Day DL, Gedgaudas E: Symposium on Nonpulmonary Aspects in Chest Radiology. The thymus. *Radiol Clin North Am* 22(3):519–38, 1984

57. De Baetselier P, Roos E, Brys L, et al: Generation of invasive and metastatic variants of a non-metastatic T-cell lymphoma by *in vivo* fusion with normal host cells. *Int J Cancer* 34(5):731–8, 1984

58. Delforge A, De Caluwe JP, Ronge-Collard E, et al: Increased levels of myeloid progenitor cells in the blood of patients with metastatic invasion of the marrow. *Scand J Haematol* 31(3):275–9, 1983

59. Dellmann H-D, Brown EM: *Textbook of Veterinary Histology*. 2nd edition. Philadelphia: Lea & Febiger, 1981

60. Dennis JW, Laferte S, Man MS, et al: Adoptive immune therapy in mice bearing poorly immunogenic metastases, using T lymphocytes stimulated *in vitro* against highly immunogenic mutant sublines. *Int J Cancer* 34(5):709–16, 1984

61. Dent LA, Finlay-Jones JJ: *In vivo* detection and partial characterization of effector and suppressor cell populations in spleens of mice with large metastatic fibrosarcomas. *Br J Cancer* 51(4):533–41, 1985

62. De Young NJ, Gill PG: Monocyte antibody-dependent cellular cytotoxicity in cancer patients. *Cancer Immunol Immunother* 18(1):54–8, 1984.

63. Dijkstra CD, Dopp EA: Ontogenetic development of T- and B-lymphocytes and non-lymphoid cells in the white pulp of the rat spleen. *Cell Tiss Res* 229:351–63, 1983

64. Drago JR, Curley RM, Sipio JC: Nb rat prostate adenocarcinoma model: metastasis. *Anticancer Res* 5(2):193–6, 1985

65. Dumont JN, Anderson E, Winner G: Some cytologic characteristics of the hemocytes of *Limulus* during clotting. *J Morph* 119:181–208, 1966

66. Dvorak HF, Senger DR, Dvorak AM: Fibrin as a component of the tumor stroma: origins and biological significance. *Cancer Metastasis Rev* 2(1):41–73, 1983

67. Dvorak HF: Thrombosis and cancer. *Hum Pathol* 18(3):275–84, 1987

68. Eikelenboom P, Kroese FGM, van Rooijen N: Immune complex-trapping cells in the spleen of the chicken. *Cell Tiss Res* 231:377–86, 1983

69. Eisenbach L, De Baetselier P, Katzav S, et al: Immunogenetic control of metastatic competence of cloned tumor cell populations. *Symp Fundam Cancer Res* 36:101–21, 1983

70. Enzinger F: A clinical and pathological staging system for soft tissue sarcomas. *Cancer* 40:1015, 1977

71. Epstein JI, Eggleston JC: Immunohistochemical localization of prostate-specific acid phosphatase and prostate-specific antigen in stage A2 adenocarcinoma of the prostate prognostic implications. *Hum Pathol* 15(9):853–9, 1984

72. Estour B, Berger N, Bancel B, et al: Immunohistochemistry of thyroglobulin by indirect immunofluorescence in thyroid cancers. *Presse Med* 13(42):25555–8, 1984

73. Ezdinii EZ, Costello WG, Kucuk O, Berard CW: Effect of the degree of nodularity on the survival of patients with nodular lymphomas. *J Clin Oncol* 5(3):413–8, 1987

74. Feneis H: Pocket Atlas of Human Antomy. (1st English edition). Stuttgart-New York: Thieme Inc, 1976

75. Fett JW, Strydom DJ, Lobb RR, et al: Isolation and characterization of angiogenin, an angiogenic protein from human carcinoma cells. *Biochemistry* 24:5480–6, 1985

76. Fidler IJ: Tumor heterogeneity and the biology of cancer invasion and metastasis. Cancer Res 38(9): 2651–60, 1978

77. Fisher B, Bauer M, Margolese R, et al: Five-year results of a randomized clinical trial comparing total mastectomy and segmental mastectomy with or without radiation in the treatment of breast cancer. *N Eng J Med* 312(11):665–73, 1985a

78. Fisher B, Redmond C, Fisher ER, et al: Ten-year results of a randomized clinical trial comparing radical mastectomy and total mastectomy with or without radiation. *N Eng J Med* 312(11):674–81, 1985b

79. Fritjofsson A, Hemmingsson A, Lindgren PG, Reinholdsson S: Preoperative staging of renal carcinoma. A methodologic comparison. *Ups J Med Sci* 90(2):101–6, 1985

80. Friedell GH, Soto EA, Kumaoka S, et al: Pathology of primary tumors and axillary lymph nodes in British and Japanese women with breast cancer. *Breast Cancer Res Treat* 3(2):165–9, 1983

81. Frost P, Kerbel RS: Immunology of metastasis. Can the immune response cope with disseminated tumor? *Cancer Metastasis Rev* 2(3):239–56, 1983

82. Fujii T: Antibody-enhanced phagocytosis of lamprey polymorphonuclear leucocytes against sheep erythrocytes. *Cell Tiss Res* 219:41–51, 1981

83. Gadaleanu V, Muresan R: Inclusions of benign nevus cells in the capsule of axillary lymph nodes in three cases of breast cancer. *Morphol Embryol* (Bucur) 30(2):137–9, 1984

84. Gasic GJ: Role of plasma, platelets, and endothelial cells in tumor metastasis. *Cancer Metastasis Rev* 3(2):99–114, 1984

85. Gatenby RA, Coia LR, Richter MP, et al: Oxygen tension in human tumors: *in vivo* mapping using CT-guided probes. *Radiology* 156(1):211–4, 1985

86. Gautam S, Deodhar SD: Inhibition of tumor growth and metastasis in mice bearing a malignant fibrosarcoma by T cell-mediated immune response to oncofetal antigens. *Am J Reprod Immunol* 3(3):141–8, 1983

87. Gianola FJ, Dwyer A, Jones AE, Sugarbaker PH: Prospective studies of laboratory and radiologic tests in the management of colon and rectal cancer patients: I. Selection of useful preoperative tests through an analysis of surgically occult metastases. *Dis Colon Rectum* 27(12):811–8, 1984

88. Gilliam M: Gel filtration of the hemolymph of the honey bee (*Apis mellifera* L.). *Separatum Experientia* 28:341, 1972

89. Gilliam M, McCaughey WF: Total amino acids in developing worker honey bees (*Apis mellifera* L.). *Separatum Experientia* 28:142, 1972a

90. Gulenchyn KY, Papoff W: Technetium-99m MDP scintigraphy. An insensitive tool for the detection of bone marrow metastases. *Clin Nucl Med* 12(1):45–6, 1987

91. Guilloteau D, Baulieu JL, Besnard JC: Medullary-thyroid-carcinoma imaging in an animal model: use of radiolabeled anticalcitonin F(ab′)2 and meta iodobenzylguanidine. *Eur J Nucl Med* 11(6–7):198–200, 1985

92. Glaves D: Correlation between circulating cancer cells and incidence of metastases. *Br J Cancer* 48(5):665–73, 1983

93. Gorelik E: Concomitant tumor immunity and the resistance to a second tumor challenge. *Adv Cancer Res* 39:71–120, 1983

94. Graus F, Rogers LR, Posner JB: Cerebrovascular complications in patients with cancer. *Medicine* (Baltimore) 64(1):16–35, 1985

95. Gregl A: Roentgen anatomy of the lymphatic system. *Z Lymphol* 9(2):59–67, 1985

96. Gupta MK, Arciaga R, Bocci L, et al: Measurement of a monoclonal-antibody-defined antigen (CA19-9) in the sera of patients with malignant and nonmalignant diseases. *Cancer* 56(2):277–83, 1985

97. Gyure LA, Styles JM, Dean CJ, et al: The shedding of viable cells into the local lymph by tumours growing in the gut of rats. *Br J Cancer* 51(3):379–82, 1985

98. Hagopian M: Unique structures in the insect granular hemocytes. *J Ultrastr Res* 36:646–58, 1971

99. Hanna N: Regulation of natural killer cell activation: implementation for the control of tumor metastasis. *Nat Immun Cell Growth Regul* 3(1):22–33, 1983

100. Harder T, Koischwitz D, Engel C: Primary tumors of the

mesentery and greater omentum. *ROFO* 139(3):274–80, 1983

101. Helle M, Krohn K: Immunohistochemical reactivity of monoclonal antibodies to human milk-fat globule with breast carcinoma and with other normal and neoplastic tissues. *Acta Pathol Microbiol Immunol Scand (A)* 94(1):43–51, 1986

102. Henson DE: Staging for cancer. New developments and importance to pathology. *Arch Pathol Lab Med* 109(1):13–6, 1985

103. Herberman RB: Possible role of natural killer cells and other effector cells in immune surveillance against cancer. *J Invest Dermatol* 83(1 Suppl):137s–40s, 1984

104. Herrmann E, Jr, Lindstrom JM, Keesey JC, Mulder DG: Myasthenia gravis – current concepts (clinical conference). *West J Med* 142(6):797–809, 1985

105. Hills BA: Surfactant as a release agent opposing the adhesion of tumor cells in determining malignancy. *Med Hypotheses* 14(1):99–110, 1984

106. Hirata H, Tanaka K: The role of blood platelet and fibrinogen in experimental metastasis in nude mice following whole body X-irradiation. *Neoplasma* 32(5):547–52, 1985

107. Hollander N: The immunotherapeutic effect of anti Lyt-1 antibodies on local and metastatic tumor growth. *Adv Exp Med Biol* 186:819–26, 1985

108. Homann B, Zenner HP, Schauber J, Ackermann R: Tumor cells carried through autotransfusion. Are these cells still malignant? *Acta Anaesthesiol Belg* 35 Suppl:51–9, 1984

109. Homo-Delarche F: Glucocorticoid receptors and steroid sensitivity in normal and neoplastic human lymphoid tissues: a review. *Cancer Res* 44(2):431–7, 1984

110. Honn KV, Onoda JM, Diglio CA, et al: Inhibition of tumor cell-platelet interactions and tumor metastasis by the calcium channel blocker, nimodipine. *Clin Exp Metastasis* 2(1):61–72, 1984

111. Hoon DS, Korn EL, Cochran AJ: Variations in functional immunocompetence of individual tumor-draining lymph nodes in humans. *Cancer Res* 47(6):1740–4, 1987

112. Hosoya T, Sakamoto A, Sakurai K, Kasai N: Vascular invasion, lymph node metastasis and extraglandula extension of well-differentiated carcinoma of the thyroid. *Gan No Rinsho* 32(1):23–6, 1986

113. Hunneshagen C: Structural characteristics of the system of lymphatic vessels in the turtle (*Pseudemys scripta elegans*). Tieraerztl Hochschule Hannover, vet med dissertation, in press

114. Hurteloup P, Armand JP, Cappelaere P, et al: Phase II clinical evaluation of doxifluridine. *Cancer Treat Rep* 70(6):731–7, 1986

115. Imam A, Drushella MM, Taylor CR, Tokas ZA: Generation and immunohistological characterization of human monoclonal antibodies to mammary carcinoma cells. *Cancer Res* 45(1):263–71, 1985

116. Inculet RI, Keller SM, Dwyer A, Roth JA: Evaluation of noninvasive tests for the preoperative staging of carcinoma of the esophagus: a prospective study. *Ann Thorac Surg* 40(6):561–5, 1985

117. Inoue Y, Nelson DS: Effect of tumor-associated macrophages on the growth of tumors in rats. *Anat J Exp Biol Med Sci* 62 (Pt 2):181–8, 1984

118. Ishizeki K, Nawa T, Tachibana T, et al: Hemopoietic sites and development of eosinophil granulocytes in the loach, *Misgurnus aguillicaudatus*. *Cell Tiss Res* 235:419–26, 1984

119. Isono K, Onoda S, Okuyama K, Sato H: Recurrence of intrathoracic esophageal cancer. *Jpn J Clin Oncol* 15(1):49–60, 1985

120. Jeglum KA: Treatment of metastasis. *Vet Clin North Am* (Small Anim Pract) 15(3):659–66, 1985

121. Johnson JT, Myers EN, Bedetti CD, et al: Cervical lymph node metastases. Incidence and implications of extracapsular carcinoma. *Arch Otolaryngol* 111(8):534–7, 1985

122. Jones JC: Hemacytopoiesis in insects. In: *Regulation of Hemacytopoiesis* AS Gordon (ed.), pp. 7–65. New York: Appleton-Century Crofts., 1970

123. Juacaba SF, McKinnell RG, Hanson WJ, Tarin D: Vascular dissemination of tumor cells in relation to temperature-dependent metastasis in frogs. *JNCI* 78(2):259–64, 1987

124. Jung S, Jung G, Tranzer A, Dorr R: Blood fibronectin changes in various neoplasms. *Presse Med* 15(5):197–8, 1986

125. Juraskova V, Drasil V, Ryabchenko NI: The radiosensitivity of lymphosarcoma cells as determined by the liver colony method. *Gen Physiol Biophys* 2(5):385–94, 1983

126. Kaiser HE: *Species Potential of Invertebrates for Toxicological Research.* University Park Press, Baltimore, 1980

127. Kaiser HE: (ed): *Neoplasms – Comparative Pathology of Growth in Animals, Plants, and Man.* Baltimore: Williams & Wilkins, 1981

128. Kaiser HE: Principles of a comparative functional histology. *Gegenbaurs morph Jahrb, Leipzig* 129(2):137–80, 1983

129. Kaiser HE: Functional Comparative Histology. 5. Communication: History of Histology. *Gegenbaurs morph Jahrb* Leipzig 131(6):815–62, 1985

130. Kalland T, Haukaas SA: Effects of diethylstilbestrol and estramustine phosphate (estracyt) on natural killer cell activity and tumor susceptibility in male mice. *Prostate* 5(6):649–60, 1984

131. Kamenov B, Kieran MW, Barrington-Leigh J, Longenecker BM: Homing receptors as functional markers for classification, prognosis, and therapy of leukemias and lymphomas. *Proc Soc Exp Biol Med* 177(2):211–9, 1984

132. Kampmeier OF: *Evolution and Comparative Morphology of the Lymphatic System.* Springfield, Illinois: Charles C. Thomas Publisher, 1969

133. Kasper N, Wolff P, Wagner R, Just H: Massive tumor embolism as the cause of acute cor pulmonale. *Z Kardiol* 74(8):482–4, 1985

134. Kato T: Tumor vascularity under hypertension induced by intravenous infusion of angiotensin II – angiographic and radionuclide angiographic observations. Gan To Kagaku Ryoho 13(4) Pt 2:1423–8, 1986

135. Kawaguchi T, Nakamura K: Cancer metastasis and blood vessels. *Gan To Kagaku Ryoho* 10(7):1569–76, 1983

136. Kehl A, Nagel GA: Significance of puncture cytology for the detection of metastases in known and unknown primary tumors from the viewpoint of the oncologist. *J Urol* 131(5):243–6, 1984

137. Keith J: An introduction to tumor immunology. *Mater Med Pol* 16(1):54–64, 1984

138. Khalmosh L, Bardychev MS: Lymphostasis of the lower extremities following the radiation or combined treatment of malignant tumors. *Med Radiol (Mosk)* 30(10):34–8, 1985

139. Khato J, Chirigos MA, Sieber SM: Antimetastatic effects of maleic anhydride-divinyl ether in rats with mammary adenocarcinoma. *J Immunopharmacol* 5(1–2):65–75, 1983

140. Khmelnitskii OK, Vasilev VN, Grintsevich II, Cheremnykh AA: Thymic carcinoids. *Vopr Onkol* 30(9):7–13, 1984

141. Kim U: On the immunogenicity of tumor cells and the pattern of metastasis. *Symp Fundam Cancer Res* 36:337–52, 1983

142. Kim U: Pathogenesis and characteristics of spontaneously metastasizing mammary carcinomas and the general principle of metastasis. *J Surg Oncol* 33(3):151–65, 1986

143. Klein FA, Smith MJ, Greenfield LJ: Extracorporeal circulation for renal cell carcinoma with supradiaphragmatic vena caval thrombi. *J Urol* 31(5):880–3, 1984

144. Klein S, de Bonaparte YP, de D'Elia I: Enhancement of the incidence of metastasis in tumor-resected mice. Influence of soluble tumor extract and splenectomy. *Invasion Metastasis* 5(5):309–16, 1985

145. Koide D, Tanino M, Yoshimatsu H: A pathologic review of thymic neoplasms. *Sangyo Ika Daigaku Zasshi* 7(4):435–52,

1985

146. Korcakova L, Pazourek J, Jarosikova T, Holub M: Large granular lymphocytes in blood of healthy donors and patients with tumors. *Neoplasma* (2):181–5, 1983

147. Koscielny S, Tubiana M, La MC, et al: Breast cancer: relationship between the size of the primary tumor and the probability of metastatic dissemination. *Br J Cancer* 49(6):709–15, 1984

148. Koya G, Chen W: Metastatic behavior of human tumor cell lines grown the nude mouse. *Nippon Rinsho* 41(10):2402–11, 1983

149. Kozlowski JM, Fidler IJ, Campbell D, et al: Metastatic behavior of human tumor cell lines grown in the nude mouse. *Cancer Res* 44(8):3522–9, 1984

150. Kradin RL, Boyle LA, Preffer FI, et al: Tumor-derived interleukin-2-dependent lymphocytes in adoptive immunotherapy of lung cancer. *Cancer Immunol Immunother* 24(1):76–85, 1987

151. Kramer P, Prins ME, Kapsenberg JG, et al: Persistent Epstein–Barr virus infection and a histiocytic sarcoma in a renal transplant recipient. *Cancer* 55(3):503–9, 1985

152. Krane RJ, deVere White R, Davis Z, et al: Removal of renal cell carcinoma extending into the right atrium using cardiopulmonary bypass, profound hypothermia and circulatory arrest. *J Urol* 131(5):945–7, 1984

153. Krug H: Quantitative DNA determinaton and its role in the prognosis of malignant tumors. *Zentralbl Allg Pathol* 130(4):333–40, 1985

154. Kudo A, Nakayama T, Shigematsu N, et al: Gallium-67 imaging in the diagnosis of malignant lymphoma. *Rinsho Hoshasen* 30 (11 Suppl):1301–9, 1985

155. Kunze E, Reckels M, Eiardt B: Hematogenous metastasis of bronchial carcinoma depending on the tumor size and the presence of lymph node metastases. *Pathologe* 6(2):71–9, 1985

156. Kurachi K, Davis EW, Strydom DJ, et al: Sequence of the cDNA and gene for angiogenin, a human angiogenesis factor. *Biochemistry* 24:5494–9, 1985

157. Lai-Fook J: The structure of the haemocytes of *Calpodes ethlius* (Lepidoptera). *J Morph* 139:79–104, 1973

158. Lanir N, Langer N, Ber R: Cloning of plasmacytoma micrometastases from spleen. *J Immunol Methods* 78(2):199–205, 1985

159. Larizza L, Schirrmacher V, Stohr M, et al: Inheritance of immunogenicity and metastatic potential in murine cell hybrids from the lymphoma ESb08 and normal spleen lymphocytes. *JNCI* 72(6):1371–81, 1984

160. Leak LV: Lymphatic capillaries in tail fin of amphibian larva: an electron microscopic study. *J Morph* 125:419–446, 1968

161. le Roux BT, Kallichurum S, Shama DM: Mediastinal cysts and tumors. *Curr Probl Surg* 21(11):1–77, 1984

162. Li XT, Hellmann K: Effect of RA233 alone and combined with radiation on experimental tumor metastasis. Part 1. *Clin Exp Metastasis* 1(1):51–9, 1983

163. Liberati AM, Puxeddu A, Biscottini B, et al: Preliminary observation on the clinical tolerance of interferon-beta in cancer patients. *Tumor* 71(1):45–9, 1985

164. Lizza EF, Farsaii A, Belis JA: Complete extrinsic occlusion of the inferior vena cava by renal cell carcinoma. *W Va Med J* 82(2):23–5, 1986

165. Logmans SC, Jobsis AC: Thyroid-associated antigens in routinely embedded carcinomas. Possibilities and limitations studied in 116 cases. *Cancer* 54(2):274–9, 1984

166. Ludwig C, Hartmann D, Landmann R, et al: Intact cellular immune response in patients with locally metastasizing breast carcinoma at the time of diagnosis. *Schweiz Med Wochenschr* 113(50):1908–11, 1983

167. Luesley DM, Monypanny IJ, Fielding JW, Chan KK: Gliomatosis peritonei associated wtih ovarian teratomas. Case report. *Br J Obstet Gynaecol* 90(7):668–70, 1983

168. Macpherson AI: The spleen: cysts and tumors. *J Appl Med* 7(5):365–7, 1981

169. Malik GB, Caylony MV, Mukerjee P: Carcinoma of the female breast: influence of some clinicopathological factors. *Indian J Cancer* 20(1A):68–73, 1983

170. Masuda F, Ohnishi T, Nakada J, et al: Lymphadenectomy for renal cell carcinoma. *Hinyokika Kiyo* 31(4):595–600, 1985

171. Mathieu D, Grenier P, Larde D, Vasile N: Portal vein involvement in hepatocellular carcinoma: dynamic CT features. *Radiology* 152(1):127–32, 1984

172. Matsunou H, Shimoda T, Kakimoto S, et al: Histopathologic and immunohistochemical study of malignant tumors of peripheral nerve sheath (malignant schwannoma). *Cancer* 56(9):269–79, 1985

173. Matsuno S, Kato S, Nakamura R, et al: Hematogenous metastasis in pancreatic cancer. *Gan No Rinsho* 31(5):537–43, 1985

174. Mattisson A, Fange R: Ultrastructure of erythrocytes and leucocytes of *Priapulus caudatus* (De Lamarck) (Priapulida). *J Morph* 140:367–72, 1973

175. Matsuzaki K, Matsuda Y, Kai H, Sugimachi K: Transnodal cancer chemotherapy for metastatic lymph nodes in rats. *Cancer Treat Rep* 71(3):235–9, 1987

176. Mazumder A, Grimm EA, Rosenberg SA: Lysis of fresh human solid tumor cells by autologous lymphocytes activated *in vitro* by allosensitization. *Cancer Immunol Immunother* 15(1):1–10, 1983

177. Mayhew E, Glaves D: Quantitation of tumorigenic disseminating and arrested cancer cells. *Br J Cancer* 50(2):159–66, 1984

178. McMillan PJ, Heidbuchel U, Vollrath U: Anomalous occurrence of immunoreactive calcitonin cells in the thymus of the rat. *Cell Tiss Res* 222:629–34, 1982

179. Mechev DS, Shishkina VV: Gamma scintigraphy of lymphatic nodes with metastatic involvement. *Med Radiol (Mosk)* 30(4):3–7, 1985

180. Mehta P: Potential role of platelets in the pathogenesis of tumor metastasis. *Blood* 63(1):55–63, 1984

181. Miettinen M, Lehto VP, Virtanen I: Antibodies to intermediate filament proteins. The differential diagnosis of cutaneous tumors. *Arch Dermatol* 121(6):736–41, 1985

182. Miles L, Wike J, Hunter N, et al: Macrophage content of murine sarcomas and carcinomas: associations with tumor growth parameters and tumor radiocurability. *Cancer Res* 47(4):1069–75, 1987

183. Moller PC, Philpott CM: The circulatory system of *Amphioxus branchiostoma floridae*. *J Morph* 139:389–406, 1973

184. Moore AV, Silverman PM, Putnam CE: Current concepts in computerized tomography of the mediastinum. *CRC Crit Rev Diagn Imaging* 24(1):1–38, 1985

185. Moskalenko IuE: Development of the circulatory function of the cardiovascular system. *Zh Evol Biokhim Fiziol* 21(1):3–12, 1985

186. Mukai M, Torikata C, Iri H, et al: Histogenesis of clear cell sarcoma of tendons and aponeuroses. An electron-microscopic, biochemical, enzyme histochemical, and immunohistochemical study. *Am J Pathol* 14(2):264–72, 1984

187. Muller-Hermelink HK, Marino M, Palestro G: Pathology of thymic epithelial tumors. *Curr Top Pathol* 75:207–68, 1986

188. Munka VL, Homza E: The drainage of lymph from the lungs in the hedgehog. *Morphologica* 18(2):111–5, 1970

189. Nair PN: A crypoto-lymphatic unit at the uvula of the monkey *Macaca fascicularis*, a light- and electron microscopic study. *Cell Tiss Res* 228(1):171–82, 1983

190. Nakagawara A, Ikeda K, Inokuchi K, et al: Deficient superoxide-generating activity and its activation of blood monocytes in cancer patients. *Cancer Lett* 22(2):157–62, 1984

191. Neuwirth M: The structure of the hemocytes of *Galleria*

mellonella (Lepidoptera). *J Morph* 139:105–24, 1973

192. Nguyen GK: Fine-needle aspiration biopsy cytology of hepatic tumors in adults. *Pathol Annu* 21 Pt 1:321–49, 1986

193. Nicoletti G, Brambilla P, De Giovanni C, et al: Colony-stimulating activity from the new metastatic TS/A cell line and its high- and low-metastatic clonal derivatives. *BR J Cancer* 52(2):215–22, 1985

194. Nicolson GL, Custead SE: Effects of chemotherapeutic drugs on platelet and metastatic tumor cell-endothelial integrity. *Cancer Res* 45(1):331–6, 1985

195. Nicolson GL: Differential growth properties of metastatic large-cell lymphoma cells in target organ-conditioned medium. *Exp Cell Res* 168(2):572–7, 1987

196. Niitsu Y, Urushizaki I: Inhibition of metastasis by anti-platelet agents:prostaglandins. *Gan To Kagaku Ryoho* 12(6):1228–34, 1985

197. Nishi M, Watanabe S: Cancer and the lymph nodes. *Gan To Kagaku Ryoho* 12(5):983–91, 1985

198. Nishi M, Nakajima T, Ohta H: Treatment of gastric cancer based on the pathological and biophysiological aspects of cancer. *Gan To Kagaku Ryoho* 13(2):180–91, 1986

199. Nomi S, Pellis NR, Kahan BD: Retardation of postsurgical metastases with the use of extracted tumor-specific transplantation antigens and cyclophosphamide. *JNCI* 73(4):943–50, 1984

200. Nowak RM, Paradiso JL (eds): *Walker's Mammals of the World*. (4th edition). Baltimore-London: The Johns Hopkins University Press, 1983

201. Obara N, Tochinai S, Katagiri C: Splenic white pulp as a thymus-independent area in the African clawed toad, *Xenopus laevis*. *Cell Tiss Res* 226:327–35, 1982

202. Oda N: Experimental studies on effects of total-body and local hyperthermia on metastases in mice. *Nippon Gaka Gakkai Zasshi* 86(2):121–31, 1985

203. Ohtsuki M, Crewe AV: Evidence for a central substructure in a *Lumbricus terrestris* hemoglobin obtained with STEM low-dose and digital processing techniques. *J Ultrastr Res* 83:312–8, 1983

204. Owe FL, Peterman GM: Neoplastic model for the differentiation of a subpopulation of lymphocytes bearing IgH-1-linked gene products. *Immunol Rev* 82:29–46, 1984

205. Pabst R, Geisler R: The route of migration of lymphocytes from blood to spleen and mesenteric lymph nodes in the pig. *Cell Tiss Res* 221:361–70, 1981

206. Pabst R, Nowara E: Organ distribution and fate of newly formed splenic lymphocytes in the pig. *Anat Rec* 202:85–94, 1982

207. Pabst R, Potschick K: Proliferation and emigration of newly formed lymphocytes from pig spleens during an immune response. *Immunology* 50:281–8, 1983

208. Pabst R, Nowara E: The emigration of lymphocytes from palatine tonsils after local labelling. *Arch Otorhinolaryngol* 240:7–13, 1984

209. Pabst R, Kaatz M, Westermann J: *In situ* labelling of bone marrow lymphocytes with fluorescein isothiocyanate for lymphocyte migration studies in pigs. *Scand J Haematol* 31:267–74, 1983a

210. Pabst R, Kamran D, Creutzig H: Splenic regeneration and blood flow after ligation of the splenic artery or partial splenectomy. *Amer J Surg*, 147:382–6, 1984a

211. Papla B, Karpiel W: A case of peritoneal gliomatosis. *Patol Pol* 34(3):325–8, 1983

212. Patterson GA, Piazza D, Pearson FG, et al: Significance of metastatic disease in subaortic lymph nodes. *Ann Thorac Surg* 43(2):155–9, 1987

213. Paul R: Comparison of fluorine-18-2-fluorodeoxyglucose and gallium-67 citrate imaging for detection of lymphoma. *J Nucl Med* 28(3):288–92, 1987

214. Perl A, Rhenso GC, Lang I, et al: Natural and lectin-dependent cell-mediated cytotoxicity in patients with SLE and metastasizing solid tumors. *Orv Hetil* 125(3):135–7, 1984

215. Pickering AD: Changes in blood cell composition of the brown trout, *Salmo trutta* L., during the spawning season. *J Fish Biol* 29:335–47, 1986

216. Pickering AD, Pottinger TG: Cortisol can increase the susceptibility of brown trout, *Salmo trutta* L., to disease without reducing the white blood cell count. *J Fish Biol* 27:611–9, 1985

217. Pui CH, Rivera G, Mirro J, et al: Acute megakaryoblastic leukemia. Blast Cell aggregates simulating metastatic tumor. *Arch Pathol Lab Med* 109(11):1033–5, 1985

218. Raczka E, Quintana A, Poggi A, Donati MB: Distribution of cardiac output during development of two metastasizing murine tumors. *Eur J Cancer Clin Oncol* 19(7):1021–9, 1983

219. Ramachandran Nair PN: A crypto-lymphatic unit at the uvula of the monkey *Macaca fascicularis*. *Cell Tiss Res* 228:171–82, 1983

220. Ramaekers F, Haag D, Jap P, Vooijs PG: Immunochemical demonstration of keratin and vimentin in cytologic aspirates. *Acta Cytol (Baltimore)* 28(4):385–92, 1984

221. Raper RF, Rogleff BR, Vandenberg RA: Subacute pulmonary hypertension due to carcinomatous microembolism. *Aust NZ J Med* 14(3):271–3, 1984

222. Robbins DS, Fudenberg HH: Editorial retrospective. Human lymphocyte subpopulations in metastatic neoplasia—six years later. *N Engl J Med* 308(26):1595–7, 1983

223. Robertson WW Jr, Janssen HF, Walker RN: Passive movement of radioactive microspheres from bone and soft tissue in an extremity. *J Orthop Res* 3(4):405–11, 1985

224. Rosenkranz L, Schroeder C: Recurrent malignant melanoma following a 46-year disease-free interval. *NY State J Med* 85(3):95, 1985

225. Rossi CR, Nitti D, Favretti F, Lise M: Regional intra-vascular and intra-lymphatic therapy of neoplastic diseases: a review. *Int Surg* 71(1):42–7, 1986

226. Rodriguez T, Rengifo E, Gavilondo J, et al: Morphologic and cytochemical study of L929 cell variants with different metastasizing ability in C3HA/Hab mice. *Neoplasma* 31(3):271–9, 1984

227. Romer F: Histology, histochemistry, polyploidy and ultra-structure of the oenocytes of *Gryllus bimaculatus* (Saltatoria). *Cytobiologie* 6(2):195–213, 1972

228. Romer F: Ultrastructural features of pterygote insect oenocytes. Verh Dtsch Zool Ges 66. Jahresversammlung. Gustav Fischer Verlag, 1973

229. Roos E, La Riviera G, Collard JG, et al: Invasiveness of T-cell hybridomas *in vitro* and their metastatic potential *in vivo*. *Cancer Res* 45(12 Pt 1):6238–43, 1985

230. Rosenow EC, Hurley BT: Disorders of the thymus. A review. *Arch Intern Med* 144(4):763–70, 1984

231. Rosenstein R: Consistency in platelet morphology in whole blood. *Am J Clin Pathol* 85(4):502–5, 1986

232. Rossleigh MA, McCarthy WH, Milton GW, et al: The role of gallium-67 studies in the management of malignant melanoma. *Med J Aust* 140(7):401–3, 1984

233. Rowland K, Brown E, Kittle CF, Reddy S: Malignant mesothelioma (clinical conference). *Med Pediatr Oncol* 13(1):40–5, 1985

234. Sainsbury JR, Farndon JR, Sherbet GV, Harris AL: Epidermal-growth-factor receptors and oestrogen receptors in human breast cancer. *Lancet* 1(8425):364–6, 1985

235. Saul SH, Kaspadia SB: Primary lymphoma of Waldeyer's ring. Clinicopathologic study of 68 cases. *Cancer* 56(1):157–66, 1985

236. Scanlon EF: James Ewing lecture. The process of metastasis. *Cancer* 55(6):1163–6, 1985

237. Scheithauer BW, Randall RV, Laws ER Jr, et al: Prolactin cell carcinoma of the pituitary. Clinicopathologic, immu-

nohistochemical, and ultrastructural study of a case with cranial and extracranial metastases. *Cancer* 55(3):598–604, 1985

238. Schelstraete K, Deman J, Vermeulen FL, et al: Kinetics of 13N-ammonia incorporation in human tumors. *Nucl Med Commun* 6(8):461–70, 1985

239. Schipp R, Flindt R: To the fine structure and innervation of the musculature of lymph hearts of amphibians (*Rana temporaria*). *Zeitschrift Anatomie and Entwicklungsgeschichte* 127:232–53, 1968

240. Schmidt EE, MacDonald LC, Groom AC: Direct arteriovenous connections and the intermediate circulation in dog spleen, studied by scanning electron microscopy of microcorrosion casts. *Cell Tiss Res* 225:543, 1982

241. Schneider ML: Morphologic prognostic criteria in endometrial cancer with special reference to nuclear grading. *Geburtshilfe Frauenheilkd* 46(5):267–77, 1986

242. Sedlarik KM, Weidenbach H, Kohler H: *In vitro* electrically activated blood – an endogenous thrombogenic substance for the blocking of arteries supplying tumors and the microcirculation of tumor tissue – an experimental study. *Z Urol Nephrol* 77(4):193–99, 1984

243. Sekine T, Suda Y: Evaluation of absolute non-curative resection in colorectal carcinoma. *Nippon Geka Gakkai Zasshi* 86(7):828–36, 1985

244. Shanahan TC, Ceglowski WS, Havas HF: Cellular changes and antitumor responses in the plasmacytoma-bearing mouse following cyclophosphamide treatment. *Cancer Res* 45(12 Pt 1):6463–70, 1985

245. Shepard JO: Computed tomography of the mediastinum. *Clin Chest Med* 5(2):291–305, 1984

246. Sipes NJ, Bregman MD, Meyskens FL Jr: Stimulation of human metastatic melanoma colony-forming cells by an acid-sensitive factor in human platelet sonicate. *Cancer Res* 45(12 Pt 1):6268–72, 1985

247. Skolnik G, Ericson LE, Bagge U: The effect of thrombocytopenia and antiserotonin treatment on the lodgement of circulating tumor cells. A vital fluorescence microscopic, electron microscopic and isotope study in the rat. *J Cancer Res Clin Oncol* 105(1):30–7, 1983

248. Skolnik G, Ivarsson L, Bagge U: The influence of antiserotonin treatment with ketanserin on the pulmonary lodgement of circulating tumor cells in normal and traumatized rats. *Eur J Cancer Clin Oncol* 19(6):843–6, 1983a

249. Skolnik G, Bagge U, Dahlstrom A, Ahlman H: The importance of 5-HT for tumor cell lodgement in the liver. *Int J Cancer* 33(4)519–23, 1984

250. Skolnik G, Bagge U, Blomqvist G, et al: Involvement of platelet-released 5-HT in tumor cell lodgement. *J Surg Res* 30(6):559–67, 1985

251. Smith VJ, Soderhall K: Induction of degranulation and lysis of haemocytes in the freshwater crayfish, *Astacus astacus* by components of the prophenoloxidase activating system *in vitro*. *Cell Tiss Res* 233:295–303, 1983

252. Soderhall K, Vey A, Ramstedt M: Hemocyte lysate enhancement of fungal spore encapsulation by crayfish hemocytes. *Dev Comp Immunol* 8:23–29, 1984

253. Sosa RE, Muecke EC, Vaughan ED Jr, McCarron JP Jr: Renal cell carcinoma extending into the inferior vena cava: the prognostic significance of the level of vena caval involvement. *J Urol* 132(6):1097–100, 1984

254. Spies RB: The blood system of the flabelligerid polychaete *Flabelliderma commensalis* (Moore). *J Morph* 139:465–90, 1973

255. Springer GF, Taylor CR, Howard DR, et al: Tn, a carcinoma-associated antigen, reacts with anti-Th of normal human sera. *Cancer* 55(3):561–9, 1985

256. Starck D: *Embryologie*. (2nd edition). Stuttgart: George Thieme Verlag, 1965

257. Stedman TL: *Stedman's Medical Dictionary*. (24th edition). Baltimore-London: Williams & Wilkins, 1982

258. Stefanini M: Enzymes, isozymes, and enzyme variants in the diagnosis of cancer. A short review. *Cancer* 55(9):1931–6, 1985

259. Stein MG, Mayo J, Muller N, et al: Pulmonary lymphangitic spread of carcinoma: appearance on CT scans. *Radiology* 162(2):371–5, 1987

260. Stein MG, Crues JV 3d, Bradley WG, Jr et al. MR imaging of pulmonary emboli: an experimental study in dogs. *AJR* 147(6):1133–7, 1986

261. Strydom DJ, Fett JW, Lobb RR, et al: Amino acid sequence of human tumor derived angiogenin. *Biochemistry* 24:5486–94, 1985

262. Takebayashi M, Nishidoi H, Kimura O, et al: Metachronous hematogenous metastasis of gastric cancer – histopathologic characteristics of gastric cancer developing of the liver, lung or bone metastasis. *Gan No Rinsho* 31(1):40–4, 1985

263. Takeda Z, Wakuya J, Maeda H, et al: A teratoma group tumor of testis with mature teratoma in metastatic foci – a case report. *Kobe J Med Sci* 31(2):73–83, 1985

264. Takekoshi T, Sakata K, Kunieda T, et al: Facilitation of tumor metastasis by operative stress and participation of cell-mediated immunity. Experimental study. *Oncology* 41(4):245–51, 1984

265. Takenaga K: Characterization of low- and high-metastatic clones isolated from a Lewis lung carcinoma. *Gann* 75(1):61–71, 1984

266. Talmadge JE: Thymosin: immunomodulatory and therapeutic characteristics. *Prog Clin Biol Res* 161:457–65, 1984

267. Talmadge JE, Uithoven KA, Lenz BF, Chirigos M: Immunomodulation and therapeutic characterization of thymosin fraction five. *Cancer Immunol Immunother* 18(3):185–94, 1984

268. Tanaka K, Fukumoto S: Role of blood platelets and prostaglandins in blood-borne metastases. *Gan To Kagaku Ryoho* 10(9):1944–7, 1983

269. Tanaka K, Fukumoto S: Cancer blood-borne metastasis and platelets. *Gan To Kagaku Ryoho* 11(12 Pt 1):2453–9, 1984

270. Tanaka T, Nakamura H, Choi S, et al: CT diagnosis of abdominal lymph node metastases in hepatocellular carcinoma. *Eur J Radiol* 5(3):175–7, 1985

271. Tarin D, Price JE, Kettlewell MG, et al: Clinicopathological observations on metastasis in man studied in patients treated with peritoneovenous shunts. *Br Med J (Clin Res)* 288(6419):749–51, 1984

272. Tavassoli M, Watson LR, Khademi R: Retention of hemopoiesis in tail vertebrae of newborn rats. *Cell Tiss Res* 200:215–22, 1979

273. Terjanian T, Kantarjian H, Keating M, et al: Clinical and prognostic features of patients with Philadelphia chromosome-positive chronic myelogenous leukemia and extramedullary disease. *Cancer* 59(2):297–300, 1987

274. Thomas J, De Wolf-Peeters C, Tricot G, et al: T-cell chronic lymphocytic leukemia in a patient with invasive thymoma in remission with chemotherapy. *Cancer* 52(2):313–7, 1983

275. Thompson CI, Kreider JW, Black PL, et al: Genetically obese mice: resistance to metastasis of B16 melanoma and enhanced T-lymphocyte mitogenic responses. *Science* 220(4602):1183–5, 1983

276. Tricot GJ, Broeckaert-Van Orshoven A, den Ottolander GJ, et al: Adult T-cell leukemia: a report on two white patients. *Leuk Res* 7(1):31–42, 1983

277. Tridente G: Immunopathology of the human thymus. *Semin Hematol* 22(1):56–67, 1985

278. Tsubura E, Yamashita T, Sone S: Inhibition of the arrest of hematogenously disseminated tumor cells. *Cancer Metastasis Rev* 2(3):223–37, 1983

279. Tsubura E, Nishikawa H, Chikata E, Yamashita T: Mecha-

nism of cancer metastasis and its inhibition – a point of view from clinical aspects. *Gan To Kagaku Ryoho* 12(6):1189–95, 1985

280. Tsuru S, Taniguchi M, Shinomiya N, et al: Augmentation of resistance against metastatic tumor cells after local administration of PSK. *Gan To kagaku Ryoho* 12(1):86–90, 1985

281. Tsutsumi Y, Ohshita T, Yokoyama T: A case of gastric carcinoma with massive eosinophilia. *Acta Pathol Jpn* 34(1):117–22, 1984

282. Vadhan-Raj S, Nathan CF, Sherwin SA, et al: Phase I trial of recombinant interferon gamma by 1-hour i.v. infusion. *Cancer Treat Rep* 70(5):609–14, 1986

283. Vallee BL, Riordan JF, Lobb RR, et al: Tumor-derived angiogenesis factors from rat Walker 256 carcinoma: an experimental investigation and review. *Experientia* 41:1–15. Birkhauser Verlag, 1985

284. van der Knaap WPW, Boerrigter-Barendsen LH, van den Hoeven DSP, Sminia T: Immunocytochemical demonstration of a humoral defence factor in blood cells (Amoebocytes) of the pond snail, *Lymnaea stagnalis*. *Cell Tiss Res* 219:291–6, 1981

285. van der Werf-Messing BH, Auerbach WM, van Putten WI: Non-seminoma testis treated by irradiation at the Rotterdamsch Radio-Therapeutisch Instituut: the risk of metastasis. *Radiother Oncol* 2(2):101–5, 1984

286. van Niekerk JL, Wobbes T, Holland R, van Haelst UJ: Malignant fibrous histiocytoma of the breast with axillary lymph node involvement. *J Surg Oncol* 34(1):32–5, 1987

287. Veksler IG, Antonenko SG, Okolot EN, Chubinskaia SG: The role of cyclic nucleotides in the development of resistance to metastases after treatment with immunomodulators. *Eksp Onkol* 6(3):52–5, 1984

288. Verhaeghe M, Laurent JC, Giaux G, Rohart J: Results of a continuous series of 761 invasive breast cancers, 408 followed more than 5 years, treated by partial mastectomy with maxillary curettage followed by irradiation. *Chirurgie* 110(4):332–42, 1984

289. Veronesi U, Cascinelli N, Greco M, et al: Prognosis of breast cancer patients after mastectomy and dissection of internal mammary nodes. *Ann Surg* 202(6):702–7, 1985

290. Villasanta U, Whitley NO, Haney PJ, Brenner D: Computed tomography in invasive carcinoma of the cervix: an appraisal. *Obstet Gynecol* 62(2):218–24, 1983

291. von Ardenne M: Fundamentals of combating cancer metastasis by oxygen multistep immunostimulation processes. *Med Hypotheses* 17(1):47–65, 1985

292. Vordermark JS, Jones BM, Harrison DH: Surgical approaches to block dissection of the inguinal lymph nodes. *Br J Plast Surg* 38(3):321–5, 1985

293. Waclawik AJ, Bogusz R, Wocjan J, et al: Metastases of medulloblastoma beyond the nervous system through a cerebrospinal fluid shunt: discussion with report of a case. *Neurol Neurochir Pol* 20(2):147–51, 1986

294. Waksal SD, Colucci G: Role of growth factors during normal and neoplastic intrathymic development. *Surv Immunol Res* 3(1):25–8, 1984

295. Wall TJ, Peters LJ, Brown BW, et al: Relationship between lymph nodal status and primary tumor control probability in tumors of the supraglottic larynx. *Int J Radiat Oncol Biol Phys* 11(11):1895–902, 1985

296. Wasserthal LT: Reciprocal functional and structural adaptations in the circulatory and ventilatory systems in adult insects. *Verh Dtsch Zool Ges*, Fischer Verlag, pp. 105–16, 1982

297. Watanabe H, Hachisuka K, Yamaguchi A, et al: A case of iliac arterial embolism after lung cancer resection. *Kyabu Geka* 38(6):484–7, 1985

298. Weiss L, Dimitrov DS: A fluid mechanical analysis of the velocity, adhesion, and destruction of cancer cells in capillaries during metastasis. *Cell Biophys* 6(1):9–22, 1984

299. Weiss L, Ward PM, Holmes JC: Liver-to-lung traffic of cancer cells. *Int J Cancer* 32(1):79–83, 1983

300. Weiss L, Dimitrov DS, Angelova M: The hemodynamic destruction of intravascular cancer cells in relation to myocardial metastasis. *Proc Natl Acad Sci USA* 82(17):5737–41, 1985

301. Welsch U, Storch V: *Comparative Animal Cytology and Histology*. London: Sidgwick & Jackson, 1976

302. Wenzel DJ: Gallium-positive tumor thrombus. *Urol Radiol* 6(1):51–3, 1984

303. Wheelock EF, Robinson MK: Biology of disease. Endogenous control of the neoplastic process. *Lab Invest* 48(2):120–39, 1983

304. Williams JC, Gusterson BA, Monaghan P, et al: Isolation and characterization of clonal cell lines from a transplantable metastasizing rat mammary tumor, TR2CL. *JNCI* 74(2):415–28, 1985

305. Wright KC, Carrasco CH, Wallace S, Stephens LC: Treatment of the rabbit V-2 carcinoma with intralesional cisplatin. *Chemotherapy* 31(1):60–7, 1985

306. Yahalon J, Eldor A, Biran S, et al: Platelet-tumor cell interaction with the subendothelial extracellular matrix: relationship to cancer metastasis. *Radiother Oncol* 3(3):211–25, 1985

307. Yamada A, Kobayashi S: Diagnosis and treatment of early esophageal carcinoma. *Zentralbl Chir* 110(22):1399–413, 1985

308. Yamamoto S, Sakata K, Kunieda T, et al: Relationship between lymphocytic cytotoxicity and phytohemagglutinin-induced lymphoblastogenesis before and after surgical tumor excision: an experimental study. *J Surg Oncol* 28(1):42–9, 1985

309. Yokoyama T, Yoshie O, Aso H, et al: Antitumor effect of human interferon-alpha A/D in mice (II). Activation of natural killer cells and suppression of metastasis. *Gan To Kagaku Ryoho* 12(3 Pt 1):510–5, 1985

310. Yoshino TP, Granath Jr WO: Identification of antigenically distinct hemocyte subpopulations in *Biomphalaria glabrata* (Gastropoda) using monoclonal antibodies to surface membrane markers. *Cell Tiss Res* 232:553–64, 1983

311. Youinou P, Zabbe C, Eveillaud C, et al: Antiperinuclear activity in lung carcinoma patients. *Cancer Immunol Immunother* 18(2):80–1, 1984

312. Yu S, Wang N, McKhann CF: The effect of immunity on pulmonary metastasis of a methylcholanthrene-induced fibrosarcoma and three of its clones. *J Surg Oncol* 27(1):51–8, 1984

313. Zachary D, Hoffmann JA: The haemocytes of *Calliphora erythrocephala* (Meig.) (Diptera). *Z Zellforsch* 141:55–73, 1973

314. Zerhouni EA, Stitik FP: Controversies in computed tomography of the thorax. The pulmonary nodule – lung cancer staging. *Radiol Clin North A* 23(3):407–26, 1985

315. Zirinsky K, Auh YH, Rubenstein WA, et al: The portacaval space: CT with MR correlation. *Radiology* 156(2):453–60, 1985

316. Zoler ML: Marshalling macrophages against metastases (news). *JAMA* 249(13):1690–1, 1695, 1983

13

IMMUNOLOGICAL CONTROL OF TUMOR METASTASES

E.L. GORELIK and R.B. HERBERMAN

INTRODUCTION

The metastatic abilities of tumor cells of the different histological types vary over a wide range. Furthermore, tumor cells of the same histological types, among individual cancer patients, also differ considerably in their potential to form distant metastases (98).

It is considered that only certain types of tumor cells are able to develop metastatic tumors in distant anatomical locations, although millions of tumor cells are constantly entering the blood stream of the tumor-bearing host. The metastatic ability of tumor cells has been said to depend on their inherent properties, which collectively determine the metastatic phenotype of the tumor cells (19, 63, 71, 92).

Although this concept is widely accepted, numerous attempts to characterize the metastatic phenotype of tumor cells have not led to the definite determination of the properties required for metastatic behavior of tumor cells.

The main results of these investigations indicate that there is no single property which can account for the metastatic ability of tumor cells. Rather, the metastatic tumor cells may be considered "the decathalon winners", possessing a series of complex properties which allow them to fulfill the metastatic cascade, including penetration into blood vessels, dissemination, extravasation and proliferation in the extravascular parenchyma of the different organs or tissues (19, 63, 71, 92). The realization of the metastatic potential depends not only on the full set of properties of the tumor cells, but also on sufficiently permissive conditions in the host. Various immunological and nonimmunological host mechanisms have been shown to influence the fate of the potential metastatic cells. Indeed, it is considered that the host's immune mechanisms could play an important role in the control of metastatic spread and growth.

IMMUNOGENICITY AND METASTATIC PROPERTIES OF TUMOR CELLS

The main evidence supporting this conclusion has come from observations that immunogenic tumors grow locally and develop huge tumor masses, but fail to form distant metastases. However, in immunosuppressed animals these tumors are able to develop numerous metastatic foci in various anatomical locations (12, 20, 59). These data indicate that: a) some tumor cells might have all of the properties required to fulfill the metastatic cascade, but the realization of their metastatic program is hampered by the presence

of antigenic determinant(s) recognized by immune mechanisms; and b) the immune response evoked against the primary tumors failed to reject the locally growing malignant tissue, but could be highly efficient against migrating, metastatic tumor cells. The results of investigations on metastatic properties of Lewis lung carcinoma (3LL) provide an illustration for such a pattern. 3LL tumor is considered weakly immunogenic and highly metastatic in syngeneic C57BL/6 mice. The 3LL tumor is even able to grow locally in allogeneic BALB/c mice as a result of low expression of $H-2K^b$ antigen, but it never develops distant metastases (31, 50–52). By transfer of the lungs of BALB/c mice bearing 3LL tumor into (BALB/c × C57B1/6) F_1 mice, it was demonstrated that 3LL tumor cells had been shed and migrated into the lungs of their allogeneic hosts, but their growth was arrested there by immune mechanisms. Furthermore, after the tumor-bearing leg of a BALB/c mouse was amputated, intravenous inoculation of 3LL cells failed to result in the formation of experimental metastases in the lungs. In contrast, when 3LL tumor cells were inoculated intravenously into normal nonimmunized allogeneic BALB/c mice, numerous lung colonies were found (52). When 3LL tumor cells were transplanted into the foot pad of immunosuppressed allogeneic mice or athymic nude mice, they grew locally and formed multiple pulmonary metastases (51). Therefore, 3LL tumor cells clearly have the potential to form pulmonary metastases in allogeneic mice. Although the immune response of allogeneic BALB/c mice was inefficient to prevent local 3LL tumor growth, it was rather efficient in controlling metastatic spread and growth of these tumor cells. Although these results are derived from an artifical experimental model, a similar pattern has been shown for immunogeneic tumors growing in syngeneic mice. Indeed, when the immunogenicity of 3LL or BL6 tumor cells was augmented by *in vitro* UV light irradiation or treatment with MNNG, the immunogeneic tumor cell variants failed to form distant metastases despite local growth in some syngeneic C57BL/6 mice. The metastatic growth was observed when these immunogeneic tumors grew in the nude mice (34, 77, 78).

IMMUNOSELECTION OF THE METASTATIC CELL POPULATION

T-cell mediated immunity appears to be mostly responsible for prevention of the metastatic dissemination from the immunogeneic tumors. Since the metastatic process takes

R. H. Goldfarb (ed.), Fundamental aspects of cancer.

place at the time when the immune response develops against the primary tumor, only shed tumor cells which can escape immune destruction have the potential to form metastatic tumors. Thus, immunoselection could participate in the formation of the metastatic cell population.

Several mechanisms could provide a selective advantage and help tumor cells to metastasize in the presence of the immune response. Numerous experimental data clearly indicate that a tumor is a heterogeneous population of malignant cells, composed of a series of related but genotypically distinct individual clones. The phenotype of these clones can be characterized in terms of their biochemical properties, cell surface markers, drug and radiation sensitivity, degree of malignancy, invasiveness and metastatic ability, and their antigenic and immunogenic properties (19, 41, 43, 58, 75, 81).

Antigenic heterogeneity of tumor cell populations might be a basis for the selection of the metastatic cells which are able to escape immune destruction. Thus, metastatic tumor cells might be antigenetically distinguishable from the parental tumor cell growing locally. Sugarbaker and Cohen (97) compared the immunogenic and antigenic characteristics of tumor cells derived from primary (P) murine methylcholanthrene-induced sarcoma and from 7 individual pulmonary metastatic foci. Three metastatic (M) tumor lines, in comparison to the P tumor, showed distinctive antigenic and immunogenic properties. Two metastatic lines were nonimmunogenic and nonantigenic, since they failed to induce immune resistance against themselves or against P tumor cells. In addition, immunization with P tumor cells did not affect the growth of these cells. Two other metastatic lines had shared common antigenic and immunogenic characteristics with P tumor; they immunized mice against themselves and against P and vice versa.

Antigenic differences between locally growing 3LL (L-3LL) and its pulmonary metastases (M-3LL) were found when normal spleen cells were sensitized *in vitro* against these tumor lines (22, 31). Spleen cells immunized against L-3LL were preferentially cytotoxic against L-3LL but less against M-3LL tumor cells. Similarly, spleen cells immune against M-3LL showed higher cytotoxic activity against M-3LL than L-3LL targets. When L-3LL and M-3LL tumor cells were admixed with immune spleen cells and inoculated into the foot pads of syngeneic mice, spleen cells immune against M-3LL, but not against L-3LL, significantly inhibited the formation of the metastatic foci in mice bearing L-3LL or M-3LL tumors (22, 31).

The antigenic specificity of the rat primary MC-induced sarcoma and its metastases was investigated by Pimm et al. (79). Using cross-immunization of rats with primary tumor or tumor lines derived from metastases into lungs, kidney, or peritoneum, it was found that primary tumor cells and tumor cells from peritoneal metastases shared common antigens, whereas metastatic cells from the lungs or kidney had distinctive antigenic specificities. Metastatic cells from the lung or kidney were able to induce protection against each other, but not against peritoneal metastatic cells (79). Intensive studies performed by Schirrmacher (1985) demonstrated that the L5178YE lymphoma (EB) and its metastatic variant ESb have different tumor-associated transplantation antigens (TATA). Cytotoxic T-lymphocytes (CTL) directed against Eb lymphoma failed to destroy the metastasizing

ESb lymphoma cells and vice versa. When ESb lymphoma cells were obtained from the metastatic deposits in the spleen and tested as target cells for the CTL, it was found that these cells were completely resistant to the cytotoxic action of the syngeneic tumor specific CTL. This immunoresistance of the metastatic cells was found to be associated with the loss of TATA. The generation of these immunoresistant TATA⁻ metastatic cells occurred with high frequency although they did not pre-exist in the parental cell population (92).

Antigen-deficient metastatic cells have been described for the hamster SV-40-induced tumors (8) and murine MDAY-D2 tumor (9).

Thus, antitumor immune response could select out the resistant metastatic tumor cells. This resistance to T-cell mediated immune destruction could be a result of selection of tumor cells with different TATA specificities or TATA⁻ tumor cell variants. The ability of T-cell mediated immunity to recognize and destroy tumor cells depends on the presence of TATA and major histocompatibility complex (MHC) antigens (10). Therefore, tumor cells could be unrecognizable by the immune system as a result of alterations in the expression of either TATA or MHC antigens.

MAJOR HISTOCOMPATABILITY ANTIGEN (MHC) ANTIGEN EXPRESSION AND METASTATIC GROWTH

Direct analysis of the cell surface characteristics of spontaneous and induced murine tumors, in regard to expression of H-2 antigens as detected by polyclonal or monoclonal antibodies, revealed numerous quantitative and qualitative alterations in the expression of class I antigens of H-2 complex (16, 26, 65).

Similar investigations performed on tumors of cancer patients demonstrated that in many tumors, HLA antigens remained undetectable or their expression was severely diminished . Almost 50% of the tumors investigated, which included melanomas, breast carcinomas, skin carcinomas and neuroblastomas, had various changes in expression of HLA-A, B, C antigens or β_2-microglobulin (11, 61, 70, 91). Ten of 11 investigated human small-cell lung cancer (SCLC) cell lines did not express at all, or expressed low levels, of class I HLA antigens or β_2-microglobulin. In contrast, almost all investigated non-small-cell lung cancer cell lines had high level of expression of β_2-microglobulin and HLA-A, B, C antigens (11). SCLC cells, in parallel with their lack of MHC antigens, exhibited rapid growth and early metastases. The degree of SCLC cells' malignancy was also associated with an amplification of the c-myc oncogene. It is of interest that SCLC cell lines with the greatest level of c-myc amplification had the lowest level of MHC antigen expression (91). In accordance with these findings, neuroblastoma cell lines which had amplification of the N-myc oncogene also demonstrated a high incidence of alteration of MHC gene expression (61). It was suggested that downregulation of MHC genes can be common aspect of malignant transformation mediated by oncogenes (11). An inverse relationship between expression of MHC class I antigen and degree of malignancy was also demonstrated for some other human tumors (91).

These alterations in MHC antigen expression on the tumor cell surface are probably not irrelevant events, but rather might provide tumor cells with the possibility to escape immune destruction. Recently, this assumption has received strong experimental support.

C3H fibroblasts were transformed *in vitro* with SV-40 virus and adapted to grow *in vivo*. Most of transformed clones failed to grow in the immunocompetent syngeneic mice if they fully expressed the H-2 antigens. Tumor cells, which were able to grow in mice, did not express H-2K^k antigens (86).

Rat or murine tumor cells transformed by human adenovirus type 12 did not express MHC class I antigens and were tumorigenic. In contrast, malignant cells transformed with adenovirus type 5 expressed MHC antigens and were rejected in the immunocompetent syngeneic host (93, 101).

The importance of MHC antigen for tumor cell immunogenicity was supported by the results of H-2 gene transfection experiments. After H-2 gene transfection, H-2 negative adenovirus type 12 transformed murine tumor cells became H-2 positive and also appeared to be highly immunogenic, since they were rejected in immunocompetent mice (101).

AKR lymphoma cells which lost H-2K^k antigens were nonimmunogenic and highly tumorigenic (16). Immunogenicity of this AKR lymphoma was completely reconstituted following transfection of the H-2K^k gene (49).

These experiments demonstrate that failure of the immune system to react against H-2-negative tumor cells is not due to the absence of TATA, but rather to the absence of MHC-associated molecules.

Changes in MHC expression might confer certain advantages to potentially metastatic cells and provide them with the possibility to form metastatic foci in different anatomic locations, even when an immune response has been evoked by the primary tumor mass. Thus, the observed antigenic differences between primary and metastatic tumor cells could be a result of differences in the expression of TATA and/or class I MHC antigens.

Although the experiments with transplantation of tumor cells into allogeneic mice suggested that metastatic cells had lower levels of MHC antigens than the primary tumor cells (3, 60), more direct experiments using specific monoclonal antibodies directed against MHC antigens allowed further investigations into the role of MHC antigens in the metastatic behavior of tumor cells. Consistent differences in expression of H-2^b antigens on the cell surface of 3LL tumor cells derived from the locally growing tumor and its pulmonary metastases were found (31). When metastatic ability and expression of both ends of H-2 complex were analyzed using numerous clones and subclones of 3LL tumor, the data demonstrated that the metastatic potential of selected clonal populations did not depend entirely on the absolute levels of class I H-2^b antigens, but rather correlated with the level of imbalance in expression of H-2K^b and H-2D^b gene products. It was concluded that a "low K^b/high D^b" phenotype is highly metastatic, whereas "low K^b/low D^b" and "high K^b/high D^b" phenotypes are nonmetastatic (13, 14).

The association between H-2 antigen expression and metastatic ability of 3LL tumor clones could be explained on the basis of immunogenicity. Clone A9, selected from 3LL tumor, expressed both H-2K^b and H-2D^b antigens and was found to be immunogenic and nonmetastatic. whereas

clone D122 expressed only H-2D^b antigens and was nonimmunogenic and highly metastatic (14).

The association between MHC gene product expression and metastatic ability was clearly demonstrated with another experimental tumor, T-10 sarcoma, induced by methylcholanthrene in a (C57BL/6J × C3HeB/FeJ) F$_1$ mouse (7, 54, 55). One would expect that this tumor should express both parental H-2 haplotypes, namely H-2^b/H-2^k antigens. Comparison of H-2 antigen expression by locally growing T-10 tumor cells (L-T10) and tumor cells derived from pulmonary metastases (M-T10) showed that L-T10 tumor cells expressed only H-2^b but not H-2^k molecules. In contrast, M-T10 expressed H-2^b and H-2^k products (7, 54). Studies of clones of the L-T10 tumor revealed that 8 out of 10 selected clones were H-2^b positive, but H-2^k negative. The other two clones expressed both H-2^b and H-2^k haplotypes and were found to be metastatic. The nonmetastatic phenotype of H-2^k negative clones appeared to be due not to their inability to proliferate in the lungs but rather to their sensitivity to immune destruction, since they were able to develop multiple metastases in immunosuppressed irradiated (450R) mice. However, metastatic cells derived from immunosuppressed mice were also H-2^k negative (54).

Detailed analysis of expression of K and D ends of both H-2^b/H-2^k haplotypes among the selected clones indicate that metastatic H-2^b/H-2^k positive clones express only H-2D^b/H-2D^k antigens, whereas K^k and K^b end molecules of these haplotypes were missing. Nonmetastatic clones as well as original L-T10 tumor cells which are H-2^b positive and H-2^k negative also did not express H-2K^b genes in addition to their lack of H-2K^k and H-2D^k products (55).

The differences in H-2 antigen expression and metastatic behavior were closely associated with the immunogenic properties of the investigated clones. T10 clones which expressed H-2D^b antigen were immunogenic and nonmetastatic, whereas clones with H-2D^b and H-2D^k antigens were nonimmunogenic and highly metastatic (56).

All these experiments indicated that the expression of some H-2 gene products on the cell surface of tumor cells influences their immunogenicity and metastatic behavior. Most direct evidence of the relationship between these parameters came from the experiments with H-2 gene transfection into T-10 tumor cells (104). Since metastatic and nonmetastatic clones did not express K^b and K^k antigens, the effect of H-2K^b and H-2K^k gene transfer on the tumorigenic, metastatic and immunogenic properties of these clones was investigated. The transfected clones became more immunogenic and lost their ability to form pulmonary metastases in the immunocompetent mice, but still produced metastases in immunosuppressed irradiated (550R) syngeneic mice (104).

Thus, the appearance of K end antigens converted metastatic tumor cells into nonmetastatic cells. In contrast, the presence of D^k antigens had the opposite effect and was observed only in the metastatic clones. The different effect of K and D end genes on the metastatic properties of tumor cells may be attributable to the different physiological functions of these molecules, with mostly immunogenic activity of the K end product and suppressogenic activity of the D^k products (54–56).

The association between class I H-2 antigen expression and metastatic behavior was also demonstrated for B16 melanoma and its sublines (34). B16F10 and BL6 sublines were selected from the B16 melanoma on the basis of their high ability to form pulmonary metastases (17). It is of interest that these selections yielded tumor cells which expressed neglectable amount of $H-2K^b$ and $H-2D^b$ antigens and also did not express β_2-microglobulin on their cell surface (28, 34). In contrast, the low metastatic parental B16 melanoma and B16F1 subline had appreciable levels of class I $H-2^b$ antigens (28). After *in vitro* treatment of H-2 negative BL6 melanoma cells with N-methyl-N-nitro-nitrosoguanidine (MNNG), the expression of $H-2K^b$ and $H-2D^b$ antigens dramatically increased. In parallel, MNNG-treated BL6 melanoma cells (termed BL6T2) became highly immunogenic and lost their metastatic ability (28, 34). However, BL6T2 melanoma cells demonstrated their metastatic potential in athymic nude mice (28).

The analysis of MHC antigen expression by human malignant cells also demonstrated substantial variability in HLA antigen expression. In addition, differences in the expression of MHC antigen among tumor cells differed between those derived from the primary and those from metastatic lesions (70, 76).

Parmiani et al. (76) showed that human melanoma cells derived from the primary and metastatic tumors expressed high and similar levels of MHC class I products, but they differed in the expression of class II HLA-DR and melanoma associated antigens. In addition, the HLA-DR molecules on the primary and metastatic melanoma cells had different physiological functions. Only DR-positive primary tumor cells were able to stimulate the autologous lymphocytes to proliferate. In addition, stimulated lymphocytes became specifically cytotoxic against autologous melanoma cells. In contrast, neither DR-positive nor DR-negative metastatic cells were able to stimulate autologous PBL. Moreover, DR-positive metastatic cells suppressed the proliferation of PBL stimulated by allogeneic cells or IL-2 (76). These findings, in parallel with prediction that tumor cells which provide suppressogenic rather than immunogenic stimuli, might have some advantages during the metastatic migration and growth.

Thus, these data demonstrate that immunogenicity of tumor cells depends not only upon the level of expression of TATA but also on MHC restricted elements. However, the expected low expression of MHC antigens by metastatic cells is not always observed.

As a general conclusion from the available data, it appears that immunogenic tumor cells can develop metastases as a result of selection of tumor cells (a) with low levels of MHC, but high TATA expression; (b) with high levels of MHC but low levels of TATA; (c) with high levels of MHC and with TATA different from the primary tumor specificity; or (d) with low levels of both MHC and TATA expression.

Although antigenic and immunogenic differences between primary and metastatic tumor cells have been demonstrated, it is impossible to extrapolate these data to all metastatic tumors. Since some tumors are nonimmunogenic, the metastatic tumor cells would not be a target for specific immune reactions and antigenic diversity between primary and metastatic tumors would not be expected. In addition, the level of immunoselective pressure should be taken into consideration when results of antigenicity and immunogenicity

of metastatic cells are analyzed. The antitumor immune response in tumor-bearing animals usually has biphasic characteristics: after the initial response, immunologic reactivity usually declines as the tumor mass increases (27, 73). In contrast, the number of tumor cells shed into the blood proportionally increases with an increase in the volume of the primary tumor (19). Thus, in advanced stages of tumor growth, the immunoselective pressure declines and more tumor cells have the potential to survive and develop metastatic tumors, regardless of their antigenic and immunogenic properties. This could also serve as an explanation for the frequent observation that there is a similarity between primary tumor cells and tumor cells derived from some individual foci, whereas other foci are antigenectically distinctive.

It should be noted that although malignant tumors can be weakly or non-immunogenic and lack the ability to induce detectable T cell-mediated immunity, other, non-T-cell-depended, immune effector mechanisms might mediate immunoselection of metastatic tumor cells. Recent experimental data indicate that, in addition to or as an alternative to specifically immune T lymphocytes, natural killer (NK) cells and/or activated macrophages might be tumoricidal and participate in the control of the metastatic spread and growth.

NATURAL CELL-MEDIATED IMMUNITY AND METASTATIC GROWTH

It was found that NK cells play an important role in the intravascular elimination of tumor cells and in the control of metastatic spread (32, 35, 37, 40, 84). This conclusion was based on the following findings:

(a) Elimination of radiolabeled tumor cells after i.v. inoculation positively correlated with the level of NK reactivity in the recipients. Nude mice with high levels of NK cell activity more efficiently eliminated tumor cell than mice of strains with lower NK reactivity (32, 37, 84). Beige mice or very young mice (3 weeks old), which have low levels of NK reactivity, showed relatively high survival of i.v. inoculated tumor cells and more metastatic foci developed in the lungs of these mice (32, 37, 99).

(b) NK cell function has been depressed by pretreatment of mice with irradiation, cyclophosphamide, β-estradiol, corticosteroids, urethane, anti-asialo GM_1 serum, or NK 1.1 or NK 1.2 antiserum. Treatment of mice with these agents also resulted in depression of tumor cell elimination, and in increased formation of experimental or spontaneous tumor metastases (32, 37, 80).

(c) The cytotoxic activity of NK cells can be stimulated by pretreatment of mice with interferon, *C. parvum*, BCG, poly I:C, MVE-2, or OK-432. In parallel, treatment of mice with these agents was associated with an increase in the clearance of radiolabeled tumor cells from the pulmonary vasculature and a decrease in the number of the detectable experimental or spontaneous metastases (33, 37, 47, 100). Furthermore, it was found that biological response modifiers increase NK-mediated antimetastatic protection by stimulation of both intravascular and extravascular organ-associated NK cells (105).

(d) More direct evidence for the involvement of NK cells

in tumor cell destruction and inhibition of metastasis formation has come from experiments with adoptively transferred NK-enriched or depleted lymphoid cell populations. NK reactivity of mice depressed by cyclophosphamide (Cy) or anti-asialo GM_1 treatment could be reconstituted by adoptive transfer of lymphoid cells. In parallel, adoptively transferred lymphoid cells were able to reconstitute the antimetastatic resistance of these mice (32, 39). Spleen cells with depleted cell activity failed to restore antimetastatic defenses in the NK-suppressed recipients (32, 39). Similarly, the depressed NK reactivity and antimetastatic resistance in rats treated with anti-asialo GM_1 serum were reconstituted by transfusion of highly purified syngeneic large granular lymphocytes, the subpopulation of cells responsible for NK activity (4).

Since NK cells can participate in the elimination of tumor cells, one might predict that tumor cells which survive and successfully metastasize would be more resistant to lysis by NK cells than tumor cells derived from local sites of tumor growth. Indeed, when the cytotoxic activity of normal spleen cells was tested against 3LL tumor cells derived from the local tumor or from spontaneous pulmonary metastases, higher resistance to lysis was found among metastatic cells (29). Furthermore, serial subcutaneous transfer of 3LL tumor cells mixed with normal spleen cells resulted in the selection of tumor cells displaying both higher resistance to the cytotoxic action of NK cells and higher metastatic ability (30). The relatively higher level of resistance to NK activity of the metastatic versus the primary tumor cells was confirmed using various experimental tumor systems (6, 102). It is of interest that the resistance of metastatic cells to NK cells was observed when the tumor cells were isolated directly from the spontaneous metastases, but this resistance disappeared after *in vitro* propagation (6).

Tumor cells derived from the experimental metastases produced by i.v. inoculation of tumor cells usually did not demonstrate resistance to NK cells (40). However, subpopulations of tumor cells or individual tumor cell clones which were selected for NK resistance produced more experimental metastases than the unselected parental tumor population when they were injected into nude mice with relatively high levels of NK cell activity. In contrast, the differences in the metastatic potential between NK-sensitive and NK-resistant tumor lines were not found when these lines were inoculated into beige or 3-week old nude mice with relatively low NK activity (40, 95).

It should be noted that although these experimental data indicate that NK resistance could be an important component of the metastatic phenotype, especially in hosts with high NK reactivity, NK resistance as well as resistance to other effector cells cannot completely account for the ability of tumor cells to metastasize. Metastatic cells have to possess a complex series of properties which permit them to fulfill the entire sequence of steps involved in the metastatic cascade.

NK CELLS AND ANTIMETASTATIC EFFECT OF ANTICOAGULANT DRUGS

The importance of NK cells in antimetastatic defense was further demonstrated when the effect of the anticoagulant agents on metastasis formation was investigated (33). For the last 20 years the mechanism of the antimetastatic effect of anticoagulants has been intensively investigated. The most widely accepted mechanism is that antiplatelet and anticoagulant drugs prevent the interaction of the factors of the hemostatic system with tumor cells and thus impair their adhesion to the endothelium of the vessels and futher extravasation (see reviews 25, 85). However, an alternative or additional possibility is that platelet aggregation and/or fibrin deposition on the surface of tumor cells might prevent their adequate recognition and lytic interaction with NK or other cytotoxic effector cells. From this hypothesis, one would predict that the antimetastatic activity of NK cells would be increased when anticoagulant drugs prevent the coating of tumor cells with platelets or fibrin, and that the antimetastatic effects of anticoagulant drugs would be augmented in animals with high NK cell activity. Conversely, one would predict that the antimetastatic effect of anticoagulants would be diminished or undetectable in animals with low NK reactivity (33). To evaluate these predictions, the antimetastatic effects of antiplatelet (prostacyclin or PGI_2) and anticoagulant drugs (heparin and warfarin) were investigated in mice with augmented or depressed NK activity. The results of these investigations indicate that the antimetastatic effects of anticoagulant or antiplatelet drugs were observed only in hosts with active NK cells, since in mice with depressed NK reactivity after anti-asialo GM_1 treatment, the antimetastatic effect of PGI_2, warfarin or heparin was abrogated. The importance of NK cells in the antimetastatic effect of anticoagulant drugs was further supported by the observation that the antimetastatic effect of the anticoagulant drugs was further potentiated by poly I:C stimulation of NK cell activity (33).

The antimetastatic effects of anticoagulants were probably mediated by the acceleration of tumor cell elimination from the lung vasculature. Using radiolabeled B16F10 or BL6 melanoma cells, this possibility was investigated by monitoring the level of residual radioactivity in the different organs and in the blood of heparin or warfarin treated mice with suppressed or augmented NK reactivity. Heparin and warfarin did not influence the NK activity of spleen cells but caused a substantial increase in the elimination of i.v.-inoculated melanoma cells. Similar effects were observed when NK cell activity was augmented by poly I:C treatment. Combined treatment of mice with anticoagulants and poly I:C had additive effects on the clearance of tumor cells from the vasculature of the lungs. In contrast, in mice treated with anti-asialo GM_1, substantial increases in the survival of the inoculated tumor cells were found and anticoagulants did not influence the survival of tumor cells. Thus, one day after inoculation of B16F10 melanoma cells into mice treated with heparin and anti-asialo GM_1, the number of surviving tumor cells was 200 times higher than in mice treated with heparin and poly I:C (33). Based on these data it was concluded that anticoagulant drugs seem to make tumor cells more vulnerable to the cytotoxic action of NK cells and increase the rate of tumor cell elimination from the blood, resulting in a decrease in metastasis formation (33). A combination of anticoagulant drugs and biological response modifiers could be particularly effective in the prevention of development of tumor metastases.

MACROPHAGES AND METASTASIS FORMATION

An increasing body of experimental data indicates that, in addition to T and NK cells, macrophages could participate in the control of the metastatic process (18, 67, 106). Activated macrophages exert *in vitro* a high level of cytotoxic and cytostatic activity against a variety of tumor cells (1, 46). Although selection of tumor cells which are completely resistant to the tumoricidal effects of macrophages is less common than selection of resistance to T and NK cells (40), heterogeneity of tumor cells in their sensitivity to lysis by activated macrophages has been documented in numerous investigations (66–68, 103, 106). The positive correlation between metastatic properties of tumor cells and their resistance to the tumoricidal action of activated macrophages, presents at least suggestive evidence for the involvement of macrophages in the elimination of potentially metastatic tumor cells.

The first *in vivo* evidence of the possible involvement of macrophages in the control of metastatic spread of tumor cells were obtained when the metastatic properties of cloned and uncloned populations of murine RAW 117 lymphosarcoma cells were investigated (82). It was demonstrated that sublines or individual clones of RAW 117 lymphosarcoma which were able to develop liver metastases had low levels of gp70 expression. The original lymphosarcoma or clones with high gp70 expression on the cell surface failed to colonize the liver in normal or nude mice. Suppression of NK cell function in these mice had no effect on antimetastatic resistance. Only when mice were treated with silica or carrageenan, agents which suppress macrophage function, RAW 117 lymphosarcoma cells were able to form metastases in the liver (82, 83). In addition, a comparison of the susceptibility of metastatic and nonmetastatic RAW 117 sublines and clones to cytotoxic and cytostatic action of activated peritoneal macrophages revealed that high metastatic potential positively correlated with high resistance to these effects of macrophages (66).

A similar association between the relative resistance to the tumoricidal action of activated macrophages and high metastatic behavior was also demonstrated with other experimental tumors such as a chemically induced murine sarcoma (68), a spontaneous mammary adenocarcinoma (106), the B16 melanoma and its highly metastatic sublines B16-B14b (66), and metastatic and nonmetastatic sublines of the mammary adenocarcinoma 13762NF (74).

It is of interest that differences in sensitivity or resistance to the tumoricidal activity of activated macrophages as well as NK cells have been found only with tumor cells isolated directly from *in vivo* growing tumors, whereas no differences in sensitivity were observed when tumor cells were tested after *in vitro* culture (74).

More direct confirmations of the potential role of macrophages in the antimetastatic defense are coming from the experiments in which the activation of macrophages with liposomes containing lymphokines or muramyl dipeptide (MDP) is associated with eradication of the established tumor metastases and survival of the treated mice (18, 21).

IMMUNOTHERAPY OF TUMOR METASTASES

Investigations of the immune mechanisms responsible for the antimetastatic defense should help to understand some of the determinants of the metastatic process and to develop approaches for the prevention and cure of metastases in patients with cancer.

An obvious therapeutic approach could combine the surgical removal of the primary tumor with immunization by the resected tumor cells, to stimulate the antimetastatic T cell mediated immunity. However, this approach has several limitations. First, spontaneously metastasizing tumors in mice are weakly- or nonimmunogenic and many or most human tumors might similarly be poorly immunogenic. Secondly, metastatic cells could be antigenically different from the primary tumor cells. In addition, the development of suppressor cells or other forms of immune depression during the primary tumor growth also could make such immunization inefficient. However, these potential obstacles might be overcome or might not occur. First, the immunogenicity of tumor cells might be substantially augmented by phenotypic modification of their cell surface and this approach has been successfully used for the treatment of postoperative murine tumor metastases (94). As discussed above, certain chemical agents such as MNNG, ethylmethanesulfonate (EMS), 5-azacytidine and UV light can be extremely efficient in the up-regulation of the immunogenicity of weakly- or nonimmunogenic tumors (5, 23, 34, 77). Secondly, antigenic differences between the primary and metastatic tumor cells are the result of the immunoselection by the immune reactions evoked by the primary tumor cells. This issue could not be relevant when the primary tumor is nonimmunogenic (and there are few expectations that metastatic cells would be antigenically different). Third, to the extent that suppressor cells are present, strategies to eliminate them are available and this would be expected to increase the efficiency of immunization (72).

Another immunotherapeutic approach is based on the stimulation of the immune system by biological response modifiers (BRMs) to augment the specific and nonspecific immune mechanisms and thereby eradicate postoperative tumor metastases. Substantial augmentation of the specific antitumor immunity by *C. parvum* or BCG has been demonstrated (37, 72). Also, BRMs could substantially augment the cytotoxic activity of NK cells and activate macrophages (44). However, this stimulation of NK activity usually is temporary, with return to preexisting levels usually within 7 days after stimulation. Furthermore, experimental animals or cancer patients usually develop hypo-responsiveness to repeated stimulation with BRMs (37, 45, 64). An understanding of the mechanisms of this hypo-responsiveness might help to develop protocols for sustained augmentation of NK cell activity and for the immunotherapy of malignant diseases.

A novel approach to activate and maintain high levels of tumoricidal activity of macrophages was proposed by Fidler (18). Multilamellar liposomes containing lymphokines or MDP were inoculated i.v. into mice, beginning at 3 days after excision of primary tumors, and repeated every 3 days for 3 weeks. Pulmonary macrophages demonstrated high levels of tumoricidal activity and this was associated wtih tumor-free survival in about 60% of the treated mice (18, 21).

Adoptive transfer of immune lymphocytes also could be an effective method for treatment of local or metastatic tumors in the experimental animals (see reviews 57, 89).

However, this approach has been limited to immunogenic tumors. Specific immune T-lymphocytes might be generated with greater frequency by utilizing immunogenic tumor cell variants produced by *in vitro* treatment of the original tumor cells by mutagens or UV irradiation. These immunogenic tumor cells could be used for *in vitro* stimulation of the autologous or syngeneic lymphocytes, with subsequent transfusion of the stimulated lymphocytes into the tumor-excised host. However, it has been reported that adoptive transfer might not be effective without elimination of T-suppressor cells by irradiation or by cyclophosphamide treatment (15, 57, 72). Such an approach was found to be rather efficient in some experimental tumor systems. Using immunogenic variant of MDAY-D2 tumor obtained after treatment with the mutagen EMS, Frost and Kerbel (23) generated specific CTL. The primary weakly immunogenic MDAY-D2 tumors were surgically removed, the tumor-excised host were pre-irradiated to eliminate suppressor cells and CTL were inoculated i.v. This resulted in complete inhibition of metastatic growth in 75% of the treated mice, with the rest of the treated mice showing prolonged survival as compared to the untreated control group.

Similarly, using an immunogenic variant of the 3LL tumor selected after *in vitro* treatment with UV light, Peppoloni et al. (78) induced immune T-lymphocytes. Eradication of the established 3LL metastases was achieved by transfusion of the immune lymphocytes into recipients pretreated with cyclophosphamide.

Discovery of the ability of the lymphokine interleukin 2 (IL-2) to propagate T cells and facilitate the generation of CTL *in vitro* opened a new possibility for adoptive immunotherapy of malignant disease (57, 87). In addition to the ability of IL-2 to increase the generation of specific CTL *in vitro* and to augment their efficiency *in vivo* against immunogenic tumors, it was found that IL-2 also was able to activate normal lymphocytes and convert them into highly cytotoxic effector cells, without apparent sensitization (57, 87). After short (3 days) culture *in vitro* in the presence of IL-2, normal lymphocytes demonstrate high level of cytotoxicity against a variety of the tumor cells, although no cytotoxicity has been found against normal cells. Human lymphocytes cultured in the presence of IL-2 were also able to destroy *in vitro* fresh tumor cells obtained from biopsy material as well as various cultured human tumor lines.

It was initially considered that the precursors of these lymphokine activated killer (LAK) cells were not NK cells, since they possess markers which characterize T cells and unstimulated NK cells had no detectable cytotoxic activity against some of the tumor target cells (36). However, numerous recent data indicate that IL-2 can also affect NK cells by stimulating their proliferation and stimulating their cytotoxic activity against NK-resistant as well as NK-sensitive tumor cells (2, 53).

Using various murine tumors it was demonstrated that spleen cells from normal mice, transferred *in vivo* after 3 days incubation with IL-2, were able to inhibit the formation of experimental metastases (69). Survival of the IL-2-activated lymphocytes *in vitro* and *in vivo* depends on the presence of IL-2. Therefore the efficacy of these lymphocytes *in vivo* depends on the *in vivo* exposure to sufficient amounts of IL-2. The antimetastatic effects of the transfused lymphocytes proportionally increased with an increase of the dose of inoculated IL-2 (69). These experiments with a wide range of doses of IL-2 became possible after the cloning of the IL-2 gene and the production of highly active recombinant IL-2 in unlimited quantity with high activity (90). This adoptive immunotherapy approach has potentially important advantages since it can utilize autochthonous lymphocytes and can be efficient against non-immunogenic tumors. However, the currently described protocols involve the transfusion of large amounts of lymphocytes and IL-2, which have substantial toxicity. In spite of this, it has opened the possibility for clinical application of adoptive immunotherapy. Rosenberg (88) reported promising preliminary results of the therapy of metastatic disease in cancer patients using the transfusion of the autochthonous lymphocytes activated *in vitro* with IL-2 and supported *in vivo* by the inoculation of the human recombinant IL-2. The immunotherapy had measurable antitumor effects in less than half of the 25 patients who had advanced disease which had failed to respond to other treatments. It seems quite possible that further investigations could make adoptive immunotherapy clinically feasible, particularly in the eradication of the tumor metastases after surgical removal of the primary tumor mass.

Another immunological approach also seems rather promising and is based on the generation of monoclonal antibodies with selectivity for tumor cells. Monoclonal antibodies could have direct antitumor effects or could be used as the vehicle for the delivery of radioisotopes, chemotherapeutic agents or toxins (48, 62, 96). Intensive clinical investigations applying monoclonal antibodies are underway and some reports demonstrate significant therapeutic efficacy of the monoclonal antibodies against metastatic deposits in the cancer patients (42, 48, 62, 96).

Recent achievements in the understanding of the role of immunological mechanisms in the antitumor and antimetastatic defenses, as well as some initial success in the application of immunological approaches for treatment of cancer patients provide hope that immunotherapy will develop into an important additional modality for treatment of cancer in man.

REFERENCES

1. Alexander P: The functions of the macrophage in malignant disease. *Annu Rev Med* 27:207–219, 1976
2. Allavena P, Klein R, Ortaldo J: Characterization of human large granular lymphocyte subpopulations: Comparison of the phenotype of NK cells and of interleukin-2-dependent progenitors of cytolytic effector cells. *Nat Immun Cell Growth Reg* 4:7–20, 1985
3. Axelrod A, Klein G: Differences in histocompatability requirements between primary tumors and their metastases. *Transpl Bull* 3:100–102, 1956
4. Barlozzari T, Reynolds C, Herberman R: *In vivo* role of natural killer cells: Involvement of large granular lymphocytes in the clearance of tumor cells in anti-asialo GM$_1$-treated rats. *J Immunol* 131:1024–1029, 1983
5. Boon T: Antigenic tumor cell variants obtained with mutagens. *Adv Cancer Res* 39:121–151, 1983
6. Brooks C, Flannery G, Wilmott N, Austin E, Kenwrick S, Baldwin R: Tumor cells in metastatic deposits with altered sensitivity to natural killer cells. *Int J Cancer* 28:191–201, 1981
7. De Baetselier P, Katzav S, Gorelik E, Feldman M, Segal S: Differential expression of H-2 gene products in tumor cells is

associated with their metastogenic properties. *Nature* 288:197–181, 1980

8. Deichman G, Kluchareva T: Loss of transplantation antigen in primary simian virus 40-induced tumors and their metastases. *J Natl Cancer Inst* 36:647–655, 1966

9. Dennis J, Donnaghue T, Kerbel R: An examination of tumor antigen loss in spontaneous metastasis. *Invasion and Metastasis* 2:111–125, 1981

10. Doherty P, Knowles B, Wettstein P: Immunological surveillance of tumors in the context of major histocompatibility complex restriction of T-cell function. *Adv Cancer Res* 42:1–65, 1984

11. Doyle A, Martin J, Fune K, Gazdat A, Carney D, Martin S, Linnoila I, Cuttitta F, Mulshine J, Bunn P, Minna J: Markedly decreased expression of class I histocompatibility antigens, protein and mRNA in human small-cell lung cancer. *J Exp Med* 161:1135–1151, 1985

12. Eccles S, Alexander P: Immunologically mediated restraint of latent tumor metastasis. *Nature* 257:52–54, 1975

13. Eisenbach L, Segal S, Feldman M: MHC imbalance and metastatic spread in Lewis lung carcinoma clones. *Int J Cancer* 32:113–120, 1983

14. Eisenbach L, Hollander N, Greenfeld L, Yakor H, Segal S, Feldman M· The differential expression of II-2K versus H-2D antigens, distinguishing high-metastatic from low-metastatic clones is correlated with the immunogenic properties of the tumor cells. *Int J Cancer* 34:567–573, 1984

15. Fefer A, Einstein A, Cheever M, Berenson J: Models for syngenic adoptive chemoimmunotherapy of murine leukemias. *Ann NY Acad Sci* 277:492–509, 1976

16. Festenstein H, Schmidt W: Variation of MHC antigenic profiles of tumor cells and its biological effects. *Immunol Rev* 60:85–127, 1981

17. Fidler I: Selection of successive tumor lines for metastasis. *Nature* 242:148–149, 1973

18. Fidler I: Therapy of spontaneous metastases by intravenous injection of liposomes containing lymphokines. *Science* 208:1469–1471, 1980

19. Fidler I, Gerstein D, Hart I: The biology of cancer invasion and metastasis. *Adv Cancer Res* 28:149–250, 1978

20. Fidler I, Kripke M: Tumor cell antigenicity, host immunity and cancer metastasis. *Cancer Immunol Immunother* 7:201–205, 1980

21. Fidler I, Poste G: Macrophage-mediated destruction of malignant tumor cells and new strategies for the therapy of metastatic disease. *Springer Semin Immunopathol* 5:161–187, 1982

22. Fogel M, Gorelik E, Segal S, Feldman M: Cell-surface antigens of tumor metastasis differ from those of the local tumor. *J Natl Cancer Inst* 62:385–388, 1979

23. Frost P, Kerbel R: Immunology of metastasis. Can the immune response cope with disseminated tumor? *Cancer Metastasis Rev* 2:239–256, 1983

24. Frost P, Kerbel R, Bauer E, Tartamella-Biondo R, Cefalu W: Mutagen treatment as a means for selecting immunogenic variants from otherwise poorly immunogenic malignant murine tumors. *Cancer Res* 43:125–132, 1983

25. Gasic G: Role of plasma platelets and endothelial cells in tumor metastasis. *Cancer Metastasis Rev* 3:99–123, 1984

26. Goodenow R, Vogel J, Linsk R: Histocompatibility antigens on murine tumors. *Science* 230:777–783, 1985

27. Gorelik E: Concomitant tumor immunity and the resistance to a second tumor challenge. *Adv Cancer Res* 39:71–120, 1983

28. Gorelik E: H-2 expression, immunogenicity and metastatic properties of BL6 melanoma cells treated with MNNG. In: *Treatment of Metastasis Problems and Prospects.* Hellmann K and Eccles S (eds.), Taylor and Francis, London, pp 355–359, 1985

29. Gorelik E, Fogel M, Feldman M, Segal S: Differences in resistance of metastatic tumor cells and cells from local tumor growth to cytotoxicity of natural killer cells. *J Natl Cancer Inst* 63:1397–1404, 1979

30. Gorelik E, Feldman M, Segal S: Selection of 3LL tumor subline resistant to natural effector cells concomitantly selected for increased metastatic potency. *Cancer Immunol Immunother* 12:105–109, 1982a

31. Gorelik E, Fogel M, De Baetselier P, Katzav S, Feldman M, Segal S: Immunobiological diversity of metastatic cells. In: *Cancer Invasion and Metastasis.* Liotta L, Hart I (eds.), Martinus Nijhoff Publ., Boston, pp 134–146, 1982b

32. Gorelik E, Wiltrout R, Okumura K, Habu S, Herberman R: Role of NK cells in the control of metastatic spread and growth of tumor cells in mice. *Int J Cancer* 30:107–112, 1982c

33. Gorelik E, Bere E, Herberman R: Role of NK cells in the antimetastatic effect of anticoagulant drugs. *Int J Cancer* 33:87–94, 1984

34. Gorelik E, Peppoloni S, Overton R, Herberman R: Increase in H-2 antigen expression and immunogenicity of BL6 melanoma cells treated with N-methyl-N'-nitro-nitrosoguanidine. *Cancer Res* 45:5341–5347, 1985

35. Gorelik E, Herberman R: Role of Natural Killer (NK) cells in the control of tumor growth and metastatic spread. In: *Basic and Clinical Immunology* 2. Herberman R (ed.), Martinus Nijhoff Publ., New York, pp 151–176, 1986

36. Grim E, Ramsey K, Mazumder A, Wilson D, Djen J, Rosenberg S: Lymphokine-activated killer cell phenomenon: II the precursor phenotype is serologically distinct from peripheral T lymphocytes memory CTL, and NK cells. *J Exp Med* 157:884–900, 1983

37. Hanna N: Role of natural killer cells in control of cancer metastasis. *Cancer Metastasis Rev* 1:45–64, 1982

38. Hanna N, Fidler I: The role of natural killer cells in the destruction of circulating tumor emboli. *J Natl Cancer Inst* 65:801–809, 1980

39. Hanna H, Burton R: Definitive evidence that natural killer (NK) cells inhibit experimental tumor metastasis *in vivo. J Immunol* 127:1754–1758, 1981

40. Hanna N, Fidler I: Relationship between metastatic potential and resistance to natural killer cell-mediated cytotoxicity in three murine tumor systems. *J Natl Cancer Inst* 66:1183–1190, 1981

41. Hauschka T: The chromosome in ontogeny and oncogeny. *Cancer Res* 21:957–974, 1961

42. Hellström K, Hellström I: Therapy of metastases by monoclonal antibodies and immunoconjugates. In: *Immune responses to metastases.* Herberman R, Wiltrout R, Gorelik E (eds.), CRC Press, Boca Raton, pp 127–138, 1986

43. Hoppner G: Tumor heterogeneity. *Cancer Res* 44:2259–2265, 1984

44. Herberman R (ed.): *NK Cells and Other Natural Effector Cells.* Academic Press, New York, 1982

45. Herberman R, Brunda M, Djeu J, Domzig W, Goldfarb R, Holden H, Ortaldo J, reynolds C, Riccardi C, Santoni A, Stadler B, Timonen T: Immunoregulation and natural killer cells. In: *Natural Killer Cells,* vol. 4, Human Cancer Immunology. Serrou B, Rosenfeld R, Herberman R (eds.), Elsevier, North Holland, Amsterdam, pp 37–52, 1981

46. Hibbs J, Charman H, Weinberg J: The macrophage as an antineoplastic surveillance cell: Biological perspectives. *J Reticuloendothel Soc* 24:549–570, 1978

47. Hoshino T, Uchida A: OK-432 (picibanil): Property, action and clinical effectiveness. In: *Clinical and experimental studies in immunotherapy.* Hoshino T, Uchid A (eds.), Excerpta Medica, Amsterdam, pp 1–19, 1984

48. Houghton A, Mintzer D, Gordon-Cardo C, Welt S, Fliegel B, Vadham S, Carswell E, Melamed M, Oettgen H, Old L: Mouse monoclonal IgG3 antibody detecting GD3 ganglioside – A phase I trial in patients with malignant melano-

ma. *Proc Natl Acad Sci USA* 82:1242–1249, 1985

49. Hui K, Grosveld F, Festenstein H: Rejection of transplantable AKR leukemia cells following MHC DNA-mediated transformation. *Nature* 311:750–752, 1984

50. Isakov N, Feldman M, Segal S: Control of progression of local tumor and pulmonary metastasis of the 3LL Lewis lung carcinoma by different histocompatibility requirements in mice. *J Natl Cancer Inst* 66:919–926, 1981

51. Isakov N, Feldman M, Segal S: An immune response against the alloantigens of the 3LL Lewis lung carcinoma prevents the growth of lung metastases but not of local allografts. *Invas Metas* 2:12–32, 1982

52. Isakov N, Katzav S, Feldman M, Segal S: Loss of expression of transplantation antigens encoded by the H-2K locus on Lewis lung carcinoma cells and its relevance of the tumor's metastatic properties. *J Natl Cancer Inst* 71:139–145, 1983

53. Itoh K, Tilden A, Kumagai K, Bolch C: Leu-11⁺ lymphocytes with natural killer (NK) activity are precursors of recombinant interleukin 2 (rIL-2)-induced activated killer (AK) cells. *J Immunol* 134:802–807, 1985

54. Katzav S, De Baetselier P, Gorelik E, Feldman M, Segal S: Immunogenetic control of metastasis formation by a methylcholanthrene-induced tumor (T10) in mice: Differential expression of H-2 gene products. *Transpl Proc* 13:742–746, 1981

55. Katzav S, De Baetselier P, Tartakovsky B, Feldman M, Segal S: Alterations in major histocompatability complex phenotypes of mouse cloned T10 sarcoma cells: Association with shifts from nonmetastatic to metastatic cells. *J Natl Cancer Inst* 71:317–324, 1983

56. Katzav S, Segal S, Feldman M: Metastatic capacity of cloned T10 sarcoma cells that differ in H-2 expression: Inverse relationship to their immunogenic potency. *J Natl Cancer Inst* 75:307–318, 1985

57. Kedar E, Weiss D: The *in vitro* generation of the effector lymphocytes and their employment in tumor immunotherapy. *Adv Cancer Res* 38:171–287, 1983

58. Kerbel R: Implications of immunological heterogeneity of tumors. *Nature* 280:358–360, 1979

59. Kim U, Baumler A, Carruthers C, Bielat K: Immunological escape mechanisms in spontaneously metastasizing mammary tumors. *Proc Natl Acad Sci* 72:1012–1016, 1975

60. Kraskovsky G, Lobko G: Alteration of the genetic structure of tumor cell population following metastasizing into the regional lymph nodes. In: Genetics of tumor growth. Turbin N, Rockitsky P, Kraskovsky G (eds.), Science and Technick, Minsk, pp 155–168, 1967

61. Lampson L, Fisher C, Whelan J: Striking paucity of HLA-A, B, C and β_2-microglobulin on human neuroblastoma cell lines. *J Immunol* 130:2471–2477, 1983

62. Levy R, Miller R: Tumor therapy with monoclonal antibodies. *Fed Proc* 42:2650–2656, 1983

63. Liotta L, Thorgeirsson U, Garbisa S: Role of collagenases in tumor cell invasion. *Cancer Metastasis Rev* 1:277–288, 1982

64. Maluish A, Ortaldo J, Conlon J, Sherwin S, Leavitt R, Strong D, Wiernik R, Oldham R, Herberman R: Depression of natural killer cytotoxicity after *in vivo* administration of recombinant leukocyte interferon. *J Immunol* 131:503–512, 1983

65. Martin W: Structural and functional alterations in H-2 antigen expression on tumor cells. *Transpl Proc* 15:2097–2100, 1983

66. Miner K, Nicolson G: Differences in the sensitivities of murine metastatic lymphoma/lymphosarcoma variants to macrophage mediated cytolysis and/or cytostasis. *Cancer Res* 43:2063–2068, 1983

67. Miner K, Klostergaard J, Granger G, Nicolson G: Differences in cytotoxic effects of activated murine peritoneal macrophages and J774 monocyte cells on metastatic variants

of B16 melanoma. *J Natl Cancer Inst* 68:507–516, 1983

68. Montovani A: *In vitro* effects on tumor cells of macrophages isolated from an early passage chemically-induced murine sarcoma and from its spontaneous metastasis. *Int J Cancer* 27:221–230, 1981

69. Mule J, Shu S, Schwarz S, Rosenberg S: Adoptive immunotherapy of established pulmonary metastases with LAK cells and recombinant interleukin-2. *Science* 225:1487–1489, 1984

70. Natali P, Bigotti A, Nicorta M, Viora M, Manfredi D, Ferrone S: Distribution of human class I (HLA-A, B, C) histocompatability antigens in normal and malignant tissues of nonlymphoid origin. *Cancer Res* 44:4679–4687, 1984

71. Nicolson G: Cancer Metastasis: Organ colonization and cell-surface properties of malignant cells. *Biochem Biophys Acta* 695:113–176, 1982

72. North R, Dye E, Mills C, Chandler J: Modulation of anti-tumor immunity: Immunobiologic approaches. *Springer Semin Immunopathol* 5:193–215, 1982

73. North R, Bursuker I: Generation and decay of the immune response to a progressive fibrosarcoma. I. Ly 1⁺2⁻ suppressor T cells down regulate the generation of Ly 1⁻2⁺ effector T cells. *j exp Med* 159:1295–1311, 1984

74. North R, Nicolson G: Heterogeneity in the sensitivities of the 13762NF rat mammary adenocarcinoma cell clones to cytolysis mediated by extra- and intratumor macrophages. *Cancer Res* 45:1453–1458, 1985

75. Nowell P: The clonal evolution of tumor cell populations. *Science* 194:23–28, 1976

76. Parmiani G, Fossoti G, Taramelli D, Anichini A, Balsari A, Gambacorti-Passerini C, Sciorelli G, Cescinelli N: Autologous cellular immune response to primary and metastatic human melanomas and its regulation by DR antigen expression on tumor cells. *Cancer Metastasis Rev* 4:7–26, 1985

77. Peppoloni E, Herberman R, Gorelik E: Induction of highly immunogenic variants of Lewis lung carcinoma tumor by ultraviolet irradiation. *Cancer Res* 45:2560–2566, 1985

78. Peppoloni S, Herberman R, Gorelik E: Reduced metastatic ability of Lewis lung carcinoma (3LL) cells treated *in vitro* with ultraviolet (UV) radiation. *Clin Exp Metastases* 5:43–56, 1987

79. Pimm M, Embleton M, Baldwin R: Multiple antigenic specificities within primary 3-methylcholanthrene-induced rat sarcomas and metastases. *Int J Cancer* 25:621–629, 1981

80. Pollack S: Direct evidence for antitumor activity by NK cells *in vivo*: Growth of B16 melanoma in anti-K 1.1 treated mice. In: NK cells and other natural effector cells. Herberman R (ed.), Academic Press, New York, pp 1347–1352, 1982

81. Poste G, Greig R: On the genesis and regulation of cellular heterogeneity in malignant tumors. *Inv Metast* 2:137–176, 1982

82. Reading C, Brunson K, Torriani M, Nicolson G: Malignancies of metastatic murine lymphosarcoma cell lines and clones correlate with decreased cell surface display of RNA tumor virus envelope glycoprotein gp70. *Proc Natl Acad Sci* 77:5943–5947, 1980

83. Reading C, Kraemer P, Miner K, Nicolson G: *In vivo* and *in vitro* properties of malignant variants of RAW 117 metastatic murine lymphoma/lymphosarcoma. *Clin Exp Metastatis* 1:135–151, 1983

84. Riccardi C, Pucceti P, Santoni A, Herberman R: Rapid *in vivo* assay of mouse NK cell activity. *J Natl Cancer Inst* 63:1041–1045, 1979

85. Rickles F, Edwards R: Activation of blood coagulation in cancer: Trousseau's syndrome revisited. *Blood* 62:14–23, 1983

86. Rogers M, Gooding L, Margulies D, Evans G: Analysis of a defect in the H-2 genes of SV40 transformed C3H fibroblasts that do not express H-2Kᵏ. *J Immunol* 130:2418–2422, 1983

87. Rosenberg S: Adoptive immunotherapy of cancer: Accom-

plishments and prospects. *Cancer Treat Rep* 68:233–248, 1984

88. Rosenberg S: Lymphokine-activated killer cells: A new approach to immunotherapy of cancer. *J Natl Cancer Inst* 75:595–603, 1985

89. Rosenberg S, Terry W: Passive immunotherapy of cancer in animals and man. *Adv Cancer Res* 25:323–348, 1977

90. Rosenberg S, Grimm E, McGrogan M, Doyle M, Kawasaki E, Koths K, Mark D: Biological activity of recombinant human interleukin-2 produced in *E Coli Science* 223:1412–1419, 1984

91. Sanderson A, Beverly P: Interferon, β_2-microglobulin and immunoselection in the pathway to malignancy. *Immunol Today* 8:211–213, 1983

92. Schirrmacher V: Cancer Metastasis: Experimental approaches, theoretical concepts and impacts for treatment strategies. *Adv Cancer Res* 43:1–73, 1985

93. Schrier P, Bernards R, Vaessen R, Houweling A, van der Erb A: Expression of class I major histocompatability antigens switched off by highly oncogenic adenovirus 12 in transformed rat cells. *Nature* 305:771–773, 1983

94. Scurnick Y, Gorelik E, Sindelar W: Reduction of metastases in murine malignancies by immunotherapy with syngeneic tumor cells treated with cholesterol hemisuccinate. *Surg. Forum* 33:396–398, 1982

95. Segal S, Kingsmore S, Gorelik E, Feldman M: Control by NK cells of the generation of lung metastases by the Lewis lung carcinoma. In: *Current concepts in human immunology and cancer immunomodulation*. Serrou B (ed.), Elsevier/North Holland Biomedical Press, Amsterdam, 227–234, 1982

96. Sell S, Reisfeld R (eds.): Monoclonal antibodies in cancer. Humane Press, Clifton, 1985

97. Sugarbaker E, Cohen A: Altered antigenicity in spontaneous pulmonary metastases from an antigenic murine sarcoma. *Surgery* 72:155–161, 1972

98. Sugarbaker E, Weingard D, Roseman J: Observations on cancer metastasis in man. In: *Tumor invasion and metastasis.* Liotta L; Hart I (eds.), Martinus Nijhoff Publishers, Hague, pp 427–465, 1982

99. Talmadge JE, Meyers KM, Prieur DJ, Starkey JR: Role of NK cells in tumor growth and metastasis in beige mice. *Nature (London)*, 284:622–624, 1980

100. Talmadge J, Adams J, Phillips H, Collins M, Lenz B, Schneider M, Chirigos M: Immunotherapeutic potential in murine tumor models of polyinosinic-polycytidylic acid and poly-L-lysine solubilized by carboxymethylcellulose. *Cancer Res* 45:1066–1072, 1985

101. Tanaka K, Isselbacher K, Khoury G, Joy C: Reversal of oncogenesis by the expression of a major histocompatibility complex class I gene. *Science* 228:26–30, 1985

102. Teale D, Rees R, Clark A, Walker J, Potter C: Reduced susceptibility to natural killer cell lysis of hamster tumors exhibiting high levels of spontaneous metastasis. *Cancer Letters* 19:221–226, 1983

103. Urban J, Schreiber H: Selection of macrophage-resistant progressor tumor variants by the normal host. *J Exp Med* 157:642–656, 1983

104. Wallich R, Bulbuc N, Hämerling G, Katzav S, Segal S, Feldman M: Abrogation of metastatic properties of tumor cells by de novo expression of H-2K antigens following H-2 gene transfection. *Nature* 315:301–305, 1985

105. Wiltrout R, Herberman R, Zhang S, Chirigos M, Ortaldo J, Green K, Talmadge J: Role of organ-associated NK cells in decreased formation of experimental metastasis in lung and liver. *J Immunol* 134:4267–4275, 1985

106. Yamamura Y, Fisher B, Harnaha J, Proctor J: Heterogeneity of murine mammary adenocarcinoma cell subpopulations. *In vitro* and *in vivo* resistance to macrophage cytotoxicity and its association with metastatic capacity. *Int J Cancer* 33:67–75, 1984

ROLE OF MACROPHAGES IN RECOGNITION AND DESTRUCTION OF METASTATIC CELLS

RAJIV NAYAR and ISAIAH J. FIDLER

INTRODUCTION

The most devastating aspect of cancer is the emergence of metastases in organs distant from the primary tumor. Metastasis has already taken place by the time many cancers are diagnosed, and therefore, despite significant advances in surgical technique and general patient care, most deaths from cancer are still due to the uncontrolled growth of metastases. There are several reasons for the failure to treat metastasis. First, in the majority of patients, by the time of diagnosis of primary malignant neoplasms, excluding skin cancers, metastasis may well have occurred and eluded detection (22). Second, metastases are typically located in different organs and may also be in different locations within the same organ. This limits the delivery of chemotherapeutic agents and effective radiation therapy to the lesions without damaging normal tissues. Third, malignant neoplasms contain multiple cell populations exhibiting tremendous biological heterogeneity. This results in the rapid emergence of metastases that are resistant to conventional therapy (26, 85).

There is now a large body of evidence for the biological heterogeneity of tumors. Cells from individual tumors exhibit phenotypic differences with respect to cell surface properties, antigenicity, immunogenicity, growth rate, karyotype, sensitivity to various cytotoxic drugs, and the ability to invade and metastasize (22, 26, 47).

This biological heterogeneity is not confined to cells in primary tumors and is equally prominent among the cells populating metastases. Indeed, many clinical observations suggest that multiple metastases proliferating in different organs or even the same organ of a cancer patient can exhibit diversity in many biological characteristics such as hormone receptors, antigenicity and immunogenicity, and sensitivity to various chemotherapeutic drugs (22, 47). The development of this heterogeneity is multifactorial. Data from our laboratory and others indicate that metastases can arise from the nonrandom spread of specialized malignant cells that preexist within a primary neoplasm (24), that some metastases can be clonal in their origin (110), that different metastases can originate from different progenitor cells (110), and that, in general, metastatic cells can exhibit a higher rate of spontaneous mutation than nonmetastatic but tumorigenic cells (13, 53).

Collectively, such data suggest that successful therapy of disseminated cancer metastases will have to circumvent the problems of neoplastic heterogeneity, development of resistance to therapy by tumor cells, and nonspecific toxicity of therapeutic regimens. An increasing body of data now suggests that the scavenger cells of the reticuloendothelial system (RES), the blood monocytes and tissue macrophages, can be "activated" to the tunoricidal state to fulfill these demanding tasks. In this chapter, we review the role of macrophages in recognition and destruction of metastatic cells. In particular, we discuss the role of the macrophages in host defense in general involving recognition of "self" from "nonself" during homeostasis, activation of macrophages to the tumoricidal state, and subsequent destruction of metastatic cells by appropriately activated macrophages under *in vitro* and *in vivo* conditions.

MACROPHAGE AND HOMEOSTASIS

Since the discovery of the lymphocyte and its pivotal role in chronic inflammatory responses and host immunity, the primitive macrophage has received far less attention than biological relevance would dictate. For well over a century, detailed microscopic studies suggested that fixed or free phagocytic mononuclear cells are associated with the processes of tissue turnover, which include tissue remodeling during embryogenesis, tissue remodeling during metamorphosis, tissue destruction and repair subsequent to injury and infection, and tissue renewal, such as the removal of damaged or senescent cells. Since most of this earlier work was based on morphological observation, it was generally accepted that the mechanism by which macrophages accomplished their tasks involved a nonsophisticated process of phagocytosis and intracellular disposal. It now appears that this is an oversimplified explanation. The macrophage, a cell remarkably well conserved in evolution, is probably one of the most versatile cells in multicellular organisms. In addition, these cells are critical to homeostasis. Animals can survive without the benefit of an intact lymphocyte system, e.g., invertebrates, athymic mice, athymic and asplenic mice, and bursectomized birds. In stark contrast, the absence of an intact macrophage system is lethal.

In invertebrate and vertebrate animals, the macrophage's primary function is to discriminate "self" from "nonself." Macrophages readily recognize, phagocytose, and dispose of effected cells, for example, senescent red blood cells, damaged cells, cellular debris, and foreign invaders. Macrophages are continuously involved in the controlled metabolism of lipids and iron and in host response to injury, that is, inflammation. They also line body cavities and hence provide the first line of defense against microbial and par-

R. H. Goldfarb (ed.), Fundamental aspects of cancer.
© 1989, Kluwer Academic Publishers, Dordrecht. ISBN 978-94-010-6980-9

asitic infections. In addition, macrophages actively participate in surveillance against foreign invaders and cancer. To accomplish this task, macrophages frequently regulate both the afferent and efferent components of the immune system (3, 15, 21, 27, 55, 112).

The mechanisms by which macrophages recognize "self" from "nonself" are now becoming better understood. Several membrane surface moieties have been implicated in the macrophage's attachment to its targets. For example, it has been shown that extracellular proteins, such as collagen, upon aging accumulate advanced glycosylation end (AGE) products, which could act as specific signals for recognition and degradation of these macromolecules (113). The biological consequences of AGE product formation on rat and human peripheral nerve myelin has also been previously investigated, and studies show that protein modification by these products promotes specific recognition and uptake by mouse macrophages (113, 114). In addition to protein modification, cell surface carbohydrates and macrophage-mediated antibody-dependent recognition mechanism occur against some tumor cells and microorganisms (15). The identification and characterization of the mannose and the Fc receptors on macrophages and its influence in carrying out the recognition of "nonself" target cells is now well recognized (1, 56, 57). The homeostatic functions of macrophages, such as removal of senescent red blood cells from circulations and of macromolecules, such as collagen, elastin, and myelin, are carried out continously. In contrast, other functions, such as participation in host defense against infection, parasites, and cancer (reviews, (23, 27)), are sporadic and appear to require the recruitment and "activation" of macrophages to defend against a challenge. Upon completion of the task, the cells may revert to the "nonactivated" state or become activated once again. "Activated macrophage" is a working definition and its use in the literature has been extended to describe a large number of macrophage characteristics that may or may not describe the increased capacity of macrophages to recognize and destroy microorganisms, parasites, or cancer cells (15, 22, 23, 48, 55). The term "activated macrophages" is therefore reserved to describe only those cells capable of lysing virus-infected or tumorigenic, but not normal, cells.

INDUCTION AND MAINTENANCE OF TUMORICIDAL PROPERTIES IN MACROPHAGES

There are two major ways of rendering macrophages tumoricidal. The first method is through interaction with specific lymphokines, diffusible molecules released by stimulated T lymphocytes (27, 60). The second method is through interaction with microorganisms or their products (3). The cellular and molecular mechanism involved in these two processes is now beginning to be understood. Present concepts of this activation process suggest that a series of phenotypic alterations are acquired in a sequential fashion for the development of tumoricidal properties. The rate of appearance or loss of a specific phenotypic alteration depends on the nature and duration of the activating factors (15, 52, 77).

Activation of macrophages by lymphokines, released by antigen and mitogen-stimulated T lymphocytes, include gamma interferon (IFN-γ) (63) and a family of lymphokines generally referred to as macrophage activation factors (MAF) (21, 23, 27, 61, 63). This process of activation requires binding of the lymphokines to a specific macrophage receptor (87). Several lines of evidence point to this. Treatment of macrophages with reagents that alter their surface properties influences the extent to which they respond to lymphokines (87). Augmentation of macrophage responses to lymphokines was observed subsequent to alteration of amino, sulphydryl, hydroxyl, or carbonyl groups on the cell surface (82). In contrast, treatment of macrophages with various proteases or with α-L-fucose decreased their response to MAF, suggesting that fucose-containing moieties could be the receptor of MAF (87, 88). Moreover, the incubation of macrophages with liposomes containing fucoglycolipids enhanced their responses to MAF, which suggests that cell surface fucoglycolipids may be the natural receptor for MAF (87). More recently, direct evidence has also been presented for the existence of cell surface IFN-γ receptors that bind IFN-γ and result in the activation of macrophages (8).

Whether the cellular alterations in lymphokine-treated macrophages resulted directly from the binding of MAF or IFN-γ to surface receptors or whether the receptor-bound material was internalized to act at an intracellular locus was not clear. In the latter case, the surface receptor would merely bind sufficient lymphokine molecules to initiate biological activity. These questions can be studied experimentally by assessing the ability to activate macrophages under conditions in which MAF or IFN-γ is allowed to bind to its surface receptor but not be internalized, or they can be studied under conditions in which the agents are introduced directly into the cell without their initial binding to surface receptors. The second possibility has been investigated by using synthetic phospholipid vesicles (liposomes) as vehicles to deliver MAF or IFN-γ directly into the intracellular matrix of the macrophages.

Lymphokines with MAF activity were obtained from cultures of mitogen-stimulated rat lymphocytes in our laboratory. These lymphokines were encapsulated within liposomes of different sizes and lipid compositions (31, 88, 102). The ability of free and liposome-encapsulated MAF to render normal murine or rat macrophages cytotoxic for tumor cells *in vitro* was compared. These studies revealed that normal rodent macrophages were rendered tumoricidal after incubation with liposome-encapsulated MAF and that the level of cytotoxicity exceeded that induced by free MAF. Control cultures of macrophages incubated with liposomes alone or with liposomes containing supernatants from normal unstimulated lymphocytes did not acquire tumor cytotoxic properties.

The activation by liposome-encapsulated lymphokine was not due to liposome-mediated alterations in the macrophage surface that enhanced their responsiveness to MAF. This was concluded from control experiments in which macrophages incubated with liposomes containing saline and suspended in medium supplemented with free concentration of MAF, which was equivalent to the MAF entrapped in the liposomes, did not acquire tumoricidal properties. Further evidence that liposome-entrapped MAF activated macrophages via an intracellular mechanism comes from activation experiments in which normal macrophages were incubated with either free MAF, or liposome-encapsulated MAF in the presence of several compounds known to inhibit MAF binding to the macrophage surface. Liposome-encapsulated MAF, but not free MAF, activated tumoricidal properties in macrophages concomitantly treated with α-L-fucosidase, which removes surface receptors for MAF, or treated with fucose-binding plant lectins (*Ulex europaeus* I and *Lotus tetragonolobus*), which compete for binding to the MAF receptor on macrophages. Moreover, populations of nontumoricidal inflammatory tissue macrophages, which were inherently unresponsive to free MAF, could be rendered tumoricidal *in vitro* by incubation with liposome-encapsulated MAF (88). Finally, liposome-encapsulated MAF activated tumoricidal properties of macrophages obtained from C3H/HeJ mice unresponsive to endotoxins, whereas free MAF did not (39). These initial investigations on the activation of tumoricidal properties in rodent macrophages by liposome-encapsulated MAF have now been expanded to a human system with equivalent results. The activation of normal, noncytotoxic human blood monocytes by human MAF does not require binding of the lymphokine to putative monocyte surface receptors (61).

The mechanism(s) by which macrophages are rendered tumoricidal through interaction with microorganisms and their structural components is different from the lymphocyte-mediated activation process. Such immunomodulators include bacteria, protozoa, and nematodes (14, 50, 58) and bacterial cell wall components such as endotoxin, lipopolysaccharide, Lipid A, and muramyl dipeptide (2, 17, 51, 54, 78, 80, 103, 111). The chemical composition of the microorganism cell wall component responsible for macrophage activation is poorly understood, and the *in vivo* use of these microorganisms is often accompanied by significant toxicity, which includes granuloma formation and allergic reaction (4). The notable exception is a low molecular weight (459), water-soluble, synthetic structural unit of mycobacteria, N-acetylmuramyl-L-alanyl-D-isoglutamine (muramyl dipeptide; MDP). This compound has potent immunopotentiating activity that can replace the intact microorganism in Freund's complete adjuvant (11, 12).

The mechanism by which MDP activates macrophages has recently been investigated in both rodent (103), and human [Fogler and Fidler, unpublished results] systems with radiolabeled muramyl peptides. The results indicate that activation of tumoricidal properties in monocytes or macrophages is not cell surface receptor mediated but results from an intracytoplasmic event following pinocytosis of the glycopeptide (103); [Fogler and Fidler, unpublished results]. This is not really surprising since, in contrast to the activation of macrophages by lymphokines, bacterial cell wall products, such as MDP, are liberated following the phagocytosis of bacteria and digestion within the macrophage lysosomes (10, 39). Therefore, under physiological conditions, MDP and other bacterial cell wall components are presented to the macrophage through an intracellular pathway. This is also in agreement with studies from several laboratories where both rodent (33, 35, 39, 81, 96, 103) macrophages can be activated following phagocytosis of liposome-encapsulated MDP.

Recently, it has been shown that the activation of tumor cytotoxic properties in macrophages by lymphokines or bacterial components need not occur independently of each other. A lymphokine such as IFN-γ (63, 64, 100) or MAF (29, 91, 102) can prime macrophages to respond to a second signal, such as endotoxin (91, 92, 102) or MDP (29, 102). Also, recent studies from our laboratory have shown that synergistic activation of tumoricidal properties in macrophages by recombinant IFN-γ and MDP can be readily achieved (32, 93, 94). Human blood monocytes and murine peritoneal exudate macrophages were activated by the combination of subthreshold amounts of MDP and recombinant IFN-γ to become tumoricidal subthreshold amounts of MDP and recombinant IFN-γ to become tumoricidal against their human or murine tumorigenic target cells (32, 93, 94). In addition, the activation of human monocytes or murine macrophages by free IFN-γ and MDP was species specific. Human IFN-γ did not activate murine macrophages and murine IFN-γ did not activate human monocytes. In both species, the activation of tumoricidal properties in macrophages by IFN-γ occurred as a consequence of intracellular interaction. This conclusion was based on data showing that liposome-encapsulated IFN-γ and MDP activated macrophages pretreated with pronase but free IFN-γ and MDP did not (32). Moreover, the encapsulation of either murine or human IFN-γ with MDP within the same liposome preparation produced synergistic activation of cytotoxic properties in both mouse macrophages and human monocytes without apparent species specificity (32). These data suggest that, at least functionally, IFN-γ consists of two separate moieties. One part may be responsible for binding to the macrophage surface to facilitate the internalization of a part or of the whole molecule. The other moiety of the IFN-γ molecule may be responsible for the intracellular activation of macrophages to the tumoricidal state, which is not species specific.

Although the above *in vitro* studies have provided a greater understanding of the mechanisms by which macrophages can be activated by pretreatment with various immunomodulators, the use of free lymphokines and microorganisms and their products for *in situ* activation of macrophages has been difficult to achieve. There are various reasons for this failure. Dilution of injected lymphokines such as IFN-γ and MAF, rapid inactivation of lymphokines caused by their binding to serum proteins, and rapid clearance of lymphokines from the circulation have led to the failure of systemically administered soluble lymphokines in achieving macrophage activation. This is not surprising since under ideal *in vitro* conditions, successful activation of human monocytes requires incubation of the monocytes with MAF for at least eight hours (61). When synthetic compounds such as MDP that are nontoxic yet capable of activating macrophage tumoricidal properties *in vitro* are used, comparable effects have not been observed *in vivo*. These observations are due in part to the findings that when administered parenterally, MDP is rapidly cleared from the body within two hours and excreted in the urine (79). As in the case of lymphokines, this brief period *in situ* is simply not sufficient to render macrophages tumoricidal, even under ideal conditions (103). Also, the adoptive transfer of macrophages, that have been activated *in vitro* has two serious shortcomings in clinical situations. First, it requires the infusion of a large number of histocompatible or autologous macrophages, and second, most intravenously injected macrophages are arrested in the capillary bed of the lung and do not reach other relevant organs. A more promising approach has therefore been the development of methods to achieve direct activation of macrophages *in situ*. In recent years, we have actively pursued methods to enhance the delivery of well-defined synthetic compounds that are relatively nontoxic yet possess immune-potentiating activity specifically to cells of the monocyte-macrophage lineage. This has been successively achieved through the use of a liposome based drug delivery system for the transport of immunomodulators to peripheral blood monocytes and tissue macrophages.

LIPOSOMES AS VEHICLES FOR DRUG DELIVERY

Various studies have demonstrated the use of liposomes as carrier vehicles for drug delivery *in vivo* (5, 41, 42, 76). There are several advantages in using liposomes to deliver drugs to macrophages.

Following intravenous administration, the majority (80–90%) of the liposomes are taken up by the the reticuloendothelial cells in the liver, spleen, lymph nodes, and bone morrow and by circulating monocytes (5, 18, 25, 27, 29, 36, 96, 98, 99). By exploiting this localization pattern, liposome-encapsulated immunomodulators can be targeted to macrophages *in vivo* (27, 98). In addition, there are several other advantages in the use of liposomes. The components of the liposomes, phospholipids, are natural constituents of all cell membranes, and they are, therefore biodegradable and non-immunogenic and have limited intrinsic toxicity (41, 65). For example, liposomes prepared from phosphatidylcholine (PC), phosphatidylserine (PS), and lysolecithin are well tolerated by mice and dogs after single or multiple intravenous injections (46). In these studies, no evidence of gross or microscopic toxicity was detected in any major organs, even after administration of high doses of these particular liposomes. Furthermore, in cancer patients, acidic liposomes consisting of PC and phosphatidylglycerol (PG) were safely distributed to organs with high reticuloendothelial activity (71). Finally, the large diversity of phospholipids allows unlimited manipulation of their biochemical and biophysical properties to tailor very specialized liposomes. For example, liposomes of different sizes and different degrees of lamellarity can be generated (109). Leakage rates of entrapped aqueous contents can be controlled by acyl chain composition of the phospholipids, surface charge, and cholesterol content in the membrane (65). Temperature and pH-sensitive liposomes have also been designed to trigger release of entrapped contents under specific conditions (107, 108), such as in the endosomal component of the cells and assays in areas of local inflammation. The use of such specialized liposomes in clinical situations has yet to be tested, because of the anatomic and physiologic barriers imposed by the circulatory system, which would limit their efficacy under *in vivo* conditions (84, 89).

As mentioned earlier, we have concentrated our efforts on the natural distribution of intravenously injected liposomes, that is, to cells of the RES and circulating monocytes. In recent reviews, it has been proposed that exploitation of this route may enhance therapeutic efficacy for a variety of parasitic, fungal, viral, and bacterial diseases (5, 66, 97).

MACROPHAGE-LIPOSOME INTERACTIONS

In order to fulfill the requirements as a drug carrier vehicle to the mononuclear phagocytes *in vivo*, several demanding criteria must be met. For example, liposomes must readily bind and be phagocytosed by phagocytic cells. They must retain their entrapped contents for a reasonable length of time and demonstrate a preferential localization to tissue other than those high in reticuloendothelial activity and the lung parenchyma since it is the major site of metastatic disease. Finally, the liposomes must have a manageable, stable shelf-life, and the preparations must be reproducible.

Methodological evaluation of different liposome preparations has revealed that macrophages are able to recognize and preferentially phagocytose certain classes of phospholipids. The inclusion of negatively charged phospholipids, PS or PG, in PC liposomes greatly enhances binding and phagocytosis of such liposomes by blood monocytes and tissue macrophages (90, 96, 98, 99). As shown in Figure 1, PC multilamellar vesicles (MLV) containing 30 mol % PS or PG are phagocytosed at rates five to ten fold faster than the pure PC MLV. Furthermore, the size of the liposomes also influences the phagocytic rate with the larger MLV (250 mm diameter) being superior to the smaller unilamellar vesicles (SUV) (< 100 nm diamter). Indeed, most cells of the RES bind liposomes containing PS or PG, since similar enhancement of phagocytosis has been shown to occur in mouse peritoneal macrophages (90), Kupffer cells of the liver (95), and human peripheral blood monocytes (62, 75). Also, under *in vivo* conditions, the lipid com-

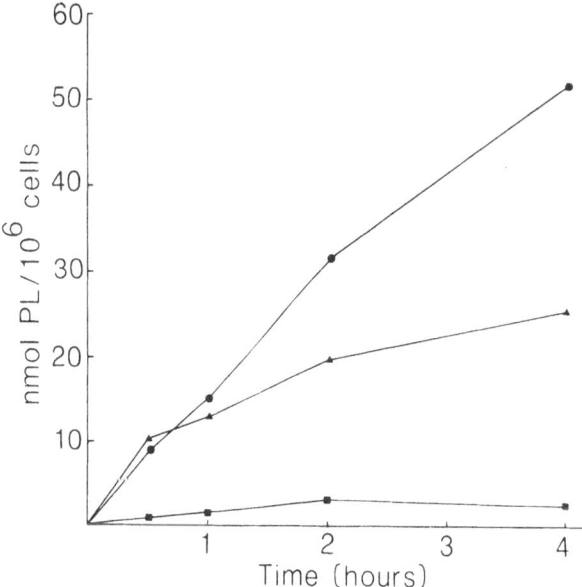

Figure 1. Phagocytosis of MLV by murine macrophages. Phagocytosis of PC, PC/PS (7:3 mol ratio), and PC/PG (7:3 mol ratio) MLV liposomes was determined by incubating 100 nmol of phospholipid with 10^5 macrophages at 37°C. Trace amounts of ^{125}I-labeled phenylpropionyl-PE was incorporated into the MLV preparations as a liposomal marker. At various times, the macrophage monolayer was washed extensively and the uptake was quantified by determining the radioactivity remaining in the wells. ■——■, PC; ●——●, PC/PS (7:3); ▲——▲, PC/PG (7:3).

position of liposomes significantly affects their distribution. Following intravenous injection, liposomes that contain negatively charged phospholipids such as PS are more efficiently arrested in the lung vasculature than the neutral PC liposomes (98). Whether such liposomes were phagocytosed by the blood monocytes was confirmed in subsequent studies in which PC/PS liposomes containing a trace of fluorescent lipid analogue were injected into tail veins of mice. After 24 hours, a period sufficient for blood monocytes to extravasate and differentiate into alevolar macrophages, fluorescent PC/PS liposomes were observed inside these cells (98).

Finally, the stability of liposomes and their entrapped contents is crucial if such vehicles are to serve effectively for delivery of the immunomodulators *in vivo*. The two aspects of stability that must be considered are leakage problems associated with the aqueous encapsulated compounds and the shelf-life and reproducibility of the liposome preparations.

Observations that low molecular weight solutes, such as MDP, leak out from the aqueous liposomal compartment of PC/PS MLV and become rapidly diluted in the external medium are disturbing, especially since serum proteins are potent induces of liposome leakage (43). To obviate this problem, the use of nonleaky lipophilic derivatives of MDP, such as muramyl tripeptide phosphatidylethanolamine (MTP-PE) (35, 36) muramyl dipeptide glyceryldipalmitate (MDP-GDP) (81), and 6-O-stearoyl MDP have been proposed (69). These compounds intercalate into the concentric phospholipid bilayers of the MLVs in a quantitative fashion, resulting in greater than 90% incorporation, as compared with 1–3% incorporation with the hydrophilic MDP (owing to aqueous space limitations). MLV containing these lipophilic immunomodulators have been shown to successfully activate the tumoricidal properties of macrophages (35, 69, 81). All of the MLV preparations produced similar levels of macrophage activation whether they were assessed by *in vitro* or *in vivo* techniques. In addition to the problem of overcoming leakage associated with water-soluble MDP, the degradation of MTP-PE incorporated into the liposomal phospholipid bilayer appears to be relatively slow (35).

The second criterion of liposomal stability involves prevention of lipid degradation due to lipid oxidation and aggregation of different liposomal preparations during storage of these preparations (101). Lyophilized preparations were the most stable over a six-month period (101). Similarly, Phillips *et al.* (81) showed that lyophilized preparations of PC/PS liposomes containing MDP-GDP were superior to PC/PS liposomes containing MDP in regard to reproducible liposomal preparations, long-term storage, and efficiency for activating macrophages.

As mentioned above, the *in situ* activation of macrophages by intravenous administration of liposomes containing MTP-PE results from the direct interaction of these liposomes with macrophages. Macrophage activation does not occur by an indirect action of the immunomodulator on T cells and subsequent release of lymphokines that activate macrophages but rather from the direct interaction with the liposomes carrying the immunomodulators (20). This conclusion is based on data from experiments in which three groups of mice with impaired T-cell function were used:

mice exposed to UV radiation, thymectomized adult mice exposed to X-rays, and athymic nude mice. Since macrophages of all three groups of mice were rendered tumoricidal by liposome-encapsulated MTP-PE but not by the control liposome preparation, the activation of macrophages occurred directly and was a thymus-independent process (20).

RECOGNITION AND LYSIS OF NEOPLASTIC CELLS BY MONOCYTES-MACROPHAGES

Macrophages activated by free or liposome-entrapped immunomodulators, such as MDP, MAF, or IFN-γ, acquire the ability to recognize and lyse neoplastic cells by a mechanism that requires direct cell-to-cell contact (6, 7, 48, 49, 73, 74). The ability of macrophages to discriminate between tumorigenic and normal cells has been studied in several systems, including syngeneic and allogenic tumors of mice, syngeneic rat tumors, and syngeneic guinea pig tumors (18, 30, 38, 44, 45, 48). Collectively, these data indicate that, at least *in vitro*, tumoricidal rodent macrophages destroy neoplastic cells by a process independent of transplantation antigens, species-specific antigens, tumor-specific antigens, cell-cycle time, and various phenotypes associated with transformation. Moreover, data obtained in various murine systems suggest that the susceptibility of tumor cells to destruction by tumoricidal macrophages is also independent of the *in vivo* biologic behavior of the tumor cells, such as invasiveness, metastatic potential, and growth rate and resistance to lysis by lymphocytes, natural killer cells, or cytotoxic drugs (review, Fidler, (22); Fidler and Poste, (27)).

Most studies on the interaction of macrophages with tumor cells have been carried out in rodent systems with isolated cultures of tumorigenic cells. Similarly, much of the work with human monocytes interacting with tumorigenic or normal cells has used isolated cultures of human target cells (61–63, 72, 104). Because metastatic cells proliferate among normal host cells, it was of interest to determine whether tumoricidal human blood monocytes could discriminate between tumorigenic and nontumorigenic allogeneic target cells under cocultivation conditions (28).

Highly purified preparation of peripheral blood monocytes isolated from normal donors were activated *in vitro* by incubation with liposomes encapsulated with human lymphokines (MAF). The cytotoxic properties of these monocytes against several tumorigenic and nontumorigenic allogeneic target cell populations were assessed under cocultivation conditions. Various combinations of three tumorigenic (A375 melanoma, HT-29 colon carcinoma, and NAT-glioblastoma) and three nontumorigenic target cell populations (lung cells, skin cells, and kidney cells) labeled with either [^{3}H]thymidine or [^{14}C]thymidine were plated onto monolayers of blood monocytes. Where possible, tumor cells with physiologically acceptable normal counterparts were paired. Both epithelial cells and fibroblasts were used as normal controls for tumors of different origins. In all combinations used, activated monocytes selectively lysed only allogeneic neoplastic cells and left nontumorigenic cells unharmed (28). Table 1 summarizes these results with cocultivation experiments done with A375 melanoma cells and normal lung cells. The selective lysis of tumorigenic cells was

Table 1. Recognition and destruction of neoplastic cells by activated human blood monocytes, (cocultivation experiments).[a]

Target cells labeled with [14C]thymidine[b]	% Cytotoxicity[c]	Target cells labeled with [3H]thymidine[b]	% Cytotoxicity[c]
A375 melanoma	53	A375 melanoma	47
Lung cells	1	–	–
–	–	Lung cells	0
A375 melanoma	36	Lung cells	1
Lung cells	0	A375 melanoma	41

[a]From Fidler and Kleinerman, 1984.
[b]Blood monocytes (10^5) were incubated for 24 hours with liposomes containing Hank's balanced salt solution (control) or liposomes containing MAF (tumoricidal) prior to the addition of radiolabeled target cells. A total of 10^4 cells labeled with either $0.5 \, \mu Ci/ml$ [3H]thymidine([3H]TdR) or [14C]thymidine([14C]TdR) were plated alone or with the monocytes. In mixed population experiments, 5×10^3 cells of each target were added into each culture well. Values are mean cmp $\pm$ SD for triplicate cultures.
[c]Percentage of cytotoxicity as compared with control monocytes and target cells ($P < 0.0001$).

not due simply to an inherent resistance of nonneoplastic cells to lysis mediated by host immune cells but was associated with activated monocytes, since both tumorigenic and nontumorigenic cells were equally susceptible to *in vitro* lysis mediated by mitogen-stimulated peripheral blood lymphocytes (28).

A severe limitation of many cancer therapies is their lack of selectivity and the resultant toxicity to the patient. Activated human blood monocytes can recognize and lyse neoplastic cells without harming normal cells. Therefore, the activation of macrophages *in situ* could be useful for the treatment of disseminated cancer.

ULTRASTRUCTURAL STUDIES OF THE INTERACTION BETWEEN ACTIVATED HUMAN MONOCYTES AND NEOPLASTIC CELLS

The interaction of control and tumoricidal human blood monocytes with allogeneic melanoma cells was analyzed by means of light microscopy, scanning and transmission electron microscopy. Activated monocytes that had phagocytosed liposomes containing MTP-PE clustered around the melanoma cells (Figure 2b) at a higher density than control monocytes (Figure 2a). This initial clustering was followed by the establishment of numerous focal points of binding, and some areas actually exhibited discontinous membranes (Figure 2c), a finding confirmed by stereophotography. After 24 hours of cocultivation, many of the target cells exhibited zones of vacuolation in the immediate vicinity of the tumoricidal monocytes (Figure 2d). This suggests that the target cell was damaged, and time course cytotoxicity studies have confirmed this.

We conclude, therefore, that the lysis of susceptible melanoma cells by human blood monocytes activated by liposomes containing immunomodulators occurs as the final step in a process that begins with direct cell-to-cell contact, damage to target cell membranes, and the development of vacuolation in the target cells (70).

RECOGNITION BY RODENT MACROPHAGES OF TUMORIGENIC CELLS WITH TEMPERATURE-DEPENDENT TRANSFORMED PHENOTYPIC CHARACTERISTICS

To determine whether any of the altered cell surface properties commonly present in virus-transformed cells provide the basis for macrophage recognition, we tested the ability of lymphokine-activated rodent macrophages to recognize and destroy target cells transformed by polyoma virus or simian virus 40 (SV-40), in which several of the cell surface characteristics associated with the transformed phenotype are only expressed at specific temperatures (30). We reasoned that if macrophages recognized target cells by a cell surface moiety that is associated with transformatiion, destruction of temperature sensitive transformed cells would occur at the permissive (33°C) but not at the nonpermissive (39°C) temperature for transformation. In these studies, we used baby hamster kidney (BHK) cells that were transformed by the ts3 mutant of polyoma virus, rat embryo 3Y1 cells transformed by a temperature-sensitive A cistron mutant of simian virus 40 (SV-40) and ts-H6-15 temperature-sensitive line of SV-40-transformed mouse 3T3 cells. All target cells were lysed *in vitro* by activated mouse or rat macrophages at both the permissive and nonpermissive temperatures for expression of the transformed phenotype. The target cells transformed by wild-type SV-40 or polyoma virus were also lysed at both temperatures. In contrast, untransformed target cells were not damaged by the macrophages. Since the macrophages killed target cells with temperature-dependent phenotypic characteristics equally well at both the temperatures, it was concluded that phenotypic characteristics of transformation such as expression of cell surface LETS proteins, Forssman antigen, surface changes for lectin agglutination, expression of SV-40 T antigen, low saturation density or density-dependent inhibition of DNA synthesis were all unlikely to contribute to the mechanism by which macrophages recognized and destroyed the transformed cells (30).

DESTRUCTION OF LUNG AND LYMPH NODE METASTASES BY THE SYSTEMIC ADMINISTRATION OF LIPOSOMES CONTAINING IMMUNOMODULATORS

These data raise the possibility that macrophages can be activated *in situ* to the tumoricidal state by systemically administered immunomodulators excapsulated in liposomes and that these activated macrophages could enhance host destruction of metastases. To test this possibility, mice bearing spontaneous metastases were injected with liposomes that contained various immunomodulators. The B16-BL6 melanoma cell line, which is syngeneic to C57BL/6 mice, was used as the model to determine the effectiveness of liposome-encapsulated materials in the treatment of metastases. After implantation in the footpad, this tumor metastasizes to lymph nodes and the lungs in more than 90% of the mice (19). C57BL/6 mice were each given an injection of melanoma cells, in the footpad and four to five weeks later, when the tumors had reached a size of 10 to 12 mm, the leg bearing the tumor, including the popliteal lymph node, was am-

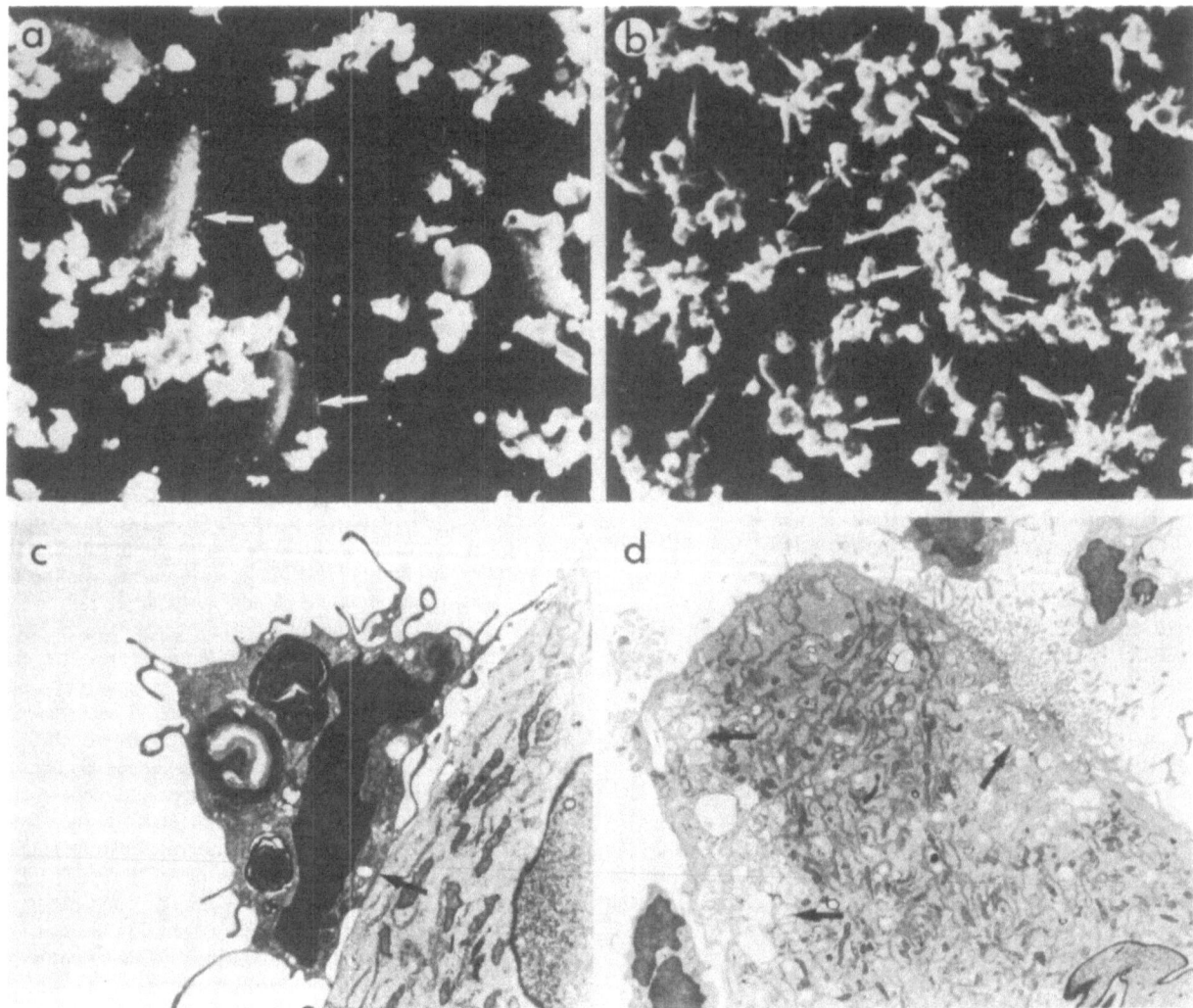

Figure 2. Scanning and transmission electron micrographs of human blood monocyte-tumor cell interaction. Scanning electron micrograph of cocultivation conditions between nonactivated monocytes and allogeneic A375 melanoma cells (2a) and between activated monocytes and A375 melanoma cells. Equal numbers of monocytes were added to both wells. Transmission electron micrograph showing monocytes with internalized liposomes adhering to the A375 melanoma cells after 24 hours of cocultivation. After 48 hours of interaction, the activated monocytes produce vacuolation in the target melanoma cell. Target cell lysis immediately follows.

putated. Three days after the amputation of the primary tumor, the mice were injected intravenously with liposomes containing immunomodulators or placebo preparations. Both test and control groups were treated twice weekly for four weeks (eight intravenous injections). Liposomes were prepared from chromatographically pure PC and PS. We have used these phospholipid liposomes as carriers because they are not toxic at the dose used (46) and because they are arrested efficiently in the lungs as well as in organs of the RES following intravenous administration.

Spontaneous metastases in the lungs and lymph nodes were well-established at the time liposome treatment began. Many individual metastases could be seen macroscopically. As shown in Figure 3, the mice treated intravenously with PBS, with free MAF, with freee MDP, or with liposomes containing PBS were dead by day 90 of the experiment, 60 days after the amputation of the tumor-bearing leg. Signifi-

cantly, 66% of mice injected intravenously with liposome-encapsulated MAF and 60% of mice injected with liposome-encapsulated MDP were alive when the experiments were terminated at 200 days. At the time of first liposome treatment, we estimate that the metastases contained 10^7 cells in this tumor system. Since the median survival time of mice injected with as few as 10 viable B16 cells (admixed with 10^6 dead cells) is 40 to 50 days (20) we speculate that the tumor burden in the successfully treated mice (alive on day 200) must have been reduced to fewer than 10 viable cells. Studies on mice treated with liposome-encapsulated MDP that have residual metastatic disease (albeit reduced compared with untreated control mice) have revealed that the tumor cells present in the lesions are still fully susceptible to destruction by activated macrophages (27, 38). Similar data on the successful treatment of other murine metastatic tumors by the systemic administration of liposomes contain-

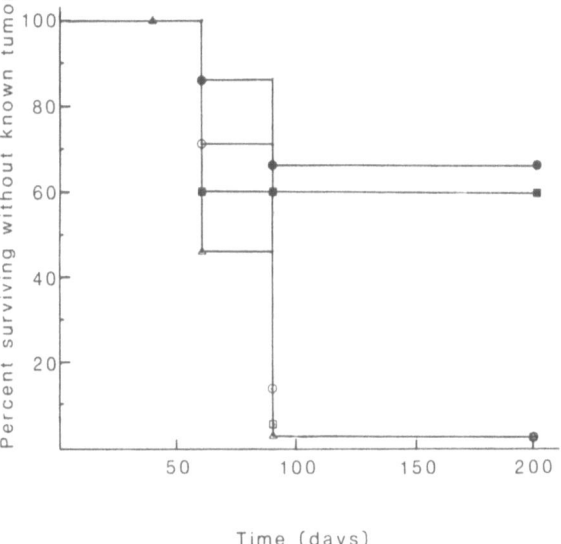

Figure 3. Treatment of spontaneous metastases by the systemic administration of liposomes containing MDP or MAF. Mice (18 to 20 mice/group) received biweekly injections for 4 weeks. △——△, control group, saline; ○——○, free MAF; ●——●, MLV containing MAF; □——□, free MDP; ■——■ MLV containing MDP, (for details see Fidler *et al.*, (36)).

ing different immunomodulators are now available (16, 36, 59, 69, 71, 81).

To enhance the efficacy of macrophage-mediated destruction of metastasis, we have combined suboptimal concentrations of a lymphokine and MDP in the same liposome preparations (29). Mice were injected intravenously with liposomes containing various dilutions of MAF, various dilutions of MDP, combinations of MAF and MDP, or control liposome dilutions of MDP, combinations of MAF and MDP, or control liposome preparations. Alveolar macrophages were harvested 24 hours later, and their antitumor activity was monitored *in vitro*. Liposomes containing combinations of MAF and MDP were most effective in generating cytotoxic properties in the lung macrophages. Moreover, this therapeutic regimen was very efficacious in the treatment of relatively large metastatic burdens. The B16 melanoma therapy experiments described above began seven days after the surgical removal of the subcutaneous (leg) melanoma when lung metastases were large, some measured greater than 1 mm in diameter (29). Liposomes were injected twice weekly for four weeks. The survival data shown in Figure 4 demonstrate that treatment with optimal doses of MDP or MAF resulted in the long-term survival (∼ 250 days) of about 30% of the mice. Neither MAF nor MDP were effective at suboptimal doses. In contrast, treatment of mice with liposomes that contained both suboptimal concentrations of MAF and MDP resulted in long-term survival (∼ 250 days) of 50% of the mice (29).

The varied response of metastases to conventional therapy is a major cause of failure in cancer treatment. Evidence that activated macrophages can recognize and destroy neoplastic cells *in vitro* without regard to their phenotypic diversity has stimulated a significant effort to develop effective approaches for the activation of macro-

phages *in situ*. Systemic administration of liposomes containing immunomodulators, such as lymphokines or MDP, has been shown to activate rodent macrophages *in situ* and to augment host destruction of spontaneous metastases (27).

Although the initial results regarding the destruction of metastases by macrophages are encouraging, it is unlikely that this approach could serve for treatment of large tumors. By the time of diagnosis, metastases are large and could contain as many as 10^9 cells. For this reason, therapeutic regimens designed to stimulate host immunity must be used in combination with other treatment modalities, such as surgery, chemotherapy, and radiotherapy in order to reduce the tumor burden. Tumoricidal macrophages can then be used to kill the few tumor cells that have survived destruction by conventional therapies.

EVIDENCE FOR THE INVOLVEMENT OF MACROPHAGES IN THE DESTRUCTION OF MELANOMA METASTASIS

The regression of established metastases following the systemic administration of liposomes containing immunomodulators was mediated by activated macrophages. This conclusion is based on several lines of evidence. First, administration of macrophage-activating agents encapsulated within PC liposomes (that are not retained in the lung) fails to activate lung macrophages, and there is no regression of lung metastases (36). Second, the treatment of tumor-bearing animals with agents that deplete macrophages (silica, carageenan, hyperchlorinated drinking water) before sys-

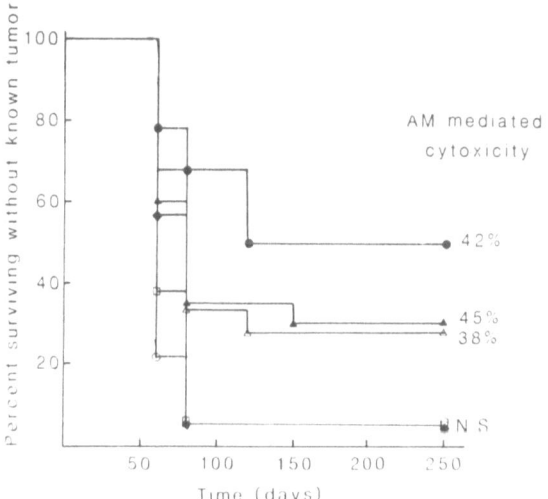

Figure 4. Treatment of spontaneous metastases by the systemic administration of liposomes containing immunomodulators. Mice (18 to 20 mice per/group) received bi-weekly injections for 4 weeks. □——□, MLV containing 1/20 MAF; ◆——◆, MLV containing 0.3 μg MDP; ○——○, MLV containing saline; ▲——▲, MLV containing 6.25 mg MDP; △——△, MLV containing 1/2 MAF; ●——●, MLV containing 0.3 μg MDP and 1/20 MAF (for details see Fidler and Schroit, (29)). AM mediated cytotoxicity was determined under *in vitro* conditions by employing appropriately treated alveolar macrophages against B16 melanoma cells (p < 0.001 N.S.; not significant (for details see Sone *et al.*, (102)).

temic therapy with liposome-encapsulated immunomodulators abrogates the effectiveness of liposome therapy (35). Third, intravenous injection of macrophages activated *in vitro* by incubation with liposomes containing MAF causes a reduction in metastatic burden comparable to that achieved by systemic administration of liposome-encapsulated activators (35). Fourth, morphologic and functional analysis of macrophages isolated from pulmonary metastases of mice injected intravenously with liposomes containing MTP-PE revealed that macrophages containing phagocytosed liposomes infiltrate and localize within pulmonary metastases. Once localized, these macrophages, but not other macrophages, are tumoricidal against the metastatic tumor cells (59).

CONCLUSIONS

The demonstration that appropriately activated macrophages can destroy tumor cells and leave normal cells unharmed has prompted an intensive search to identify agents that can render these cells tumoricidal *in vivo*. In addition, liposomes can be a useful carrier system to deliver the immunomodulators to the monocyte-macrophage system *in vivo*. The passive localization of liposomes in the peripheral circulation to phagocytic reticuloendothelial cells provides an effective mechanism for targeting liposome-entrapped materials to macrophages and monocytes. This mechanism has been exploited to deliver lymphokines and well-defined synthetic MDP to macrophages *in situ*. As a result, activation of macrophages has been achieved *in vivo* with significant success in treating metastases in model systems. The optimal conditions for systemic therapy with liposome-encapsulated immunomodulators and its efficacy alone or in combination with other cancer therapeutic regimens in treating metastases are currently being defined. As with other cancer therapies, the optimal application of activated macrophages in the destruction of metastatic cells would require combining them with other antitumor agents. The most likely role for tumoricidal macrophages is probably in the destruction of residual micrometastases after treatment with conventional therapeutic regimens.

ACKNOWLEDGMENTS

This research was sponsored by a grant from Ciba-Geigy, Ltd, Basel, Switzerland. Rajiv Nayar is a postdoctoral fellow of the Medical Research Council of Canada. We thank Dr. Corazon Bucana for providing the electron micrographs and Mrs. Carol Kakalec and Marfield Dodd-Johnson for editing and typing of this manuscript.

REFERENCES

1. Alderman EM, Fudenberg HH, Lovins RE: Isolation and characterization of an age-related antigen present on senescent human red blood cells. *Blood* 50:341–349, 1981
2. Alexander P, Evans R: Endotoxin and double stranded RNA render macrophages cytotoxic. *Nature* 232:76–78, 1971
3. Allison AC: On the role of mononuclear phagocytes in immunity against viruses. *Prog Med Virol* 18:15–31, 1974
4. Allison AC: Mode of action of immunological adjuvants *J Reticuloendothel Soc* 26:619–630, 1979
5. Alving CR: Delivery of liposome-encapsulated drugs to macrophages. *Pharmacol Ther* 22:407–424, 1983
6. Bucana C, Hoyer LL, Hobbs B, Breesman S, McDaniel M, Hanna MG Jr: Morphological evidence for the translocation of lysosomal organelles from cytotoxic macrophages into the cytoplasm of tumor target cells. *Cancer Res* 36:4444–4458, 1976
7. Bucana CD, Hoyer LC, Schroit AJ, Kleinerman E, Fidler IJ: Ultrastructural studies of the interaction between liposome-activated human blood monocytes and allogeneic tumor cells *in vitro Am J Pathol* 112:101–111, 1983
8. Celede A, Gray PW, Rinderknecht E, Schreiber R: Evidence for a gamma-interferon receptor that regulates macrophage tumoricidal activity. *J Exp Med* 160:55–62, 1984
9. Chapes SK, Tompkins WAF: Cytotoxic macrophages induced in hamsters by vaccinia virus: Selective cytotoxicity for virus-infected targets by macrophages collected late after immunization. *J Immunol* 123:303–309, 1979
10. Chapes SK, Haskill S: Role of *Corynebacterium parvum* in the activation of peritoneal macrophages. I. Association between intracellular *C. parvum* and cytotoxic macrophages. *Cell Immuno* 70:65–75, 1982
11. Chedid L, Audibert F, Johnson AG: Biological activities of muramyl dipeptide, a synthetic glycopeptide analogous to bacterial immunoregulating agents. *Prog Allergy* 26:63–105, 1978
12. Chedid L, Audibert F: Recent developments concerning muramyl dipeptide, a synthetic immunoregulating molecule. *J Reticuloendothel Soc* 26:631–641, 1979
13. Cifone MA, Fidler IJ: Increasing metastatic potential is associated with increasing genetic instability of clones isolated from murine neoplasms. *Proc Natl Acad Sci USA* 78:6949–6952, 1981
14. Cleveland RP, Meltzer MS, Zbar B: Tumor cytotoxicity *in vitro* by macrophages from mice infected with *Mycobacterium bovis* strain BCG. *JNCI* 52:1887–1895, 1974
15. Cohn Z: The activation of mononuclear phagocytes: Fact, fancy, future. *J Immunol* 121:813–861, 1978
16. Deodhar SD, Barna BP, Edinger M, Chiang T: Inhibition of lung metastases by liposomal immunotherapy in a murine fibrosarcoma model. *Biol Response Mod* 1:27–34, 1982
17. Doc WF, Henson PM: Macrophage stimulation by bacterial lipopolysaccharides. *J Exp Med* 148:544–556, 1978
18. Fidler IJ: Recognition and destruction of target cells by tumoricidal macrophages. *Isr J Med Sci* 14:177–191, 1978
19. Fidler IJ: Therapy of spontaneous metastases by intravenous injection of liposomes containing lymphokines. *Science* 208:1469–1471, 1980
20. Fidler IJ: The *in situ* induction of tumoricidal activity in alveolar macrophages by liposomes containing muramyl dipeptide is a thymus-independent process. *J Immunol* 127:1719–1720, 1981
21. Fidler IJ: The MAF dilemma. *Lymphokine Research* 3:51–54, 1984a
22. Fidler IJ: The evolution of biological heterogeneity in metastatic neoplasms. In: GL Nicolson, L Milas (eds.), *Cancer Invasion and Metastasis: Biologic and Therapeutic Aspects*, pp 5–27. New York Raven Press. 1984b
23. Fidler IJ: The generation of tumoricidal activity in macrophages for treatment of established metastases. *Symp Fundam Cancer Res* 36:421–437, 1984c
24. Fidler IJ, Kripke ML: Metastasis results from preexisting variant cells within a malignant tumor. *Science* 197:893, 1977
25. Fidler IJ, Fogler WE: Activation of tumoricidal properties in macrophages by lymphokines encapsulated in liposomes.

Lymphokine Research 1:73–77, 1982

26. Fidler IJ, Hart IR: Biological diversity in metastatic neoplasms: Origins and implications. *Science* 217:998–1003, 1982

27. Fidler IJ, Poste G: Macrophage-mediated destruction of malignant tumor cells and new strategies for the therapy of metastatic disease. *Springer Semin. Immunopathol* 5:161–174, 1982

28. Fidler IJ, Kleinerman ES: Lymphokine-activated human blood monocytes destroy tumor cells but not normal cells under cocultivation conditions. *Journal of Clinical Oncology* 2(8):937–943, 1984

29. Fidler IJ, Schroit AJ: Synergism between lymphokines and muramyl dipeptide encapsulated in liposomes: *In situ* activation of macrophages and therapy of spontaneous cancer metastasis. *J Immunol* 133(1):515–518, 1984

30. Fidler IJ, Roblin RO, Poste G: *In vitro* tumoricidal activity of macrophages against virus-transformed lines with temperature-dependent transformed phenotypic characteristics. *Cell Immunol* 38:131–146, 1978

31. Fidler IJ, Sone S, Fogler WE, Barnes ZL: Eradication of spontaneous metastases and activation of alveolar macrophages by intravenous injection of liposomes containing muramyl dipeptide. *Proc Natl Acad Sci USA* 78:1680–1684, 1981

32. Fidler IJ, Fogler WE, Kleinerman ES, Saiki I: Abrogation of species specificity for activation of tumoricidal properties in macrophages by recombinant mouse or human gamma interferon encapsulated in liposomes. *J Immunol* 136:4289–4296, 1985.

33. Fidler IJ, Raz A, Fogler WE, Hoyer LC, Poste G: The role of plasma membrane receptors and the kinetics of macrophage activation by lymphokines encapsulated in liposomes. *Cancer Res* 41:495–504, 1981

34. Fidler IJ, Raz A, Fogler WE, Kirsh R, Bugelski P, Poste G: The design of liposomes to improve delivery of macrophage-augmenting agents to alveolar macrophages. *Cancer Res* 40:4460–4466, 1980

35. Fidler IJ, Barnes Z, Fogler WE, Kirsh R, Bugelski P, Poste G: Involvement of macrophages in the eradication of established metastases following intravenous injection of liposomes containing macrophage activators. *Cancer Res* 42:496–501, 1982

36. Fidler IJ, Fogler WE, Tarcsay L, Schumann G, Braun DG, Schroit AJ: Systemic activation of macrophages and treatment of cancer metastases by liposomes containing hydrophilic or lipophilic muramyl dipeptide. In: *Advances in Immunopharmacology*, 2:235–253, Oxford Pergamon Press. 1983

37. Fidler IJ, Sone S, Fogler WE, Smith D, Braun DG, Tarcsay L, Gisler RJ, Schroit AJ: Efficacy of liposomes containing a lipophilic muramyl dipeptide derivative for activating the tumoricidal properties of alveolar macrophages *in vivo*. *J Biol Response Mod* 1:43–55,1982

38. Fogler WE, Fidler IJ: Nonselective destruction of murine neoplastic cells by syngeneic tumoricidal macrophages. *Cancer Res* 45:14–18, 1985

39. Fogler WE, Talmadge J, Fidler IJ: The activation of tumoricidal properties in macrophages of endotoxin responder and nonresponder mice by liposome-encapsulated immunomodulators. *J Reticuloendothel Soc* 33:165–174, 1983

40. Fogler WE, Wade R, Brundish DE, Fidler IJ: Distribution and fate of free and liposome-encapsulated [³H]nor-muramyl dipeptide and [³]muramyl tripeptide phosphatidylethanolamine in mice. *J Immunol* 135(2):1372–1377, 1985

41. Gregoriadis G, Allison AC: (eds): *Liposomes in Biological Systems*. Wiley Interscience, New York, 1974

42. Gregoriadis G, Neorungen DE, Hunt R: Fate of liposome-associated agents injected into normal and tumor-bearing rodents. *Life Sci* 21:357–370, 1977

43. Guo LSS, Hamilton RL, Georke J, Weinstein JN, Havel RJ: Interaction of unilamellar liposomes with serum lipoproteins and apolipoproteins. *J Lipid Res* 21:993–1003, 1980

44. Hamilton TA, Fishman M: Characterization of the recognition of target cells sensitive or resistant to cytolysis by activated rat peritoneal macrophages. *J Immunol* 127:1702–1706, 1981

45. Hamilton TA, Fishman M: Characterization of the recognition of target cells sensitve to or resistant to cytolysis by activated macrophages. *Cell Immunol* 68:155–164, 1982

46. Hart IR, Fogler WE, Poste G, Fidler IJ: Toxicity studies of liposome-encapsulated immunomodulators administered intravenouslyl into dogs and mice. *Cancer Immunol Immunother* 10:157–164, 1981

47. Heppner G: Tumor heterogeneity. *Cancer Res* 214:2259–2265, 1984

48. Hibbs JB Jr: Discrimination between neoplastic and non-neoplastic cells *in vitro* by activated macrophages. *JNCI* 53:1487–1492, 1974a

49. Hibbs JB Jr: Heterocytolysis by macrophages activated by Bacillus Calmette-Guerin: Lysosome exocytosis into tumor cells. *Science* 184:468–1474, 1974b

50. Hibbs JB, Lambert LH, Remington JS: Macrophage-mediated nonspecific cytotoxicity: Possible role in tumor resistance. *Nature New Biol* 235:48–50, 1972

51. Hibbs JB, Taintor RR, Chapman HA, Weinberg JB: Macrophage tumor killing: Influence of the local environment. *Science* 197:279–282, 1977

52. Hibbs JB Jr, Weinberg JB, Chapman HA: Modulation of the tumoricidal function of activated macrophages by bacterial endotoxin and mammalian macrophage activation factor. *Adv Exp Med Biol* 121 B:433–53, 1979

53. Hill RP, Chambers AF, Ling V, Harris JF: Dynamic heterogeneity: Rapid generation of metastatic variants in mouse B16 melanoma cells, *Science* 224:998–1001, 1984

54. Juy D, Chedid L: Comparison between macrophage activation and enhancement of nonspecific resistance to tumors by mycobacterial immunoadjuvants. *Proc Natl Acad Sci USA* 72:4105–4109, 1975

55. Karnovsky ML, Lazdins JK: Biochemical criteria for activated macrophages. *J Immunol* 121:809–812, 1978

56. Key MMB: Mechanism and removal of senescent cells by human macrophages *in situ*. *Proc Natl Acad Sci USA* 72:3521–3525, 1975

57. Key MMB: Cells, signals and receptors: The role of physiological autoantibodies in maintaining homeostasis. *Adv Exp Med Biol* 129:171–200, 1980

58. Keller R, Jones VE: Role of activated macrophages and antibody in inhibition and enhancement of tumor growth in rats. *Lancet* 2:847–849, 1971

59. Key ME, Talmadge JE, Fogler WE, Bucana C, Fidler IJ: Isolation of tumoricidal macrophages from lung melanoma metastases of mice treated systematically with liposomes containing a lipophilic derivative of muramyl dipeptide. *JNCI* 69:1189–1198, 1982

60. Kleinerman ES, Fidler IJ: Production and utilization of human lymphokines containing macrophage-activating factor (MAF) activity. *Lymphokine Research* 2:7–12, 1983

61. Kleinerman ES, Schroit AJ, Fogler WE, Fidler IJ: Tumoricidal activity of human monocytes activated *in vitro* by free and liposome-encapsulated human lymphokines. *J Clin Invest* 72:304–315, 1983a

62. Kleinerman ES, Erickson KL, Schroit AJ, Fogler WE, Fidler IJ: Activation of tumoricidal properties in human blood monocytes by liposomes containing lipophilic muramyl tripeptide. *Cancer Res* 43:2010–2014, 1983b

63. Kleinerman ES, Zicht R, Sarin PS, Gallo RC, Fidler IJ: Constitutive production and release of a lymphokine with

macrophage-activating factor activity distinct from gamma-interferon by a human T-cell leukemia virus-positive cell line. *Cancer Res* 44:4470–4475, 1984

64. Kleinschmidt WJ, Schultz RM: Similarities of murine gamma interferon and the lymphokine that renders macrophages cytotoxic. *J Interferon Res* 2:291–299, 1982

65. Knight CA (ed): *Liposomes from physical structure to therapeutic applications.* Elsevier/North Holland, Amsterdam, 1981

66. Koff WC, Fidler IJ: The potential use of liposome-mediated antiviral therapy. *Journal of Antiviral Research* 5(3):179–190, 1985

67. Koff WC, Showalter SD, Hampar B, Fidler IJ: Protection of mice against herpes simplex type 2 infection by liposomes containing muramyl tripeptide. *Science* 228:495–497, 1985

68. Koff WC, Fidler IJ, Showalter SD, Chakrabarty MK, Hampar B, Ceccorulli LM, Kleinerman ES: Human monocytes activated by immunomodulators in liposomes lyse herpes virus infected but not normal cells. *Science* 224:1007–1009, 1984

69. Lopez-Berestein G, Mehta K, Mehta R, Juliano RL, Hersh EM: The activation of human monocytes by liposome-encapsulated muramyl dipeptide analogues. *J Immunol* 130:1500–1504, 1983

70. Lopez-Berestein G, Kasai L, Rosenblum MG, Haynie T, Johns M, Glenn H, Mehta R, Mavligit GM, Hersh EM: Clinical pharmacology of ^{99m}Tc-labeled liposomes in patients with cancer. *Cancer Res* 44:375–378, 1984a

71. Lopez-Berestein G, Milas L, Hunter N, Mehta K, Eppstein D, VanderPas MA, Mathews TR, Hersh EM: Prophylaxis and treatment of experimental lung metastases in mice after treatment with liposome encapsulated 6-O-steroyl-N-acetyl muramyl-L-aminobutyryl-D-isoglutamine. *Clin Exp Metastasis* 2(2):366–367, 1984

72. Mantovani A, Jerrells TR, Dean JH, Herberman R: Cytolytic and cytostatic activity on tumor cells of circulating human monocytes. *Int J Cancer* 23:18–27, 1979

73. Marino PA, Adams DO: Interaction of Bacillus Calmette-Guerin-activated macrophages and neoplastic cells *in vitro*: I. Conditions of binding and its selectivity. *Cell Immunol* 54:11–25, 1980a

74. Marino PA, Adams DO: Interaction of Bacillus Calmette-Guerin-activated macrophages and neoplastic cells *in vitro*: II. The relationship of selective binding to cytolysis. *Cell Immunol* 54:26–35, 1980b

75. Mehta K, Lopez-Berestein G, Hersh EM, Juliano RL: Uptake of liposomes and liposome-encapsulated muramyl dipeptide by human peripheral blood monocytes. *J Reticuloendothel Soc* 32:155–164, 1982

76. Nicolau C, Paraf A (eds.): *Liposomes, drugs and immunocompetent cell functions,* London: Academic Press, 1981

77. North RJ: The concept of the activated macrophages. *J Immunol* 121:806–809, 1978

78. Pace JL, Russell SW: Activation of mouse macrophages for tumor cell killing: I. Quantitative analysis of interactions between lymphokine and lipopolysaccharide. *J Immunol* 126:1863–1867, 1981

79. Parant M, Parant F, Chedid L, Yapo A, Petit JF, Lederer E: Fate of the synthetic immunoadjuvant, muramyl dipeptide (^{14}C-labelled) in the mouse. *Int J Immunopharmacol* 1:35–41, 1979

80. Peu G, Polentarutti N, Sessa C, Mangioni C, Mantovani A: Tumoricidal activity of macrophages isolated from human ascitic and solid ovarian carcinomas: Augmentation by interferon, lymphokines and endotoxin. *Int J Cancer* 128:143–152, 1981

81. Phillips NC, Mora ML, Chedid L, Lefrancier P, Bernard JM: Activation of tumoricidal activity and eradication of experimental metastases by freeze-dried liposomes containing a new lipophilic muramyl dipeptide derivative. *Cancer Res* 45:128–134, 1985

82. Piessens WF, Remold HG, David JR: Increased responsiveness to macrophage-activating factor (MAF) after alteration of macrophage membranes. *J Immunol* 118:2078–2082, 1977

83. Poste G: The tumoricidal properties of inflammatory tissue macrophages and multinucleate giant cells. *Am J Pathol* 96:595–606, 1979

84. Poste G: Liposome targeting *in vivo*: Problems and opportunities. *Biology of the Cell* 47:19–38, 1983

85. Poste G, Fidler IJ: The pathogenesis of cancer metastasis. *Nature* 283:139–146, 1979

86. Poste G, Kirsh R: Rapid decay of tumoricidal activity and loss of responsiveness to lymphokines in inflammatory macrophages. *Cancer Res* 39:2582–2590, 1979

87. Poste G, Kirsh R, Fidler IJ: Cell surface receptors for lymphokines. *Cell Immunol* 44:71–88, 1979a

88. Poste G, Kirsh R, Fogler W, Fidler IJ: Activation of tumoricidal properties in mouse macrophages by lymphokines encapsulated in liposomes. *Cancer Res* 39:881–892, 1979b

89. Poste G, Bucana C, Raz A, Bugelski P, Kirsh R, Fidler IJ: Analysis of the fate of systematically administered liposomes and implications for their use in drug delivery. *Cancer Res* 42:1412–1422, 1982

90. Raz A, Bucana C, Fogler WE, Poste G, Fidler IJ: Biochemical, morphological and ultrastructural studies on the uptake of liposomes by murine macrophages. *Cancer Res* 41:487–494, 1981

91. Ruco LP, Meltzer MS: Macrophage activation for tumor cytotoxicity: Development of macrophage cytotoxic activity requires completion of a sequence of short-lived intermediary reactions. *J Immunol* 121:2035–2042, 1978a

92. Ruco LP, Meltzer MS: Macrophage activation for tumor cytotoxicity: Tumoricidal activity by macrophages from C3H/HeJ mice requires at least two activation stimuli. *Cell Immunol* 41:35–46, 1978b

93. Saiki I, Fidler IJ: Synergistic activation by recombinant mouse gamma-interferon and muramyl dipeptide of tumoricidal properties in mouse macrophages. *J Immunol* 135:684–688, 1985

94. Saiki I, Sone S, Fogler WE, Kleinerman ES, Lopez-Berestein G, Fidler IJ: Synergism between human recombinant gamma interferon and muramyl dipeptide encapsulated in liposomes for activation of antitumor properties in human blood monocytes. *Cancer Res* 45(12):6188–6193, 1985

95. Scherphof G, Roerdink F, Dijkstre J, Ellens H, Dezander R, Wisse E: Uptake of liposomes by rat and mouse hepatocytes and Kupffer cells. *Biol Cell* 47:47–85, 1983

96. Schroit AJ, Fidler IJ: Effects of liposome structure and lipid composition on the activation of the tumoricidal properties of macrophages by liposomes containing muramyl dipeptide. *Cancer Res* 42:161–167, 1982

97. Schroit AJ, Fidler IJ: The use of activated macrophages for the destruction of heterogeneous metastases. In: Honn KV (ed). *Mechanisms of metastases.* Martinus Nijhoff Publishers, Amsterdam, 1985

98. Schroit AJ, Galligioni E, Fidler IJ: Factors influencing the *in situ* activation of macrophages by liposomes containing muramyl dipeptide. *Biology of the Cell* 47:87–94, 1983a

99. Schroit AJ, Hart IR, Madsen J, Fidler IJ: Selective delivery of drugs encapsulated in liposomes: Natural targeting to macrophages involved in various disease states. *J Biol Response Mod* 2:97–100, 1983b

100. Schultz RM: Synergistic activation of macrophages by lymphokine and lipopolysaccharide: Evidence for lymphokine as the primer and interferon as the trigger. *J Interferon Res* 2:459–466, 1982

101. Shulkin PM, Seltzer SS, Davis MA, Adams DF: Lyophilized liposomes: A new method for long term vesicular

storage. *J Microencapsulation* 1:73–80, 1985

102. Sone S, Fidler IJ: Synergistic activation by lymphokines and muramyl dipeptide of tumoricidal properties in rat alveolar macrophages. *J Immunol* 125:2454–2460, 1980

103. Sone S, Fidler IJ: *In vitro* activation of tumoricidal properties in rat alveolar macrophages by synthetic muramyl dipeptide encapsulated in liposomes. *Cell Immunol* 57:42–50, 1981

104. Sone S, Tsubura E: Human alveolar macrophages: Potentiation of their tumoricidal activity by liposome-encapsulated muramyl dipeptide. *J Immunol* 129:1313–1317, 1982

105. Sone S, Poste G, Filder IJ: Rat alveolar macrophages are susceptible to free and liposome-encapsulated lymphokines. *J Immunol* 124:2197, 1980

106. Sone S, Matsuura S, Ogawara M, Tsubura E: Potentiating effect of muramyl dipeptide and its lipophilic analog encapsulated in liposomes on tumor cell killing by human monocytes. *J Immunol* 132:2105–2110, 1984

107. Straubinger RM, Duzgunes N, Papahadjopoulos D: pH-Sensitive liposomes mediate cytoplasmic delivery of encapsulated macromolecules. *FEBS Lett* 179:148–154, 1985

108. Sullivan SM, Huang L: Preparation and characterization of heat-sensitive immunoliposomes. *Biochim Biophys Acta* 812:116–126, 1985

109. Szoka FC, Papahadjopoulos D: Comparative properties and methods of preparation of lipid vesicles (Liposomes). *Annu Rev Biophys Bioeng* 9:467–508, 1980

110. Talmadge JE, Wolman SR, Fidler IJ: Evidence for the clonal origin of spontaneous metastases. *Science* 217:361–363, 1982

111. Taniyama T, Holden HT: Direct augmentation of cytolytic activity of tumor-derived macrophages and macrophage cell lines by muramyl dipeptide. *Cell Immunol* 48:369–374, 1979

112. Van Furth R: *Mononuclear phagocytes in immunity, infection, and pathology.* Blackwell Scientific Publications, Oxford, 1975

113. Vlassara H, Brownlee M, Cerani A: High-Affinity-receptor-mediated uptake and degradation of glucose-modified proteins: A potential mechanism for the removal of senescent macromolecules. *Proc Natl Acad Sci USA* 82:5588–5592, 1985

114. Vlassara H, Brownlee M, Cerani A: Accumulation of diabetic rat peripheral nerve myelin by macrophages increases with the presence of advanced glycosylation end products. *J Exp Med* 160:197–207, 1984

METASTASES FROM METASTASIS: CLINICAL RELEVANCE IN HUMAN CANCER

JOHN D. CRISSMAN

INTRODUCTION

Successful management and cure of cancer is to a large degree achieved by control of the primary tumor. Effective treatments are directed towards localized therapies such as surgery and radiation. By definition, these therapies ablate or destroy tumors that are confined to an anatomical distribution amenable to surgical resection or to an achievable field of radiation. These cancer therapies represent the standard of cancer care and have been used effectively for nearly a century. When surgery and radiation were introduced to treat malignant disease, cures were reported in an appreciable number of cases for the first time. The development of techniques successful in cancer cure resulted in major efforts to refine surgical procedures and produce sophisticated radiation therapy equipment. Concurrent with the evolution of improved therapies to treat and cure malignant disease was an improved understanding of the biology of cancer. More specifically, the effects of surgery and radiation on malignant tumors were addressed along with the relationship of treatment modalities to improved patient survival.

The evolution of sophisticated surgical techniques, improvement in patient preparation, anesthesia, and postoperative support have resulted in the capability for more extensive and radical cancer operations with little increase in mortality. It has been hypothesized that if cures result from excision of the primary tumor, and in some patients resection of regional lymph nodes, then more extensive resections would presumably remove additional malignant disease, enhancing the patients' chances of survival. Likewise, improvements in radiation therapy resulted in more aggressive therapy with higher doses of radiation to larger treatment fields. The development and subsequent application of radical therapies encompassing greater amounts of tissue resulted in greater morbidity and some, but not major improvements in patient survival (14). However, the ability to successfully eradicate the primary neoplasm and, in many instances, local or regional spread of tumor improved dramatically. Most likely, it was the improved local and regional control of malignant neoplasms that accounted for the observed increase in survival. The prevailing concept of the spread of malignant neoplasms was that a progression of metastases occurred. First, the primary tumor metastasized to regional lymph nodes draining the tumor; secondly, additional metastases spread to lymph nodes along the lymphatic circulation with the eventual development of systemic metastases. This prevailing theory of cancer spread was championed by Halsted and formed the basis for cancer therapy for many generations. Unfortunately, the removal of increasing volumes of normal tissue, or radiating larger fields, did not translate to significant improvement in survival. Clinical cancer specialists ultimately became aware that the development of micrometastases prior to the clinical diagnosis and initiation of therapy had become the single most important reason for treatment failure. Improvements in surgical procedures and the expansion of radiation fields resulted in acceptable local tumor control, and patients without pre-existing metastases were cured of their disease. However, the improvements in locally directed therapies had little impact on the distant metastases. The initial concept that cancer metastasized in a stepwise fashion was questioned, along with the concept that improved treatment required more radical procedures "chasing" the spread of the malignant neoplasm. The recognition of the significance of metastases in treatment failures led to a reversal of the trend to excise large amounts of normal tissue as well as to expose the primary tumor to ionizing radiation. The extensive experience in adequately controlling primary (and regional) disease has been well defined. Current treatments minimize the removal and injury to adjacent normal noncancerous tissues. The maintenance of local cancer control is being actively investigated.

Recent advances in our understanding of the biology of tumor invasion and metastasis has also led to major shifts in the philosophy of cancer treatment. Clinicians now realize that approximately 50% of patients diagnosed with cancer will have distant metastases at the time of diagnosis (14). Obviously, these microscopic sites of tumor spread are not clinically detectable. This readily explains why radical therapies directed at the primary tumor do not improve survival for this subgroup of patients. The factors responsible for early metastasis in some cancers, while others fail to metastasize after reaching large proportions, is poorly understood. Malignant neoplasms represent a wide diversity of cell types. There exists considerable heterogeneity in phenotypic expression for factors contributing to invasion of host stroma, penetration of blood and lymph vessels and establishment of regional lymph node and/or distant metastases. Some malignancies have the inherent capacity to invade and metastasize early in their evolution. Other neoplasms only develop these capabilities after a considerable growth interval. Some invasive tumors, such as basal cell carcinoma, rarely develop the mechanisms required for blood or lymph vessel invasion and successful metastases.

The efficiency of local therapy is well established and both surgery and radiation are effective modalities for the control

R. H. Goldfarb (ed.), Fundamental aspects of cancer.
© 1989, Kluwer Academic Publishers, Dordrecht. ISBN 978-94-010-6980-9

of both local tumors and regional lymph node metastases. Undoubtedly, the current challenge is the effective treatment of that large percentage of cancer patients who have developed metastases prior to diagnosis and who cannot be cured by local therapies. In the past two decades, toxic chemotherapy has been the foremost systemic therapy available, and it has been used after distant metastases have proliferated sufficiently for clinical recognition. Improvements in chemotherapy regimens have increased its use in patients with a high likelihood of having distant metastases, referred to as adjuvant therapy. Impressive success with chemotherapy in the treatment of childhood tumors and acute leukemias has been achieved. In the adult population, germ cell tumors of the testes and Hodgkin's disease are likewise curable by systemic chemotherapy even after metastases have developed. Unfortunately, the majority of adult solid tumors arise from epithelial structures and these carcinomas remain relatively resistant to currently available cytotoxic drugs.

After successful ablation of the primary tumor, and in some instances regional metastases, the patient will either survive, or if previously undetected metastases have occurred, the patient will eventually die of disseminated cancer (1). With time, more and more metastases will become clinically evident. This increasing tumor burden will eventually reach lethal proportions, resulting in the patient's death. The major question that this chapter addresses is the source of these multiple tumor metastases. Are they primarily a result of numerous micrometastases originating from the primary tumor, exhibiting varying growth rates or the ability to remain viable but dormant for protracted periods? Or in the alternative, are the initial and presumably limited numbers of metastases capable of continued proliferation, ultimately developing the same biologic characteristics of their parent tumors, such as the capacity to invade normal tissue, infiltrate blood and lymph vessels, and develop second generation metastatic deposits, metastases from metastases (Figure 1)? The latter has not been a popular explanation for the progression of cancer to the development of a lethal body burden. The rationale for resisting this latter concept is not clear. It may be due to the prevalent tradition of emphasizing locally directed therapies. Understandably, the success achieved with local therapies has led to a myopic focus on treatment of the primary tumor with a concurrent de-emphasization of the role or importance of metastases, at least, in part out of frustration at the lack of therapy effectiveness for those patients with disseminated tumor deposits. As previously mentioned, the explanation that all or most of the foci of the disseminated tumor arise from the primary tumor is unlikely. The amount and distribution of cancer in patients with lethal tumor burdens is so extensive that it is difficult to believe that widespread metastasis does not result from a sequence of metastasizing metastases, or a metastatic cascade. The presence of widespread metastases, all originating from the primary tumor, is not consistent with the results of autopsies on cancer patients (5). In many instances, only rare microscopic metastases are found in patients previously diagnosed with cancer who die of unrelated diseases. Some of these patients are free of metastases and would presumably be cured of their cancers. Other patients have rare and focal deposits of metastases. These metastases would unquestionably progress to wide-

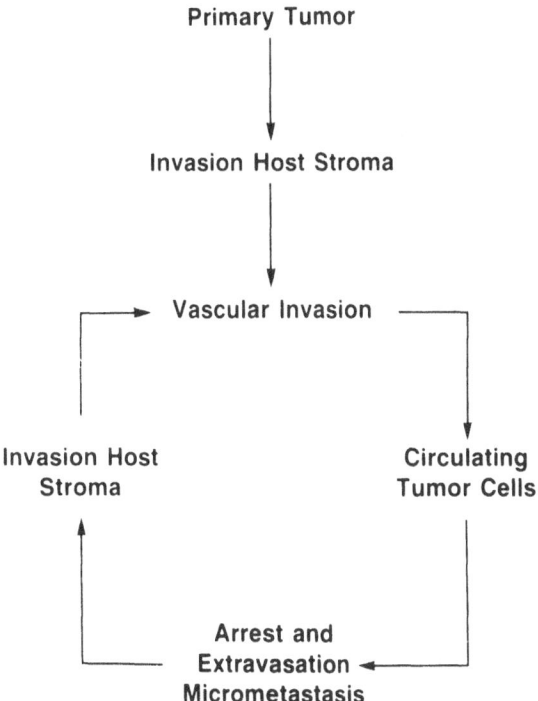

Figure 1. Scheme of the metastatic cascade. Once extravasation and establishment of metastasis occurs, the same sequence is observed in the primary tumor as initiated. This leads to the continuation of the metastatic cascade with "metastases from metastases".

spread disease and eventual death from lethal body burdens of tumor. These observations strongly suggest that a cascade of metastases from metastases is instrumental in the evolution of lethal body burdens of tumor. Admittedly, this does not prove the importance of the role of metastases from metastases in tumor progression, but suggests that a metastatic cascade does exist and is an important contributor to the development of lethal amounts of tumor in patients dying of cancer.

AUTOPSY STUDIES

Evaluation of the distribution of metastases in a large series of autopsies performed at the Roswell Park Memorial Institute has provided provocative data regarding the mechanisms of tumor dissemination. Several studies have been reported and invariably reach similar conclusions (16–18). These autopsy studies evaluate the distribution pattern of metastases in a series of specific types of cancer occurring in different sites. The basic question that these studies address is, are there specific "generalizing sites" of metastases invariably present when metastases are found at a more distant and less common site of metastasis? For example, does carcinoma of the breast always metastasize to the lung when metastases are found in the central nervous system? This does appear to be the situation as evaluated in 647 autopsies of patients dying of disseminated breast carcinoma (16). Similar conclusions were reached in several additional similar studies of the patterns of metastatic spread of tumors of the kidney and prostate (17) and the digestive tract (18). This data was interpreted as secondary or a cascade of metastases occurring from key "generalizing sites" which are invariably present before the secondary metastasis can develop. These statistical analyses of autopsies were interpreted to mean that metastases from metastases was a prominent factor in tumor dissemination in cancer progression. However, in a re-evaluation of these studies, the statistical analyses were severely criticized by statisticians from the same institution (2), clouding the value of the interpretation of these autopsy studies.

The data presented by Weiss (21) comparing the patterns of metastases for squamous cell carcinomas of the upper and lower esophagus and adenocarcinomas of the upper and lower rectum represents one of the best human models for unravelling the sequence in which human carcinomas metastasize. The neoplasms from the upper rectum and lower esophagus have a venous drainage to the portal vein through the liver and into the hepatic venous circulation. The neoplasms from the lower rectum and upper esophagus have venous drainage into the vena caval system and directly to the lungs, bypassing the portal venous system. For neoplasms of the upper rectum and lower esophagus, lung metastases were seldom observed in the absence of liver metastases. This is similar to the observations originally reported by Willis (23) and is interpreted to mean that the liver metastases represent a "generalizing site" which is the source for the secondary tumors subsequently developing in the lung (metastases from metastases). Admittedly, autopsy studies represent only one observation in a dynamic sequence of events, usually in advanced disease. However, the data is suggestive that a sequential series of metastases occur and represents one of the early arguments supporting the presence of a metastatic cascade leading to lethal body burdens in human cancer.

EXPERIMENTAL ANIMAL MODELS FOR METASTASES FROM METASTASES

The release of tumor cells into the circulation by pulmonary metastases was the first step in proving that metastases retained the capacity to form metastases (10). Three animal tumors were studied by inducing lung metastases from "primary" tumors produced by injection of tumor cells into thigh muscles of the hind leg. Once pulmonary metastases were expected to have developed, the legs were amputated effectively ablating the primary tumor. The lung metastases which were invariably present were allowed to grow (4–6 weeks depending on the tumor line) and blood was removed from the left ventricle of the mice. The blood was immediately injected via the tail vein into syngeneic mice. Pulmonary tumors developed in a majority of the injected mice, confirming the presence of tumor cells in cardiac blood draining the pulmonary metastases. The observations from these early experiments were the first of a series of observations documenting the capability of metastases to invade host tissue and release tumor cells into the circulation.

An effort to produce metastases from metastasis was attempted using a model incorporating organ fragment implantation in syngeneic animals (15). The hypothesis tested was that the tumor cells released in the blood draining the pulmonary metastases were capable of forming metastases in the tissue implants placed after removal of the "primary"

tumors. The primary tumors were produced by injection of tumor cells into the hind leg of the animal. Fragments of kidney, lung and spleen from newborn mice were implanted in two groups of adult mice. The first group received implants 48 hours after intramuscular injection of tumor cells to produce the "primary" tumor and the second group received implants 48 hours after amputation of the hind legs when the tumors that were of sufficient size to insure the presence of pulmonary metastases. Metastases to the implanted newborn organ tissues were found only in animals with intact "primary" intramuscular tumors. The mice implanted with organ fragments after amputation of the "primary" tumor failed to produce metastases to the implanted tissues from the pre-existing pulmonary metastases. This important study failed to confirm that tumor cells released into the circulation from pulmonary metastases were capable of developing secondary metastases in the implanted tissues.

The use of parabiotic animals allowed the demonstration of metastases from metastases for the first time in an animal model (9). Pulmonary metastases were established from foot pad injected "primary" tumors with subsequent amputation once the leg tumors had reached appropriate size, insuring the presence of lung metastases. The animals with lung metastases were then joined in a parabiotic fashion to non-tumor bearing syngeneic "guest" mice. Many of the guest or recipient animals subsequently developed lung metastases. This clearly documented the capacity of the pulmonary metastases in the donor animals to release tumor cells into the circulation and to develop secondary metastases. The use of the parabiotic animal clearly demonstrated that the circulating tumor cells were capable of successful arrest and extravasation and the development of metastases from metastases.

Our interest in the tumor dissemination and the metastatic cascade led to the development of an animal model of metastases from metastases which did not require the use of parabiotic joining of animals. Our ultimate objective was to develop an intact model to evaluate methods to interrupt the metastatic cascade (3). It was our hypothesis that the reason (15) did not find metastases from metastasis after transplantation of newborn organ tissue to animals with lung metastases was that the implanted organs were not exposed to the circulating tumor cells released from pulmonary metastases for a sufficient period for the development of secondary metastases.

We elected to use the B16 amelanotic melanoma tumor because of its rapid proliferation, ease of transplantation and its characteristic predilection to metastasize to lung tissue. Pulmonary metastases were induced both by tail vein injection of tumor cells and by the development of foot pad tumors. In both groups, the expected number of pulmonary metastases was purposely minimized. This was done by titrating the minimum number of tumor cells injected via the tail vein that would still produce lung colonies in most of the animals. Amputation of the foot pad was performed as early as possible to produce a minimal number of lung metastases in this model (4). The minimization of the number of lung tumors allowed longer animal survival, which, in turn, lengthened the period of observation for the development of metastases from the pulmonary tumors to the implanted fetal organ tissues. The fetal organ tissues were implanted

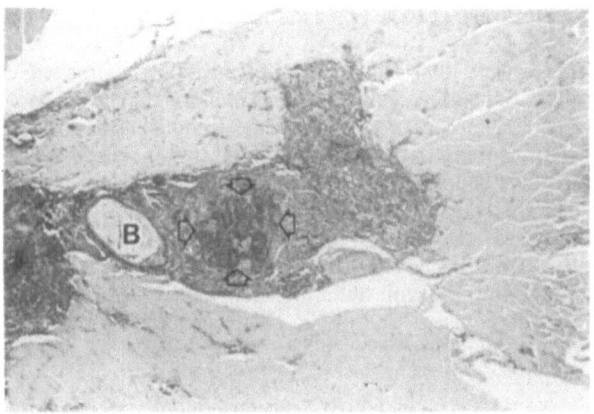

Figure 2. Low magnification microphotograph of the implanted fetal lung. The lung contains a dilated bronchial structure (B) and atelectatic lung tissue. Skeletal muscle surrounds the implanted lung tissue. In the center is a focus of metastatic B16a melanoma outlined by arrows.

3–5 days post I.V. injection or leg amputation and the animals survived an average of 42–45 days. Sacrifice and histologic evaluation of the thoracic lung and fetal transplanted tissue was carried out on day 35 post-implantation of fetal tissues to insure consistent evaluation of all animals prior to animal death from lethal lung burdens of tumor (Figures 2, 3). The B16 amelanotic melanoma metastasizes primary to lung tissue, and animals die of extensive pulmonary tumor resulting in respiratory insufficiency. This model has uniformly resulted in a high frequency of documented metastases from metastases. Both the I.V. injection of tumor cells and the production of foot pad tumors have developed metastatic tumors in approximately 75% of the animals (4). It is of interest that invariably the metastases from metastases occurred in implanted fetal lung tissue and only rarely in ovary or testes. It was not observed in any of the other

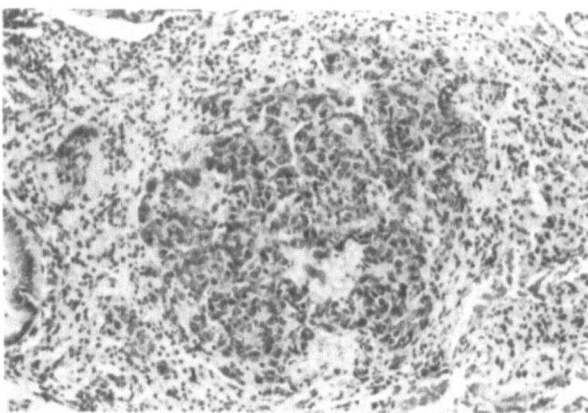

Figure 3. This high magnification of Figure 2 demonstrates the details of the metastatic B16a melanoma from the thoracic lung metastasis. The surrounding lung tissue does not contain air as the fetal animal never established respiration. The metastatic tumor is obvious from the increased cell size and nuclear pleomorphism.

control tissues, confirming the specificity of B16a melanotic melanoma for the development of lung metastases.

A study of two tumor systems using high and low metastatic variants revealed non-linear development of lung tumor metastases, suggesting metastases of metastases in the lungs of intact animals (12). This study resulted from previous observations that the absolute number of tumor lung colonies developing in the tumor lines tested varied depending on when the experiment was terminated. The numbers of lung colonies found immediately after tail vein injection was small but rapidly increased with longer intervals prior to evaluation of the pulmonary tumor colonies. This observation suggested that the increased numbers of lung tumors present in long-term experiments might represent secondary metastases. Both of the highly metastatic tumor lines tested resulted in a marked increase of lung colonies after an initial period of 16–17 days. Animals evaluated 10 and 14 days post intravenous injection of highly metastatic tumor cells produced 20–40 lung surface tumor colonies. Animals evaluated 18 and 22 days after tumor cell injection had greater than 200 lung surface colonies present. This data was interpreted that the highly metastatic cell line variants produce a second wave of metastases (from the initial lung colonies) after 15–17 days. This observation did not apply to the low metastatic cell line variants which developed fewer lung colonies after tumor cell injection, and further, did not result in the marked increase in lung tumors during the period of the experiment. These experiments support the concept of metastases from metastases, in this case within a single organ. In view of the specificity of selected tumors for certain organs, these observations may have important clinical significance. The observation of intraorgan metastases is one explanation for the success of our attempts to develop a model for metastases from metastases while the earlier attempts by Sugarbaker and colleagues (15) were not. The minimization of the number of lung tumors in both the tail vein and foot pad models resulted in longer survival periods as compared to survival periods when large numbers of lung tumors were produced in the first group of metastases. The longer the animal survives, the greater is the opportunity for the pulmonary tumor colonies to proliferate and to release increasing numbers of tumor cells into the circulation. When large numbers of pulmonary tumors are present initially, the development of the wave of secondary metastases results in massive pulmonary tumor and respiratory death before metastases can be observed in the implanted fetal lung tissue. We also found that the implanted fetal lung required between two and three weeks to re-establish sufficient blood flow for circulating tumor cells to implant. In addition, 7 to 10 days for proliferation of the metastases in the implanted fetal lung is needed for the tumors to reach sufficient size so as to be easily identified on histologic sections.

A complex model demonstrating metastases from lung tumor colonies has recently been described (13). Lung tumor colonies were produced by tail vein injection of KHT sarcoma cells and the lungs were radiated at various times to sterilize the lung colonies. Secondary metastases to the ovaries and kidneys were found only if the irradiation was carried out four or more days after tumor cell injection. Radiation to the lung prior to four days not only sterilized the lung tumors, but the animals failed to develop tumors in either the kidneys or ovaries. These animals were followed up to 120 days. Animals receiving thoracic irradiation after the four-day-period developed increasing frequencies of metastases in the kidneys and ovaries, with 100% of the animals developing metastases after a 16 day interval before lung irradiation. This model also supports the notion that metastases retain their ability to contribute to the formation of additional metastases. While this model introduces the variable of radiation, it appears to represent a simple and reproducible model of metastases from metastases in an intact animal.

CLINICAL IMPLICATIONS

The ability of metastases to invade host tissue, release tumor cells into the circulation, and produce secondary or metastases from metastases is well established in animal models. Unfortunately, the majority of observations regarding mechanisms of the kinetics of tumor dissemination in humans relies heavily on autopsy data. The extensive data from the Roswell Park Memorial Institute autopsy studies supports but does not prove the thesis that a metastatic cascade exists and is important in human cancer. Conversely, the evidence that metastatic tumors do not retain their capacity to contribute to the metastatic cascade is weak or non-existent. There is little or no evidence to suggest that once a tumor metastasizes the tumor looses its ability to continue to invade and metastasize.

Tumor cell dormancy has been hypothesized as an alternative explanation to the metastatic cascade (22). Growth restraint or tumor cell dormancy is dependent on a number of factors including: 1) inherent properties of the tumor cells and the presence (or absence) of growth related factors, 2) failure of development of vascular beds required to support tumor growth, and 3) immunologic, primarily cell-mediated, factors interfering with tumor cell proliferation. The possibility that multiple foci of metastatic tumor can originate from the primary cancer cannot be proved or disproved at this time. The possibility that varying growth rates (or degrees of dormancy) of micrometastases account for the numerous metastases usually associated with lethal tumor burdens in human cancer cannot be discounted. However, the animal models used to demonstrate tumor dormancy are highly artificial and not analogous to the clinical situation.

The examples of human cancer most commonly cited as possible situations wherein tumor dormancy accounts for clinical observations are breast carcinomas and melanomas (22). The observation of late "recurrences" of tumor, often after the arbitrary five year hiatus, are most commonly cited as examples of tumor cell dormancy. However, it is well known that both of these two neoplasms have a wide range of growth rates in which slow growing tumors may not reach sufficient size for clinical recognition for many years, often greater than the traditional five-year-interval for evaluating survival (8). Breast carcinomas are notorious for their great variability in growth rates and the clinical observations cited as potential examples of tumor cell dormancy are better explained by the great variation in the measured growth rates of these two unpredictable human tumors.

TUMOR HETEROGENEITY

The concept that malignant neoplasms are comprised of cells with heterogenous features is well documented. One of the first demonstrations of the heterogenous nature of malignant neoplasia was the variability of tumor cells to metastasize (7). Tumor heterogeneity is a complex subject, and accordingly, I will confine my comments to the variation of metastases of cell lines within a tumor. This classic experiment demonstrated that cell lines could be isolated from animal tumors with differing frequencies of metastases formation. These and other similar experiments altered many of the entrenched tenets of tumor biology. It was concluded that cell lines possessing different biologic behavior could be isolated from heterologous cell mixtures present in the primary tumors. It was thought that through selection pressures, cell lines with greater resistance to chemotherapy, higher propensity for metastasizing, etc., could evolve from the apparently heterologous cell populations constituting most tumors. The concept of dynamic tumor properties introduced an era of great pessimism in cancer therapy (6). It was feared that the presence of a successful metastasis implied the emergence of a cell line with increased capacity to metastasize. It was argued that those cells which had developed the capability to form metastases would continue to express this new found talent and rapidly disseminate throughout the host. These observations create strong arguments favoring the role of metastases from metastases in the progression of human cancer. Other than the demonstration of metastases from metastases in the animal models cited, this additional characteristic strongly suggests that the development of a successful metastasis leads to a continuation of the process, the metastatic cascade.

However, these observations have not been universal for all animal tumor lines studied (20). In a series of four animal tumors, it was found that B16 melanoma and KHT osteosarcoma metastases gave rise to increased numbers of metastases when transplanted to syngeneic animals. In contrast, the opposite was observed for Lewis lung carcinoma and T241 carcinomas, the original primary tumor had a higher rate of metastases than cells from the metastases when transplanted to subsequent animals. This observation is in keeping with the great variability encountered in human cancer. Not only is there considerable variation in the growth rates or doubling times of human neoplasms, but considerable variation exists in their capacity to metastasize. For the most part, human cancers that metastasize are most likely to continue to do so in keeping with Fidler's observations. However, this is not universal and great variability is observed between growth rates and presumably the propensity to metastasize amongst human cancers, as well as within the multiple metastases observed in an individual patient.

RESECTION OF TUMOR METASTASIS

Admittedly, the salvage or cure of patients with single or limited numbers of metastases is low. However, several small series of patients have been studied in which one or more lung metastases have been surgically resected (11, 19). Once the primary tumor is adequately controlled and a single or limited number of lung metastases are evident without evidence of other metastases, the patient is a candidate for surgical resection of the metastases. Without question, patients fulfilling these criteria are few, but the survival rates for these selected patients are encouraging. In general, several important lessons can be learned from these studies. The type of primary tumor is important, with better survivals found in those patients exhibiting tumors tending to metastasize primarily to lung, such as sarcomas or neoplasms that are relatively slow growing, for example, renal cell carcinomas. In general, the slow growing metastases are more amenable to resection. Those patients with the longest interval to the appearance of the metastases exhibit the best survivals post-resection (19). The ability to successfully remove one or more metastases and still achieve a cure is an important observation. Unfortunately, in the overwhelming majority of patients developing tumor metastases, cure is not possible, and these patients invariably die of disseminated metastases. The overwhelming evidence suggests that much of the eventual tumor burden results from metastases arising from metastatic tumor deposits. Once a metastasis has developed, there is considerable evidence to suggest that not only is the metastasis capable of metastasizing but that it may have an increased capacity to do so. However, this latter observation is not absolute as demonstrated by the successful resection of metastases in occasional patients.

SUMMARY

The animal model data clearly defines the existence and to some degree, the importance of metastases from metastasis. There is little question that a metastatic cascade exists although its relative contribution in achieving lethal body burdens of tumor is not clearly documented. The data regarding metastases from metastasis in human cancer is less well understood for obvious reasons. The arguments about the mechanisms of tumor dissemination, the role of dormancy, and variable growth rates of micrometastases remain unsettled. In spite of the increasing body of knowledge demonstrating that many metastatic animal tumors are even more prone to metastasize, the concept of metastases from metastasis remains unpopular with clinical oncologists. Alternatives are commonly argued, but evidence suggesting that metastatic cancers are not capable of continuing the sequence of invasion and metastasis has yet to be proven.

The best positive data suggesting that human cancers disseminate in a stepwise fashion is from the autopsy studies documenting "generalizing sites". Admittedly, this is circumstantial evidence but we are limited in our ability to make controlled observations, and the clinical cancer patient is not a good model for studying tumor progression. The occasional argument that metastases from metastasis is not of great importance and that all metastases arise from the primary tumor and exhibit varying degrees of "dormancy" cites evidence propounded upon questionable animal models. While tumor dormancy or, more likely, heterogenous growth rates may play a role in the clinical recognition of disseminated tumors, the more obvious explanation for tumor progression is metastases arising from existing metastases. Our current knowledge of tumor biology and the conclusive data from animal models unequivoc-

ally supports a major role for metastases from metastasis in the dissemination of human cancer.

REFERENCES

1. Cairns J: The treatment of diseases and the war against cancer. *Scientific American* 253:51–59, 1985
2. Colombano SP, Reese PA: The cascade theory of metastatic spread: Are there generalizing sites? *Cancer* 46:2312–2314, 1980
3. Crissman JD: Is there clinical relevance for therapies which disrupt the metastatic cascade? In: *Hemostatic Mechanisms and Metastasis*, KV Honn and BF Sloane, eds., Martinus Nijhoff, Boston, pp. 1–14, 1984
4. Crissman JD, Honn KV, Sloane BF: Metastasis from metastases: An animal model. In: *Treatment of Metastasis*: Problems and Prospects, K Hellmann and SA Eccles, eds., Taylor and Francis, London, pp. 211–214, 1985
5. Fallon RH, Roper CL: Operative treatment of metastatic pulmonary cancer. *Ann Surg* 166:263–265, 1967
6. Fidler IJ: Tumor heterogeneity and the biology of cancer invasion and metastasis. *Cancer Res* 38:2651–2660, 1978
7. Fidler IJ, Kripke ML: Metastasis results from pre-existing variant cells within a malignant tumor. *Science* 197:893–895
8. Gullino PM: Natural histories of breast cancer progression from hyperplasia to neoplasia as predicted by angiogenesis. *Cancer* 39:2697–2703, 1977
9. Hoover HC, Ketcham AS: Metastasis of metastases. *Am J Surg* 130:405–411, 1975
10. Ketcham AS, Ryan JJ, Wexler H: The shedding of viable circulating tumor cells by pulmonary metastases in mice. *Ann Surg* 169:297–299, 1969
11. Ramming KP, Holmes EC, Skinner DG, Morton DL: Surgery for pulmonary metastases: The UCLA approach. Chapter 20, pp. 252–259, 1978
12. Raz A: The demonstration of non-linear development of experimental lung tumor metastases. *Clin Exp Metastasis* 2:5–13, 1984
13. Siemann DW, Mulcahy RT: Characterization of growth and radiation response of KHT tumor cells metastatic from lung to ovary and kidney. *Clin Exp Metastasis* 2:73–81, 1984
14. Sugarbaker EV: Cancer metastasis: A product of tumor-host interactions. *Current Problems in Cancer* 3:1–59, 1979
15. Sugarbaker EV, Cohen AM, Ketcham AS: Do metastases metastasize? *Ann Surg* 174:161–166, 1971
16. Viadana E, Bross IDJ, Pickren JW: An autopsy study of some routes of dissemination of cancer of the breast. *Br J Cancer* 27:336–340, 1973
17. Viadana E, Bross IDJ, Pickren JW: The metastatic spread of kidney and prostate cancers in man. *Neoplasm* 23:323–332, 1976
18. Viadana E, Bross IDJ, Pickren JW: The metastatic spread of cancers of the digestive system in man. *Oncology* 35:114–126, 1978
19. Vincent RG, Choksi LB, Takita H, Gutierrez AC: Surgical resection of the solitary pulmonary metastasis. In: *Pulmonary Metastasis*, L. Weiss and H. Gilbert, eds., G.K. Hall and Co., Boston, Chapter 18, pp. 232–242, 1978
20. Weiss L, Holmes JC, Ward PM: Do metastases arise from pre-existing subpopulations of cancer cells? *Br J Cancer* 47:81–89, 1983
21. Weiss L, Voit A, Lane WW: Metastatic patterns in patients with carcinomas of the lower esophagus and upper rectum. *Invas Metastasis* 4:47–60, 1984
22. Wheelock EF, Robinson MK: Biology of disease. Endogenous control of the neoplastic process. *Lab Invest* 48:120–138, 1983
23. Willis RA: *The spread of tumors in the human body*. Churchill, London, pp. 167–183, 1934

16

TREATMENT RESEARCH IN CANCER

GREGORY A. CURT and BRUCE A. CHABNER

INTRODUCTION

The steady progress being made in cancer treatment has a growing impact on a growing number of different kinds of cancer and on national cancer survival statistics. This is reflected in a substantial increase in five-year survival for *all* Americans diagnosed with cancer since the passage of the National Cancer Act in 1971 (34). One of every two Americans diagnosed with cancer this year will be cured, and yet the challenge for cancer prevention, diagnosis, and treatment remains enormous.

An estimated one-third of Americans born this year will eventually develop a serious cancer. Cancer remains the second leading cause of death in the United States and claimed an estimated 482,000 lives in 1986. The urgent priority or improved cancer diagnosis, prevention, and treatment is obvious.

However, medical research has already made significant inroads in a number of different kinds of cancer. For example, as shown in Table 1, advances in the treatment of cancer with drugs (chemotherapy) has led to significant long-term disease-free survival for patients with specific cancers (5). In addition, the demonstration that drugs given to cancer patients at high risk for relapse (so-called "adjuvant chemotherapy") can improve survival stands out as one of the major achievements of the decade. Already these studies, performed throughout the United States by the Clinical Cooperative Groups of the NCI, have shown significant improvement in survival for patients with breast cancer (16, 17, 32), and ongoing studies are showing positive trends in cancers that were previously thought to be very poorly responsive to drugs, such as colon cancer, rectal cancer, and adenocarcinoma of the lung. If adjuvant chemotherapy in these tumors were to be applied to patients nationwide, many thousands of lives could be saved each year, as shown in Table 2.

A major task, however, is to move effective therapy from the setting of the clinical trial to its routine application in medical practice. Review of the NCI SEER data base, which reviews cancer patient survival for 10% of the American population, indicates that many cancer patients do not now receive the best available treatments. This transfer of technology represents a major challenge for NCI to achieve its goal of reducing cancer mortality by 50% of today's rate by the year 2000. Thirty percent of this reduction is expected to accrue from improved treatment of cancer patients. Overall, if every patient with cancer in the United States were to receive the best treatment available today, there would be an

immediate 105 improvement in five-year survival, and this would save 40,000 lives each year (15).

To facilitate the transfer of treatment research advances to the community, the NCI has undertaken a number of unique and important initiatives, as shown in Table 3.

The accomplishments and discoveries of the past decade have clearly shown that advanced malignancies of certain types, primarily those affecting the younger population, can be cured with systemic therapies. It is difficult to overemphasize the importance of this observation, which provided the confidence to undertake a systematic search for therapies for the more common, and more refractory, solid tumors of the respiratory and digestive tracts. Fortunately, new developments in basic research have created unparalleled opportunities to treat these tumors. Major scientific breakthroughs are forthcoming from the NCI's major commitment to research in basic cancer biology and have led to the characterization of the surface features of tumor cells isolated from patients with cancer, the identification of growth factors that control tumor proliferation and oncogenes, a better understanding of how cancer cells spread throughout the body (the process of metastasis), the elucidation of the biochemical and genetic changes that lead to drug resistance, and the description of the cells and growth factors that control the immune response to tumors. New perspectives and a more complete understanding of the cancer process have been growing with unprecedented speed, and there has never been a time of greater opportunity to apply what has already been learned in the laboratory to the innovative and successful treatment of patients with cancer. The efficient translation of basic research advances to the clinic is demonstrable in studies undertaken during the past year in treatment research, most notably very promising studies involving the immunotherapy of cancer and the development of drugs to treat the many manifestations of AIDS. Together with clinical application of research findings in cancer prevention and improved cancer diagnosis, prospects are increasingly favorable for achieving the eradication of cancer.

The NCI's prime commitment to basic research has contributed substantially to the explosion in biotechnology that has placed the United States firmly in the lead of innovative biomedical research worldwide. Importantly, spin-offs in basic cancer research have led to promising areas of research in unrelated scientific disciplines. Immunosuppressive agents developed by the NCI's drug development program have become essential in organ transplantation programs. The worldwide discovery of human retroviruses as a cause

R. H. Goldfarb (ed.), Fundamental aspects of cancer.

Table 1. Change in prognosis for patients with advanced malignancy 1973–1985.

	Long-term disease-free survival	
Type of cancer	1973	1985
Acute lymphocytic leukemia	30%	60%
Hodgkin's diseases	50%	65%
Diffuse lymphoma	5%	65%
Testicular cancer	10%	80%
Choriocarcinoma	80%	90%
Childhood sarcomas	50%	90%
Breast (Stage II) postmenopausal	64%	73%
Small-cell lung cancer (limited stage)	5%	33%

of cancer in man (1, 13) has led to a search for similar viruses capable of causing other ailments such as autoimmune diseases and multiple sclerosis. Identification of such viruses would have profound clinical ramifications in the prevention and treatment of diseases other than cancer. Gene-splicing techniques, so critical for the availability of large quantities of genetically pure biologics (such as TNF and interleukin II) were pioneered by investigators of basic cancer biology. Already these techniques have been commercially extended to the synthesis of recombinant human insulin and recombinant human growth hormone and used in the treatment of patients with serious metabolic diseases. In addition, the recent discovery of oncogenes and a better understanding of their role not only in cancer causation but also normal growth and development will have unprecedented applications across biologic disciplines.

The NCI has also efficiently applied advances in pharmacology, immunology, physics, and biology to patient treatment. For example, the NCI is unique within government in administering a large and successful program in drug development, to be discussed later. This national resource has been rapidly mobilized for the development of new drugs for the treatment of acquired immunodeficiency syndrome (AIDS), recently declared the number one health priority of the United States by the Secretary of Health and Human Services. Already, promising antiviral agents such as suramin and 5-azidothymidine dideoxycytine, dideoxyadenosine, and dideoxyinosine have been identified by the NCI.

For much of its support of clinical treatment research, the NCI supports a number of integrated clinical cooperative groups that perform cancer treatment research under the cooperative agreement mechanism (24). Each group is or-

Table 2.

Disease	Improvement in 5-year survival with adjuvant therapy (%)	Number of lives saved
Breast (stage 2) (2, 6)	15%	5,147
Colon (stage C) (33)	15%	8,120
Rectum (B₂ and C) (14)	20%	3,792
Lung-adeno-stage III (18)	19%	4,900
Total		21,959

Table 3. NCI initiative to transfer treatment advances to the community.

Program	Purpose
Physician Data Query (PDQ) Computer Data Base	Provides up-to-date treatments for over 100 cancers
	Lists NCI-supported clinical studies by disease and geographic location
	Lists physicians who specialize in cancer treatment by speciality (medical oncology, surgery, and radiation)
	Available to all physicians with access to a personal computer or medical library
Cooperative Group Outreach Programs Cancer Center Outreach Programs Community Clinical Oncology Programs	Extend the perimeter of the national network of cancer treatment programs into the community
	Serve as vehicles for continuing education of community physicians of the rapidly improving treatment options for patients with cancer
Office of Cancer Communications Cancer "Hot Line" (1-800-4-CANCER)	Provides patients themselves with understandable and current advice on cancer treatment options so as to expedite informed decision-making by patients and their families
Minority Satellite Supplement Program	Finds minority institutions to allow access of patients to ongoing cancer treatment trials. This is an important initiative since cancer survival among minorities has lagged behind improvements seen in the U.S. population

ganized to provide the optimal structure for clinical researchers to collaborate in the design of large-scale clinical trials and to accrue patients most effectively for testing of new and promising cancer therapies. The groups differ in their tumor type of interest (for example, emphasis on tumors responsive to radiotherapy), in their age group of interest (pediatric versus adult cancer), or may have multimodality broad-based programs of research (national or regional groups). For each cancer site there may be several different ongoing trials that test the efficacy of chemotherapy, immunotherapy, radiation therapy, and surgery. These trials are identified as individual treatment programs or protocols. The NCI reviews and funds approximately 600 new protocols per year that continue to add new patients and follow patients over time.

The cooperative agreement mechanism provides considerable flexibility by permitting integration of basic cancer biology, pathology, surgery, diagnostic radiology, radiation therapy, and medical oncology. The clinical cooperative groups have proven to be enormously efficient in providing timely answers to scientific questions that require large numbers of patients, for studies of less common tumor types, or in those clinical situations for which subgroup analysis is essential. More recently, collaboration between clinical cooperative group trials has increased, and these "intergroup studies" can provide even greater efficiency. The pooling of scientific talents, patient resources, and statistical expertise results in a powerful investigative instrument on an unparalleled scale.

The intramural NCI clinical program at the National Institutes of Health and Navy Medical Center campuses in Bethesda and the Frederick Cancer Research Facility in Frederick, Maryland, complement this national clinical trials network. In the intramural program, NCI scientists have pioneered new treatments for AIDS, curative regimens for patients with lymphomas and testicular and ovarian cancer, and new biological treatments using monoclonal antibodies and adoptive immunotherapy. These programs are described under the sections on preclinical and clinical treatment research.

PRECLINICAL TREATMENT RESEARCH

Drug development – application of the advances in tumor biology

The majority of patients with cancer will have either obvious or occult tumor metastases at the time of diagnosis (28). While surgery and radiotherapy are powerful tools in the control of local disease, they are limited in the successful management of patients with widespread malignancy. What is needed are systemic treatments that are able to kill tumor cells selectively. Prior to developments in chemotherapy there were no effective treatments for patients with metastatic cancer.

In recognition of the need for better systemic cancer treatment, the NCI's new-drug program was mandated by Congress in 1955 (35). In the 33 years since the launch of this program, the NCI has discovered 50% and screened 75% of the commercial drugs available to physicians in the U.S. for the treatment of cancer (9). In addition, the NCI supported the developmental clinical studies for *all* of these agents. The success of this program provided the impetus for a dramatic expansion of cancer treatment research in academia and industry in the 1970s and early 1980s.

Although the mission of the NCI new-drug program – discovery of improved agents for the treatment of metastatic malignancy – has remained unchanged, its direction has responded significantly to current scientific opportunities. For example, because of scientific collaboration with the private-sector pharmaceutical industry, there has been a shift in emphasis in drug analog development, such that much of this work is now done by private-sector expertise.

It is often possible to synthesize analogs of active anticancer compounds that retain antitumor activity with considerably less toxic side effects for the patient. Research in this area has led to improved platinum compounds (such as carboplatin, introduced into clinical trial in 1978, that has less kidney and nerve toxicity than the parent drug, cisplatin) and anthracyclines (such as mitoxantrone, introduced into trials in 1980, that has potentially less cardiac toxicity than the parent drug, adriamycin) (24). In both cases, these analogs were developed by private industry with NCI guidance. Because beginning research with chemical structures with known efficacy in the treatment of human malignancy represents a relatively low-risk area of drug development, this approach has become particularly attractive to pharmaceutical houses. Increasingly, NCI has collaborated with industry to see that this important work continues, offering to test primary analogs in its preclinical and clinical system while concentrating its own resources on new lead development. Thus, while the new-drug program budget at NCI has been reduced by 50% since 1980, there has been no reduction in either output or creativity.

New drug-screening programs

During this early period of drug development, research focused on a single feature of the cancer cell – its ability to proliferate and grow in an uncontrolled fashion. The target molecule for these agents was DNA, the building block of genetic material within the cell. Now, other factors recently discovered to be involved in uncontrolled proliferation (such as oncogenes and growth factors) may be inhibited with entirely new classes of drugs. In addition, as shown in Table 4, other unique features of the cancer cell can be attacked as the processes of metastasis and differentiation are further unraveled.

Drug development efforts as presently planned at the NCI will encompass both a revamped screening effort that will examine 8,000 compounds per year and a biologically tar-

Table 4. The biologic basis for cancer therapy.

Cancer cell feature	Target molecule	Drug
Metastasis	Collagenase	Inhibitor
	Laminin	Fragments or analogs
Failure to differentiate	Protacyclin	Inducers
	Protein kinase	Phorbol ester
	Growth factor receptor	Vitamin A
	Cell surface antigens	Monoclonal antibodies
Uncontrolled proliferation	DNA	Antimetabolites
		Alkylating agents
		Intercalators
		Hormones
	Oncogenes	Methyphosphonatin
		Oligonucleosides
		Anti-RNA
	Growth factors	Monoclonal antibodies

geted discovery effort. New anticancer drugs have commonly been screened for antitumor activity against highly proliferative and drug-sensitive mouse leukemias. While this approach has been successful in the identification of drugs that can cure rapidly proliferating human leukemias and lymphomas, more effective therapies are required for patients with the more common slowly growing solid tumors such as cancers of the lung, breast, ovary, and colon. Advances in the ability to grow human cancer cells in culture have made new screening programs a high priority of the NCI new-drug program.

In the last years, a major reorientation of the drug development program was initiated. This effort, the *Lung Cancer Drug Discovery Project*, utilizes a bank of human lung cancers grown in culture as the initial screen to identify new drugs specifically useful for the treatment of patients with lung cancer. This cancer was chosen as highest priority for several reasons:

● Lung cancer is the leading cause of cancer death among men in the United States. Since 1953, lung cancer rates have increased 172% among men and 256% among women.
● Drug therapy to date has had limited effectiveness against lung cancer.
● The availability of multiple human lung cancer cell lines.

The use of actual cancer cells derived from patients as a drug-screening device has a number of appealing advantages:

● This approach can select new drugs that are preferentially activated by cancer cells to kill tumor while sparing normal tissues.
● The use of cell lines is cost effective, as it is adaptable to automation. For the equivalent cost of a single mouse study, information on many different cell lines of different tumor types (human, lung, colon, ovary, breast, brain) can be obtained.
● Since assays can be performed in micro-titer plates, only a small amount of drug is necessary. This allows for the efficient screening of natural-product compounds that, although highly promising, are available initially only in small quantities. Lead compounds derived from entirely new sources (fungi, algae, and marine organisms) can thus be effectively screened.
● Data from the Lung Cancer Drug Discovery Program efforts can be appropriately expanded into screening for new drugs useful in the treatment of other solid tumors such as colon, ovary, breast, and central nervous system malignancies.

This initiative is currently being implemented at the NCI's Frederick Cancer Research Facility in Frederick, Maryland.

Acquired immunodeficiency syndrome (AIDS) drug development

The discovery of human T-cell leukemia/lymphoma virus III (HTLV III) as the cause of AIDS by NCI scientists in 1983 has now allowed the preclinical and clinical development of agents capable of inhibiting the growth of the virus in AIDS patients. The promise of effective AIDS drug therapy rests firmly on advances in basic cancer biology:

● The discovery, isolation, characterization, and cloning of interleukin-II (T-cell growth factor) by Robert Gallo of NCI and T. Taniguchi of Japan allowed propagation of normal human T lymphocytes (the target of the AIDS virus) in tissue culture (31).
● The isolation by Samuel Broder of NCI of a T-cell clone that is easily infected with the AIDS virus now allows for rapid laboratory screening of drugs or other agents that may be useful in the treatment of AIDS.

The NCI screen initially identified several drugs that were able to inhibit infection of T cells in culture: suramin azidothymidine dideoxycytine, dideoxyionosine, and dideoxyadenosine. Both of these agents were initially tested in AIDS patients in the NCI intramural program and clinical trials subsequently expanded in NCI-supported extramural trials. The preliminary results of these clinical trials are quite encouraging, with both inhibition of viral outgrowth and improvement in immune parameters observed in a number of patients.

The National Cancer Institute and the National Institute of Allergy and Infectious Diseases (NIAID) have now developed a collaboration for the joint development of drugs, vaccines and biologics for the treatment and cure of AIDS. For example, with NIAID co-sponsorship, the NCI is planning the formation of National Cooperative Drug Discovery Groups (NCDDG) for identification of new anti-AIDS drugs. These groups, modeled after the NCDDGs for cancer drug development, can call on the best national expertise in medicinal chemistry, immunology, virology, and pharmacology from academia, government, and the private sector for the rational development of new treatment strategies in AIDS.

Growth factor antagonists – disrupting cancer's control of its own proliferation

Research advances into the new biology of cancer have demonstrated that cancer cells are uniquely able to determine their own destiny by secreting specific growth factors. Again, these most basic of biologic observations are being translated into new treatments for cancer patients.

Tumor cells are able to produce and secrete growth-promoting factors that are capable of either stimulating their own proliferation directly or alter their environment to provide a selective growth advantage (Table 5). These

Table 5. Growth factors related to cell transformation.

Growth factor	Biologic activity	Molecular weight	Cloned
Insulin-like growth factors (I and II)	Somatomedin activity, mitogen	7,500	yes
Epidermal growth factor	Mitogen, promotes keratinization	6,200	yes
Platelet-derived growth factor	Supports cell growth, characteristic agent	28,000	yes
Transforming growth factor	Promotes anchorage-independent growth	22,000	yes

Table 6. Growth factors as targets for treatment intervention.

Strategy	Example
Monoclonal antibodies to growth factors	Anti-bombesin monoclonal antibodies
Monoclonal antibodies to growth factor receptor	Anti-TAC monoclonal antibodies
Analogs of growth factors	Laminin fragments
Block receptor action	Protein kinase C

growth factors can be classified as endocrine, paracrine, or autocrine growth factors.

Endocrine growth factors such as insulin and sex hormones are secreted by normal glandular tissue into the circulation to effect the growth of distant cells; paracrine growth factors stimulate the growth of adjacent cells without entering the circulation. Of greatest interest are autocrine growth factors that stimulate the proliferation of the same cancer cell that makes the substance. All three types of factors have been found to stimulate tumor cell growth in certain situations.

For example, one can make cells estrogen independent by transvecting them with oncogenes that stimulate secretion of the same peptides that promote the proliferation of estrogen-dependent breast cancer cells (20). Marc Lippman of NCI has shown that the growth factors secreted by the transvected cells can support the growth of estrogen-dependent cells (19). These novel growth factors are being characterized and represent a unique therapeutic target for inactivation by monoclonal antibodies (8). In addition, these basic observations provide an explanation for development of hormone resistance and heterogeneity of clinical response in women with breast cancer.

Tumor cells are also capable of altering their environment by secreting paracrine growth factors. For example, angiogenesis factor is a secreted peptide that causes the growth of blood vessels into a cancer to provide nutrients (10, 21). Agents capable of inhibiting production of angiogenesis factor or blocking its effect may be capable of reversing the control of the cancer over the host's normal tissues. Current treatment research is aimed at developing steroidal and heparin antagonists of human blood vessel formation.

In the most direct demonstration of control over their own growth, cancer cells are also capable of secreting autocrine growth factors. For example, small-cell lung cancer in man secretes a small molecular weight protein called *bombesin* (7). Small-cell lung cancer also has receptors for this protein so that *bombesin* secreted by the tumor stimulates its own growth. Monoclonal antibodies have now been raised against bombesin, and administration of these antibodies to animals inoculated with human small-cell lung cancer blocks this autocrine effect and controls the growth of the tumor. A clinical trial of antibombesin monoclonal antibodies in lung cancer patients will begin shortly in the NCI intramural program.

Overall, as shown in Table 6, the demonstration that growth factors play an important role in the growth and proliferation of some cancers offers an entirely new approach to the development of effective treatments for patients with metastatic malignancy.

Control of metastasis – a major obstacle to cancer cure

As has already been noted, patients die not from their primary tumor (which can often be removed surgically) but rather from spread of the cancer to distant vital organs. As the process of metastasis is better understood, rational ways of intervening to prevent tumor spread become increasingly possible.

For example, researchers have shown that the aggressiveness of cancers in patients, including their ability to metastasize, is related to the expression of oncogenes, portions of DNA present in every cell that control the ability of cells to proliferate. While oncogene expression is part of normal growth and development, overexpression or amplification of these genes can result in uncontrolled cellular proliferation. Cancer researchers have already identified more than 20 human oncogenes and are characterizing the products of oncogene expression. Already it has been shown that overexpression or amplification of oncogenes confers a poor prognosis in patients with small-cell lung cancer or neuroblastoma (23). Prevention of oncogene expression (e.g., with a new class of drugs called differentiating agents) or inhibition of the oncogene products themselves (such as inhibitors or protein kinase enzymes) has the potential to reverse malignant cells into more normal cells incapable of spreading and killing patients. As part of an effort that focuses on the inhibition of oncogenes as a therapeutic thrust, the NCI has established a National Cooperative Drug Discovery Group to explore this area of high priority basic research, which has tremendous potential for treatment application. This consortium, funded under the cooperative-agreement mechanism, brings together the best medicinal chemists, molecular biologists, and pharmacologists from academia, government, and industry. Few, if any, institutions have the critical mass of expertise to approach this opportunity from a multidisciplinary perspective. However, the NCDDG represents an innovative funding instrument where the whole is greater than the sum of its parts.

The metastatic process itself is being unraveled. It is known that cancer spread is a complex process that requires tumor cells to survive in the circulation, attach to vessel walls, penetrate the vessel, and grow at a distant site. Each of these steps potentially can be blocked to prevent the spread of tumor. For example, immunoaugmentative strategies potentially could stimulate the patient's natural ability to search out and destroy tumor cells while they are still circulating. Other approaches are currently being assessed to inhibit the processes of attachment and penetration.

It has now been demonstrated that tumor cells attach to invade basement membrane that blocks their spread by recognizing a structural protein called laminin (25). Cancer cells that lack the laminin receptor are unable to attach to the vessel wall. Indeed, the importance of laminin receptors in patients' tumor specimens has already been demonstrated in patients with breast cancer. Analysis of primary tumors from patients' breasts has shown that the greater the number of laminin receptors present on the tumor itself, the greater the likelihood that the patient will have documented spread beyond the breast. Thus the assay for laminin in primary tumor specimens may useful in predicting which patients are most likely to benefit from adjuvant forms of systemic treatment. It is now possible to block attachment in one of two ways:

1. block the laminin receptor on the tumor with cloned fragments of laminin itself, or
2. cover laminin itself using specific monoclonal antibodies, thus preventing cellular attachment.

Both of these approaches have already been successful in totally inhibiting tumor cell spread in experimental animals, and clinical trials using laminin fragments to prevent cancer metastasis are scheduled to begin this year.

Finally, the process of cancer cell penetration of the normal vessel wall requires that the malignant cell digests the basement membrane by secreting specific enzymes such as collagenases and proteases (22). Drugs such as certain forms of heparin and prostaglandin inhibit these enzymes and so prevent spread of the cancer beyond the perimeter of the primary tumor. Again, these drugs are being developed using new animal metastasis models.

CLINICAL TREATMENT RESEARCH

Biological response modifiers – the fourth modality of cancer treatment

As has already been detailed, recent advances in basic cancer biology research now offer the promise of increasingly specific and directed treatments that exploit the fundamental differences between normal and malignant cells. Seminal research in the area deals with *biological response modifiers* that are rapidly joining surgery, radiotherapy, and chemotherapy as the fourth modality of cancer treatment. Biological response modifiers fall into two categories:

1. Cellular products that have direct antitumor effect
2. Chemical and biological agents that can effect host resistance mechanisms that may be involved in the control of growth or metastasis of cancer.

The first category of biologicals, those with direct toxicity to tumor cells, has already been discussed in the context of monoclonal antibodies to growth factors or labeled with toxic substances (radionucleotides, toxins, or anticancer drugs). In addition, a novel agent in this category of biologics – tumor necrosis factor (TNF) – has recently been described and characterized. Again, the clinical application of this basic research discovery has been possible only because of recent advances in molecular biology.

Tumor necrosis factor (TNF)

In the early 1970s, NCI-supported scientists discovered that serum from mice pretreated with tuberculosis extracts and endotoxin could destroy certain mouse tumors. This discovery led to 15 years of research designed to determine what was present in the serum that killed tumors, to extract and purify the active component, and to use this component in the treatment of patients with cancer (26). These early investigations of TNF revealed that it was capable of killing a large variety of tumor cells from mouse and man in experimental systems. In other words, there was no restriction of activity of TNF from any species of animal to the cancers arising in that species. Importantly, normal cells from the same animal species were spared, and little toxicity was seen

in mice treated with this natural substance. However, because the material was difficult to synthesize and purify in large quantities, animal studies were limited and trials in patients unlikely.

However, advances in molecular biology set the stage for explosive advances in this area. Two new technologies were used: 1) amino and sequencing, where precise structural formulations can be determined, and 2) recombinant DNA techniques, also known as gene splicing, that allowed the genes that control the production of a particular protein to be inserted into a cell, directing the machinery of the recipient cell to produce the desired product in almost unlimited quantities. In this way, large quantities of recombinant human TNF have become available, allowing scientists to study TNF in detail (30). In every respect, from the destruction of tumor cells in test tubes to the cure of experimental animals with sensitive tumors, TNF is an exciting new biological that does not rely on the host immune system for cancer cell kill. Clinical trials with TNF are now under way.

Immune stimulation therapies/adoptive immunotherapy

Other biological destroy malignant cells by boosting the host's immune system. These agents include the interferons, interferon inducers, lymphokines, and macrophage-activating factors. Again, the techniques of recombinant DNA technology and gene splicing have allowed cancer clinicians to bridge the gap between laboratory and patient bedside. For example, recombinant techniques made cloned, pure interferon available in large quantities at a tenth of the cost of the natural product. Already, interferon has shown 50 percent response rates for heavily pretreated patients with nodular lymphoma and cutaneous T-cell lymphomas (11). In addition, virtually all patients with hairy-cell leukemia respond to even exquisitely low doses of interferon. The reasons for this unparalleled sensitivity of a human cancer to a single biological are under intense investigation and may expand the clinical use of the interferons in other cancers.

Preclinical studies also indicate that combinations of biologics or biologics in combination with tumor-differentiating agents may be even more selectively effective in the same way that drug combinations have already cured thousands of patients with leukemias and metastatic solid tumors.

Adoptive immunotherapy. Yet another promising immunologic approach to the treatment of patients with cancer is adoptive immunotherapy, a treatment pioneered by Dr. Steven Rosenberg in the NCI intramural program (27). Adoptive immunotherapy is the transfer to the tumor-bearing host of active immunologic cells with antitumor activity that can mediate antitumor effects. Possible advantages of this entirely new approach to cancer treatment are that it does not require full immunocompetence of the host, it can easily be used with other therapies (such as surgery, radiotherapy, and chemotherapy), and it has a high specificity of effect with potentially less toxicity and immunosuppression.

As developed by NCI scientists, adoptive immunotherapy involves the removal of the patient's own white cells and incubation with interleukin-II (T-cell growth factor). Interleukin-II, also discovered by NCI scientists, allows the growth of normal T cells (killer cells) *in vitro*. The activated killer cells are able to lyse fresh human tumors (but not normal cells) directly. When transferred to patients in combination with high doses of interleukin-II, these activated killer cells are able to seek out and selectively destroy cancer cells throughout the patient's body. Already this approach, recently published in The New England Journal of Medicine, has resulted in impressive responses in patients with heavily pretreated, poor-prognosis cancers (29). The activity of this regimen was already confirmed in six extramural trials, and the FDA has agreed to the use of IL-2/LAK for primary treatment of renal cell cancer and melanoma at cancer centers throughout the U.S. Again, this novel and effective new treatment for cancer patients would not have been possible before the cloning of the gene for interleukin-II. Recombinant DNA technology has once more provided cancer physicians with sufficient quantities of immunologically pure materials to bridge the gap between laboratory and bedside.

Especially exciting is the fact that adoptive immunotherapy in combination with active chemotherapy cures experimental animals in situations where either modality, in and of itself, is ineffective. Thus, biological response modifiers in concert with surgery, chemotherapy, and radiotherapy are becoming the fourth modality of cancer treatment.

Diagnostic imaging and radiation therapy – application of new technology to cancer diagnosis and treatment

DIAGNOSTIC IMAGING

Diagnostic imaging has made spectacular technological advances during the past decade. Computer tomography (CT) scanning has radically improved the ability of physicians to diagnose cancer during its earliest, most curable stages. The NCI is supporting basic and applied research in spectroscopy and physics to carry imaging technology forward to the next generation of instrument sophistication.

Magnetic resonance imaging. Magnetic resonance imaging (MRI) is a major breakthrough in the imaging field, providing anatomic information not previously available to physicians. The sensitivity of MRI has the potential to improve patient treatment planning by surgeons and radiotherapists and accurately assess tumor response to treatments. The NCI is supporting clinical research to compare the relative indications for CT versus MRI in specific patient-care areas. This work will permit the safe and cost-effective translation of this technology to the clinic.

At the basic level of magnetic resonance research, investigators have now used sodium and phosphorus imaging techniques to distinguish malignant from benign tumors solely on their imaging characteristics. This represents a major breakthrough that may eventually allow specific tissue diagnosis without need for surgical biopsy.

Other pioneering imaging techniques can now give physicians information on function in addition to structure. For example, positron-emission-tomography (PET) scanning is capable of assessing nutrient utilization in cancers versus surrounding normal tissues, providing a sensitive index of a cancer's functional response to treatment in an individual patient.

RADIATION THERAPY

New technologies have also been seminal in radiation therapy research, a powerful weapon in the treatment of localized cancer.

Particle beam therapy. Radiation therapy using particles (neutrons, protons, and helium lows) promises superior dose localization and sparing of normal tissues contiguous with the tumor as a radiologic advantage in being able to kill oxygen-deprived tissues, such as large tumors. Clinical research in this area has shown superiority in the treatment of prostate and salivary gland tumors.

Hyperthermia. Hyperthermia (heating tumor tissue) is not only capable of killing cancer cells directly, but also sensitizes these cells to the effects of both radiation and chemotherapy. While clinical studies have shown that superficial cancers (such as cancers of the skin or eye) are quite responsive to single heating, a major obstacle in extending these studies has been the inability to heat deep-seated cancers in a controlled fashion. New hyperthermia systems using electromagnetic radiation (radio frequency and microwave) and ultrasound are addressing current clinical limitations at the basic research level.

Photodynamic therapy. Certain dyes (such as hematoporphyrins) are preferentially accumulated and retained by cancer cells. When excited by light from a laser source, these dyes are activated into forms that can effectively kill cells. Basic research in photodynamic therapy is progressing at a rapid rate. A specific di-hematoporphyrin ester with an affinity for plasma lipoproteins has been identified as an active tumor-localizing component of hematoporphyrins and the actual mechanism of hematoporphyrin-light cytotoxicity unraveled. Clinical studies on cancer patients using photodynamic therapy have confirmed activity of the treatment in lung, head, neck, bladder, and eye cancers. Simple techniques for uniformly distributing light within a body cavity using lipid emulsions may also make this approach applicable to patients with ovarian cancer, mesothelioma, or other cancers confined to the abdominal or thoracic cavities.

Clinical trials

NCI-supported clinical treatment trials are effectively bringing the advances of basic cancer biology into the arena of clinical cancer medicine. Today, over 5,000 cancer physicians involved in NCI studies follow 75,000 patients annually and see an additional 200,000 patients with cancer each year. The NCI is unique within NIH both in developing new anticancer drugs using the contract mechanism and in its support of a nationwide network of cancer centers, outreach programs, community clinical oncology programs and cooperative groups for clinical trials. This network provides rapid and effective transfer of cancer treatment research advances from laboratory to clinic.

For much of its support of clinical treatment research, the NCI supports a number of integrated clinical cooperative groups that perform cancer research under the cooperative-agreement mechanism. This mechanism provides the maximum flexibility for clinical trials in cancer treatment. Within broad parameters, each group may pursue research approved by its members, who are the Nation's pre-eminent experts in a particular disease or treatment, and by NCI. Recently, collaboration between cooperative clinical trial groups has increased and the resulting "intergroup studies" can provide even greater efficiency. The pooling of scientific talents, patient resources, and statistical expertise results in a clinical trial instrument of unprecedented strength for solving problems in pediatric cancers, interferon therapy of lymphoma, new hormonal therapy for prostate cancer, and studies in bone marrow transplantation. Selected intergroup studies include:

Intergroup Study	Treatment Strategy
Prostate cancer intergroup study	Investigate the role of complete pharmacologic androgen oblation in prostate cancer treatment using newly available hormone agonists and anti-androgens
Colon cancer intergroup study	Investigate the role of combined adjuvant chemotherapy and immunotherapy in patients with advanced-stage, but potentially curable, colon cancer
Head and neck cancer intergroup studies	Investigate innovative combination of surgery, radiotherapy, and chemotherapy for patients with poor-prognosis, potentially curable cancers
Melanoma intergroup study	Compare surgical approaches to loco-regional disease
Acute leukemia intergroup study	Investigate the role of differentiating agents and novel ara-C treatments in patients with acute leukemia

The cooperative groups uniquely disseminate new approaches to cancer treatment to a broad patient population. The cooperative groups can definitively answer important questions, such as the role of adjuvant therapy in selected diseases. The positive adjuvant treatment studies in breast cancer, rectal cancer, colon cancer, and adenocarcinoma of the lung have the potential of saving thousands of lives each year. In addition, the recent National Surgical Adjuvant Breast Project Cooperative Group trial, involving thousands of women nationwide, confirmed that breast-sparing surgery in combination with radiotherapy is a rational alternative to mastectomy for women with breast cancer. Thus, alternatives to standard mastectomy can be offered for the treatment of the most common cancer in American women.

Other cooperative trials are investigating the prognostic significance of cytogenetic and immunohistochemical correlations for patients with leukemia and lymphoma. These sophisticated biomarkers are allowing treatments to be custom-designed for patients with good- or poor-prognosis disease. Bone marrow transplantation, which allows the use of higher and potentially curative drug doses to be given to patients, is also being studied by the cooperative groups. Review of the promising results of biological response modifiers has led to critical studies for new research in chronic myelogenous leukemias, hairy-cell leukemia, and non-Hodgkin's lymphomas. In addition, a definitive trial of the role of BCG for the prevention of recurrence of superficial bladder cancer is planned.

Finally, in an attempt to interface between laboratory and clinic using effective drug combinations, patient studies are planned to develop clinical trials based on biochemical modulation. That is, clinical trials will be undertaken to test whether combinations of drugs based on laboratory demonstration of interaction at the biochemical pathway level produce similar perturbations in the patient's cancer and result in improved therapeutic results.

Laying the foundation for curative therapy of advanced malignancy

Curative single agent chemotherapy
  Choriocarcinoma – methotrexate – 1957[1,2]
  Burkitt's lymphoma – cytoxan – 1963[3]
Curative combination chemotherapy
  Acute lymphocytic leukemia – early 1960s[4]
  Hodgkin's disease – 1970[5]
  Diffuse histiocytic lymphoma – 1974[6]
  Testicular cancer – 1975[7,8]
Combined modality therapy
  Pediatric sarcomas – 1970s[9]
Adjuvant therapy
  Breast cancer (premenopausal) – 1970s[10]

---

[1] Zubrod CG, Schepartz S, Leiter J et al: The chemotherapy program of the National Cancer Institute: History, analysis and plans. *Cancer Chemotherapy Rep* 50:349, 1961

[2] Hertz R, Lewis J, Lipsett MB: Five years experience with chemotherapy of metastatic trophoblastic diseases in women. *AM J Obstet Gynecol* 86:808, 1963

[3] Oettgen HF, Clifford P, Burkitt D: Malignant lymphoma involving the jaw in African children: Treatment with alkylating agents and actinomycin D. *Cancer Chemotherapy Rep* 28:25, 1963

[4] Frei E, Freireich EJ: Progress and perspectives in the chemotherapy of acute leukemia. *Advances in Chemotherapy* 2:269, 1965

[5] DeVita V, Serpick A, Carbone PP: Combination chemotherapy in the treatment of Hodgkin's disease. *Am Intern Med* 73:881, 1970

[6] Schein PS, Chabner BA, Canellos GP et al: Potential for prolonged disease-free survival following combination chemotherapy of non-Hodgkin's lymphoma. *Blood* 43:81, 1974

[7] Einhorn LH, Donohue JP: Cis-diammunedichloroplatinum, vinblastine and bleomycin combination chemotherapy in disseminated testicular cancer. *Ann Int Med* 87:293, 1977

[8] Samuels ML, Johnson DE, Holoye PY: Continuous intravenous bleomycin therapy with vinblastine in Stage III testicular neoplasia. *Cancer Chemotherapy Rep* 59:563, 1975

[9] Green DM, Jaffe N: Progress and controversy in the treatment of childhood rhabdomyosarcoma. *Cancer Treat Rep* 5:7, 1978

[10] Bonadonna G, Rossi A, Valagussa P et al: Combination chemotherapy as an adjuvant treatment in operable breast cancer. *N Engl J Med* 294:405, 1976

REFERENCES

1. Beem PA, Schechter GP, Jaffe ES et al: Clinical cause of retrovirus-associated adult T-cell lymphoma in the United States. *N Engl J Med* 309:257–264, 1983
2. Bonadonna G, Brusamolino E, Valaguessa P et al: Combination chemotherapy as an adjuvant in operable breast cancer. *N Engl J Med* 294:405–410, 1976
3. Broder S: Personal communication, 1986
4. Cadman E, Heiman R, Davis L: Enhanced 5-fluorouracil nucleotide formation after methotrexate administration: explanation for drug synergism. *Science* 205:1135–1137, 1979
5. Chabner BA, Fine RL, Allegra CJ et al: Cancer chemotherapy: progress and expectations. *Cancer* 54:2599–2608, 1984

6. Cummings FJ, Gray R, Davis TE et al: Adjuvant tamoxifen treatment of elderly women with stage II breast cancer. *Ann Intern Med* 103:324–329, 1985

7. Cuttitta F et al: Bobesin-like peptides can function as autocrine growth factors in small cell lung cancer. *Nature* 316:823–826, 1985

8. Davidson N, Wilding G, Lippman ME, Gelmann EP: Isolation of estrogen regulated cDNA clones from human breast cancer cell. *Proc Amer Soc Clin Onc Res* 33:577, 1985

9. Driscoll JS: The preclinical new drug research program of the National Cancer Institute. *Cancer Treat Rep* 68:63–76, 1984

10. Folkmann J, Langer R, Linhardt R et al: Angiogenesis inhibition and tumor regression caused by heparin or a heparin fragment in the presence of cortisone. *Science* 221:719–725, 1983

11. Foon KA et al: Recombinant leukocyte A interferon in the treatment of non-Hodgkin's lymphoma, chronic lymphocyte leukemia, and cutaneous T-cell lymphoma. In Zoon KC, Naguchi PD, Liu TY (Eds.), *Interferon: Research, Clinical Application, and Regulatory Consideration.* Elsevier Science Publishing Co., New York, pp. 219–227, 1984

12. Frei E: Pharmacology in cancer. In Burchenal JA, Oettgen HF (Eds.), *Achievements, Challenges and Prospects for the 80s.* Lippincott, Philadelphia, pp. 371–385, 1981

13. Gallo RC, Wong-Staal F: Retroviruses as etiologic agents of some animal and human leukemias and lymphomas as tools for elucidating the molecular mechanisms of leukemogenesis. *Blood* 30:545–557, 1982

14. Gastrointestinal Tumor Study Group: Prolongation of the disease-free interval in surgically treated rectal carcinoma. *N Engl J Med* 312:1465–1472, 1985

15. Greenwald P, Sondik EJ: Cancer control objectives for the nation 1985–2000. U.S., Department of Health and Human Services, Public Health Service, National Institutes of Health, National Cancer Institute, Monograph II. *NIH* 86-2880, 1986

16. Henderson IC: Chemotherapy of breast cancer. *Cancer* 51:2553–2562, 1983

17. Henderson IC, Canellos GP: Medical progress: cancer of the breast. *N Engl J Med* 302:17–30, 78–90, 1980

18. Holmes EC, Hill LB, Gail M: A randomized comparison of the effects of adjuvant therapy on resected stages II and III non-small cell cancer of the lung. *Lung Cancer Study Group Annals Surgery* 22:335–341, 1985

19. Huff KK, Kaufman D, Gabby KH, Spencer EM, Lippman ME, Dickson RB: Secretion on an insulin-like growth factor I-related protein by human breast cancer cells. *Cancer Res* 46(9):4613–19, 1986

20. Kasid A, Lippman ME, Papageorge AG et al: Transvection of

21. Langer R, Corn H, Vacenti J et al: Control of tumor growth in animals by infusion of an angiogenesis inhibitor. *Proc Natl Acad Sci USA* 77:4331–4335, 1980

22. Liotta LA, Thorgeirsson VP, Gabrisa S: Role of collagenases in tumor cell invasion. *Cancer Metab Rev* 1:227–288, 1982

23. Little CD, Nau MM, Carney DN et al: Amplification and expression of the *c-myc* oncogene in human lung cancer cell lines. *Nature* 306:194–196, 1983

24. Marsoni S, Wittes R: Clinical development of anticancer agents – a National Cancer Institute perspective. *Cancer Treat Rep* 68:77–85, 1984

25. Murray JC, Liotta LA, Rennard SI, Martin GR: Adhesion characteristics of murine metastatic and nonmetastatic tumor cells *in vitro. Cancer Res* 40:347–351, 1980

26. Prendergast JS, Old LJ: Tumor necrosis factor. *Proc Natl Acad Sci USA* 80:5397–5481, 1983

27. Rosenberg SA: Adoptive immunotherapy of cancer: accomplishments and prospects. *Cancer Treat Rep* 68:233–255, 1984

28. Rosenberg SA: Principles of surgical oncology in cancer. In *Principles and Practice of Oncology*, DeVita VT, Hellman S, Rosenberg A. (Eds.), Lippincott, Philadelphia, pp. 215–226, 1985

29. Rosenberg SA: Observations on the systemic administration of autologous lymphokine-activated killer cells and recombinant interleukin-2 to patients with metastatic cancer. *N Engl J Med* 313:1485–1492, 1985

30. Sugarman BJ et al: Recombinant human tumor necrosis factor alpha: effects on proliferation of normal and transformed cells *in vitro. Science* 230:943–945, 1985

31. Taniguchi T, Matsui H, Fugita T et al: Structure and expression of a cloned cDNA for human interleukin-2. *Nature* 302:305–310, 1983

32. Tormey DC, Weinberg VE, Holland JF et al: Randomized trial of five- and three-drug chemotherapy and chemoimmunotherapy in women with operable node positive breast cancer. *J Clin Oncol* 1:138–145, 1983

33. Unpublished data, North Central Cooperative Group

34. Young JL, Percy CL, Asire AJ et al: *Surveillance, Epidemiology, End Results: Incidence and Mortality Data 1973–1977*, Monograph #57. Washington, D.C., U.S. Government Printing Office, 1–187, 1981

35. Zubrod CG: Origins and development of chemotherapy research at the National Cancer Institute. *Cancer Treat Rep* 68:9–20, 1984

v-ras DNA into MCE-7 human breast cancer cells bypasses dependence on estrogen for tumorigenicity. *Science* 228:725–728, 1986

CHEMOTHERAPY FROM ANIMALS TO MAN

TAKAO OHNUMA and JAMES F. HOLLAND

INTRODUCTION

Cancer chemotherapy has now produced a cure in at least 12 categories of human cancer. In addition, major tumor regression and prolongation of survival have been accomplished in a significant number of disease categories (20, 21). The considerable success made, to date, in the area of clinical cancer chemotherapy convinces us that this is indeed one of the most efficacious approaches in the control of human cancer.

Major progress in chemotherapy research requires new drugs, new schedules and new techniques of drug administration in an effort to eradicate entire neoplastic diseases in man.

Evidence has proven that it is most effective to initiate treatment with a given drug or drug combination after establishing the most appropriate method of drug administration. Establishing the best method of drug administration can be derived through toxicological studies by exploring different dosage schedules, by comparing a broad variety of predecessor compounds and by making correla-

tions between clinical observations and pharmacological data. This phase of drug development is called phase I clinical trial (Table 1). Thus, the phase I trials are the initial human testing of new anticancer agents which were shown to be active in experimental animals and other screening systems. Phase I trials are also considered for combinations of agents and for combined modalities. It is common that during phase I study, subject to the feasibility of appropriate methodology, drug concentrations are measured and pharmacokinetic parameters are obtained. These studies will give information on the bioavailability, plasma clearance, biotransformation and excretion of the parent compounds, as well as active and inactive metabolites.

The end results of such a study will be the establishment of an optimal dose schedule applicable for therapeutic trials (phase II and III trials) in relation to risk factors and preexisting organ dysfunctions of patients. The dose schedule which will ultimately be used in therapeutic trials is determined at the conclusion of phase I studies. This is based on the toxicity patterns encountered, pharmacological rationale and from the practical applicability of the schedule.

Table 1. Stages in the clinical testing of new anticancer agents

Stage	Objectives	Patient population studied
Phase I	(1) To determine the maximally tolerated dose (MTD) To determine dose-limiting toxicity To determine degrees and parameters of toxicity To establish proper dose schedules (2) To determine bioavailability, plasma clearance, biotransformation and excretion (3) (To record therapeutic effects)	(See text)
Phase II	(1) To determine therapeutic effects in a panel of human tumors (2) To determine toxicity in relationship to therapeutic effects	(1) Histologically confirmed diagnosis of malignancy (2) No longer amenable to conventional therapy (3) Disease category must be uniform and sample size adequate
Phase III	(1) To compare the therapeutic effects to existing standard therapy (2) To compare toxicity to existing standard therapy	(1) Histologically confirmed diagnosis of malignancy (2) Usually previously untreated (3) Disease category must be uniform and sample size adequate (4) Controls are usually randomized occasionally historical
Phase IV	(1) To integrate into primary treatment in combination with other modalities (2) To determine toxic effects in the integrated regime (to monitor longterm effects)	(1) Histologically confirmed malignancy (2) Disease category must be uniform and sample size adequate (3) Controls are usually randomized

R. H. Goldfarb (ed.), Fundamental aspects of cancer.

In this chapter, we reviewed the procedures of phase I trials, together with our past experience.

GENERAL APPROACH FOR PHASE I STUDY

The main objectives of a phase I study of an anticancer agent are to determine: (a) the degrees and parameters of structural, functional and chemical effects on the host of the regimen under investigation, (b) the maximally tolerated dose (MTD), (c) the dose-limiting toxicity, (d) the recommended Phase II dose and (e) if possible, the apparent optimally effective dose schedule.

Phase I trials of anticancer agent are conducted in patients with disseminated cancers and leukemias for whom standard treatment either does not exist or has proven ineffective. While drugs are given in a phase I trial with therapeutic intent, the primary goal is to define the quantitative and qualitative characteristics of the drug's acute and subacute toxicities, and in so doing, to determine a biologically active dose which is tolerable for every patient.

In a broader sense, phase I studies of anticancer agents encompass: (a) new drug classes and new analogues of existing known agents, (b) new combination regimens (including combinations with biochemical modifiers), (c) new dose schedules, (d) new surgery plus chemotherapy, (e) new radiotherapy plus chemotherapy, (f) new chemotherapy plus immunotherapy and (g) new chemotherapy plus bone marrow transplantation (set A).

The MTD for patients with acute leukemia is often substantially higher than that for solid tumors (*vide infra*). Similarly, the MTD is often higher in children than in adults (30). Therefore, for a phase I study of anticancer agents at least 4 different target populations (solid tumors, leukemia, adult and children) must be considered. Thus, for phase I development of each drug, any subcategory in set A must be tested on 4 different target populations.

The basic approach of a phase I trial involves a new agent and a defined population of patients with solid tumors and/or leukemia.

ANTICANCER AGENTS

Drugs to be selected for phase I trials are characterized by a new structure with high promise of therapeutic activity based upon experimental therapeutics in murine tumors and in human xenografts or *in vitro* colony assay using human tumor cells, or by being an analogue of a clinically active parent compound with higher therapeutic index in preclinical studies, or by being a compound from a foreign country where clinically promising activity has been demonstrated.

For the past 30 years, comprehensive preclinical toxicological protocols have been developed at the National Cancer Institute to provide data of immediate relevance to initial trials in man (9, 23, 55, 89, 106, 107). More than 10,000 compounds/year are selectively acquired and screened against murine tumor models. In the United States the National Cancer Institute plays a central role in the development of anticancer agents. Other cancer institutions, universities and pharmaceutical industries also carry out extensive drug development programs.

Candidate compounds are those active against such experimental tumors of uniform and predictable behavior as leukemia P388, L1210, Lewis lung carcinoma, CD8F1 mammary carcinoma, colon 26 and 38 carcinomas and B_{16} melanoma. Since screening of chemicals in experimental animal system is intended primarily not to miss active compounds, there has been a considerable number of phase I agents shown to be active in murine tumor, but failed to demonstrate therapeutic efficacy in man. Possible explanations for this false positive have been offered (44, 56). Dose schedules and response criteria used in animal screens are different from those in man and these differences clearly amount for the false positives. Yet several clinically important drugs, including doxorubicin and cisplatin, were indeed identified through this procedure. In addition, drugs active against human colon (CX-1), breast (MX-1) or lung xenograft (LX-1) growing in athymic mice are of interest. In general, the responses to chemotherapy of different types of human tumors transplanted in nude mice are reported to resemble those observed in clinical investigations (29, 87, 103). There are exceptions, however, to these rules. Good examples of the latter are the high efficacy of glutamine antagonists in human tumor xenografts without substantiated activity in clinical testing (26, 96, 100).

Furthermore, drugs which induce interferon, which inhibit oncogenic viral multiplication, which produce differentiation or which have some other unique characteristics perhaps not demonstrable in experimental tumor systems (e.g., good penetration into cerebrospinal fluid), should be potential candidates. Included on this list are such biological materials as interferon, interleukin II, lymphotoxins, macrophage-derived toxins and immunotoxins.

Phase I combinations

For phase I combinations of anticancer agents, where at least one phase I agent is included, the following theoretical considerations can be made (92):

(1) Pharmacologic factors

In order for a drug administered by mouth or intravenously to reach the "target site(s)" within the neoplastic cell, the agent must pass through a number of barriers. Examples of combinations in attempts to increase membrane permeability of a prime agent include the use of amphotericin B (49, 58) and vincristine (4, 31, 113). (It should be noted, however, that in the latter case, further studies failed to confirm therapeutic synergism of vincristine followed by methotrexate (5, 13, 14, 46).). Synergistic antitumor activity can also be expected when one agent (a) interferes with the enzymatic destruction of an active compound, e.g., cytosine arabinoside plus tetrahydrouridine (62) and cordycepin plus 2′deoxycorformycin (43); (b) produces a delay in the excretion of an anticancer agent, e.g., 5-fluorouracil plus thymidine (78); (c) improves the conversion of anticancer agents to active metabolites, e.g., cytosine arabinoside plus uridine (66), and (d) improves the binding of anticancer agents to target molecules (104).

(2) Toxicologic factors

Toxicologic factors may be involved in two different ways in the design of combination chemotherapy. First, agents characterized by differing toxicities to various host tissues may be used in a mixture without reducing the optimal doses of each drug, e.g., doxorubicin plus bleomycin (3, 18) and doxorubicin plus cisplatin (6, 85, 98, 108). This allows the toxicity to the population of tumor cells to be intensified without significant increase in damage to any single tissue of the host. Such a practice is exemplified in many of the active multi-drug combinations used in man.

Knowledge of the precise mechanism of action of an anticancer agent allows the addition of a second compound to provide an element of selective antineoplastic action by reducing the toxicity of the first drug for susceptible normal tissue without significantly altering carcinostatic potency. The use of leukovorin rescue following high-dose methotrexate is a prime example of this consideration (2, 67, 99).

(3) Cell kinetic consideration

There is an ordered sequence of cellular activities during the cell cycle. Certain parameter, such as the replicative synthesis of DNA and the event of mitosis, are restricted to specific phases of the cell cycle. Many others, including the synthesis of RNA and proteins, occur continuously throughout the cycle. Since most anticancer agents exert their principal effects at the molecular level on nucleic acids and/or the pathways involved in their fabrication, the efficacy of these drugs is correlated with changes in their biochemical target sites. This conveys a degree of specificity not only for actively proliferating cells, but also in many cases for a particular phase of the cell cycle.

With this in mind, 2 therapeutic approaches have been considered. One is a synchronization of cells by 1 drug followed by treatment with a phase or cycle specific drug so that a greater cell kill can be accomplished. The second approach is a recruitment. When a bulk of tumor is killed by a cycle non-specific drug, the regrowth of tumor will be accompanied by an increased dividing fraction, or an increased number of cells in a specific cycle vulnerable to cycle specific agents. Although a number of clinical trials using dose regimens with cell kinetic considerations were reported to show increased efficacy, in a majority of cases synchronization or recruitment of tumor cells *in vivo* has not yet been demonstrated.

(4) Biochemical considerations

Earlier, Sartorelli (91) suggested 3 biochemical considerations for the combination of chemotherapeutic agents: (a) sequential, (b) concurrent and (c) complimentary. Our clinical experience of a combination of pyrazofurin and azacytidine is an example of the concurrent inhibition (11).

Recently, in addition to combinations which use two active anticancer agents, the biochemical modulation of anticancer agents by non-anticancer agents has, as exemplified by the use of amphotericin B and leucovorin above, gained interest. Our experiences with 5-fluorouracil plus thymidine (78), based on the work by Martin and Stolfi (57) 5-fluorouracil plus leucovovin (n) based on the work by Bruckner and Waxman (111) and cytosine arabinoside plus uridine (66, 86) belong to this category. Encouraging results in the treatment of colorectal cancer with 5-fluorouracil and leucovorin were confirmed by others (53).

PATIENT SELECTION AND ELIGIBILITY

For the selection of eligible patients, all of the following criteria must be met:

(1) Patients must have a microscopically confirmed diagnosis of cancer or leukemia.

This criteria is obvious for clinical trials of anticancer agents. The approaches to patients with solid tumors and those with leukemia should obviously differ. Since in most chemotherapeutic agents, myelosuppression is the main dose-limiting toxicity, patients with leukemia, who already have preexisting abnormalities in marrow function are unevaluable for hematological toxicity. Our approach has been to limit the dose escalation of phase I agents to patients with solid tumors. Only after myelosuppression is found to be the single most obvious toxicity, we can proceed to leukemic patients for further dose escalation because the recommended dose is often higher in these patients. Dose escalation in leukemic patients is also useful in identifying non-hematological toxicity because much higher doses are conventionally given in a deliberate attempt to produce marrow aplasia. This is exemplified in our experience in neocarzinostatin (75), amsacrine (32) and mitroxantrone (34, 83). In mitroxantrone studies, after reaching the MTD of $6.8 \, mg/m^2/dx5$ (and a recommended dose for phase II study of $4.2 \, mg/m^2/dx5$) in patients with solid tumors, doses were further escalated from 8 to $20 \, mg/m^2/dx5$ in patients with leukemia. We identified mucosal toxicity and greater frequency of infectious complications as dose-limiting, non-hematological toxicities (83). Candidate compounds for phase I study in leukemic patients include those with marrow toxicity, especially leukopenia, as the major, and ideally only, toxicity in patients with solid tumors; analogs of compounds with known high efficacy in leukemia; and those identified as having antileukemic effects in foreign clinical studies. It is yet to be determined whether all active antileukemic agents can be classified as differentiation-inducing agents.

(2) Patients must be staged by conventional methods and must be found to have disseminated or locally advanced disease not amenable to curative-intent therapy with surgery and/or radiotherapy or any other form of known effective therapy including chemotherapy.

This criterion holds true not only from the point of view of patients' welfare, but also ethically and legally. Indeed, this category of patients, those with maximal prior radiotherapy and chemotherapy, constitute a majority of patient population for phase I study.

It is pointed out that this patient population also produces problems in the interpretation of phase I data. It is known that patients who were exposed to the maximal doses of large numbers of myelosuppressive agents as well as untreated patients cannot tolerate new myelosuppressive phase I agents, and the recommended dosage for phase II study obtained from such patients would be lower as compared to those obtained from patients with no prior chemotherapy. This was amply demonstrated in many of the chemotherapeutic agents we studied, (e.g., amsacrine, indicine N-oxide, and mitroxantrone). With advances in adjuvant therapy, it is expected that the chemotherapy will be given progressively more often to patients with no prior chemotherapy or radiotherapy. Phase I studies sometimes fail to recommend a dosage as high as eventually could be tolerated in such patients. In order to clarify this point, one may have to enter, at the end of dose-escalation, patients with no or minimal prior therapy. They include (a) previously untreated patients with drug-sensitive tumors in whom cure or major survival benefit cannot be expected from currently available anticancer agents (e.g., carboplatin in previously untreated head and neck carcinoma) and (b) previously untreated patients with tumors not responsive to "standard" anticancer agents (e.g., renal cell carcinoma).

Similarly, the identification of toxicity of new analogues may pose a problem if the patient had already been exposed to the maximal cumulative doses of the parent compound (e.g., the phase I study of rubidazone in patients who had received doxorubicin). They would be unduly exposed to a high risk of toxicity or the toxicity might become apparent much earlier. We saw that vindesine-induced neurological toxicity was enhanced in patients with prior exposure to vincristine (68).

A recall phenomenon is another problem when patients with prior chemotherapy or radiotherapy are exposed to new phase I agents. This is exemplified in our own experience where pyrazofurin-induced skin toxicity was found to be more pronounced in the previously irradiated skin (70).

Based on response to currently available agents, human tumors have been classified as curable, subcurable and precurable (41). Curable tumors include choriocarcinoma, acute lymphoblastic leukemia, Burkitts's tumor, Wilms' tumor, Hodgkin's disease, testicular cancer, certain stages of embryonal rhabdomyosarcoma and Ewing's tumor, and the best series of patients with osteogenic sarcoma. Subcurable tumors include acute myelocytic leukemia, large cell lymphoma, breast cancer, localized small cell lung cancer, and ovarian cancer. Precurable cancers constitute advanced head and neck cancer, non-small cell lung cancer, advanced cancers of the gastrointestinal tract, metastatic renal cell cancer and metastatic melanoma. Basically, patients available for phase I study with curable tumor are heavily pretreated and those with subcurable tumors are less heavily treated. Theoretically, patients with precurable disease, in whom survival is not increased by currently available treatment can, be entered to phase I studies before "standard treatment".

(3) Patients must have a performance satus (PS) of 3 or less in Zubrod scale or at least 40% on the Karnofsky scale.

Zubrod and Karnofsky classifications of PS are shown in Table 2. It is noted that Zubrod scale 3 or less corresponds to Karnofsky's scale of more than 40 points. The PS is an important prognostic factor in certain disease categories where the correlation between PS and life expectancy has been found (1, 47). Similarly, the PS was correlated with tolerance to surgery, to aggressive chemo/radiotherapy (59) and to response rate (60). The most widely cited study correlating the pretreatments PS and survival is that by Stanley (101), where median survivals of patients with inoperable lung cancer were 24, 23 = 27, 14 = 21, 7 = 9 and 3 = 5 weeks for patients with Zubrod PS scale of 0, 1, 2, 3 and 4, respectively. The patients with Zubrod scale 3 may mean those with a survival as short as 7 weeks. This life expectancy should be construed as a compromise assuming that patients will recover from subacute toxicity (e.g., myelosuppression) within this time-span and be analyzable. Such a short survival is, however, not optimal for identification of delayed toxicitiy (e.g., doxorubicin-induced cardiotoxicity) and it is recognized that this is the major limit-

Table 2. Performance status scale.

Zubrod performance status scale

Grade	Description
0	Fully active, able to carry out all predisease activities without restriction.
1	Restricted in physically strenuous activity but ambulatory and able to carry out work of a light or sedentary nature.
2	Ambulatory and capable of all self-care, but unable to carry out any work activities; up and about 50% or more of waking hours.
3	Capable of only limited self-care, confined to bed or chair 50% or more of waking hours.
4	Completely disabled; cannot carry on any self-care; totally confined to bed or chair.

Karnofsky performance scale

Point	Activity status	Description
100	Normal activity	Normal, with no complaints or evidence of disease.
90		Able to carry on normal activity, but with minor sign or symptoms or disease present.
80		Normal activity, but requiring effort; sign and symptoms of disease more prominent.
70	Self-care	Able to care for self, but unable to carry on other normal activities.
60		Able to care for most needs but requires occasional assistance.
50		Considerable assistance required, along with frequent medical care; some self-care still possible.
40	Incapacitated	Disabled and requiring special care and assistance.
30		Severely disabled; hospitalization required, but death from disease not imminent.
20		Extremely ill; supportive treatment, hospitalized care required.
10		Imminent death.
0		Dead.

Comparison of Zubrod scale and Karnofsky scale

Zubrod	Karnofsky	Bried definition
0	100	asymptomatic.
1	80–90	symptomatic, but fully ambulatory.
2	60–70	symptomatic and in bed less than 50% of the day.
3	40–50	symptomatic and in bed more than 50% of the day, but not bedridden.
4	20–30	bedridden.

ing factor of currently accepted procedures for phase I clinical trials.

It may be added that the PS does not correlate with survival for all disease categories. It is well known that patients having ovarian cancer with Zubrod scale 4 from intestinal obstruction can live for months with parenteral nutritional support. Similarly, patients with neurological injury (e.g., sacral chondrosarcoma) with Zubrod scale 4 live for many months. Recently, the uses and limitations of the PS scales were defined and the problems inherent in their application were reviewed (82).

Alternative to the PS is a practice of estimating survival. However, both PS and survival estimates are imperfect in estimating actual patient survival. Development of new criteria which incorporates other factors such as disease categories, nutritional status and biochemical abnormalities are desired.

(4) Patients must have normal liver, renal and bone marrow functions, unless otherwise indicated by the specifics of the leukemia or pharmacokinetic protocol.

The initial cohort of patients should have normal major organ function, especially normal bone marrow function (not applicable to leukemias) and normal functions for major excretory or inactivation systems, kidney and liver. The normal bone marrow function which can be arbitrarily defined as a WBC of more than $4000/\mu l$ with normal differentials and platelets of more than $100,000/\mu l$, has been satisfactory in Phase I trials. Although marrow reserve can be more precisely defined by marrow stimulation studies using either endotoxin or ethiocholanolone, and a correlation between the degree of marrow reserve and marrow toxicity can be made, the marrow reserve studies have not been common as a prerequisite for phase I studies. The reasons for this are that if marrow toxicity were recognized at a specific dose level, a lower dose by 1 or 2 steps can safely be tested in patients with suspected compromised marrow reserve (extensive prior chemotherapy and/or radiotherapy, or neoplastic involvement of the bone marrow). It is not necessary to use any cut-off point for hemoglobin/hematocrit levels. Blood transfusion can be given prior to the start of trials to exceed the hemoglobin/hematocrit level which produces symptoms. Those who require frequent transfusions cannot be analyzed for toxicity to erythropoiesis.

In the later part of the study, it has been customary to cautiously enter patients with bone marrow involvement with tumors or marrow dysfunction from prior exposure to myelosuppressive agents at lower than "current" dose levels, in order to test the effects of the drug on compromised marrow function. In so doing, we have shown that such drugs as dichloromethotrexate (25) and bleomycin (79) can be well-tolerated in patients with mild to moderate marrow dysfunction. Similarly, we found entry of patients with mild to moderate impairment of hepatic and/or renal function provided useful clinical toxicity data. This is exemplified in our experience with vindesine, wherein patients with preexisting hepatic dysfunction developed more hematological toxicity and neurotoxicity (68), an observation consistent with known excretion of this class of compounds through the liver (19). These patients are also useful candidates for pharmacokinetic studies, in order to evaluate changes in pharmacokinetic parameters vs. clinical toxicity. Such information is of critical value in the eventual application of drugs in therapy.

By the same token, patients with significant third fluid space accumulations should not be entered in the early phase of the study because the third fluid space may act as a reservoir for a certain drug (e.g., methotrexate), thus possibly exposing the patient to increased toxicity. In the latter phase of the study, however, patients with significant third fluid space will be deliberately entered at lower dosages of 1 or 2 steps to evaluate the effects of third space on clinical toxicity. We have shown such third space effects for mit-

oguazone dihydrochloride (40), neocarzinostatin (75) and carboplatin (52).

The concept in evaluating the influence of preexisting major organ dysfunction can be extended to dysfunctions other than the ordinary organ systems of drug excretion and metabolism. This is exemplified by a trial of carboplatin in patients with preexisting cisplatin-induced peripheral neuropathy and ototoxicities, showing that repeated cycles of carboplatin were tolerated in such patients (74). Mitroxantrone was given to patients who had received full cardiotoxic threshold doses of doxorubicin. They were monitored with serial ventricular ejection fraction assessment as well as selected endomyocardial biopsies. While these approaches require diligent monitoring of candidate patients by experienced clinical investigators, only through such an approach can useful information, not otherwise obtainable, become available.

(5) Patients' concurrent medication must be under the complete control of the investigator.

The effects of an anticancer agent may be modified by prior or concurrent administration of other non-anticancer agents. An improved therapy is sometimes possible by judicious use of concurrent medications as described in the previous section. Anticancer Agents, *Phase I combinations*. However, serious adverse effects may also result from drug interaction. Interactions of anticancer agents with other drugs can be conveniently classified as: (a) direct chemical or physical interaction, (b) interaction during intestinal absorption, (c) interaction at plasma or blood transport sites, (d) interaction at the cellular receptor site, (e) interaction by accelerated or inhibited metabolism, (f) altered acid-base balance leading to changes in drug distribution and renal clearance, (g) alterations of renal function that influence rates of renal excretion, (h) alterations in cellular transport mechanisms, and (i) alterations in cellular biochemical pathways and drug resistance (15).

Nitrogen mustard and many of its derivatives are highly reactive compounds. Thus, direct chemical inactivation in physical mixtures of drugs in infusion solutions is a likely problem. Doxorubicin precipitates in a syringe containing heparin; for simultaneous administration of these 2 agents 2 intravenous lines are needed. Patients who are on continuous infusion of parenteral nutrition or those receiving Amphotericin B daily as a 6 hour infusion pose a problem when one wishes to study a drug by continuous infusion schedule just for mechanical reasons.

Procarbazine, a monoamine oxidase inhibitor is known to interact with (a) alcohol, causing antabuse-like reactions; (b) central nervous system depressants synergistically; (c) hypoglycemic agents, increasing hypoglycemia; (d) levodopa, causing hypertensive crisis (nullified by carbidopa); (e) meperidine, causing hypertension or hypotension and coma; (f) symphathomimetic amines, causing hypertensive crises and (g) tricyclic antidepressants, causing hyperpyrexia and convulsions (10).

Mithramycin, given for the treatment of hypercalcemia, may produce thrombocytopenia which may be interpreted to be a result of the concurrent phase I agent. Lorazepam, given as an antiemetic, may produce lethargy, which may be mistakenly considered from the concurrent phase I agent.

Methotrexate absorption may be profoundly altered by concomitant use of antibiotics which suppress gastrointestinal microbial flora (114). Methotrexate is transported on serum albumin, and both aspirin and sulfonamides are known to displace this drug and, thereby, to alter free drug levels and drug toxicity (22). Cellular transport of specific drugs may be altered by other drugs. One example of this appears to be the inhibition of methotrexate transport across cell membranes by L-asparaginase (61).

Allopurinol, a potent xanthine oxidase inhibitor, can profoundly affect the metabolism of 6-mercaptopurine. Clinically, this effect results in markedly augmented toxicity when the 2 drugs are used in combination, and it is, therefore, necessary to decrease the dose of 6-mercaptopurine to 25% of the usual amount (8).

We have shown that the inhibitory effects of certain anticancer agents are influenced by the presence of human serum albumin (104, 105), and such agents as salicylate, dicloxacillin and sulfisoxazol displaced albumin binding of dichloromethotrexate, thereby producing increasing biological effects *in vitro* (64). These observations clearly indicate the need to examine concurrent medication for the administration of agents known to have a high affinity to serum albumin.

(6) Patients must give signed, informed consent, indicating that they are aware of the investigational nature of the studies involved.

When a research procedure is carried out on a patient, the clinical investigator must inform the patient (or a responsible relative or guardian, if the patient or subject is not competent to act on his own behalf) that the patient is a participant in a research study and the investigator must obtain a signature on a written consent form.

Basic Elements of Informed Consent contain the following, as specified in Federal Register Vol. 46, #17, January 27, 1981: (a) a statement that the study involves research, an explanation of the scope, aims and purposes of the research and the procedures to be followed (including identification of any treatment or procedures which are experimental) and the expected duration of the subject's participation; (b) a description of any foreseeable risks or discomfort to the subject; (c) a description of any benefits to the subject or to others which reasonably may be expected from the research; (d) a disclosure of appropriate alternative procedures or courses of treatment, if any, that might be advantageous to the subject; (e) a statement describing the extent, if any, to which confidentiality of records identifying the subject will be maintained (The patient should be informed that his/her medical record may be inspected by sponsoring agencies); (f) for research involving more than minimal risk, an explanation as to whether any medical treatments are available if injury occurs, and, if so, what they consist of, or where further information may be obtained; (g) an explanation of whom to contact for answers to pertinent questions about the research and research subject's rights, and whom to contact in the event of a research-related injury to the subject; and (h) a statement that participation is voluntary, refusal to participate will involve no penalty or loss of benefits to which the patient is otherwise entitled, and the patient may discontinue participation at any time without penalty or loss of benefits to which the patient is otherwise entitled.

When appropriate, one or more of the following elements of information will also be provided to each patient: (a) a statement that the particular treatment or procedure may involve risks to the patient which are currently unforeseeable; (b) anticipated circumstances under which the patient's participation may be terminated by the investigator without regard to the patient's consent; (c) any additional costs to the patient that may result from participation in the research; (d) the consequences of a patients's decision to withdraw from the research and procedures for orderly termination of participation by the patient; (e) a statement that significant new findings developed during the course of the research which may relate to the patient's willingness to continue participation will be provided to the patient and (f) the approximate number of patients involved in the study.

(7) Patients must have no previous myelosuppressive anticancer therapy for at least 4 weeks and must have recovered from the toxic effects of prior treatment.

This is an important criterion in order to differentiate between delayed toxicity from prior therapy and acute or subacute toxicity from a phase I agent under study; and to preclude the possibility of toxicity arising from additive or synergistic effects of prior therapy and a phase I agent under study. However, several exceptions to this criterion must be considered. First, drug-induced alopecia (e.g., doxorubicin-induced), which may last as long as 6 months before full recovery, but is of minor importance for toxicological evaluation, can be excluded. Second, when there is a patient with leukemia in relapse who satisfies all other eligibility criteria except this one and who has rapidly increasing leukemic white cell count, a waiting period of 4 weeks is not logically justified if myelosuppressive effects are expected from that particular phase I agent. In addition, if prior anticancer therapy involves radium implant, hormonal treatment and such anticancer agents as nitrosourea which produce prolonged effects on bone marrow, a longer waiting period may be required.

(8) Protocol must specify a patient's age range; consideration of sex is not usually necessary.

As stated earlier the tolerance by children to chemotherapeutic agents differs from that of adults. While for the majority of drugs evaluated no major differences in tolerance were noted between adults and children when the drugs were given on a mg/m^2 basis, a commonly accepted impression that children generally tolerate drugs better than adults may be too simplistic. Thus, the ratio of tolerance for children over adults ranged from 83% for dihydrogalactitol to 200% for cyclocytidine and more than 220% for ICRF 187 (30). Pharmacokinetics of several drugs were shown to be different for children compared to adults (97, 109). It is essential, therefore, if children and adults are entered in the same protocol that they should be studied and analyzed separately. This does not preclude, in certain drugs, studies in children in association with pediatric oncologic colleagues after studies have been initiated in adults (e.g., vinca alkaloid analogues for the treatment of acute lymphoblastic leukemia).

In certain chemotherapy protocols, the upper limits of age was customarily set at 60 years (e.g., protocols for the treatment of acute myelocytic leukemia) because of lesser tolerance to myelosuppressive agents and expected higher toxicity. With the increasing life span in man and the better supportive care now available, it is possible to remove this upper age limit for the study of phase I agents. It is advisable, however, to analyze the data including age as a variable if sufficient patient population is available. This is of particular interest if pharmacokinetic methods are available. Geriatric pharmacokinetics have not yet been carried out extensively in the cancer chemotherapy field.

In certain chemotherapeutic agents, sex differences in toxicity have been recognized in experimental animals. For example, in animal study of acivicin, female CDF1 mice showed evidence of 3-fold increased sensitivity to the toxic effects of the compound than did males (16). Our clinical study of acivicin (100) and those by others failed to confirm this observation in man. In general, no chemotherapeutic agents are known to be tolerated differently in men and women. Dacarbazine is shown to be less effective in men for the treatment of cutaneous melanoma; however, no clear differences in tolerance or pharmacokinetics between men and women have been reported.

INITIAL (STARTING) DOSE

To determine the initial dose in man, all drugs in the chemotherapy program at the National Cancer Institute were studied both in the rhesus monkey and the beagle dog employing a standard toxicological protocol. Routinely, half the animals were sacrificed 1 day or 1 week after the last treatment for pathologic examination, while the other animals were allowed at least 45 days following the last treatment to recover from drug effects or to demonstrate signs of delayed toxicity.

Based on these large animal toxicological studies, *Toxic Dose Low* (TDL) – that dose which is just able to produce pathologic alterations in clinical, hematological, chemical or morphological parameters; by definition, doubling this dose produces non-lethality – was established in large animals for single-dose and 5 consecutive daily treatments. Studies in dogs and monkeys were also utilized to obtain information on the major organ toxicity in both species. Attempts were made to determine the predictability and reversibility of acute or delayed toxic effects and to compare the consistency of quantitative and qualitative observations within and between the species. The influence of dosage schedule on drug toxicity was also evaluated.

The initial clinical doses were, thus, decided as a fraction of the defined toxic dose, and for the past several years it has been customary to start at one-third the TDL, expressed in mg/m^2, of the most sensitive large animal. The use of the 1/3 TDL as a safe initial clinical dosage has been confirmed (36, 84).

Important questions have, however, been raised concerning such preclinical toxicology protocols. To what extent do they provide useful information concerning safety in the clinical introduction of a new antitumor agent? Is it possible to streamline the preclinical toxicologic program with respect to time and monetary expenditure? Should other approaches be investigated? Such questions led the National Cancer Institute to a reexamination of the preclinical toxicological protocols and phase I clinical data.

Overall, the combined large animal screen did predict a useful population of the total spectrum of qualitative toxicities inherent in a new compound: however, these correct predictions were accomplished at the cost of a high percentage of false positives, particularly for renal and hepatic toxicity (93, 94). There were several possible explanations of the high incidence of overprediction. For determination of all possible qualitative toxicities inherent in a given compound, the drugs had to be given at severely toxic, sometimes lethal-dose levels. This was particularly true for the prediction of hematological, liver and neurological toxicity. This stands in contrast to a phase I clinical trial where the study is terminated when the first dose-limiting toxicity is encountered. In addition, there appeared to be definite differences in organ system sensitivity to drug toxicity among the 3 species. Man may or may not show toxicity in an organ system predicted to be susceptible by the animal studies; moreover, this toxicity may be expressed in a different specific clinical or chemical parameter. It was also observed that the adverse reaction may appear in man at a greater or lesser dosage level than in the animal, or it may follow a different order of appearance in relation to the total spectrum of qualitative toxicity inherent in the compound. These data have shown that there is no real advantage using large animal species instead of rodents (90).

It became increasingly clear that murine-defined toxic doses were predictable for human dose (28, 36, 90). The distribution of the ratio of the MTD in man over 1/6 LD$_{10}$ (lethal dose in 10% of the animals) in mice and that of the ratio of the MTD in man over 1/3 TDL in dog was found to be very similar (90). Using 1/10 LD$_{10}$ in mice or the lowest of 1/6 LD$_{10}$ in micee and 1/3 TDL in dogs, a similar number of dose-escalation steps in phase I clinical trials were required when escalation schemes were based on the Fibonacci series (84).

In the current system, implemented in 1981, a dose response curve of a new drug is developed in mice. The LD$_{10}$, LD$_{50}$ and LD$_{90}$ are determined for daily $\times$ 1 and daily $\times$ 5 schedules, and the reproducible dose that is lethal in 10% of tested animals (LD$_{10}$) is hence used to establish an initial dose for clinical trials. This dose is further tested for toxicity in dogs prior to its use in humans. To maximize safety when administering an unknown compound in humans, 10% of the LD$_{10}$ in rodents is selected for the initial human dose. While correlation of toxic effects on rapidly dividing normal tissue (marrow and gastrointestinal tract) between rodents, dogs, monkeys and man is good, correlation of other toxic effects is not as consistent. Therefore, routine pathologic examination of rodent tissue is not performed prior to clinical testing. The validity and safety of this approach were recently confirmed (38).

EXPRESSION OF DRUG DOSING

Various expressions of drug dosing are listed in Table 3. Chemotherapeutic agents are currently being given nearly exclusively on a mg/kg or mg/m^2 basis. The expression of drug dosing using m^2 of body surface is the most popular because it gives a clear advantage in conversion of animal data to man and better correlations between adults and children's doses.

We looked into the suitability of other expressions of drug dosing. For example, we tested administration of drugs on moles or millimoles/m^2 basis (an unpublished trial in treatment using high dose methotrexate). This expression is ideal

Table 3. Expression of drug dosing.

	Advantage	Disadvantage
1. Tablespoonful, teaspoonful		
2. Ounce, grain, tablet		
3. ml or mg		
4. mg/kg		
5. mg/m^2	(1) Animal toxicological data can be coverted to man (2) Correlates with cxt (3) Better for children	(1) Need nomogram (2) Tends to overdose obese or elderly patients
6. moles/m^2	(1) Easier to evaluate pharmacokinetic data (2) Easier to evaluate analogs (3) Direct comparison of *in vitro* and *in vivo* data may be possible (4) In accord with direction of SI	(1) Unfamiliar; calculation errors (2) mg/m^2 is needed for transfer of animal data to man
7. moles/TBW	(1) Ideal for drugs which distribute to TBW	(1) Difficult to estimate TBW (2) Probably not useful for drug not distributed to TBW
8. moles of free drug/m^2	(1) More precise expression of biological activity	(1) Amount of free drug may vary depending on concentration of binding protein
9. biological unit/m^2	(1) Probably most nearly ideal	(2) Parameters of biological effect must be defined

TBW, total body water.

when pharmacological data are given on a molar basis. Thus, it appears to make more sense to give 6.6×10^{-3} moles/m^2 instead of 3 gm/m^2 of methotrexate and to say that the 24 hour methotrexate plasma level is 10^{-6} M. Consequently, we also tested administration of drugs as moles/liter of total body water (TBW), based on a calculation of TBW using creatinine clearance. The advantage of this method is that the expression is ideal for a compound that has an initial distribution volume equal to TBW, when one wishes to do concurrent pharmacological study. There are other expressions of drug-dosing such as expressions based on a free-drug concentration for a drug with high-protein binding affinity (104) or the use of units based on biological activity (e.g., bleomycin).

ROUTE OF ADMINISTRATION

Drugs may be administered orally (po), intravenously (iv), intraarterially (ia), intracavitally or intrathecally. The primary role of chemotherapy is the systemic treatment; oral and iv administration are the primary routes to be studied initially. While oral administration is the preferred route, initial clinical trials usually begin with the iv route because of the uncertainty of absorption by the alimentary tract. Indeed, the majority of anticancer agents are commonly given intravenously.

If animal pharmacology data of a new compound shows excellent bioavailability orally, then its oral administration can be studied in man only after the completion of the study using the iv route. In clincal trials of oral administration, concurrent pharmacological studies for bioavailability are essential.

DOSE SCHEDULES

Determination of an optimal schedule is important in any drug. This is exemplified by the fact that cytosine arabinoside has almost no activity on iv bolus, but is active as a continuous infusion schedule. In current practice, phase I agents are mainly tested using 4 different schedules: (a) single iv bolus every 3 weeks, (b) daily iv bolus $\times 5$, (c) weekly, and (d) continuous infusion, with the premise that, any drug not active in any of these 4 schedules is clinically inert. This has been the case for most of the drugs being explored. On the basis of clinical and pharmacological rationale other dose schedules may be explored (Table 4). In order to test the pharmacological rationale that a drug with high affinity for serum albumin should be given frequently as an iv bolus (as many iv antibiotics are given), we tested dichloromethotrexate iv bolus every 6 hours. A twice-weekly schedule of bleomycin was based on experience reported in foreign trials. In a reevaluation of mitoguazone, we tested

Table 4. Dose schedules for Phase I clinical trials.

"Standard" schedule
Single dose, iv bolus* every 3 weeks
Daily iv bolus* $\times 3$, $\times 5$, $\times 10$
Weekly
Continuous infusion

"Alternative" schedule	
iv bolus every 6 hours	e.g., Dichloromethotrexate (64)
iv bolus twice weekly	e.g., Bleomycin (79)
2 hr, 24 hr and 120 hr infusion	e.g., Mitoguazone (40)
6 hr infusion daily $\times 10$	e.g., Homoharringtonine (54)

* Include short infusion up to 1 hour.

Table 5. Examination of different dose schedules.

	Tolerance	Dose-limiting toxicity	Biological activity is likely: To be related to	Not related to	Ref
Vindesine	bolus = 24 hr infusion	Hematological	Total dose given[a]	Peak concentration or exposure time	68
Maytansine	bolus = 24 hr infusion	Hematological	Total dose given	Peak concentration or exposure time	12
Carboplatin	bolus = 24 hr infusion	Hematological	Total dose given	Peak concentration or exposure time	52
Neocarzinostatin	2 hr < 24 hr	Acute reaction vs. Hematological (mucosal)	Peak concentration Exposure time (?)	Exposure time	75
Mitoguazone	30 min < 24 hr < 120 hr	Neuromuscular vs. Mucositis	Peak concentration Exposure time (?)[b]	Exposure time	40
Phosphonacetyl L-aspartate	24 hr > 120 hr	Mucositis	Exposure time	Peak concentration	39
Homoharringtonine	6 hr < 24 hr	Cardiovascular vs. Hematological	Peak concentration Exposure time (?)	Exposure time	54

[a] cxt may be identical irrespective of infusion time.
[b] Increased tolerance with prolonged infusion may be due to rapid elimination or inactivation of the drug.

a short (30 min) infusion and 120 hour infusion biweekly. A six hour infusion of homoharringtonine was tested, based on Chinese data showing that a bolus dosing produced cardiovascular complications.

We find that the exploration and comparison of 2 or more schedules by a single investigator are an important method of obtaining information on the biological and pharmacological characteristics of a particular compound. Our experience in exploration of 2 or more schedules of phase I agents and likely pharmacologic explanations are summarized in Table 5. We tested vindesine and maytansine by weekly bolus and 24-hour infusion schedules. Both schedules were tolerated equally and dose-limiting toxicities were similar. From these data it may be suggested that the biological activity of these compounds is related to a total dose or to a component of a total dose given, and not related to a peak concentration or to the exposure time. Pharmacokinetic study of vindesine concurrently carried out in the phase I study confirmed our clinical impression (76). In contrast, in the case of neocarzinostatin we demonstrated that by increasing the infusion time from 2 hours to 24 hours, 3 to 4 times more doses of the drug were tolerated and the dose-limiting toxicity was shifted from "acute reaction"

to hematological toxicity (75). This observation suggests that the acute reaction is peak-concentration related and that the drug is rapidly eliminated or inactivated. Phosphonacetyl L-aspartate was found to be different in that the drug was less tolerated when infusion time was increased. This suggested that the exposure time rather than the peak concentration is important for the development of dose-limiting mucosal toxicity; we confirmed this pharmacologically (69).

In this context it is stated that the current art of pharmacokinetics is insufficient to explain all clinical toxicologic data. This is especially true if we attempt to correlate pharmacokinetic data of a short duration (e.g., 1–2 days) with incidious late developing complications. In our experience the pharmacokinetic data alone from bleomycin (72), pyrazofurin (77) and vindesine (76) were insufficient to explain degrees of pulmonary, cutaneous and neurologic toxicities, respectively.

When pharmacological data are available, one may be able to propose a new rational schedule. Our current thoughts along this line are illustrated in Table 6. If a drug has a short plasma half-life or short effects on a biochemical target, the drug can be given daily or even more often. If the

Table 6. Pharmacological data and proposal of schedule.

Plasma half life or effects on biochemical target	short	daily × 5, × 10; every 6–8 hours
	long	weekly, every 6 weeks
Phase or cycle specificity	yes	infusion
	no	bolus
Plasma binding	high	bolus
	low or no	bolus or infusion
Immunological	yes	daily schedule or infusion rather than weekly
Toxicity related to peak serum concentration		infusion

plasma half-life is prolonged or the effects on a biochemical target are long lasting, the drug may be given at longer intervals. The drug with phase or cycle specificity should be infused so that the cells coming to the specific phase or the cycle can be affected sequentially. Drugs with no phase or cycle specificity can be given as a bolus. If a drug has a high protein binding and the binding is time-dependent, a bolus administration at frequent intervals (e.g., every 6 hours) rather than continuous infusion may be evaluated. If a drug is immunogenic, as we have experienced in phase I trials of asparaginase (71, 73, 81), it should be given as a short daily course rather than weekly. Peak serum concentration-related toxicity is also apparent. We have shown that neocarzinostatin's acute toxicity is probably peak dose-related. Doxorubicin's cardiac toxicity was also thought to be peak-drug-concentration-related, and infusional treatment is being carried out (51).

DOSE ESCALATION

As a general rule, at least 3 patients are entered at the initial dose level. The second and third patients enter the study after a lapse of at least 1 week after entry of the first patient. Such spaced entry is followed in order to diminish the risk of toxic effects for each subsequent patient. After observing the course of 3 patients at the initial dose level, a subsequent cohort of patients can be entered and escalated at progressively higher dose levels if no dose-limiting toxicities are observed from the "current" dose. It is our practice that, during the initial period of dose escalation, no patient should have major organ dysfunctions or third space fluid and should be subject to meticulously close clinical observation. The first patient on any dose level should always be treated as an inpatient.

In the past, it was customary not to escalate the dose in the same patient during a phase I trial because of the difficulty that follows when it comes to interpreting the complex functions of dose, prior exposure, duration of exposure and cumulative toxicity with respect to subsequent findings. However, as we have gained experience our earlier practice was found to be not only impractical, but also non-economical. This is particularly true when the initial human dose is too low and produces no toxicity. For economy of study, for the information to be gained about the influence of prior drug exposure, for information about tolerated dose in a

patient not affected by a lower dose, for potential therapeutic activity and for the psychological influence on the patient, cautious escalation of dose in the same patients after a sufficient interval was found to be useful.

When a patient reaches a level which produces dose-limiting toxicity, subsequent patients can be treated at a dose 1 step lower, in order to differentiate dose level-related toxicity from time-related or cumulative dose-related toxicity. At toxic levels, more than 3 patients per dose schedule are required to further define the parameter of toxicity.

When a patient reaches a level which produces dose-limiting toxicity, several alternative paths can be considered. If the toxicity involved life-threatening complications (e.g., severe leukopenia with sepsis, anaphylaxis, renal shut-down or death) no further entry of patients to that level should be made. Instead, additional patients will be entered at a 1 step lower dose. The number of patients to be entered at the lower level depends on additional experience with life-threatening toxicity at that dose level. Only after confirmation that the lower dose is safe and that it does not produce dose-limiting toxicity, will the dose be escalated to an intermediary dose level. When the intermediary dose has been proven safe the dose can be escalated step-wise to and beyond the level which was life-threatening, intitially. When the dose-limiting toxicity was not life-threatening, more patients should be entered to that level for confirmatory purposes. Depending on the variability of the data, the number of patients to be entered will be determined. When the variability of toxicity is uncertain, one can deliberately enter previously heavily treated and previously untreated patients, patients with third fluid space and patients without third fluid space as well as patients with mild to moderate hepatic and renal dysfunctions. With this approach, one can delineate exact risk factors. One of our unique observations was that hypoalbuminemia was a major risk factor for dichloromethotrexate (64) and this was confirmed by others (112).

The methods of drug escalation we have used are listed in Table 7. Drug dose may be escalated by simple arithmetic progression from n to 2n, 3n, 4n,.... We used this cautious escalation in the study of maytansine because quantification of dose-limiting neurotoxicity was difficult and uncontrollable diarrhea, dehydration and death had been reported from other institutions using other schedules. The same holds true with mitoguazone where the biologically active dose and toxic dose were very close. Probably a more com-

Table 7. Does escalation of single agents experienced by the author.

1. Arithmetic progression n, 2n, 3n, 4n, 5n. . .	e.g., Maytansine (12), Mitoguazone (40)

2. Modified Fibonacci search scheme
    n, 2n, 3.3n, 5n, 7n, 9n, 12n. . .(33.3%)
	e.g., Amsacrine (32), Bleomycin (79), Indicine N-oxide (80),
	    Neocarzinostatin (75), Vindesine (68)

3. Fibonacci search scheme n, 2n, 3n, 5n, 8n, 13n. . .(61.8%)	e.g., Acivicin (100), Phosphonacetyl L-aspartate (69)
4. Geometric progression n, 2n, 4n, 8n, 16n. . .(100%)	e.g., Alanosine (35), Dichloromethotrexate (25), Mitoxantrone (34)
5. Modified geometric progression n, 2n, 4n, 6n, 9n. . .	e.g., Carboplatin (52)
6. Logarithmic progression n, 10n, 100n . . .	e.g., Asparaginase (71)

logarithmic escalation (100, 1000, 10,000 iu/kg of asparaginase).

Figure 1 illustrates the dose escalation schemes we tested and analyses of the human MTD of 12 diverse phase I compounds (84) at the National Cancer Institute. The number of steps required to reach the MTD by the most popular modified Fibonacci search scheme varied from 2 to more than 12, or from 2n to more than 49n and the median was 7 steps or 12n. A new analysis using the murine LD_{10} as a human starting dose again confirmed the safety with a median of 5 steps and a range of 0–15 to reach the MTD (38). When we compare what we know about the MTD in man with these various escalation schemes, we note no major advantage or disadvantage of one schedule over the other, except in extreme cases of arithmetic or logarithmic progression. A dose reached in 7 steps in the modified Fibonacci search scheme is reached at the 6th step in the original Fibonacci search scheme. In a more recent protocol, we tested "100% × 2 then 50% increments" (modified geometric progression) for the ease of remembering the dose (e.g., carboplatin) (52). Our current position is that there is no need to adhere to a single escalation scheme. Drugs with steep dose-toxicity curves such as mitoguazone, drugs which produce dose-limiting neurotoxicity such as maytansine or vindesine, and drugs with cumulative effects should have a gentle and cautious escalation scheme. On the other hand, drugs with high TDH/TDL ratio (or high LD_{90}/LD_{10} ratio) and drugs where specific rescuing agents are available may be escalated more rapidly. Recently, dose escalation based on pharmacokinectic data in murine LD_{10} and human pharmacokinetic data from starting dose (1/10 murine equivalent LD_{10}) has been suggested (17).

Our experiences with dose escalations in combinations are summarized in Table 8. In the study of pyrazofurin plus azacytidine we attempted to escalate the 2 drugs alternately. In the study of amsacrine plus cisplatin, the 2 drugs were simultaneously escalated, and in the combination of thymidine plus 5-fluorouracil, we made the former a constant and escalated the latter. In retrospective analyses of our small series, we found it easier to delineate the biological effects of the target compound, using method 3. We believe and ideal escalation in combination is the escalation of one drug against a constant second drug, and this can be sequentially studied for each drug. This approach appears best-suited for the exploration of biochemical modulating agents, as discussed in the earlier section. In our work with 5-fluoro-

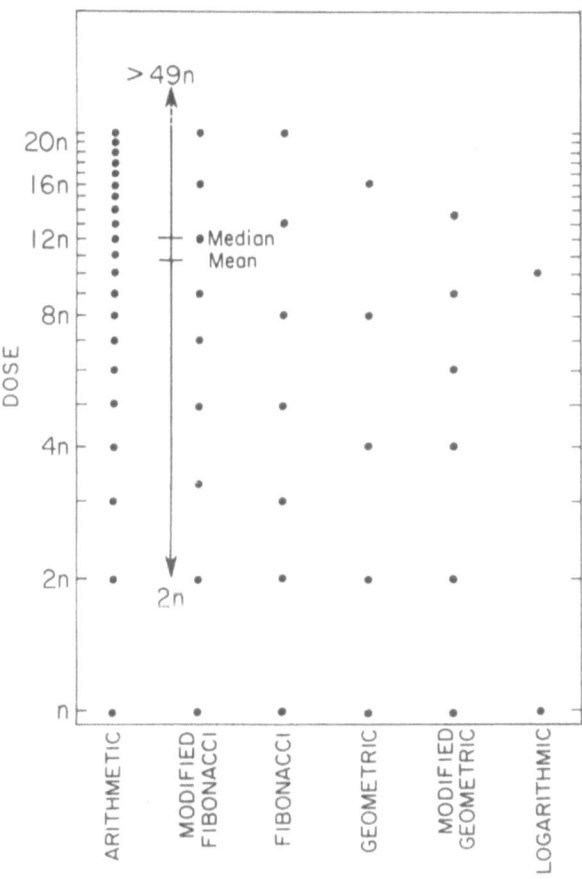

Figure 1. The relationship between the dose steps required to reach the human MTD and the various dose escalation schemes. In evaluating 12 phase I agents Penta et al (84) showed that by using the modified Fibonacci search scheme, it took from 2 to more than 12 steps to reach the MTD. This means that, if the starting dose (1/3 TDL) was n, then the human MTD was between 2n and over 49n. The median was 12n, or 7 steps to reach the MTD with the modified Fibonacci Search scheme. (For the calculation of the mean, actual available numbers were used).

mon method of escalation is a modified Fibonacci search scheme, in which the initial increment is 100%. The increment is then gradually decreased to a more gentle 33%. We used this escalation in a number of phase I agents. The original Fibonacci search scheme gave a somewhat steeper escalation with a final constant increment of 61.8%. A much steeper dose escalation can be achieved by geometric progression with a constant increment of 100%. We carried out this steep escalation in the study of dichloromethotrexate, alanosine and mitoxantrone. In the case of dichloromethotrexate, this escalation was possible because clinical toxicity was known from earlier clinical data and because it was our intention to combine dose escalation with leucovorin rescue. The steep escalation of alanosine was tested, based on dog data which showed a high TDH/TDL ratio of 800%. Similarly, mitoxantrone was escalated rapidly in our daily × 5 schedule becuase of known MTD from a single dose study. In one exceptional circumstance, we pursued a

Table 8. Dose escalation of phase I combinations experienced by the author.

(1) Drug A	n, n, 2n, 2n, 3n, 3n . . .
Drug B	p, 2p, 2p, 3p, 3p, 4p . . .
	e.g., Pyrazofurin and Azacytidine (11)
(2) Drug A	n, 2n, 3n . . .
Drug B	p, 2p, 3p . . .
	e.g., Amsacrine and Cisplatin (33)
(3) Drug A	n, n, n, n . . .
Drug B	p, 2p, 3.3p, 5p . . .
	e.g., 5-Flourouracil and Thymidine (78)
(4) Drug A	n, n, n, n, 2n, 3n, 5n. . .
Drug B	p, 2p, 3p, 5p. .xp, xp, xp. . .

uracil plus thymidine we were able to extrapolate our *in vitro* data to man.

The problem we face in a combination is that the different doses of 2 drugs in equitoxic combinations may not give equitherapeutic efficacy. This problem has to be resolved through a disease-oriented phase II study. The development of *in vitro* combination studies applicable to the clinical setting is desired.

ASSESSMENT OF DRUG COURSE FOR TOXICITY EVALUATION

For the precise determination of the nadir and recovery of drug-induced toxicity, the patient should ideally be evaluated through daily physical examination, daily blood counts, and daily chemistries, with chest X-rays and EKG's at frequent intervals until complete recovery of toxicity, which may require as much as 6 months for certain drugs (e.g., doxorubicin-induced alopecia). Certain biochemical and histological injuries may, however, never recover completely (e.g., bleomycin-induced pigmentation, doxorubicin-induced cardiomyopathy). In contrast, drug-induced toxicity can be recognized within a few minutes (e.g., asparaginase-induced anaphylaxis) to a few hours (e.g., cisplatin-induced vomiting).

Customarily, we examine inpatients daily and outpatients at least weekly for 3 weeks or until recovery from both acute and subacute toxicities (e.g., acute cutaneous reaction, gastrointestinal, central nervous system, hematological, biochemical and constitutional toxicities) with frequent examinations of blood counts and biochemical profiles. If analogs of a compound with known specific organ toxicity are being tested, specific relevant studies are also frequently performed. If any drug-induced toxicities are suspected in patients currently on study, new patients on the study will be more carefully evaluated to determine whether these suspected toxicities are reproducible. Examples of specific studies we carried out include EEG determinations prior to and after treatment with acivicin (100); urinary amino acid determinations prior to and after administration of neocarzinostatin (75); audiogram and urinary creatine clearance for carboplatin (52); and diligent monitoring of vital signs and ECG during homoharringtonine administration (54).

While it would be convenient and "clean" to consider patients followed for less than 21 days unevaluable, we feel that this approach is inappropriate in phase I studies. Patients who die "early" require special attention to assess whether their demise was related to drug administration. Patients followed less than 1 week should be evaluated for acute toxicity (e.g., nausea and vomiting, anaphylactic reaction, etc.), but not for subacute and chronic toxicities. Ordinarily assessment of hematological toxicity, specifically leukopenia (granulocytopenia) and thrombocytopenia, is performed only for those who have reached the nadir of toxicity, which occurs in most myelosuppressive agents within 2–4 weeks.

Since hematological toxicity is numerically definable, it has been our customary procedure that drugs with hematological toxicity that is dose-limiting will be followed until recovery of WBC and until platelet count is above the lowest normal range (usually WBC more than 4000/μl and platelets more than 100,000/μl). Some other toxicities are less definable and may require a prolonged period of follow-up. For chronic toxicities, usually those which last more than 2 months, we cannot set an arbitrary cut-off point and follow the patients as long as they are available for follow-up, in attempts to clarify reversibility of the chronic toxicity. Therefore, the follow-up period is dependent upon the period required for recovery from the major toxicity in question.

In some institutions patients become eligible only after receiving a minimum of 2 courses. This is a pitfall: a convenient method to eliminate poor risk patients who could not live long enough to receive 2 courses; it may invite bias to the toxicity evaluation because of artificial selection of the patient population.

TOXICOLOGICAL EVALUATION

The prime purpose of phase I study is the evaluation of toxicity in man. This is detailed below.

(i) It is ideal to daily observe clinical toxicity of all patients under study on an inpatient basis. Outpatient observation on phase I drugs not only puts risks on patients through unexpected toxicity, but also often misses the real nadir of toxicity. On the other hand, inpatient observation in the early phases of the study are often uneconomical and impractical because toxicity may never appear. Our current practice is to have patients path, with the initial dose and a leading dose, hospitalized and observed daily for 3–7 days, and if a method is available, for as long as material for pharmacological evaluation is required. After discharge, the patients are closely monitored through office and/or clinic visits, oncology nurse surveillance and telephone conversations. Additional patients at the same dose level may be treated as outpatients if the patient with the leading dose continues to tolerate it without major toxicity. At sufficient toxic levels, all patients will be observed as inpatients, or if they live close to the hospital, in the most appropriate fashion (e.g., blood counts 3 times a week).

(ii) Uniform criteria of toxicity grading are ideal for computation of data from different institutions for comparison purposes. The toxicity criteria recently developed at the National Cancer Institute is listed in Table 9. Grades 0, 1, 2, 3 and 4 correspond to none, moderate, slight, severe and life-threatening toxicity, respectively.

Several important considerations should be given to the toxicity criteria. First, it should be emphasized that a mild vomiting presumed to be well tolerated by an ordinary patient may be life-threatening in those with head and neck cancer with trismus or pharyngeal stenosis due to neoplastic involvement, because these patients may drown from vomitus. Second, it should be noted that the toxicity grading usually does not address dose-limiting nature. For example, BUN of 45 which is 2+ or moderate toxicity after asparaginase is reversible and of no major consequence, whereas BUN of 40 after cisplatin should be of major importance. Similarly, cisplatin produces usually intractable vomiting and will be recorded as severe; but it is recognized that severe (3+) vomiting is of lesser importance than 2+ or moderate nephrotoxicity. Similarly, "mild" pulmonary toxicity after bleomycin should be a serious problem be-

Table 9. Toxicity criteria proposed by the National Cancer Institute (1984).

	0	1	2	3	4
Leukopenia					
WBC × 10³	≥ 4.5	3.0–4.5	2.0–2.9	1.0–1.9	< 1.0
Gran × 10³	≥ 1.9	1.5–1.8	1.0–1.4	0.5–0.9	< 0.5
Thrombocytopenia	≥ 130	90–129	50–89	25–49	< 25
PLT × 10³					
Anemia					
HGB (gm%)	11.0	9.5–10.9	< 9.4	Not included	Not included
HCT (%)	≥ 32.0	28–31.9	< 28	Not included	Not included
Hemorrhage (non-surg)					
Clinical	None	Mild No transfusions	Gross, 1–2 units blood	Gross, 3–4 units blood	Massive, > 4 units blood
Infection					
Clinical	None	No active Rx	Requires active Rx	Debilitating	Life-threatening
Nausea/vomiting	None	Nausea only	Controllable	Intractable	Not included
Diarrhea					
Clinical	None	Semi-solid stools	Watery < 4 × daily	Watery > 4 × daily	Hemorrhagic, ehydration, electrolyte imbalance
Stomatitis					
Clinical	None	Erythema, screness	Ulcers, can eat	Ulcers, can't eat	Ulcers with hemorrhage & necrosis
Liver					
Bilirubin	< 1.25 × N	1.25–2.5 × N	2.6–5.0 × N	5.1–10.0 × N	> 10.0 × N
SGOT	< 1.25 × N	1.25–2.5 × N	2.6–5.0 × N	5.1–10.0 × N	> 10.0 × N
Alk. phos.	< 1.25 × N	1.25–2.5 × N	2.6–5.0 × N	5.1–10.0 × N	> 10.0 × N
Clinical	Not included	Not included	Not included	Pre-coma	Hepatic coma
Renal					
BUN	≤ 20	21–40	41–60	> 61	Not included
Creatinine	< 1.25 × N	1.25–2.5 × N	2.6–5.0 × N	5.1–10.0 × N	> 10.0 × N
Creatinine Cl.	N	0.75–0.99 × N	0.50–0.74 × N	0.25–0.49 × N	< 0.25 × N
Proteinuria	None	1+	2+ –3+	4+	Not included
Hematuria	None	Microscopic	Gross	Gross plus clots	Obstructive urooathy
Other GI					
Esophagus	None	Mild fibrosis, no pain, slight difficulty with solid food	Fibrosis, mild pain Semi-solid food only	Severe fibrosis, severe pain, liquid only, dial-ation required	Necrosis, fistual, perforation
Alopecia					
Clinical	No loss	Mild loss	Pronounced	Not included	Not included
Respiratory					
Symptoms	None	Mild or transient dyspnea	Dyspnea on exertion	Requires inter-mittent oxygen	Requires continuous O₂ or assisted ventilation
Function	Normal	25–50% decrease in DCO or VC	> 50% decrease in DCO or VC	Not included	Not included
X-ray	Normal	Linear streaking	Bilateral, opacifi-cation < 50% lung vol	Opacification 50–70%	Opacification > 75%
Cardiac					
heart	Normal	ST-T changes, sinus tachycardia > 110 at rest	Atrial arrhythmias, unifocal PVC's	Mild CHF Multifocal PVC's	Intractable CHF, ventricular tachycardia
Pericardial	Normal	Asymptomatic EKG suggestive of pericarditis	Symptomatic no tap required	Effusion requiring taps or constrictive pericarditis not requiring surgery	Tamponade or constrictive peri-carditis re-quiring peri-cardectomy
Neurologic					
strength	Normal	Mild weakness	Moderate weakness	Severe weakness	Paralysis
Reflex & sensory	Normal	Decreased DTR's mild paresthesia, mild constipation	Absent DTR's marked paresthesia marked constipation	Disabling sense loss, severe pain, obstipa-tion bladder dysfunc.	obstipation requiring surgery bladder included
Skin & subcutaneous skin (excluding surg. wounds)	Normal	Erythema, macules, papules, pigmentation; slight atrophy, nail changes	Dry desquamation vesiculation phlebitis	Ulceration moist desquamation severe pain	Exfoilation necrosis requiring surgery

Table 9. cont. Toxicity criteria proposed by the National Cancer Institute (1984)

	0	1	2	3	4
Other side effects fever (°C)	None	37.5–38	> 38	> 40, or with chills	Fever with hypotension
Allergy	None	Transient rash	Urticaria, broncho-spasm not needing parenteral therapy	Serum sickness, bronchospasm requiring parenteral therapy	Anaphylaxis

* Gran, granulocytes; N, normal range; DCO, diffusion capacity of carbon monoxide; VC, vital capacity; PVC, premature ventricular contraction.

cause of the often irreversible nature of the toxicity. Thus, the reversibility rather than the grade, should be considered an important factor of toxicity. While it is often difficult to identify chronic toxicity in phase I study, every effort should be made to identify late developing or cumulative toxicities by prolonged observation. Ideal candidate-patients for such study include those with slowly growing-tumors and those who are responding to the treatment.

Toxicities are classified according to the time of appearance:

(a) Acute toxicity: The toxicity developed soon after the drug was administered, ranging from immediately after the drug was administered (anaphylaxis, nausea and vomiting) to 1 week (hemolysis, diarrhea).

(b) Subacute toxicity: Toxicity developed between 1 and 3 weeks after the drug was administered (e.g., leukopenia, granulocytopenia, thrombocytopenia, stomatitis).

(c) Chronic (Delayed) toxicity: The toxicity developed after the third week of drug administration (e.g., skin and nail pigmentation).

(d) Cumulative toxicity: The chronic or delayed toxicity developing only after repeated dosing (e.g., doxorubicin-induced cardiomyopathy).

In the current practice of phase I clinical trials, emphasis is being made on rapid dose escalation, identification of acute and subacute toxicities and of the MTD, as well as the proposal of phase II dose in the shortest possible time using the least number of evaluable patients. While this approach is sound and economical, several additional considerations can be raised.

"Good risk" "poor risk" categorization

Phase I study requires determination of the rate, degree and duration of toxicity parameters. Since a drug may in the future be given to patients with preexisting organ dysfunction, it is required in phase I study to establish drug effects in patients with already impaired organ function. Since it is not always possible systematically to recruit patients with preexisting "signal" organ dysfunction for a dose level under study, a recommended dose derived from phase I study tends to be imprecise. It has been customary to give a recommended phase II dose based on "good risk" and "poor risk" categories. Since risk factors differ for each drug, we believe good risk and poor risk categorization is imprecise and thus unsatisfactory. It has been our routine procedure to analyze as many possible risk factors as possible in attempts to single out specific risk factors for specific

drugs, as related to clinically observed toxicities. This is exemplified in our evaluation of 12 possible risk factors in attempts to explain unexpectedly increased toxic manifestations in certain patients exposed to neocarzinostatin (75). In search of risk factors for dichloromethotrexate we found that patients with hypoalbuminemia developed increased hematological toxicity (64).

As has been the case with high-dose administration of methotrexate, pharmacokinetic data may presage clinically important toxicities. However, it is also clear that the current art and precision of pharmacokinetics are unsatisfactory in explaining all the toxicities. Here again, entry of patients with preexisting organ dysfunction for empirical observation may be as important.

Identification of chronic, delayed or cumulative toxicity

This is the most neglected area in phase I trials of anticancer agents. It has been argued that this category of toxicity can best be identified in phase II or III studies. Indeed, if there is no therapeutic activity, the drug will not be given repeatedly, and thus, identification of chronic toxicity would be unnecessary. While this argument is accurate for a majority of phase I compounds (because of a lack of therapeutic activity), this concept cannot be applied to analogue development. Anthracycline analogues shown to have no cardiomyopathic effects in animals, new bleomycin analogues without pulmonary toxicity and new cisplatin analogues without renal toxicity will be given repeatedly for a prolonged period of time. In such instances, attempts to delineate a new dose-limiting toxicity are the responsibility of phase I investigators. This concept is analogous to attempts to define non-hematological, dose-limiting toxicities in patients with leukemia after identification of myelosuppression as a major dose-limiting toxicity in patients with solid tumors. While a well-prepared, well-conducted phase II study will be able to provide this information, major emphasis of the phase II study is the identification of therapeutic effects, and detailed toxicological description is often lacking in phase II literature.

Histological study and post-mortem examination

Attempts are being made to obtain information on the histological abnormalities produced by phase I agents through biopsy and post-mortem examinations. During the phase I study of phosphonacetyl L-aspartate, we carried out serial skin punch biopsies in patients on-study to characterize cutaneous toxicities (39). Cardiac biopsies have now become routine for the development of anthracycline analogues. In contrast, we find histological data from routine post-mortem examinations difficult to interpret because of the exposure of the patient to various and often numerous chemotherapeutic agents. This exposure could preclude the attribution of a specific toxicity to any one particular drug. However, when certain toxicities are reproducibly seen (e.g., pulmonary toxicity from bleomycin), however, every attempt should be made to obtain permission for histological evaluation of the lesion in question.

ESTABLISHMENT OF THE MAXIMALLY TOLERATED DOSE (MTD) AND RECOMMENDED DOSE FOR THERAPEUTIC TRIALS.

The assumption underlying all phase I escalation procedures is that anticancer agents must be given at or near the MTD. Therefore, the goal of a phase I trial is to define the highest dose that can safely be delivered to a patient since this dose will also be the one that has the best chance of being active (55). This approach reflects the difficulties in establishing a clear-cut measurable end-point for drug's therapeutic activity. Since the induction of response is not always assured and is not usually an event that is immediately recognizable, attainment of toxicity is the only assurance that at least a biologically active dose was delivered.

This approach is justified since the relationship between dose and response is linear in a majority of studies; the higher the administered dose, the more probable are the antitumor effects (27, 45, 50), or the longer is the duration of response (37).

More recently, data suggesting the possibility that response does not continue to increase linearly as the dose approaches the MTD were presented both at laboratory (63) and clinical level (1). Further study in this area is needed before current practice of phase I evaluation is to be modified.

The definition of the MTD in large animals (dogs or monkeys) has varied from one toxicity report to another. Freireich et al (28) considered the MTD as the highest dose killing none of the animals under investigation. Homan (42) and Schein (93) defined the MTD as the dose producing only minimal reversible toxicity. In rodents, LD_{10} is considered the MTD. The definition of the MTD in man may vary greatly according to the individual investigator criteria, the selection of patient, the type of disease to be treated, and the quality of supportive care available. We define the MTD in a given schedule as the highest tolerable dose at which level toxicity is predictable, treatable and reversible. The MTD may be established on a single dose or on a cumulative dose repeatedly given at a lower level than the MTD established in a single dose. Patients with leukemia need a different definition. Since patients with leukemia receive large doses of drug to produce marrow aplasia, hematological toxicity becomes irrelevant and the MTD will be non-hematological. Clinically, the MTD can conveniently be decided as a dose which produces severe (3+) toxicity in 10% of good risk patients (see Table 9 for the definition of severe and life-threatening toxicities). The present method of 3-patient dose

Table 10. Sample size necessary to detect toxicity in at least one patient at a desired confidence level.

Desired confidence of detecting toxicity in at least 1 patient at specified dose level	True incidence of toxicity At specified dose level (P)			
	0.10	0.15	0.20	0.25
≥80%	16	10	8	6
≥90%	22	15	11	9
≥95%	29	19	14	11

evaluation, 25 patients per drug, cannot, however, ascertain the MTD in a biostatistically meaningful term based on the following considerations:

Statistical Consideration for the Determination of the MTD

The conventional method of procedure, which will be adhered to in our experimental design, is of the escalation of dose level following 3 consecutive "successes" at a given dose level (that is, 3 consecutive administrations without intolerable toxicity). While 3 successes are significantly different from 3 "failures" (intolerable toxicity) at a p value of 0.05 (Fisher's exact permutation test), there is a greater than 50% chance of accepting a drug as safe at a particular level even if the true incidence of untoward toxicity is as great as 20%. To be 80% confident of discovering a toxic effect at a given dose level, if the true incidence of toxicity is 20% it would require at least 8 patients treated at that level. That is, if the true incidence of intolerable toxicity were indeed 20%, there would be approximately an 80% chance of seeing at least 1 toxic occurrence in the first 8 patients treated (the actual probability is 83.2%), leaving a less than 20% chance of accepting that dose as "safe" if it were not. To be more than 95% sure of identifying a toxic dose (if the true incidence of toxicity is 20%), it would require 14 patients per dose level. Such calculations are based on the binomial distribution; where P is the probability of failure and the probability of n consecutive successes is $(1-P)^n$; Table 10 shows the sample sizes necessary to detect specified levels of toxicity. Therefore, to be confident at the $p = 0.05$ level of identifying a toxic drug level even as high as 25%, we would require 11 patients per dose level prior to escalation.

It may be possible that a single untoward toxicity occurs for a reason that would not be expected to occur again in a long series (e.g., anaphylaxis). In order not to disqualify this dose level as safe it may be advantageous to allow at least 2 occurrences of toxicity before rejecting this as unsafe (especially if the first 1 is of a rare type). Table 11 shows the sample sizes necessary to detect specified levels of toxicity using this scheme. Using this scheme, for example, if we detect toxicity in 1 or less of 18 patients then we can reject the hypothesis (at the 0.10 level) that the true incidence of toxicity is greater than 20%.

Both of these schemes require not only a large number of patients, but also represent an unethical practice. A reasonable approach to this problem, therefore, and our current practice, is as follows:

Table 11. Sample size necessary to detect toxicity in at least two patients at a desired confidence level.

Desired confidence of detecting toxicity in at least 2 patients at specified dose level	True incidence of toxicity At specified dose level (P)			
	0.10	0.15	0.20	0.25
≥ 80%	29	19	14	11
≥ 90%	38	25	18	15
≥ 95%	46	30	22	18

(a) Therapy should be initiated at an estimated safe level (*vide supra*).

(b) After 3 consecutive successful administrations, the dose level may be escalated, treating 3 consecutive patients at the next dose level, and so on.

(c) When any 1 of 3 patients in a certain dose level develops moderate degrees of toxicity additional patients will be entered. The number of patients to be entered will depend on the parameters of toxicity. When a toxicity such as leukopenia, which is numerically definable and quite constant is seen in a total of 6 to 10 patients it will be evaluated before escalation to a new dose based on the above Table. In contrast, peripheral neuropathy and other incidences less quantifiable as toxicities must be evaluated more carefully and more than 6 to 10 patients may be required to make certain that we are not seeing the MTD.

(d) At the first episode of severe or life-threatening toxicity (see Table 9 for definitions), that dose level will be suspended.

(e) Additional cases will then be treated at a dose step immediately below the level associated with the intolerable toxicity or the dose in-between: the number of such cases may be chosen from the Table 10, specifying a desired degree of confidence and an estimated percentage of "acceptable" toxicity. The entry of 8 good-risk patients at that new dose level without severe or life-threatening toxicity can reject the hypothesis that the dose is the MTD at a probability of less than 0.2.

(f) If factors of importance to drug metabolism or patient response are confounding in the experience at the toxic dose level, a cautious return to or toward the higher dose level may also be appropriate.

These procedures would assure both a desirable rate of dose escalation and a specified degree of confidence in the safety of the chosen maximal dose level. Several other important factors should be considered when attempts at determining the MTD are made. (a) As described earlier, if myelosuppression is dose-limiting in patients with non-hematological neoplams, the MTD may be different for patients with hematological neoplasms. In such cases, the non-hematological, dose-limiting toxicity may decide the MTD for patients with hematological neoplasms. (b) The MTD obtained in a phase I trial in advanced, cachectic, biochemically distorted patients with cancer may be too low in a phase II trial. We have, therefore, attempted on several occasions to grade the toxicity based on performance status, risk factors or disease categories (68, 75, 100). Depending on the drug studied, increased toxicities were correlated well with major organ dysfunction and prior exposure to certain chemotherapeutic agents. (c) The MTD for children is often

different than that in adults (*vide supra*). For this reason, the MTD for children should be developed independently. There are no clear data available on whether different age ranges in adult patients produce different MTDs, although clinical experience suggests that those over age 60 have less resiliency to injury from drugs. (d) It is important to determine, as has been discussed earlier, if there is a cumulative MTD in repeated courses (e.g., anthracycline cardiotoxicity) in phase I trials, in order to avoid late developing, fatal complications during phase II study. We have tested this question in weekly courses of maytansine in patients with very slow-growing tumors (12). It was concluded that the dose-limiting neurotoxicity is related to the total cumulative dose and to the starting dose. Thus, a cumulative dose of 6 mg/m^2 at weekly doses ranging from 0.4 to 1.3 mg/m^2 by iv bolus and 1 or 2 doses at 1.4 mg/m^2 produced severe neurologic toxicity. As a more recent example we have attempted to delineate the cumulative MTD of carboplatin (74).

Recommended Dose for Therapeutic Trial.

After establishment of the MTD, it is desirable to propose a recommended dose for therapeutic trial. Since we do not wish to propose severe toxicity in 10% of patients, recommended phase II doses are usually lower than the MTD. The recommended dose should produce predictable, moderate, reversible toxicity in the majority of patients, and should be a dose 1 step lower than MTD or a dose close to that. One cannot recommend a dose that has not been clinically tested which is between these steps. As experience accumulates from phases II and III trials, the eventual dose levels may, of course change.

Experience indicates that whenever a drug has dose-limiting side effects other than myelosuppression, its transition into phase II has often been compromised. An analysis of 31 drugs entered in phase I evaluation by the National Cancer Institute shows that whenever a drug has myelosuppression alone as the dose-limiting toxicity, it had a high probability of undergoing full phase II study; however, when other organ toxicity was dose-limiting, only 25% of the drugs proceeded to full phase II study (55). Evaluation of the remainder of drugs was restricted by either the National Cancer Institute or lack of investigator interest. The main reason for these difficulties related largely to the uncertainty regarding reversibility of acute major organ damage. In addition, even if organ damage turned out to be reversible, medical support during the periods of organ failure was either extremely intensive and costly (kidney, central nervous system), or technically unsatisfactory (liver), and was not seen as feasible or justifiable by most investigators in the context of a clinical experiment.

This dilemma appears to have no easy solution. In this context, the development of platinum coordination complexes is noteworthy. In order to overcome dose-limiting nephrotoxicities, 2 approaches were made; one was to develop anti-nephrotoxic regimens (e.g., hydration, hypertonic saline) and the other to develop non-nephrotoxic analogues (e.g., carboplatin). It is conceivable that it will take years of research before a new drug is perfected.

Table 12. Mathematical expression of the definition of response (modified from ref. 75)

Complete response (remission, regression) (CR)

$$\sum_{i=1}^{n} a_i(t)b_i(t) = 0$$

Partial response (PR)

$$\sum_{i=1}^{n} a_i(t)b_i(t) \bigg/ \sum_{i=1}^{n} a_i(0)b_i(0) \leqslant 0.5$$

and $a_i(t)b_i(t)/a_i(0)b_i(0) \leqslant 1.25$ for all i

and $n(t) \leqslant n(0)$.

Improvement (IMP), < PR or minimal response (MR)

$$0.5 < \sum_{i=1}^{n} a_i(t)b_i(t) \bigg/ \sum_{i=1}^{n} a_i(0)b_i(0) \leqslant 0.75$$

and $a_i(t)b_i(t)/a_i(0)b_i(0) \leqslant 1.25$ for all i

and $n(t) \leqslant n(0)$.

Stale disease (SD)

$$\sum_{i=1}^{n} a_i(t)b_i(t) \bigg/ \sum_{i=1}^{n} a_i(0)b_i(0) \leqslant 1.0 \pm 0.25$$

and $a_i(t)b_i(t)/a_i(0)b_i(0) \leqslant 1.25$ for all i

and $n(t) \leqslant n(0)$.

Progressive disease (PD)

$$\sum_{i=1}^{n} a_i(t)b_i(t) \bigg/ \sum_{i=1}^{n} a_i(0)b_i(0) \geqslant 1.25$$

and/or $n \geqslant n_0 + 1$

THERAPEUTIC ACTIVITY

Observation of therapeutic activity, by definition, is not required in a phase I study. We recognize the need and importance of observing this activity, however. This is based on the following reasons:

(a) Recognition of therapeutic activity means that a therapeutically active schedule has now been established in the phase I study and can be adopted in the phase II study.

(b) Recognition of therapeutic activity encourages phase II study investigators to work on the drug.

(c) Recognition of the therapeutic activity in certain disease categories serves to set up phase II and III studies of those particular disease categories.

(d) Responding patients can be observed for a prolonged period of time for possible chronic or cumulative toxicity.

In order to recognize even a minor response, "stable disease" status produced after the drug in patients with progressive disease should be considered of possible interest. It is, therefore, our current practice to include criteria of response in phase I protocols. Indeed, a recent analysis by the National Cancer Institute revealed that a drug shown to have therapeutic activity during the phase I trial had a better chance of being an active drug (24).

We devised the mathematical expression of therapeutic criteria commonly practiced for the evaluation of patients with solid tumors (75) (Table 12), where a and b are the longest and the widest perpendicular diameters of a tumor area. "a(0)b(0)" is the measurement on day 1, "a(t)b(t)" that after exposure to a drug or drugs under study. "Complete response (regression)" means the disappearance of an entire tumor area. "Partial response (regression)" is defined as more than a 50% decrease in the sum of the tumor areas. "Improvement" is synonymous with "Minimal Response" or "less than PR" and the decrease from the initial total tumor area is less than 50%, but more than 25%.

There are 2 recent developments in this area worthy of consideration: One is a proposal of new criteria for tumor response set forth by Warr *et al* (110) and the other focuses on the issue of the quality of life.

In the study by Warr *et al* simulated tumor nodules, pulmonary metastases on chest X-rays, malignant neck nodes and enlarged livers were each measured by a group of 8 physicians. Measurements of identical lesions were then compared to obtain an estimate of measurement error for each type of lesion evaluated. There was an increased false categorization of partial response for smaller simulated nodules. Larger errors were evident when using the current definition of disease progression requiring only a 25% increase in area. It has been concluded that many published trials have used criteria that are subject to large errors. Based on these results the authors have proposed the response criteria shown in Table 13.

The new criteria will require a test of time to determine whether it can correlate better for survival than the currently used one. Nevertheless, whether this new criteria is applicable to clinical testing of new anticancer agents is uncertain because phase I study investigators' goal is not to miss the active dose schedule during phase I trials, rather than obtain a precise documentation of response and survival prolonga-

Table 13. Response criteria proposed by Warr *et al* (110).

Criteria	Suggested changes
Progression	Redefine as a 100% increase in area* of any measurable lesion, or the appearance of new lesions.
Minimal response	This term should be abandoned.
Partial response	Redefine as a 50% decrease in area* of all index lesions recorded at two consecutive assessments at least 1 month apart. No new lesions should occur. Require a minimum duration† of 3 months. Require index lesions to have an initial mean diameter of 2 cm.
Complete remission	Require disappearance of all evidence of disease recorded at two consecutive assessments at least 1 month apart. Require a minimum duration† of 3 months.

---

* For malignant hepatomegaly replace "area" with sum of measurements of the liver edge below the costal margin in the midline and MCL. the distance of the liver edge below the costal margin in the midline or MCL must exceed 5 cm in order to use hepatic disease as a marker of response.

† Duration of response is the interval between start of treatment and the last assessment at which response criteria are satisfied.

tion. It is more likely that with this new proposal "a hint of activity" would be overlooked or ignored.

Recently, the quality of life in cancer patients became a major issue. Quality of life ranges from a psychological dysfunction due to the surgical loss of a breast, an organ endowed with self-dignity of a woman, to a comatose cancer patient on a respirator, where the decision of discontinuation of supportive care must be made. It has been shown that the quality of life can decrease by therapeutic intervention, in spite of tumor regression (88). It is, therefore, important for physicians to assess toxicity carefully, not only from a standpoint of whether it is expected or unexpected toxicity or how it influences the next dose of treatment, but also with regard to degree to which the toxicity may impact upon the patient's quality of life. This issue is especially important in the care of patients who are being treated for palliation without expectation of cure (since a transient decrease in quality of life might be justified in order to achieve a cure).

While the quality of life issue cannot be stressed more in the treatment of cancer, it cannot be used as an endpoint for the evaluation of a phase I agent; as the determination of the MTD is not compatible with the quality of life issue. Nevertheless, phase I study investigators are required to preserve the best quality of life expected for the patient on study, even with widespread tumor and in the presence of palliative interventions.

CONCLUSION AND PROSPECT

In this chapter the procedures used for transition of anticancer agents from animal to man is described in some detail. The procedure of antineoplastic drug development in man was largely an empirical effort. The procedures described here emphasize progressive improvements over the years in making them more scientific and rational: backed by animal data, pharmacological information and statistical input.

Recently, Staquet *et al* assessed the clinical predictability of the National Cancer Institutes' tumor panel for 69 anticancer agents. They reported that the correlation of screening and clinical results was low and that a modified approach using lesser numbers of animal tumor panel would have been sufficient. Based on their computer aided analyses, they proposed a new 3-stage strategy; P388 prescreen; screening with the B16, L1210 and MX-1 systems; and the 3rd stage screen with Co38, Lewis lung carcinoma and CX-1 (102). These observations will likely influence the current drug screening protocols at the animal level (106).

We have shown earlier the advantage of using human cell lines rather than animal cells for toxicological studies (65). Only recently, the use of a panel of human tumor cell lines to screen active anticancer agents has begun. The National Cancer Institute is currently working on development of a new *in vitro* screening model based on the use of established tumor cell lines. This model has been conceived as a "disease oriented" one in which panels of tumor cell lines are used to represent disease types (95). Automated growth inhibition assays compatible with large-scale screening are being evaluated for use in this model. In contrast, the important role of murine tumor model in optimizing dosage and administration schedules, and its potential for developing new combination chemotherapy has recently been emphasized (56).

At the clinical level concurrent pharmacokinetic studies will play an increasingly important role in obtaining a better understanding of drug clearance and elimination. Pharmacological approach during phase I trials has recently been described (48).

The goal of these studies is the establishment of optimal dose schedules for therapeutic studies (Phase II and Phase III studies), which will be applicable to cancer patients in good and poor risk.

In the years to come it is likely that laboratory investigation in animals, human tumor cells *in vitro*, as well as pharmacological data at the cellular level will have an increasingly important role. Areas of pharmacology more likely to be involved in the future will include (a) comparative pharmacokinetics in animals and man, (b) age related pharmacokinetics (pediatric pharmacokinetics and geriatric pharmacokinetics), (c) pharmacokinetics in patients with organ dysfunction, (d) pharmacokinetics of active metabolites within tumor cells and (e) determination (intensity and duration) of inhibition of intracellular target macromolecules.

The use of computers has become an integral part in the conduct of phase I trials. The computer not only provides better handling of data for hematological and biochemical nadirs within an institution, but promotes better communication between sponsoring agencies and hospitals in an on-line fashion for the timely transfer of data generated along the conduct of clinical trials. In addition, data on pharmacokinetic parameters in multi-compartment open models are commonly generated through the use of computers. It is expected that with the computerization of the entire hospital, necessary data will be generated and transferred to sponsoring agencies directly from the hospital, hematology and chemistry laboratories as well as from the pharmacy.

With the rapid expansion of availability of biologically-generated anticancer agents (biological response modifiers) obtained through new biotechnology (e.g., interferons, interleukin II, cell-mediated toxins and immunotoxins), this category of anticancer agents rather than cytotoxic chemicals will become a new source of phase I study. Since it is expected that for these agents the MTD and the optimal dose will differ considerably, new concepts and methodologies, including immunological and biological approaches, must be developed for the determination of the phase II dose. The best dose schedules of these agents will be developed based on the maximal biological response of the host rather than mere pharmacokinetic parameters. In this context the procedures for phase I study are constantly evolving, both conceptually and methodologically. Certainly, we are entering a new era in the therapeutic research of human cancer.

ACKNOWLEDGMENT

We thank Dr. L. Norton for the development of statistical consideration for the determination of the maximally tolerated dose.

REFERENCES

1. Aisner J, Alerto P, Bitran J, Comis R, Daniels J, Hansen H, Ikegami H, Smyth J: Role of chemotherapy in small cell lung

cancer: a concensus report of the International Association for the Study of Lung Cancer Workshop. *Cancer Treat Rep* 67:37–43, 1983

2. Ambinder EP, Perloff, Ohnuma T, Biller H, Holland JF: High dose methotrexate followed by citrovorum factor reversal in patients with advanced cancer. *Cancer* 43:177–182, 1979

3. Barlow JJ, Piver MS, Chuang JT, Cortes EP, Ohnuma T, Holland JF: Adriamycin and bleomycin alone and in combination in gynecologic cancers. *Cancer* 32:735–743, 1973

4. Bender RA, Bleyer WA, Frisby SA, Oliverio VT: Alteration of methotrexate uptake in human leukemia cells by other agents. *Cancer Res* 35:1305–1308, 1975

5. Bender RA, Nichol AP, Norton L, Simon RM: Lack of therapeutic synergism between vincristine and methotrexate in L1210 murine leukemia *in vivo. Cancer Treat Rep* 62:997–1003, 1978

6. Briscoe KE, Pasmantier M, Ohnuma T, Kennedy BJ: Cis-diammine dichloroplatinum (II) (NSC-119875) and adriamycin (NSC-123127) in treatment of advanced ovarian cancer. *Cancer Treat Rep* 62:1363–1366, 1979

7. Bruckner HW, Ohnuma T, Hart R, Jaffrey I, Spigelman M, Ambinder E, Storch JA, Wilfinger C, Goldberg J, Biller H, Holland JF: Leucovorin (LV) potentiation of 5-fluorouracil (FU) efficiency and potency. *Proc Am Assoc Cancer Res* 23:111, 1982

8. Calabresi P, Parks RE, Jr: Alkylating agents, antimetabolites, hormones and other antiproliferative agents. In *The Pharmacological Basis of Therapeutics*. 4th ed., (Eds.) Goodman LS, Gilman A. Macmillan, New York, pp. 1348–1395, 1970

9. Cancer Chemotherapy National Service Center. An outline of procedures for preliminary toxicology and pharmacologic evaluation of experimental cancer chemotherapeutic agents. *Cancer Chemother Rep* 37:1–37, 1964

10. Casciato DA, Lowitz BB: *Manual of bedside oncology*, Little, Brown and Co., Boston, Toronto, p. 54, 1983

11. Chahinian AP, Ohnuma T, Greenfield D, Holland JF: Sequential combination of pyrazofurin and 5-azacytidine in patients with acute myelocytic leukemia and carcinoma. *Oncology* 38:7–12, 1981

12. Chahinian P, Nogeire C, Ohnuma T, Greenberg M, Sivak M, Holland JF: Phase I study of weekly maytansine given as iv bolus or 24 hour infusion. *Cancer Treat Rep* 63:1953–1960, 1979

13. Chello PL, Sirotnak FM: Increased schedule-dependent synergism of vindesine versus vincristine in combination with methotrexate against L1210 leukemia. *Cancer Treat Rep* 65:1049–1053, 1981

14. Chello PL, Sirotnak FM, Dorick DM, Moccio DM: Schedule-dependent synergism of methotrexate and vincristine against murine L1210 leukemia. *Cancer Treat Rep* 63:1889–1894, 1979

15. Cline MJ, Haskel CM: *Cancer Chemotherapy*, 2nd edition, W.B. Saunders, Philadelphia, p. 19, 1975

16. Clinical Brochure AT-125, NSC 163501, Investigational Drug Branch, Division of Cancer Treatment, NCI, April 1979

17. Collins JM, Zaharko DS, Dedrick RL, Chabner BA: Potential roles for preclinical pharmacology in phase I clinical trials. *Cancer Treat Rep* 70:73–80, 1986

18. Cortes EP, Shedd D, Albert DJ, Ohnuma T, Hreschyshyn M: Adriamycin and bleomycin in advanced cancer. *Proc Am Assoc Cancer Res & ASCO* 13:66, 1972

19. Culp HW, Daniels WD, McMahon RE: Disposition and tissue levels of [^{3}H] vindesine in rats. *Cancer Res* 37:3053–3056, 1977

20. DeVita VT, Jr: *Principles of Chemotherapy.* In *Cancer. Principles & Practices of Oncology*, 2nd edition (Eds.), DeVita VT, Jr, Hellman S, Rozenberg SA, J.B. Lippincott,

Philadelphia, pp. 257–285, 1985

21. DeVita VT, Jr, Henney JE, Hubbar SM: Estimation of the numerical and economic impact of chemotherapy in the treatment of cancer. In *Cancer. Achievements, Challenges and Prospects for the 1980's* (Eds.), Burchenal JH, Oettger HF, Grune & Stratton, New York, pp. 859–880, 1981

22. Dixon RL, Henderson ES, Rall DP: Plasma protein binding of methotrexate and its displacement by various drugs. *Fed Proc* 24:454, 1965

23. Driscoll JS: *The preclinical new drug research program of the National Practice of Oncology*, 2nd edition (Eds.), DeVita VT, Jr, Hellman S, Rosenberg SA. J.B. Lippincott, Philadelphia, pp. 257–285, 1985

24. Estey E, Hoth D, Simon R, Marsoni S, Leyland-Jones B, Wittes R: Therapeutic response in phase I trials of antineoplastic agents. *Cancer Treat Rep* 70:1105–1115, 1986

25. Fernbach BR, Takahashi I, Ohnuma T, Holland JF: Clinical and laboratory reevaluation of dichloromethotrexate. *Recent Results in Cancer Res* 74:56–64, 1980

26. Fleishman G, Yap H-Y, Murphy WK, Bodey G: Phase II trial of acivicin in advanced metastatic breast cancer. *Cancer Treat Rep* 67:843–844, 1983

27. Frei E III, Canellos GP: Dose: a critical factor in cancer chemotherapy. *Am J Med* 69:585–594, 1980

28. Freireich J, Gehan EA, Rall DP, Schmidt LH, Skipper HE: Quantitative comparison of toxicity of anticancer agents in mouse, rat, hamster, dog, monkey and man. *Cancer Chemother Rep* 4:219–244, 1966

29. Giovanella BC, Stehlin JS Jr, Williams LJ, Lee SS, Shepard RC: Heterotransplantation of human cancers into nude mice. A model system for human cancer chemotherapy. *Cancer* 42:2269–2281, 1978

30. Glaubiger DL, von Hoff DD, Holcenberg JS Kamen B, Pratt C, Ungerleider RS: The selective tolerance of children and adults to anticancer drugs. *Front Radiat Ther Oncol* 16:42–49, 1982

31. Goldman ID, Fyfe M-J: The mechanism of action of methotrexate. II. Augmentation by vincristine of inhibition of deoxyribonucleic acid synthesis by methotrexate in Ehrlich ascites tumor cells. *Mol Pharmacol* 10:275–282, 1974

32. Goldsmith MA, Bhardwaj S, Ohnuma T, Greenspan EM, Holland JF: Phase I study of mAMSA in patients with solid tumors and leukemia. *Cancer Clin Trials* 3:197–202, 1980

33. Goldsmith MA, Holland JF, Ohnuma T, Hart R, Greenspan EM: Phase I evaluation of mAMSA and cisplatin (DDP) combination. *Proc Am Assoc Cancer Res & ASCO* 21:360, 1980

34. Goldsmith MA, Ohnuma T, Jaffrey IH, Greenspan EM, Holland JF: Phase I study of mitoxantrone on a daily × 5 schedule. *Am J Clin Oncol* 7:567–570, 1984

35. Goldsmith MA, Ohnuma T, Spigelman M, Greenspan EM, Holland JF: A phase I study of L-alanosine. *Cancer* 51:378–380, 1983

36. Goldsmith MA, Slavik M, Carter SK: Quantitative prediction of drug toxicity in humans from toxicology in small animals. *Cancer Res* 35:1354–1364, 1975

37. Gralla RJ, Casper ES, Kelsen DP, Braun DW Jr, Dukeman ME, Martini N, Young CW, Golby RB: Cisplatin and vindesine combination chemotherapy for advanced carcinoma of the lung: a randomized trial investigating two dosage schedules. *Ann Int Med* 95:414–420, 1981

38. Grieshaber CK, Marsoni S: Relation of preclinical toxicology to findings in early clinical trials. *Cancer Treat Rep* 70:65–72, 1986

39. Hart RD, Ohnuma T, Holland JF: Initial clinical study with N-(phosphonacetyl)-L-aspartic acid in patients with advanced cancer. *Cancer Treat Rep* 64:617–624, 1980

40. Hart RD, Ohnuma T, Holland JF, Bruckner HW: Phase I reevaluation of methyl-glyoxal bis-guanylhydrazone. *Cancer Treat Rep* 66:65–71, 1982

41. Holland JF: Breaking the cure barrier. *J Clin Oncol* 1:75–90, 1983
42. Homan ER: Quantitative relationships between toxic doses of antitumor chemotherapeutic agents in animals and man. *Cancer Chemo Rep* 3:13–19, 1972
43. Johns DG, Adamson RH: Enhancement of the biological activity of cordycepin (3′-deoxyadenosine) by the adenosine deaminase inhibitor 2′-deoxycoformycin. *Biochem Pharmacol* 25:1441–1444, 1976
44. Johnson RK, Goldin A: The clinical impact of screening and other experimental tumor studies. *Cancer Treat Rep* 68:63–76, 1984
45. Jones RB, Holland JF, Bhardwaj S, Norton L, Wilfinger C, Strashun A: A Phase I–II study of intensive-dose adriamycin for advanced breast cancer. *J Clin Oncol* 5:172–177, 1987
46. Kano Y, Ohnuma T, Okano T, Holland JF, Goldsmith MA: Schedule–dependent synergism and antagonism of methotrexate (MTX) and vincristine (VCR) combinations *in vitro*. *Proc Am Assoc Cancer Res* 24:270, 1983
47. Kansal V, Omura GA, Soong S: Prognosis in adult acute myelogenous leukemia related to performance status and other factors. *Cancer* 38:329–334, 1976
48. Kovach JS: Pharmacokinetic studies of anticancer agents during phase I trials. In *Pharmacokinetics of Anticancer Agents in Humans* (Eds.), Ames MM, Powis G, Kovach JS, Elsevier Science, Amsterdam, New York, Oxford, pp. 433–462, 1983
49. Kuwano M, Kamiya T, Endo H, Komiyama S: Potentiation of 5-fluorouracil, chromomycin A_3 and bleomycin and amphotericin B or polymyxin B in transformed fibroblastic cells. *Antimicrob Agents Chemother* 3:580–584, 1973
50. Lazarus HM, Herzig RH, Graham-Pole J, Wolf SN, Philips GL, Strandjord S, Hurd D, Forman W, Golden EM, Coccia P, Gross S, Hergig GP: Intensive melphalan chemotherapy and cryopreserved autologous bone marrow transplantation for the treatment of refractory cancer. *J Clin Oncol* 1:359–367, 1983
51. Legha SS, Benjamin RS, MacKay B, Ewer M, Wallace S, Valdivieso M, Rasmuse SL, Blumenschein GR, Freireich EJ: Reduction of doxorubicin cardiotoxicity by a prolonged continuous intravenous infusion. *Ann Int Med* 96:133–139, 1982
52. Leyvraz S, Lassus M, Ohnuma T, Holland JF: A phase I study of carboplatin (CBDCA) in patients with advanced cancer, intermittent iv bolus and 24 hour infusion. *J Clin Oncol*, 3:1385–1392, 1985
53. Madajewicz S, Petrelli N, Rustum YM, Campbell J, Herrera L, Mittelman A, Perry A, Creaven PJ: Phase I–II trial of high dose calcium leucovorin and 5-fluorouracil in advanced colorectal cancer. *Cancer Res* 44:4667–4669, 1984
54. Malamud SC, Ohnuma T, Coffey V, Paciucci PA, Wasserman LR, Holland JF: Phase I study of homoharringtonine (HHT) in 10 day schedule: 6 hr infusion daily vs continuous infusion. *Proc Am Assoc Cancer Res* 25:179, 1984
55. Marsoni S, Wittes R: Clinical development of anticancer agents – a National Cancer Institute perspective. *Cancer Treat Rep* 68:77–85, 1984
56. Martin DS, Balis E, Fisher B, Frei E, Freireich EJ, Heppner G, Holland JF, Houghton JA, Houghton PJ, Johnson RK, Mittelman A, Rustum Y, Sawyer RC, Schmid FA, Stolfi RL, Young CW: Role of murine tumor models in cancer treatment research. *Cancer Res* 46:2189–2192, 1986
57. Martin DS, Stolfi RL: Thymidine enhancement of antitumor activity of 5-fluorouracil against advanced murine (CD8F1) breast carcinoma. *Proc Am Assoc Cancer Res & ASCO* 18:126, 1977
58. Medoff G, Valeriote F, Lynch RG, Schlessinger D, Kobayashi GS: Synergistic effect of amphotericin B and 1,3-bis(2-chloroethyl)-1-nitrosourea against a transplantable AKR leukemia. *Cancer Res* 34:974–978, 1974
59. Moertel CG, Schutt AJ, Hahn RG, Reitmeier RJ: Effects of patient selection on results of phase II chemotherapy trials in gastrointestinal cancer. *Cancer Chemother Rep* 58:257–259, 1974
60. Mountain CF: Biologic, physiologic and biochemical determinations in surgical therapy for lung cancer. In *Lung Cancer: Clinical Diagnosis and Treatment*, (Ed.) Straus MJ, Grune and Stratton, New York pp. 185–198, 1977
61. Nahas A, Capizzi R: Inhibition of *in vitro* uptake of methotrexate by L-asparaginase in L5178Y murine leukemia cells. *Proc Am Assoc Cancer Res* 12:63, 1971
62. Neil GL, Moxley TE, Manak RC: Enhancement by tetrahydrouridine of 1-α-D-arabinofuranosylcytosine (cytarabine) oral activity in L1210 leukemia mice. *Cancer Res* 30:2166–2172, 1970
63. Norton L, Simon R, Tansman L, Holland JF: Non-monotonic dose response to chemotherapy of murine B_{16} melanomia. *Proc Am Assoc Cancer Res* 22:226, 1981
64. Ohnoshi T, Ohnuma T, Brown JC, Cohen S, Holland JF: Clinical and laboratory studies of dichloromethotrexate given every 6 hours. *Proc Am Assoc Cancer Res & ASCO* 22:353, 1981
65. Ohnuma T, Arkin H, Minowada J, Holland JF: Differential chemotherapeutic susceptibility of human T-lymphocytes and B-lymphocytes in culture. *J Natl Cancer Inst* 60:749–752, 1978
66. Ohnuma T, Arkin H, Takahashi I, Andrejczuk A, Roboz J, Holland JF: Biochemical bases of the differential susceptibility of malignant immune cells to asparaginase and to cytosine arabinoside. In *Molecular Interactions of Nutrition and Cancer*. Proc 34th Annual Symposium of Fundamental Cancer Res. M.D. Anderson Hospital and Tumor Institute, (Eds.) Arnott MS, Van Eys J. Raven Press, NY, pp. 105–121, 1982
67. Ohnuma T, Biller H, Kopel S, Holland JF: High dose methotrexate and leucovorin in patients with head and neck cancer. *Proc Am Assoc Cancer Res & ASCO* 19:350, 1978
68. Ohnuma T, Greenspan EM, Holland JF: Initial clinical study of vindesine. *Cancer Trest Rep* 61:389–394, 1977
69. Ohnuma T, Hart R, Roboz J, Andrejczuk A, Holland JF: Clinical and pharmacological studies with phosphonacetyl-aspartate (PALA). *Proc Am Cancer Res & ASCO* 20:344, 1979
70. Ohnuma T, Holland JF: Initial clinical study with pyrazofurin. *Cancer Treat Rep* 61:389–394, 1977
71. Ohnuma T, Holland JF, Freeman A, Sinks LF: Biochemical and pharmacological studies with asparaginase in man. *Cancer Res* 30:2297–2305, 1970
72. Ohnuma T, Holland JF, Masuda H, Waligunda JA, Goldberg GA: Microbiological assays of bleomycin: inactivation, tissue distribution and clearance. *Cancer* 33:1230–1239, 1974
73. Ohnuma T, Holland JF, Meyer P: Erwinia carotovora asparaginase in patients with prior anaphylaxis to asparaginase from *E. coli*. *Cancer* 30:376–381, 1972
74. Ohnuma T, Leyvraz S, Coffey V, Biller H, Muggia F, Holland JF: Carboplatin: activity in patients with head and neck (H&N), renal cell (RC) and ovarian carcinomas. *Proc Am Assoc Cancer Res* 25:179, 1984
75. Ohnuma T, Nogeire C, Cuttner J, Holland JF: Phase I study with neocarzinostatin: tolerance to two hour infusion and continuous infusion. *Cancer* 42:1670–1679, 1978
76. Ohnuma T, Norton L, Andrejczuk A, Holland JF: Pharmacokinetics of vindesine given as an iv bolus and 24 hour infusion in man. *Cancer Res Res* 45:464–469, 1985
77. Ohnuma T, Roboz J, Shapiro M, Holland JF: Pharmacological and biochemical studies of pyrazofurin in man. *Cancer Res* 37:2042–2049, 1977
78. Ohnuma T, Roboz J, Waxman S, Mandel E, Martin DS, Holland JF: Clinical and pharmacological effects of thymidine plus 5-fluorouracil. *Cancer Treat Rep* 64:1169–1177, 1980
79. Ohnuma T, Selawry OS, Holland JF, DeVita VT Jr, Shedd

DP, Hansen HH, Muggia FM: Clinical study with bleomycin: tolerance to twice weekly dosage. *Cancer* 30:914–922, 1972

80. Ohnuma T, Sridhar KS, Ratner LH, Holland JF: Phase I study of indicine N-oxide in patients with advanced cancer. *Cancer Treat Rep* 66:1509–1515, 1982

81. Ohnuma T, Rosner F, Levy RM, Cuttner J, Moon JH, Silver RT, Blom J, Falkson G, Burmingham R, Glidewell O, Holland JF: Treatment of adult leukemia with asparaginase. *Cancer Chemother Rep* 55:269–275, 1971

82. Orr ST, Aisner J: Performance status assessment among oncology patients: a review. *Cancer Treat Rep* 70:1423–1429, 1986

83. Paciucci PA, Ohnuma T, Cuttner J, Silver RT, Holland JF: Mitoxantrone in patients with acute leukemia in relapse. *Cancer Res* 43: 3919–3922, 1983

84. Penta JS, Rozencweig M, Guarino AM, Muggia FM: Mouse and large animal toxicology studies of twelve anticancer agents: relevance to starting dose for phase I clinical trials. *Cancer Chemother Pharmacol* 3:97–101, 1979

85. Perloff M, Ohnuma T, Holland JF, Kennedy BJ, Curtis Mills R: Adriamycin ad diamminedichloroplatinum in advanced prostatic carcinoma. *Proc Am Assoc Cancer Res & ASCO* 18:333, 1977

86. Perlow L, Ohnuma T, Andrejczuk A, Shafir M, Strauchen J, Holland JF: Pharmacology and toxicology of a seven day infusion of 1-α-D-arabinofuranosylctosine plus uridine in dogs. *Cancer Res* 45:2572–2577, 1985

87. Polvsen CO: Status of chemotherapy, radiotherapy, endocrine therapy and immunotherapy studies of human cancer in nude mice. In *Nude Mouse in Experimental and Clinical Research* (Eds.), Fogh J, Giovanella BC, New York, Academic Press, Inc., pp. 437–456, 1978

88. Presant CA: Quality of life in cancer patients. *Am J Clin Oncol* 7:527–573, 1984

89. Prieur DJ, Young OM, Davis RD, Cooney DA, Homan ER, Dizon RL, Guarino AM: Procedures for preclinical toxicologic evaluation of cancer chemotherapeutic agents: Protocols of the laboratory of toxicology. *Cancer Chemother Rep, Part 3,* 4:1–30, 1973

90. Rozencweig M, von Hoff DD, Staquet MJ, Schein PS, Penta JS, Goldin A, Muggia FM, Freireich EJ, DeVita VT Jr: Animal toxicology for early clinical trial with anticancer agents. *Cancer Clin Trials* 4:21–28, 1981

91. Sartorelli AC: Combination chemotherapy with actinomycin-D and ribonuclease: an example of complimentary inhibition. *Nature* 203:877–879, 1964

92. Sartorelli AC, Creasey WA: Combination chemotherapy. In *Cancer Medicine* 2nd edition, (Eds.), Holland JF, Frei E III, Lea & Febiger Philadelphia, pp. 720–730, 1982

93. Schein PS: Preclinical toxicology of anticancer agents. *Cancer Res* 37:1934–1937, 1977

94. Schein PS, Davis RO, Carter SK, Newman J, Schein DR, Rall DP: The evaluation of anticancer drugs in dogs and monkeys for the prediction of qualitative toxicities in man. *Clin Pharmacol Ther* 11:3–40, 1970

95. Shoemaker RH: New approaches to antitumor drug screening: the human tumor colony-forming assay. *Cancer Treat Rep* 70:9–12, 1986

96. Sklaroff RB, Casper ES, Magil GB, Young CW: Phase I study of 6-diazo-5-oxo-L-norleucine (DON). *Cancer Treat Rep* 64:1247–1251, 1980

97. Sladek NE, Priest J, Doeder D, Mirocha CJ, Pathre S, Krivit W: Plasma half-life and urinary excretion of cyclophosphamide in children. *Cancer Treat Rep* 64:1061–1066, 1980

98. Sridhar KS, Holland JF, Brown JC, Cohen J, Ohnuma T: Doxorubicin and cisplatin in the treatment of apudomas. *Cancer* 55:2634–2637, 1985

99. Sridhar KS, Ohnuma T, Biller H, Holland JF, Ambinder EP, Barba J: Combination chemotherapy with high dose methotrexate, bleomycin and cisplatin in the management of head and neck carcinoma. *Am J Clin Oncol* 8:55–60, 1985

100. Sridhar KS, Ohnuma T, Chahanian AP, Holland JF.: Phase I study of acivicin in patients with advanced cancer. *Cancer Treat Rep* 67:701–703, 1983

101. Stanley KE: Prognostic factors for survival in patients with inoperable lung cancer. *J Natl Cancer Int* 65:25–32, 1980

102. Staquet MJ, Byar DP, Green SB, Rozencweig M: Clinical predictivity of transplantable tumor systems in the selection of new drugs for solid tumors: rationale for a three-stage strategy. *Cancer Treat Rep* 67:753–765, 1983

103. Steel GG, Courtnay VD, Peckham MJ: The research to chemotherapy of a variety of human tumor xenografts. *Brit J Cancer* 47:1–13, 1983

104. Takahashi I, Ohnuma T, Kavy S, Bhardwaj S, Holland JF: Interaction of human serum albumin in anticancer agents *in vitro. Brit J Cancer* 41:602–608, 1980

105. Takahashi I, Ohnuma T, Holland JF: Comparison of biological effects of dichloromethotrexate and methotrexate on human leukemia cells in culture. *Cancer Res* 39:1264–1268, 1979

106. Venditti JM: The National Cancer Institute antitumor drug discovery program, current and future prospectives: A commentary. *Cancer Treat Rep* 67:767–772, 1983

107. Venditti JM, Wesley RA, Plowman J: Current NCI pre-clinical antitumor screening *in vivo.* Results of tumor panel screening, 1976–1982, and future directions. In: *Advances in Pharmacology and Chemotherapy*, New York, Academic Press, vol. 20, 1984

108. Vogel S, Ohnuma T, Perloff M, Holland JF: Combination chemotherapy with adriamycin and cis-diamminedichloroplatinum in patients with neoplastic diseases. *Cancer* 38: 21–26, 1976

109. Wang YM, Sutow WW, Sullivan MP, Romsdahl M: Preliminary studies of age and disease effects on pharmacokinetics of MTX following high dose MTX-CF therapy in children. *Proc Am Assoc Cancer Res & ASCO* 19:381, 1978

110. Warr D, McKinney S, Tannock I: Influence of measurement error on assessment of response to anticancer chemotherapy: proposal of new criteria to tumor response. *J Clin Oncol* 2:1040–146, 1984

111. Waxman S, Bruckner H: Enhancement of 5-fluorouracil antimetabolic activity by leucovorin, menadione and or -Tocophenol. *Eur J Cancer Clin Oncol* 18:685–692, 1982

112. Wheeler RH, Natale RB, Roshon SG, Baker SR: A phase I–II trial of cisplatin and dichloromethotrexate in squamous cell cancer of the head and neck. *J Clin Oncol* 2:831–835, 1984

113. Zager RF, Frisby SA, Oliverio VT: The effects of antibiotics and cancer chemotherapeutic agents on the cellular transport and antitumor activity of methotrexate in L1210 murine leukemia. *Cancer Res* 33:1670–1676, 1973

114. Zaharko DS, Bruckner H, Oliverio VT: Antibiotics alter methotrexate metabolism and excretion. *Science* 166:887–888, 1969

18

THERAPY OF METASTASIS IN ANIMAL MODELS

VINCENT A. POLLACK

INTRODUCTION

Recent advances in diagnostic methods and surgical techniques have led to increased success in the control of primary human neoplasms. With rare exceptions, neoplastic tissue which develops from, and is confined to, the site of origin no longer comprises a life-threatening clinical condition. However, the process of metastasis, the growth of tumor cells in organs distant from the site of origin, is responsible for the vast majority of deaths in clinical neoplastic disease and represents one of the greatest medical challenges in this century.

The purpose of this review is to discuss those aspects of cancer metastasis which have been shown, in animal models, to be amenable to pharmacologic intervention and to focus attention on the utility of animal models for the discovery of new chemotherapeutic agents with activity against established micro- and macro-metastatic disease.

Transplantable tumor systems in animals, principally murine hosts, have long been recognized as essential and important components of the discovery process for anticancer agents (reviewed by (16, 21, 45, 53, 132)). Unlike spontaneous and carcinogen-induced primary tumors, transplantable tumors induce relatively rapid, synchronous tumor growth in recipients with frequencies of metastatic spread which can be standardized and, therefore, render these systems useful for routine screening for anti-tumor agents (48, 152). Transplanted tumors have been observed to be more sensitive to chemotherapy than similar autochthonous (133, 158) or virus-induced tumors (13, 44).

There are, however, discrepancies between animal tumors and human neoplasia (16, 65). Research on animal tumors deals primarily with tumors of short latent periods (i.e., days to weeks) and rapid growth, whereas human tumors are primary (autochthonous) with long latent periods (i.e., years) and grow slowly. In humans, carcinomas predominate (14), tumors are of low immunogenicity and antigenicity (116, 135), and metastases are common (7, 69, 138), whereas sarcomas and leukemias are studied most frequently in animals (123), tumors are of high antigenicity (64, 65) and metastases are uncommon, usually regional (6). Tumors occur most frequently in humans in the aged, or in early childhood; hosts are often debilitated, histoincompatible, and have a longer life span. Experimentation with healthy, young, inbred animals is much more easily accomplished. None of these differences is common to all animal models and yet no model is without some of them. Fortunately, the

major differences between animal models and human neoplasia represent features which are desirable for experimental manipulation and standardization of screening systems (i.e., accessible sites for tumor implantation and monitoring, high antigenicity and rapid course) (46).

Of greater importance than the dissimilarities between the discovery methods and clinical neoplastic disease is the finding of correlations between the chemotherapeutic responses of patients and the sensitivity of transplantable murine tumor systems. In an early study (26), the chemotherapeutic response of the L1210 mouse leukemia correlated with the clinical responses in patients with acute lymphocytic leukemias for a number of anticancer agents. Since then, there have been numerous published correlations of this nature (reviewed by (47, 151)). Though sufficient clinical data on responses to newer agents have not yet been obtained, a wide variety of drugs in routine clinical usage have established the clinical predictivity of the transplantable murine tumor systems (136). Moreover, the use of allometric concepts has facilitated the quantitative prediction of clinical drug toxicity from data gathered in small and large animals (27, 49).

A large body of experimental and clinical data indicate that cells of malignant neoplasms, though they may originate from a single cell (17), represent a mosaic of phenotypic properties. Cells comprising both animal and human tumors have been found to differ with respect to their metastatic potential, immunogenicity, antigenic properties, growth rates, karyotypes, metabolic characteristics, pigment production and radiosensitivity (reviewed by Fidler and Hart, (23)). Clones isolated from solid tumors demonstrate remarkable diversity in sensitivity to cytotoxic drugs (5, 55, 62). Trope (1975) isolated metastases of the Lewis lung carcinoma (3LL) and found that they were more sensitive *in vitro* to vinblastine and melphalan than were cells from *sc* tumors. Using the B16 melanoma, K-1735 melanoma, UV2237 fibrosarcoma and the human A375 melanoma, Tsuruo and Fidler (145) found wide differences in sensitivity to several cytostatic agents *in vitro* between the parental tumor cells, selected variants and spontaneous metastases. Cloned subpopulations of the RIF-1 sarcoma showed marked differences in sensitivity to X-irradiation and cytotoxic drugs and no correlation was noted with ploidy values or metastatic capabilities (122). Using the human tumor colony-forming assay and several agents Tanigawa et al. (142) found heterogeneity amongst individual metastases as well as between the metastases and the primary tumors. The

R. H. Goldfarb (ed.), Fundamental aspects of cancer.

studies of Talmadge et al. (140) suggest that the cellular heterogeneity for chemosensitivity can develop rapidly even within a metastasis of clonal origin.

Collectively, these observations are consistent with the hypothesis of Nowell (112) that the genetic instability inherent to neoplastic cells is not confined to solid tumors but is extended in tumor progression to metastatic tumor foci. Since metastatic tumor cells comprise a small, pre-existing subpopulation of primary neoplasms (18), the usefulness of drug sensitivity tests involving primary or solid tumors seems unclear. More importantly, the implications of these findings to clinical oncology may in part explain cancer deaths resulting from metastases which do not respond to conventional treatment. Though means exist whereby metastatic variants can be recovered from primary tumor specimens by selection in athymic mice (119) this technique may not be feasible for routine clinical usage. For these reasons, emphasis in this review is confined to the effects of pharmacologic agents on nascent or established metastases, though by necessity this will involve the neglect of many excellent studies of antitumor agents in non-metastatic systems.

CYTOSTATIC AGENTS

Perhaps the most straightforward, and certainly the oldest, approach to therapy of cancer is the use of agents which selectively kill or prevent the replication of tumor cells. Indeed cytostatic agents represent the majority of drugs in current usage in clinical oncology.

One of the most thoroughly studied drugs in animal models is the polyfunctional alkylating agent cyclophosphamide. Its utility in surgical adjuvant chemotherapy for increasing life span has been shown in spontaneous mammary tumors (77), 3LL (51, 84, 85) and is associated with a substantial reduction in pulmonary metastases, lung colony assay (51). Enhancement of the effects of cyclophosphamide have been noted in combination therapy with other cytostatics (reviewed by Schabel, (132); Merker et al. (105)), the angiometamorphic agent ICRF-159 (90) and the anticoagulant phenprocoumon (67); additive effects have been shown in conjunction with local tumor hyperthermia (161) and X-irradiation (144). This agent is active against experimental (iv-induced) metastases of 3LL (114) and B16 melanoma (141). Reports of enhanced lung metastases in animals dosed prior to iv tumor challenge (10, 150) may be due to its impairment of host resistance (immunotoxicity) rather than acceleration of the metastatic process (106). No enhancement of spontaneous metastases was observed (10). A study of perioperative adjuvant chemotherapy has indicated that the sequence and interval of chemotherapy and surgery is critical for maximal reduction of residual micrometastases (25). The structurally related iphosphamide, though less toxic, is not so potent as cyclophosphamide for therapy of spontaneous 3LL metastases (13, 51).

Cis-platinum, a metal complex with significant antitumor and antimetastatic activities, is synergistic with perhaps the widest spectrum of antitumor agents and has recently been reviewed (126).

The nitrosoureas (especially BCNU, CCNU and MeCC-NU) represent alkylating agents with very broad spectrum

antitumor activity. Effective therapy producing long-term survivors occurred in experimental 3LL metastasis (114) and post-surgical micrometastatic disease in the B16, C3H mammary adenocarcinoma, colon 26 carcinoma (53, 132) and 3LL (105) where surgery or chemotherapy alone were ineffective. In these systems, synergism with cyclophosphamide, cis-platinum and 5-fluorouracil was noted (105, 132).

Other alkylating agents, though less often studied in metastatic tumor systems, are nitrogen mustard (mechlorethamine), melphalan and chlorozotocin, which produced substantial increased life span in mice bearing experimental 3LL metastases (114). BCNU and melphalan in conjunction with other cytostatic agents and surgery produced substantial reductions in pulmonary metastases in the MS-2 system (42).

Several antimetabolites have been shown to be effective agents against established micrometastatic disease in animal models. The first compound to have indicated the synergistic effects of surgery and chemotherapy was 6-mercaptopurine in the mammary adenocarcinoma 755 (134) and in spontaneous mammary tumors (77). The pyrimidine antagonist 5-fluorouracil has broad spectrum antimetastatic effects, being active in the 3LL (79), B16-BL6 and C26-NL17 colon adenocarcinoma systems (146). Therapy of experimental 3LL metastases producing increased life span has been shown for 6-thioguanine, 5-fluorouracil, floxuridine, cytosine arabinoside, 5-azacytidine during testing with the tumor panel of the National Cancer Institute (48).

Growth arrest of both experimental and spontaneous 3LL metastases occurred with the phosphodiesterase inhibitor isobutylmethylxanthine (IBX) which appears to require normal cells for its cytostatic effects on malignant cells (82).

An interesting agent, tiazofurin, with a broad dosage range and little toxicity produced long-term survivors of experimental 3LL metastases (124). Moreover, therapy of intracerebrally implanted 3LL suggested that the compound effectively crossed the blood-brain barrier.

The antibiotic adriamycin (doxorubicin) has broad spectrum antimetastatic activity in animal models (reviewed by Carter, (11)) and has been used successfully in surgical adjuvant polychemotherapy (53, 90, 105). Synergistic effects with ICRF-159 were observed in the MS-2 sarcoma when both agents were administered prior to, but not after, surgery (42).

One of the major obstacles to effective chemotherapeutic algorithms is dose-limiting toxicity. Concerted efforts to discover compounds with improved margins of safety have not met with great success. Nevertheless, it is conceivable that novel forms of drug delivery systems may circumvent this difficulty. Encapsulation of cytotoxic agents in multilamellar lipid vesicles (liposomes), patterned after encapsulated lymphokines (see next section), offers the promise of greatly reduced toxicity and, in some cases, greater efficacy. Therapy of iv-induced metastases has been demonstrated for encapsulated MeCCNU (80), cytosine arabinoside (121), and adriamycin (28).

BIOLOGICAL RESPONSE MODIFIERS

A second, major approach to therapy of cancer has involved

the activation of host antitumor defenses (i.e., biological response modification). It is clear from examination of the results of adoptive transfer of specifically sensitized cells and passive transfer of immune globulin (reviewed by Kedar and Weiss, (86) and Rosenberg and Terry, (127), respectively) that there are a variety of endogenous tumoricidal mechanisms. Nevertheless, it is also clear that these factors may have been effectively exhausted or paralyzed at the onset of tumor dissemination, such that the control of metastatic tumor growth would necessitate stimulation of immune responses most probably by combinations of immune modulators. Since there are more than one hundred immunomodulators currently being developed as cancer therapeutants, a comprehensive discussion of these is beyond the scope of this review, which is restricted to those agents with confirmed activity against micro- and macro-metastatic disease.

Perhaps the most frequently studied and most potent stimulants of immune responses can be found in microbial products and particularly among the actinomycetes. In early work, viable *Mycobacterium bovis* (Bacillus Calmette-Guerin, BCG) was employed in intratumoral injection of dermal implants of the guinea pig line 10 hepatocarcinoma and resulted in regression of the dermal tumors and eradication of regional lymph node metastases (56, 162). Killed cells of another actinomycete, *Corynebacterium parvum*, were used in conjunction with surgery of primary 3LL tumors to dramatically reduce pulmonary metastases (128); the treatment of post-surgical micrometastases with *C. parvum* has been shown in the 3LL, Dunn osteosarcoma and B16 systems (31). Use of viable or whole killed cells was supplanted by efforts to identify the most active subcellular fractions of these and other organisms. Regression of primary tumors and regional lymph node metastases was accomplished with cell wall skeletons of BCG (163), mycobacterial RNA (109) and synthetic subfractions such as muramyl dipeptide (MDP) and trehalose dimycolate (TDM) (160).

Systemic administration of pleuripotent tumor antigen-nonspecific immunomodulators was then employed in metastatic tumor systems with a variety of agents. Microbial subcellular fractions, such as the BCG cell wall (139), *Nocardia rubra* cell wall (83), levan (94) and schizophyllan (159) were shown to be potent agents against established micrometastatic disease in animal systems. Plant extracts such as krestin (PS-K) (149) and lentinan (125) were also effective in this context. Moreover, several synthetic agents were found to be effective against established micrometastatic disease and these include thiabendazole (100), akyllysophospholipids (8), azimexon (137), maleic anhydride divinyl ether (107), pyrimidinones (108), and poly (I,C)-LC (141).

A novel means for biological response modification employs liposomes for selective delivery of potent, though labile, activators to mononuclear phagocytes. Multilamellar lipid vesicle (MLV) encapsulating the lymphokine macrophage activation factor, MAF (19), muramyl tripeptide, MTP-PE (87), or the synergistic combination of MAF-MDP (24) selectively activated macrophages *in vitro* and elicited cytotoxic alveolar macrophages in systemically treated mice. These liposome preparations induced therapy of post-surgical micrometastases as assessed by lung colony assay and in survival studies. In a similar manner, liposome-encapsulated C-reactive protein prolonged survival of mice bearing post-surgical metastases of the T241 sarcoma (15).

The use of liposomes for selective delivery of substances to macrophages constitutes a unique approach to therapy of metastasis. It is not inconceivable that the therapeutic effects of encapsulated cytostatic agents (mentioned earlier) may be due in part to delivery of internalized liposomes to tumor cells *in situ* by mononuclear phagocytes.

An important requisite to immune potentiation is the ability of the tumor-bearing host to respond in an immunologically specific manner. Despite the common belief that tumors in relevant animal models are non-immunogenic (reviewed by Hewitt, (64, 65)), active specific immunotherapy using vaccines composed of inactivated tumor cells and potent immunomodulators (adjuvants) has shown considerable progress in eradication of disseminated tumors. In an early study, Proctor et al. (120) combined irradiated hepatoma cells with *C. parvum* and immunized the rat hosts after surgical excision of the primary tumor; reductions of lung metastases were noted at necropsy whereas facilitation or suppression of metastases occurred with the use of tumor cells alone. In a series of carefully controlled experiments, Hanna and coworkers identified the important parameters of vaccine composition (i.e, tumor cell preparation and inactivation, adjuvant-tumor cell ratios, etc.) and optimized the BCG-tumor cell vaccine therapy using survival studies in the guinea pig L10 hepatocarcinoma system (57, 58, 115). An important aspect of vaccination is the demonstration of synergistic effects of immunotherapy and chemotherapy in animals with disseminated micrometastatic disease (88). Furthermore, the pathogenic complications associated with the use of a viable microorganism in tumor-bearing hosts can be prevented (59). The utility of vaccine therapy in weakly immunogenic tumor systems has been confirmed using adjuvants such as *C. parvum* (117), BCG (98) and BCG cell walls (2).

Recent advances in passive immunotherapy have revived interest in this field where the results of earlier studies (reviewed by Rosenberg and Terry, (127)) inspired very cautious optimism. The benefit of adoptive transfer of sensitized cells for therapy of micrometastases was shown in B16 by Wang and coworkers (153, 154) who used xenogenic immune RNA extracted from the lymphoid tissue of immunized guinea pigs to sensitize mouse lymphocytes *in vitro*. More recently, remarkable results were obtained through the adoptive transfer of syngeneic lymphocytes in a manner which avoids xenogeneic substances. Successful immunotherapy of post-surgical micrometastases was achieved by adoptive transfer of lymphocytes activated *in vitro* by interleukin-2 (IL-2) (104). Therapeutic effects of these lymphokine activated killer (LAK) cells was augmented by concurrent IL-2 therapy (110, 111).

Treatment of established micrometastases through replacement therapy with endogenous substances has been shown for interferon type 1 (43), thymostimulin, TP-1 (89) and tumor necrosis serum (155).

Though in its infancy, an area of investigation with exciting promise is the use of monoclonal antibodies or antibody-toxin conjugates (immunotoxins) for localization or treatment of metastatic tumor foci (reviewed by Baldwin and Pimm (3)). Using xenogeneic immune globulin, Lozzio et al. (99) produced a significant reduction of systemic metastases of the human K-562 leukemia cells in athymic-asplenic mice. Selective delivery to metastases has been shown for radiolabelled antibody (156) and for daunomycin-immunoglobulin conjugates; lymph node metastases were retarded or completely abolished by a monoclonal antibody conjugated to the A chain of abrin (78).

SELECTIVE ANTIMETASTATIC AGENTS

A third approach to the control of metastatic disease is directed to inhibition of those processes of tumor and host origin which lead to dissemination of tumor cells, but involves agents with neither direct cytocidal effects or activation of host antitumor defenses, and have been collectively termed "selective antimetastatic agents" (39).

Since much is known of the altered hemostatic status of animals and humans with malignant neoplasms, it is not surprising that agents affecting blood coagulation, platelet aggregation and fibrin-fibrinolytic systems were the earliest examples of selective agents. Kolenich et al. (92) described the inhibition of metastasis by heparin, warfarin and aspirin in the mouse BW10232 adenocarcinoma system. Heparin was shown to prevent lung metastases in a number of tumor systems, including the 3LL, B16 mouse tumors and WAG/ Rij and ETC-5 tumors of rats (101). However, interest in heparin waned when it was observed that this agent caused an intravascular redistribution of tumor cells and enhanced metastasis in extrapulmonary, extrathoracic sites (12, 101). Warfarin, on the other hand, exerts more significant and reproducible effects. In experimental metastasis, pretreatment with warfarin caused a reduction in lung colony counts in the KHT sarcoma (10), 3LL (68, 102, 118) and B16 systems (102). Prevention of spontaneous metastasis has been observed in the MCA-1 and T241 fibrosarcomas (75, 76) as well as 3LL (67, 118). The mechanism of warfarin action may not be due primarily to its anticoagulant effect, but the induction of vitamin K deficiency (67, 68). Gorelik et al. (50) have suggested that a possible explanation may be that of warfarin-induced exposure of blood-borne tumor cells to destruction by natural killer (NK) cells.

Hypofibrinogenemia produced by Arvin, an enzyme purified from the venom of the Malayan viper (*Agkistrodon rhodostoma*) prevented metastasis of the V2 carcinoma in rabbits (157) and experimental metastasis of 3LL and B16 tumors (103). In contrast to these results, Hagmar (54) found that defibrination with Arvin enhanced the metastases of the MCG1-SS sarcoma and the B16 melanoma.

The selective antimetastatic effects of a number of platelet aggregation inhibitors have been described, due to early studies in aspirin-treated animals (29, 92). The synthetic agent ticlopidine prevented lung metastasis formation after iv tumor challenge in the B16 and 3LL tumors as well as the AH130 rat hepatoma systems (4, 91). Prevention of iv-induced metastases and therapy of post-surgical metastases, assessed by lung colony counts was demonstrated in the B16 and 3LL systems by Bando et al. (4) using ticlopidine, diltiazem, dipyridamole and trapidil. Forskolin, a diterpene plant extract, inhibited the formation of experimental B16-F10 metastases in pre-treated mice (1). The synthetic agent RA233, though showing little effect alone, substantially reduced lung metastases when combined with X-irradiation and then surgery of the primary B16 and 3LL tumors (96, 97).

A potent endogenous inhibitor of platelets is prostacyclin (PGI2) which inhibited lung metastases of the amelanotic B16 melanoma (B16a) when administered in conjunction with the phosphodiesterase inhibitor theophylline immediately prior to iv tumor challenge (70, 72). Nafazatrom, which stimulates endogenous PGI2 biosynthesis, prevents experimental and spontaneous metastases when applied shortly before or during the intravascular phase of B16a metastasis (71).

In general, it appears that potent, synthetic inhibitors of platelet aggregation can substantially reduce lung metastases when administered during tumor dissemination. The observations of treatment of post-surgical micrometastases (4) are unique and, once confirmed, may provide exciting new areas for investigation.

The angiometamorphic compound ICRF-159 (Razoxane) is a synthetic agent with interesting and unique properties (reviewed by Herman et al., (63)). ICRF-159 prevented spontaneous 3LL metastasis (60) and inhibited iv-induced metastasis (48). Though this compound is cytotoxic *in vitro* (93), it appears to exert its action *in vivo* by "normalizing" the structure and integrity of the blood vessels within tumors (81, 95), resulting in a reduced rate of escape of malignant cells into the blood-stream. Broad spectrum antimetastatic activity has been observed with ICRF-159 (reviewed by Herman et al., (63)).

Pharmacologic intervention of tumor angiogenesis is the proposed mechanism for the antimetastatic effects of protamine (143). A substantial reduction in the volume, though not necessarily the number, of lung metastases was observed in both experimental and spontaneous 3LL metastases, as well as the Walker 256 carcinoma and B16 melanoma (143).

Triazene derivatives and N-diazoderivatives of amino acids are classical examples of selective antimetastatic agents. Reduction of experimental metastasis and prevention of spontaneous metastases have been achieved by triazenes (e.g., dacarbazine [DTIC] and BRL 51308) (39, 66, 130) and by N-diazoglycine derivatives (e.g., DGA) (35–37). Therapy of post-surgical micrometastases produced significantly increased life span (131). Cytotoxic effects on primary and metastatic tumors has been excluded as a mechanism of *in vivo* action (34). It is postulated that these agents prevent metastases by inhibiting tumor cell entry into the bloodstream, possibly by inhibiting proteases responsible for tumor invasion (39), but the mechanism of *in vivo* action has yet to be fully described.

A diverse array of protease inhibitors have been shown to have substantial, if somewhat variable, effects on metastasis formation. Aprotinin (trasylol) prevented spontaneous 3LL metastasis (3), but enhanced metastases in another study (148). Leupeptin inhibited blood-borne lung metastases of the Yoshida hepatomas AH7974 and AH100B (129) but had no effect on spontaneous metastasis (33). A nonspecific protease, aurintricarboxylic acid, ATA, prevented spontaneous 3LL metastases (36) and an extract of the salivary gland of the leech (*H. ghiliani*) inhibited pulmonary metastases and increased the clearance of radiolabelled tumor cells in the T241 system (30). Endogenous neutral proteases extracted from leukocytes (33) and splenocytes (39) prevented spontaneous metastases. These studies utilized the lung colony assay as an endpoint and the effects of these agents on survival of tumor-bearing animals has yet to be determined. Of particular importance is the demonstration by

Ossowski and Reich (113) that inhibition of plasminogen activator, through the use of anti-urokinase immune globulin, completely inhibited the outgrowth of the human HEp3 epithelial micrometastases in the embryonated egg. Collectively, these studies suggest that inhibition of proteases regulating tumor invasion may in future become important targets for therapy of micrometastases.

The effects of calcium channel blockers have only recently been studied in metastasizing tumor systems. While these agents may selectively enhance the effectiveness of cytostatic agents (61), they appear to have independent antimetastatic activity. Nifedipine alone prevented metastases of the amelanotic B16 (72). Recently, Tsuruo et al., (147) used verapamil to prevent experimental and spontaneous metastases in the B16-BL6 melanoma and C26-NL17 colon carcinoma systems. The combined effects of independent therapeutic activity and possible synergy with cytostatic agents render the calcium channel blockers an interesting area for further study.

ACKNOWLEDGMENTS

The author wishes to express his gratitude to J.V. Hersh for information sciences and to M. DeMaio, D.E. Sloan and P. Goodwin for their help, suggestions and critical reviews of this chapter.

REFERENCES

1. Agarwal KC, Parks RE Jr: Forskolin: A potential antimetastatic agent. *Int J Cancer* 32:801–804, 1983
2. Ashley MP, Zbar B, Hunter JT, Rapp HJ, Sugimoto: Adjuvant-antigen requirements for active specific immunotherapy of microscopic metastases remaining after surgery. *Cancer Res* 40:4197–4203, 1980
3. Baldwin RW, Pimm MV: Antitumor monoclonal antibodies for radio-immunodetection of tumors and drug targeting. *Cancer Metastasis Rev* 2:89–106, 1983
4. Bando H, Yamashita T, Tsubura E: Effects of antiplatelet agents on pulmonary metastases. *Gann* 75:284–291, 1984
5. Barranco SC, Ho DHW, Drewinko B, Romsdahl MM, Humphrey RM: Differential sensitivities of human melanoma cells grown *in vitro* to arabinosylcytosine. *Cancer Res* 32:2733–2736, 1972
6. Bartlett GL, Kreider JW, Purnell DM: Immunotherapy of cancer in animals: Models or muddles? *J Natl Cancer Inst* 56:207–210, 1976
7. Beahrs OH, Carr DT, Rubin P (Eds.): *Manual for staging of cancer*, 1977: Report of American Joint Committee for cancer staging and end results reporting. American Joint Committee, Chicago, IL, 1977
8. Berdel WE, Bausert WR, Weltzien JU, Modolell ML, Widman KH, Munder PG: The influence of alkyl-lysophospholipids and lysophospholipid-activated macrophages on the development of metastasis of 3-Lewis lung carcinoma. *Eur J Cancer* 16:1199–1204, 1980
9. Carmel RJ, Brown JM: The effect of cyclophosphamide and other drugs on the incidence of pulmonary metastases in mice. *Cancer Res* 37:145–151, 1977
10. Carter SK: Adriamycin: A review. *J Natl Cancer Inst* 55:1265–1274, 1974
11. Chan SY, Pollard M: Metastasis-enhancing effect of heparin and its relationship to a lipoprotein factor. *J Natl Cancer Inst* 64:1121–1125, 1980
12. Chirigos MA, Moloney JB, Humphreys SR, Mantel N, Goldin A: Response of a virus-induced murine lymphoid leukemia to drug therapy. *Cancer Res* 21:803–811, 1961
13. Corsi A, Calabresi F, Greco C: Comparative effects of cyclophosphamide on Lewis lung carcinoma. *Br J Cancer* 38:631–633, 1978
14. Cutler SJ, Young JL Jr, (Eds.): *Third National Cancer Survey: Incidence data. Natl Cancer Inst Monogr* 41:1–454, 1975
15. Deodhar SD, James K, Chiang T, Edinger M, Barna BP: Inhibition of lung metastasis in mice bearing a malignant fibrosarcoma by treatment with liposomes containing human C-reactive protein. *Cancer Res* 42:5084–5088, 1982
16. Detre SI, Davies AJS, Conners TA: New models for cancer chemotherapy. *Cancer Chemother Rep* 5:133–143, 1975
17. Fialkow PJ: Clonal origin of human tumors. *Biochim Biophys Acta* 458:283–310, 1976
18. Fidler IJ, Kripke ML: Metastases results from preexisting variants cells within a malignant tumor. *Science* 197:893–895, 1977
19. Fidler IJ: Therapy of spontaneous metastases by intravenous injection of liposomes containing lymphokines. *Science* 208:1469–1471, 1980
20. Fidler IJ, Sone S, Fogler WE, Barnes ZL: Eradication of spontaneous metastases and activation of alveolar macrophages by intravenous injection of liposomes containing muramyl dipeptide. *Proc Natl Acad Sci USA* 78:1680–1684, 1981
21. Fidler IJ, Barnes Z, Fogler WE, Kirsh R, Bugelski P, Poste G: Involvement of macrophages in the eradication of established metastases following intravenous injection of liposomes containing macrophage activators. *Cancer Res* 42:496–501, 1982
22. Fidler IJ, Berendt M, Oldham RK: The rationale for and design of a screening procedure for the assessment of biological response modifiers for cancer treatment. *J Biol Response Modif* 1:15–26, 1982
23. Fidler IJ, Hart IR: The development of biological diversity and metastatic potential in malignant neoplasms. *Oncodev Biol Med* 4:161–176, 1982
24. Fidler IJ, Schroit AJ: Synergism between lymphokines and muramyl dipeptide encapsulated in liposomes: *In situ* activation of macrophages and therapy of spontaneous cancer metastases. *J Immunol* 133:515–518, 1984
25. Fisher B, Gunduz N, Saffer EA: Influence of the interval between primary tumor removal and chemotherapy on kinetics and growth of metastases. *Cancer Res* 43:1488–1492, 1983
26. Frei E III: Comparisons of activities of antitumor agents in selected human and rodent tumor systems. *Cancer Chemother Rep* 16:19–24, 1962
27. Freireich EJ, Gehan EA, Rall DP, Schmidt LH, Skipper HE: Quantitative comparison of toxicity of anticancer agents in the mouse, rat, hamster, dog, monkey, and man. *Cancer Chemother Rep* 50:219–244, 1966
28. Gabizon A, Goren D, Fuks Z, Meshorer A, Barenholz Y: Superior therapeutic activity of liposome-associated adriamycin in a murine metastatic tumour model. *Br J Cancer* 51:681–689, 1985
29. Gasic GJ, Gasic TB, Murphy S: Anti-metastatic effect of aspirin. *Lancet* ii:932–933, 1972
30. Gasic GJ, Viner ED, Budzynski A, Gasic GP: Inhibition of lung tumor colonization by leech salivary gland extracts from *Haementeria ghiliani. Cancer Res* 43:1633–1636, 1983
31. Gatenby P, Basten A: A mouse model for immunotherapy of osteosarcoma. II. *Corynebacterium parvum* therapy. *Cancer Immunol Immunother* 8:103–111, 1980
32. Giraldi T, Kopitar M, Sava G: Antimetastatic effect of a leukocyte intracellular inhibitor of neutral proteases. *Cancer Res* 37:3834–3835, 1977a
33. Giraldi T, Nisi C, Sava G: Lysosomal enzyme inhibitors and

antimetastatic activity in the mouse. *Eur J Cancer* 13:1321–1323, 1977

34. Giraldi T, Houghton PJ, Taylor DM, Nisi C: Antimetastatic action of some triazene derivatives against the Lewis lung carcinoma in mice. *Cancer Treat Rep* 62:721–725, 1978
35. Giraldi T, Guarino AM, Nisi C, Baldini L: Selective antimetastatic effects of N-diazoacetylglycine derivatives in mice. *Eur J Cancer* 15:603–607, 1979
36. Giraldi T, Guarino AM, Nisi C, Sava G: Antitumor and antimetastatic effects of benzenoid triazenes in mice bearing Lewis lung carcinoma. *Pharmacol Res Commun* 12:1–11, 1980
37. Giraldi T, Sava G, Nisi C: Mechanism of the antimetastatic action of N-diazoacetylglycinamide in mice bearing Lewis lung carcinoma. *Eur J Cancer* 16:87–92, 1980
38. Giraldi T, Sava G, Kopitar M, Brzin J, Turk V: Neutral proteinase inhibitors and antimetastatic effects in mice. *Eur J Cancer* 16:449–454, 1980
39. Giraldi T, Sava G: Selective antimetastatic drugs (review). *Anticancer Res* 1:163–174, 1981
40. Giraldi T, Sava G, Kopitar M, Brzin J, Suhar A, Turk V: Antimetastatic effects and tumor proteinase inhibition by spleen intracellular inhibitors of neutral proteinases. *Eur J Cancer* 17:1301–1306, 1981
41. Giraldi T, Sava G, Cuman R, Nisi C, Lassiani L: Selectivity of the antimetastatic and cytotoxic effects of 1-p-(3,3-dimethyl-1-triazeno)benzoic acid potassium salt, (+/− 1,2-di(3,5-dioxopiperazin-1-yl)propane, and cyclophosphamide in mice bearing Lewis lung carcinoma. *Cancer Res* 41:2524–2528, 1981
42. Giuliani F, Di Marco A, Casazza AM, Sava G: Combination chemotherapy and surgical adjuvant chemotherapy on MS-2 sarcoma and lung metastases in mice. *Eur J Cancer* 15:715–723, 1979
43. Glasgow LA, Kern ER: Effect of interferon administration on pulmonary osteogenic sarcomas in an experimental murine model. *J Natl Cancer Inst* 67:207–212, 1981
44. Glynn JP, Moloney JB, Chirigos MA, Humphreys SR, Goldin A: Biological interrelationships in the chemotherapy of Moloney virus leukemia. *Cancer Res* 23:269–278, 1963
45. Goldin A, Johnson RK, Venditti JM: Preclinical characterization of candidate antitumor drugs. *Cancer Chemother Rep* 5:21–81, 1975
46. Goldin A, Johnson RK, Venditti JM: Usefulness and limitations of murine tumor models for the identification of new antitumor agents. *Antibiot Chemother* 28:1–7, 1980
47. Goldin A, Kline A, Sofina ZP et al: Experimental evaluation of antitumor drugs in the USA and USSR and clinical correlations. *Natl Cancer Inst Monogr* vol. 55, 1980
48. Goldin A, Venditti JM, MacDonald JS, Muggia FM, Henney JE, DeVita VT Jr: Current results of the screening program at the Division of Cancer Treatment, National Cancer Institute. *Eur J Cancer* 17:-129–142, 1981
49. Goldsmith MA, Slavik M, Carter SK: Quantitative prediction of drug toxicity in small and large animals. *Cancer Res* 35:1354–1364, 1975
50. Gorelik E, Bere WW, Herberman RB: Role of NK cells in the antimetastatic effect of anticoagulant drugs. *Int J Cancer* 33:87–94, 1984
51. Greco C, Corsi A, Caputo M, Cavallari A, Calabresi F: Cyclophosphamide and iphosphamide against Lewis lung carcinoma: Evaluation of toxic and therapeutic effects. *Tumori* 65:169–180, 1979
52. Greco C, Calabresi F, Caputo M, Corsi A, Saachi A, Zupi G: Adriamycin effect on the Lewis lung carcinoma. Comparison between the original line and its derivative subline. *Eur J Cancer* 16:1251–1255, 1980
53. Griswold DP Jr: The potential for murine tumor models in

surgical adjuvant chemotherapy. *Cancer Chemother Rep* 5:187–204, 1975
54. Hagmar B: Defibrination and metastasis formation: Effects of arvin on experimental metastases in mice. *Eur J Cancer* 8:17–28, 1972
55. Hakansson L, Trope K: On the presence within tumors of clones that differ in sensitivity to cytostatic drugs. *Acta Pathol Microbiol Scand* 82:35–40, 1974
56. Hanna MG Jr, Zbar B, Rapp HJ: Histopathology of tumor regression and intralesional injection of *Mycobacterium bovis*. I. Tumor growth and metastasis. *J Natl Cancer Inst* 48:1441–1455, 1972
57. Hanna MG Jr, Peters LC, Fidler IJ: The efficacy of BCG-induced tumor immunity in guinea pigs with regional and systemic malignancy. *Cancer Immunol Immunother* 1:171–177, 1976
58. Hanna MG Jr, Peters LC: Specific immunotherapy of established visceral micrometastases by BCG-tumor cell vaccine alone or as an adjunct to surgery. *Cancer* 42:2613–2625, 1978
59. Hanna MG Jr, Pollack VA, Peters LC, Hoover HC: Active specific immunotherapy of established micrometastases with BCG plus tumor cell vaccines: Effective treatment of BCG side effects with isoniazid. *Cancer* 49:659–664, 1982
60. Hellmann K, Burrage K: Control of malignant metastases by ICRF 159. *Nature* 224:273–275, 1969
61. Helson L: Calcium channel blocker enhancement of anticancer drug cytotoxicity: A review. *Cancer Drug Deliv* 1:353–361, 1984
62. Heppner GH, Dexter DL, De Nucci T, Miller F, Calabresi P: Heterogeneity in drug sensitivity among tumor cell subpopulations of a single mammary tumor. *Cancer Res* 38:3758–3763, 1978
63. Herman EH, Witiak DT, Hellmann K, Waravdeker VS: Biological properties of ICRF-159 and related bis-(dioxopiperazine) compounds. *Adv Pharmacol Chemother* 19:249–290, 1982
64. Hewitt HB: Choice of animal tumors for experimental studies of cancer therapy. *Adv Cancer Res* 27:149–200, 1978
65. Hewitt HB: Animal tumor models and their relevance to human tumor immunology. *J Biol Resp Modif* 1:107–119, 1982
66. Heyes J: Antimetastatic effect of 4-carboxy-5-(3,3-dimethyl-1-triazene)-2-methylimidazole. *J Natl Cancer Inst* 53:279–280, 1974
67. Hilgard P: Experimental vitamin K deficiency and spontaneous metastases. *Br J Cancer* 35:891–892, 1977
68. Hilgard P, Maat B: Mechanism of lung tumour colony reduction caused by coumarin anticoagulation. *Eur J Cancer* 15:183–187, 1979
69. Holland JF, Frei E III: *Cancer Medicine*. Lea & Febiger. Philadelphia, PA, 1982
70. Honn KV, Cicone B, Skoff A: Prostacyclin: A potent antimetastatic agent. *Science* 212:1270–1272, 1981
71. Honn KV: Prostacyclin/thromboxane ratios in tumor growth and metastasis, p. 733, In Powles TJ, Bockman RS, Honn KV, Ramwell PW (Eds.) *Prostaglandins in Cancer*, Alan Liss, Inc. New York, NY, 1982
72. Honn KV: Inhibition of tumor cell metastasis by modulation of the vascular prostacyclin/thromboxane A2 system. *Clin Exp Metastasis* 1:103–114, 1983
73. Honn KV, Onoda JM, Diglio CA, Sloane BF: Calcium channel blockers: Potential antimetastatic agents. *Proc Soc Exp Biol Med* 174:16–19, 1983
74. Hoover HC Jr, Ketcham AS: Decreasing experimental metastasis formation with anticoagulation and chemotherapy. *Surg Forum* 26:173–174, 1975
75. Hoover HC Jr, Ketcham AS: Techniques for inhibiting tumor metastases. *Cancer* 35:5–14, 1975

76. Hoover HC Jr, Jones D, Ketcham AS: The optimal level of anticoagulation for decreasing experimental metastases. *Surgery* 79:625–630, 1976

77. Humphreys SR, Mantel N, Goldin A: Chemotherapy and surgery of spontaneous tumors in mice. *Eur J Cancer* 2:1–7, 1966

78. Hwang KM, Foon KA, Cheung PH, Pearson JW, Oldham RK: Selective antitumor effect of L10 hepatocarcinoma cells of a potent immunoconjugate composed of the A chain of Abrin and a monoclonal antibody to a hepatoma-associated antigen. *Cancer Res* 44:4578–4586, 1984

79. Iigo M, Hoshi A, Nakamura A, Kuetani K: Antineoplastic effect of orally administered 1-alkyl carbamoyl derivatives of 5-fluorouracil on *sc* implanted Lewis lung carcinoma and B16 melanoma. *Cancer Treat Rep* 63:1895–1899, 1979

80. Inaba M, Yoshida N, Tsukagoshi S: Preferential action of liposome-entrapped 1-(2-chloroethyl)-3-(4-methylcyclohexyl)-1-nitrosourea on lung metastasis of Lewis lung carcinoma as compared with the free drug. *Gann* 72:341–345, 1981

81. James SE, Salsbury AJ: Effect of (+/−)-1,2-bis(3,5-dioxopiperazin-1-yl)propane on tumor blood vessels and its relationship to the antimetastatic effect in the Lewis lung carcinoma. *Cancer Res* 34:839–842, 1974

82. Janik P, Assaf A, Bertram JS: Inhibition of growth of primary and metastatic Lewis lung carcinoma cells by the phosphodiesterase inhibitor isobutylmethylxanthine. *Cancer Res* 40:1950–1954, 1980

83. Kagawa K, Yamashita T, Tsubura E, Yamamura Y: Inhibition of pulmonary metastasis by *Nocardia rubra* cell wall skeleton, with special reference to macrophage activation. *Cancer Res* 44:665–670, 1984

84. Karrer K, Humphreys SR: Continuous and limited courses of cyclophosphamide (NSC-26271) in mice with pulmonary metastasis after surgery. *Cancer Chemother Rep* 51:439–449, 1967

85. Karrer K, Humphreys SR, Goldin A: An experimental model for studying factors which influence metastasis of malignant tumors. *Int J Cancer* 2:213–223, 1967

86. Kedar E, Weiss DW: The *in vitro* generation of effector lymphocytes and their employment in tumor immunotherapy. *Adv Cancer Res* 38:171–287, 1983

87. Key ME, Talmadge JE, Fogler WE, Bucana C, Fidler IJ: Isolation of tumoricidal macrophages from lung melanoma metastases of mice treated systemically with liposomes containing a lipophilic derivative of muramyl dipeptide. *J Natl Cancer Inst* 69:1189–1198, 1982

88. Key ME, Brandhorst JS, Hanna MG Jr, Synergistic effects of active specific immunotherapy and chemotherapy in guinea pigs with disseminated cancer. *J Immunol* 130:2987–2992, 1983

89. Klein AS, Shoham J: Effect of the thymic factor, thymostimulin (TP-1), on the survival rate of tumor-bearing mice. *Cancer Res* 41:3217–3221, 1981

90. Kline I: Potentially useful combinations of chemotherapy detected in mouse tumor systems. *Cancer Chemother Rep* 4:33–43, 1974

91. Kohga S, Kinjo M, Tanaka K, Ogawa H, Ishihara M, Tanaka N: Effects of 5-(2-chlorobenzyl)-4,5,6,7-tetrahydrothieno[3,2-C]pyridine hydrochloride (ticlopidine), a platelet aggregation inhibitor, on blood-borne metastasis. *Cancer Res* 41:4710–4714, 1981

92. Kolenich JJ, Mansour EG, Flynn A: Haematological effects of aspirin. *Lancet* ii:714, 1972

93. Lazo JS, Ingber DE, Sartorelli AC: Enhancement of experimental lung metastases by cultured cells treated with (+/−)-1,2-bis(3,5-dioxopiperazin-lyl) propane (ICRF-159). *Cancer Res* 38:2263–2270, 1978

94. Leibovici J, Sinai Y, Wolman M, Davidai G: Effects of high-molecular weight levan on the growth and spread of lymphoma in AKR mice. *Cancer Res* 35:1921–1925, 1975

95. LeServe AW, Hellmann K: Metastases and the normalization of tumor blood vessels by ICRF-159: A new type of drug action. *Br Med J* 1:597–601, 1972

96. Li X-T, Hellmann K: Effect of RA233 alone and combined with radiation on experimental tumour metastasis. Part 1. *Clin Exp Metastasis* 1:51–59, 1983

97. Li X-T, Hellmann K: Antitumour effect of RA233 alone and combined with radiotherapy. *Clin Exp Metastasis* 1:181–190, 1983

98. Liotta LA, Catanzaro PJ, Kleinerman J: Reduction of metastatic rate by immunotherapy: A comparison of the immunogenic properties of metastasizing tumor cells versus tumor cells in the primary mass. *J Surg Oncol* 11:59–64, 1979

99. Lozzio BB, Machado EA, Lozzio CB, Mitchell J, Wust CJ: Immunotherapy of metastases of human neoplastic cells grown in immunodeficient mice. *Cancer Immunol Immunother* 12:135–140, 1982

100. Lundy J, Lovett EJ III, Wolinsky SM, Conran P: Immune impairment and metastatic tumor growth. The need for an immunorestorative as an adjunct to surgery. *Cancer* 44:945–951, 1979

101. Maat B: Extrapulmonary colony formation after intravenous injection of tumour cells into heparin-treated animals. *Br J Cancer* 37:369–376, 1978

102. Maat B: Selective macrophage inhibition abolishes warfarin-induced reduction of metastasis. *Br J Cancer* 41:313–316, 1980

103. Maat B, Hilgard P: Anticoagulants and experimental metastases: Evaluation of antimetastatic effects in different model systems. *J Cancer Res Clin Oncol* 101:275–283, 1981

104. Mazumder A, Rosenberg SA: Successful immunotherapy of natural killer-resistant established pulmonary melanoma metastases by intravenous adoptive transfer of syngeneic lymphocytes activated *in vitro* by interleukin 2. *J Exp Med* 159:495–507, 1984

105. Merker PC, Wodinsky I, Cantor ML, Venditti JM: Effectiveness of clinically active antineoplastic drugs in a surgical-adjuvant chemotherapy treatment regimen using the Lewis lung (LL) carcinoma. *Int J Cancer* 21:482–489, 1978

106. Milas L, Malenica B, Allegretti N: Enhancement of artificial lung metastases in mice caused by cyclophosphamide. I. Participation of host impairment of host antitumor resistance. *Cancer Immunol Immunother* 6:191–196, 1979

107. Milas L, Hersh EM, Hunter N: Therapy of artificial and spontaneous metastases of murine tumors with maleic anhydride-divinyl ether-2. *Cancer Res* 41:2378–2385, 1981

108. Milas L, Hersh EM, Stringfellow DA, Hunter N: Studies of the antitumor activities of pyrimidinone-interferon inducers. I. Effect against artificial and spontaneous lung metastases of murine tumors. *J Natl Cancer Inst* 68:139–145, 1982

109. Millman I, Scott AW, Halbherr T, Youmans AS, Youmans GP: Mycobacterial ribonucleic acid: Comparison with mycobacterial cell wall fractions for regression of murine tumor growth. *Infect Immun* 14:929–933, 1976

110. Mule JJ, Shu S, Schwarz SL, Rosenberg SA: Adoptive immunotherapy of established pulmonary metastases with LAK cells and recombinant interleukin-2. *Science* 225:1487–1489, 1984

111. Mule JJ, Rosenstein M, Shu S, Rosenberg SA: Eradication of a disseminated syngeneic mouse lymphoma by systemic adoptive transfer of immune lymphocytes and its dependence upon a host component(s). *Cancer Res* 45:526–531, 1985

112. Nowell PC: Clonal evolution of tumor cell populations. *Science* 194:23–28, 1976

113. Ossowski L, Reich E: Antibodies to plasminogen activator inhibit tumor metastasis. *Cell* 35:611–619, 1983

114. Ovejera AA, Johnson RK, Goldin A: Growth characteristics

and chemotherapeutic response of intravenously implanted Lewis lung carcinoma. *Cancer Chemother Rep Pt 2* 5:111–125, 1975

115. Peters LC, Brandhorst JS, Hanna MG Jr: Preparation of immunotherapeutic autologous vaccines from solid tumors. *Cancer Res* 39:1353–1360, 1979

116. Piessens WF: Evidence for human cancer immunity. A review. *Cancer* 26:1212–1220, 1970

117. Pimm MV, Baldwin RW: *C. parvum* immunotherapy of transplanted rat tumours. *Int J Cancer* 20:923–932, 1977

118. Poggi A, Mussoni L, Kornblith L, Ballabio E, DeGaetano G, Donati MB: Warfarin enantiomers, anticoagulation, and experimental tumour metastasis. *Lancet* i:163–164, 1978

119. Pollack VA, Fidler IJ: Use of young nude mice for selection of subpopulations of cells with increased metastatic potential from nonsyngeneic neoplasms. *J Natl Cancer Inst* 69:137–141, 1982

120. Proctor J, Rudenstam CM, Alexander P: Increased incidence of lung metastases following treatments of rats bearing hepatomas with irradiated tumour cells and the beneficial effect of *Corynebacterium parvum* in this system. *Biomedicine* 19:248–252, 1973

121. Rahman YE, Patel KR, Cerny EA, Maccoss M: The treatment of intravenously implanted Lewis lung carcinoma with two sustained release forms of 1-beta-D-arabinofuranosylcytosine. *Eur J Cancer* 20:1105–1112, 1984

122. Reeve JG, Wright KA, Twentyman PR: Response to X-radiation and cytotoxic drugs of clonal subpopulations of different ploidy and metastatic potential isolated from RIF-1 mouse sarcoma. *Br J Cancer* 47:841–848, 1983

123. Roberts DC, Barton M: Research using transplanted tumours of laboratory animals: A cross-referenced bibliography-IX., Imperial Cancer Research Fund, London, England, 1972

124. Robins RK, Srivastava PC, Narayanan VL, Plowman J, Paull KD: 2-beta-D-ribofuranosylthiazole-4-carboxamide, a novel potential antitumor agent for lung tumors and metastases. *J Med Chem* 25:107–108, 1982

125. Rose WC, Reed FC III, Siminoff P, Bradner WT: Immunotherapy of Madison 109 lung carcinoma and other murine tumors using lentinan. *Cancer Res* 44:1368–1373, 1984

126. Rosenberg B: Fundamental studies with cisplatin. *Cancer* 55:2303–2316, 1985

127. Rosenberg SA, Terry WD: Passive immunotherapy of cancer in animals and man. *Adv Cancer Res* 25:323–388, 1977

128. Sadler TE, Castro JE: Effects of *Corynebacterium parvum* and surgery on the Lewis lung carcinoma and its metastases. *Br J Surg* 63:292–296, 1976

129. Saito D, Sawamura M, Umezawa K, Kanai Y, Furihata C, Matsushima T, Sugimura T: Inhibition of experimental blood-borne metastasis by protease inhibitors. *Cancer Res* 40:2539–2542, 1980

130. Sava G, Giraldi T, Lassiani L, Nisi C: Mechanism of the antimetastatic action of dimethyltriazenes. *Cancer Treat Rep* 63:93–98, 1979

131. Sava G, Giraldi T, Lassiani L, Nisi C: Antimetastatic action and hematologic toxicity of p-(3,3-dimethyl-1-triazene) benzoic acid potassium salt and 5-(3,3-dimethyl-1-triazeno) imidazole-4-carboxamide used as prophylactic adjuvants to surgical tumor removal in mice bearing B16 melanoma. *Cancer Res* 44:64–68, 1984

132. Schabel FM Jr: Surgical adjuvant chemotherapy of metastatic murine tumors. *Cancer* 40:558–568, 1977

133. Scholler J, Philips FS, Sternberg SS, Bittner JJ: A comparative study of chemotherapeutic agents in spontaneous mammary adenocarcinomas of mice in transplants of recent origin. *Cancer* 9:240–251, 1956

134. Shapiro DM, Fugmann RA: A role for chemotherapy as an adjunct to surgery. *Cancer Res* 17:1098–1101, 1957

135. Southam CM: Evidence for cancer-specific antigens in man. *Progr Exp Tumor Res* 9:1–39, 1967

136. Staquet MJ, Byar DP, Green SB, Rozencweig M: Clinical predictivity of transplantable tumor systems in the selection of new drugs for solid tumors: Rationale for a three-stage strategy. *Cancer Treat Rep* 67:753–765, 1983

137. Stylos WA, Chirigos MA, Papademetriou V, Lauer L: The immunomodulatory effect of BM 12.531 (azimexon) on normal and tumored mice: *In vitro* and *in vivo* studies. *Immunopharmacol* 2:113–132, 1980

138. Suen KC, Lau LL, Yermakov V: Cancer and old age. An autopsy study of 3,535 patients over 65 years old. *Cancer* 33:1164–1168, 1974

139. Sukumar S, Hunter JT, Yarkoni E, Rapp HJ, Zbar B, Lederer E: Efficacy of mycobacterial components in the immunotherapy of mice with pulmonary tumor deposits. *Cancer Immunol Immunother* 11:125–129, 1981

140. Talmadge JE, Benedict K, Madsen J, Fidler IJ: Development of biological diversity and susceptibility to chemotherapy in murine cancer metastases. *Cancer Res* 44:3801–3805, 1984

141. Talmadge JE, Adams J, Phillips H, Collins M, Lenz B, Schneider M, Chirigos M: Immunotherapeutic potential in murine tumor models for polyinosinic-polycytidylic acid and poly-L-lysine solubilized by carboxymethylcellulose. *Cancer Res* 45:1066–1072, 1985

142. Tanigawa N, Mizuno Y, Hashimura T, Honda K, Satomura K, Hikasa Y, Niwa O, Sugahara T, Yoshida O, Kern DH, Morton DL: Comparison of drug sensitivity among tumor cells within a tumor, between primary tumor and metastases, and between different metastases in the human tumor colony-forming assay. *Cancer Res* 44:2309–2312, 1984

143. Taylor S, Folkman J: Protamine is an inhibitor of angiogenesis. *Nature* 297:307–312, 1982

144. Travis EL, Reinartz G, Chu AM, Down JD, Fowler JF: Effect of cyclophosphamide or X-rays on spontaneously occurring metastases from tumors transplanted into the tails of mice. *Cancer Res* 41:1803–1807, 1981

145. Tsuruo T, Fidler IJ: Differences in drug sensitivity among tumor cells from parental tumors, selected variants, and spontaneous metastases. *Cancer Res* 41:3058–3064, 1981

146. Tsuruo T, Yamori T, Nakanuma K, Hori K, Kawabata H, Tsukagoshi S, Sakurai Y: Spontaneous metastasis of highly metastatic variants of mouse tumors and the effects of drugs on the metastasis. *Gann* 75:557–563, 1984

147. Tsuruo T, Iida H, Makishima F, Yamori T, Kawabata H, Tsukugoshi S, Sakurai Y: Inhibition of spontaneous and experimental tumor metastasis by the calcium antagonist verapamil. *Cancer Chemother Pharmacol* 14:30–33, 1985

148. Turner GA, Weiss L: Analysis of aprotinin-induced enhancement of metastasis of Lewis lung tumors in mice. *Cancer Res* 41:2576–2580, 1981

149. Usui L, Urano M, Koike S, Kobayashi Y: Effect of PS-K, a protein polysaccharide, on pulmonary metastases of a C3H mouse squamous cell carcinoma. *J Natl Cancer Inst* 56:185–187, 1976

150. Van Putten LM, Kram LKJ, van Dierendonck HHC, Smink T, Fuzy M: Enhancement by drugs of metastatic lung nodule formation after intravenous tumor cell injection. *Int J Cancer* 15:588–595, 1975

151. Venditti JM: Pre-clinical drug evaluation: Rationale and methods. *Semin Oncol* 8:349–361, 1981

152. Venditti JM, Wesley RA, Plowman J: Current NCI preclinical antitumor screening, 1976–1982, and future directions. *Adv Pharmacol Chemother* 20:1–20, 1984

153. Wang BS, Onikul SR, Mannick JA: Prevention of death from metastases by immune RNA therapy. *Science* 202:59–60, 1978

154. Wang BS, Steele G, Mannick JA, Fallon M, Onikul SR: *In vivo* effects and parallel *in vitro* cytotoxicity of splenocytes

harvested from treated or control C57BL/6J mice after adjuvant immunotherapy of pulmonary metastases using xenogeneic RNS specific to B16 murine melanoma. *Cancer Res* 39:1702–1707, 1979

155. Watanabe N, Niitsu Y, Sone H, Neda H, Yamauchi N, Urushizaki I: Inhibitory effect of tumor necrosis serum on the metastasis of B-16 mouse melanoma cells. *Gann* 76:989–994, 1985

156. Weinstein JN, Steller MA, Keenan AM, Covell DG, Key ME, Sieber SM, Oldham RK, Hwang KM, Parker RJ: Monoclonal antibodies in the lymphatics: Selective delivery to lymph node metastases of a solid tumor. *Science* 222:423–426, 1983

157. Wood S, Hilgard PH: Arvin-induced hypofibrinogenemia and metastasis formation from blood-borne cancer cells. *Johns Hopkins Med J* 133:207–213, 1973

158. Woolley DW, Stewart JM: Permanent cure of some spontaneous mammary cancers of mice with analogs of 1,2-dimethyl-4,5-diaminobenzene. *Biochem Pharmacol* 11:1163–1173, 1962

159. Yamamoto T, Yamashita T, Tsubara E: Inhibition of pulmonary metastasis of Lewis lung carcinoma by a glucan, schizophyllan. *Invasion Metastasis* 1:71–84, 1981

160. Yarkoni E, Lederer E, Rapp HJ: Immunotherapy of experimental cancer with a mixture of synthetic muramyl dipeptide and trehalose dimycolate. *Infect Immun* 32:273–276, 1981

161. Yerushalmi A, Hazan G: Control of Lewis lung carcinoma by combined treatment with local hyperthermia and cyclophosphamide: Preliminary results. *Isr J Med Sci* 15:462–463, 1979

162. Zbar B, Bernstein ID, Bartlett GL, Hanna MG Jr, Rapp HJ: Immunotherapy of cancer: Regression of intradermal tumors and prevention of growth of lymph node metastases after intralesional injection of living *Mycobacterium bovis. J Natl Cancer Inst* 49:119–130, 1972

163. Zbar B, Ribi E, Meyer T, Azuma I, Rapp HJ: Immunotherapy of cancer: Regression of established intradermal tumors after intralesional injection of mycobacterial cell walls attached to oil droplets. *J Natl Cancer Inst* 52:1571–1577, 1974

GLOSSARY

MONINA D. PELINA

Adamantinoma: ameloblastoma; adamantoblastoma; multilocular cyst of jaw; epithelial odontome

Additional care requirement: pyschology, recreation, sexual therapy, special care for the terminally ill

Adenocystic carcinoma: cylindroma

Adenolymphoma: papillary cystadenoma lymphomatosum; oncocytoma; Warthin's tumor; branchioma; orbital inclusion cyst; branchiogenic adenoma

Adjuvant cancer treatment: supplemental therapies to main cancer therapies such as surgery, chemo- or radiotherapy, important for the stimulation of body strength

Adrenocorticotropic hormone* (M): present in abnormal amounts in patients with all types of lung cancer

Adverse effects of treatment: cardiac and pulmonary toxicity, gonadal dysfunction, loss of hair, nausea and vomiting, oral complications

African lymphoma: Burkitt's tumor

Ameloblastic fibroma: soft odontome

Anaplasia: reversion of cells to an embryonic, immature, or undifferentiated state; degree usually corresponds to malignancy of tumor

Angiofollicular lymph node hyperplasia: lymph nodal hamartoma; follicular lympho-reticuloma; angiomatous lymphoid hamartoma; benign giant lymphoma

Angiogenesis factors: factors (compounds) promoting the development of blood vessels; in oncology, produced by growing neoplasms

Angioreticuloma: hemangioblastoma; hemangioendothelioma (Cushing and Bailey)

Angiosarcomas: angioendotheliomas, angioblastic sarcomas

Antigens: substances which elicit a cellular or humoral immune response

Anthropology: study of the interrelationships of biological, cultural, geographical, and historical aspects of human populations. Anthropology is a basic science to oncologic epidemiology.

Antioncogene therapy: therapy directed at the genes which induce cancer growth

Bacteriology: study and science of bacteria; a specialized branch of microbiology. The best known plant tumor, crown gall disease is produced by *Bacterium tumefaciens*.

Basal-cell carcinoma: rodent ulcer; Jacob's ulcer; Basalzellenkrebs of Krompecher

B-cells: lymphocytes produced by the bone marrow

Benign chondroblastoma: cartilage-containing giant-cell tumor; calcifying giant-cell tumor; epiphyseal chondromatous giant-cell tumor

Benign cutaneous melanoma: pigmented nevus

Benign giant-cell synovioma: myeloid tumor; xanthoma; villonodular synovitis; tumeur à myeloplaxes

Benign nodular hyperplasia: benign prostatic hypertrophy; chronic lobular prostatitis

Benign osteoblastoma: giant osteoid osteoma; osteogenic fibroma

Biologicals and biological response modifiers: molecules that alter biological responses the host-molecule's tumor interaction; important in immunotherapy

Biophysics: hybrid science involving the methods and ideas of physics and chemistry to study and explain the structures of living organisms and the mechanics of life processes.

Bone marrow transplantation: removal of bone marrow portions of patients which are later reintroduced into the body after destruction of the patient's bone marrow, i.e. treatment for leukemia.

Botany: basics of botany are important for the evaluation of plant tumors in comparison to animal and human tumors

Breast cyst fluid protein: glycoprotein first isolated from breast cysts; useful for detecting recurrent and metastatic neoplasms

Bronchiolar carcinoma: alveolar-cell carcinoma, alveolar-cell tumor; pulmonary adenomatosis; bronchio-alveolar carcinoma

Bronchoscopy: visual investigation of the bronchi with a bronchoscope

Calcifying epithelial ondontogenic tumor: adenoid adamantoblastoma (Thoma and Goldman)

Calcitonin* (M): hypocalcemic factor synthesized by the thyroid C cells and is elevated in association with medullary carcinoma of the thyroid

Capillary hemangioblastoma: von Hippel's disease, von Hippel-Lindau disease

Carcinoembryonic antigen* (M): glycoprotein specific for adenocarcinomas of the digestive tract but also present in the endodermal tissues during the first two trimesters of embryonic and fetal development

Carcinoerythemia: (carcinoma cell leukemia) floating distribution of cancer cells in the circulatory system of terminal cancer patients

Carcinogen: any agent that incites development of a carcinoma or any other type of malignancy

Carcinoma: malignant neoplasm arising from epithelial tissue

Carcinoma in situ: a true malignant tumor of squamous or glandular epithelium in which no invasion of underlying or adjacent structures has occurred

Carcinoma of the kidney: hypernephroma; Grawitz tumor; malignant nephroma

Carcinoid (argentaffinoma): potentially malignant tumor of the argentaffin cells of the stomach and intestine

Carcinoid syndrome: a complex of symptoms arising from the metastasis of a carcinoid tumor to the liver

Carcinoid tumors (gastrointestinal tract): enterochromaffinoma, argentaffinoma; karcinoid tumor (Obendorfer)

Carotid body tumor: juxta-carotid chemodectoma; nonchromaffin paraganglioma; potato tumor

Cavernous angioma: cavernoma

Celioscopy: visual examination of the peritoneum with an endoscope; also known as peritoneoscopy

Chemotherapy: (see respective chapters on treatment) treatment of neoplasms, especially secondary tumors with cytostatica

Cholangiohepatocarcinoma: hepatobiliary cancer

"Chondroma" or Chondromatous hamartoma: chondroadenoma

Choriocarcinoma: chorioepithelioma

Chorioepithelioma or choriocarcinoma: choriopapillary trophocarcinoma (Friedman and Di Rienzo); the only carcinoma without stroma

Chromosome rearrangements: changes occurring in the sequence of the chromosomal units

Chronobiology: study of the effect of time on living systems

Clear-cell hidroadenoma: clear-cell papillary carcinoma; clear-cell myoepithelioma

Clear-cell tumor: adenocarcinoma with clear cells (hypernephroid of ovary; mesonephric tumor)

Clinical trials: arrangement of therapeutic regimen

Colloid cysts of the third ventricle: paraphyseal cysts; suprasellar cysts; neuroepithelial cysts

Colonoscopy: examination of the inner surface of the colon through visual means, i.e. colonoscope

Colony stimulating factors: group of functionally related glycoprotein effectors (CSF; also called macrophage- and granulocyte-inducing protein (MGI)) necessary for the development of hematopoietic precursor cells into mature macrophages and granulocytes

Colorectal carcinoma antigen (M): tumor-associated antigen useful for monitoring patients with colorectal cancer and for detecting recurrences

Comparative Pathology: Branch of pathology comparing diseases in different species

Complications, acute: such as nausea, vomiting, oncologic emergencies

Complications, chronic: such as paraneoplastic syndromes, impairments of body functions, cachexia

Computed tomography (CT): computer synthesizing x-ray technique designed to obtain anatomical information from examination of the cross sectional plane of the body; primary imaging tool for detection of central nervous system neoplasms

Congenital mesoblastic nephroma of infancy: leiomyomatous hamartoma of the kidney

Craniopharyngioma: adamantinoma of the pituitary; suprasellar cyst; suprasellar epidermoid cyst; Rathke's pouch tumor, ameloblastoma

Creatinine kinase* (M): enzyme catalyzing the transfer of phosphate phosphocreatine to yield creatine and ATP; also, useful as tumor marker for lung, breast, and prostate carcinoma

Cystic hyperplasia: Brodie's benign cystic disease; cystophorus desquamative epithelial hyperplasia; Schimmelbusch's disease; fibroadenosis (Atkins); maladie cystique de Reclus; Semb's fibroadenomatosis cyst

Cytology: branch of biological science dealing with the structure, behavior, growth, and reproduction of cells and the function and chemistry of cells and cell components

Cytotoxic anti-tumor agents: compounds detrimental to the growth of neoplastic cells

Desmoid tumor: desmoma; desmoid fibromatosis

Differentiation: In the case of neoplasms, differentiation constitutes specialization of a tissue or organ to perform inferiorly a particular function, but accompanied by characteristic morphologic changes simulating the parent tissue

Differentiation antigens: tumor associated antigens that reflect distinctive stages of differentiation in subpopulations of cells in normal adult tissue

Differentiation control: use of small effector molecules (i.e. retinoids) in the regulation of induced differentiation of cancer cells

Digital radiography/fluoroscopy: examination of the tissues and deep structures of the body by x-ray through use of the fluoroscope

Diktyoma: medulloepithelioma

Direct spread of neoplasms: neoplastic spread in which the spreading cells remain connected to the primary tumor

Dysgerminoma: seminoma; alveolar carcinoma; embryonal carcinoma with lymphoid stroma (Ewing); large cell carcinoma; gonocytoma (Teilum)

Embryology: study of the development of the organisms from the zygote or fertilized egg. Important for the study of embryonal and mixed tumors, teratomas included and for such problems as tumor regression.

Embryonal carcinoma (Scully and Parham): embryoma; teratocarcinoma; trophocarcinoma (Friedman and Di Rienzo)

Embryonic tumors (of liver): embryonal mixed tumor; embryonic hepatoma; hepatoblastoma

Emergencies: CNS emergencies, metabolic, superior vena cava syndrome, surgical, urologic

Endodermal sinus tumor: yolk-sac tumor

Endoscopy: examination of the interior of a hollow organ or channel with a special instrument (endoscope)

Epidermoid cysts: cholesteatoma (misnomer)

Epithelioma adenoides cysticum: trichoepithelioma

Esophagoscopy: inspection of the interior of the esophagus, using an endoscope

Fibroblastoma (Mallory, Penfield): meningioblastoma (Oberling)

Fibroma: non-osteogenic fibroma; non-ossifying fibroma; metaphyseal fibrous defect (Hatcher)

Follicular adenocarcinoma: angioinvasive carcinoma or malignant adenoma

Follicular lymphoma: Brill-Symmers disease; lymphoid follicular reticulosis (Robb-Smith); giant follicular lymphadenopathy (Symmers); giant lymph follicle hyperplasia (Brill, Baehr, and Rosenthal)

Foreign body carcinogenesis: neoplastic development initiated or promoted by compounds (i.e. environmental) foreign to the host

Ganglioneuroma: ganglioma; sympathicocytoma

Ganglioneuroblastomas: malignant ganglioneuromas

Genetics: science concerned with biological inheritance and the resemblances and differences among related individuals. Genetic facts are involved, at least, in certain human neoplasms, and certain animal and plant neoplasms have a genetic basis.

Geography: science dealing with the description of land, sea, and air and the distribution of plant and animal life, including humans.

Geology: study or science of earth, its history, and its life as recorded in the rocks; includes the study of the geologic features of an area, such as the geometry of rock formations, weathering, erosion, and sedimentations. Stratigraphy, the sequence of the layers of sediments is determined by fossil content.

Germinoma: atypical teratoma; pinealoma

Giant-celled glioblastomas: monstrocellular; gigantocellular glioblastoma; spongioblastoma ganglioides

Giant osteoid osteoma (Dahlin): benign osteoblastoma (Jaffe); osteogenic fibroma (Lichtenstein)

Growth factors: compounds fostering cell growth

Hemangioendothelioma: angiosarcoma

Hemangioma of the placenta: chorioangioma

Heterogeneity of neoplastic cells: neoplastic cell aggregates distinguished by differences in their ability to metastasize, location site of metastasis, resistance to chemotherapy, and aggressiveness of growth; major impedance to effective cancer therapy.

Histology: study of the structure and chemical composition of animal and plant tissues as related to their function. The basic science for determination and diagnosis of neoplasms.

Hodgkin's paragranuloma: early Hodgkin's disease (Jackson); benign Hodgkin's disease (Harrison); indolent Hodgkin's disease (Symmers); reticular lymphoma (Lumb); lymphoreticular medullary reticulosis (Robb-Smith)

Human tumor-specific antigens: antigens specific to particular tumors

Hyperthermia: treatment of neoplasms with restricted increase of tissue temperature

Immunology: division of biological science concerned with the native or acquired resistance of higher animal forms and humans to infection with microorganisms and distribution of neoplastic cells, foreign bodies, etc.

Immune response: reaction of the body to antigens

Immunity changes: processes occurring during cancer development which may increase the risk of infection

Immunosuppression: decrease in immune response

Initiators of chemical carcinogenesis: chemical compounds able to induce cancer growth

Inorganic Chemistry: science dealing with the study of noncarbon compounds

Insulin family of growth factors: Insulin-based growth promoting substances

Intraoperative endoscopy: exploration of the inner surface of a hollow organ during surgery

Intraoperative radiotherapy: radiation therapy applied to inoperable neoplasms exposed during surgery

Invasion of neoplasms: growth of a malignant neoplasm into surrounding tissues, causing destruction of those tissues

Ionizing radiation: particles with sufficient energy to produce ionization directly in their passage through a substance

Irreversible toxic changes during carcinogenesis: non-revertant processes occurring during the latter stages of carcinogenesis

Juvenile aponeurotic fibroma: calcifying fibroma

Kaposi's disease: idiopathic multiple hemorrhagic sarcoma

Keratoacanthoma: Molluscum sebaceum; Molluscum pseudocarcinomatosum

Lactic dehydrogenase (M): tetramer catalyzing the oxidation of lactate to pyruvate; also, may be used as a marker for germ cell cancers

Laparoscopy: exploration of the abdomen utilizing a type of endoscope, specifically, a laparascope

Laser therapy: surgical treatment of tissue with a narrow beam of coherent, monochromatic light of concentrated energies

Leiomyoma: myoma; fibroid; fibromyoma

Lipid-bound sialic acid* (M): heterogeneous mixture of gangliosides, sialolipids, and sialoglycoprotein, functional as a tumor marker for particular neoplastic diseases, such as Hodgkin's disease, melanoma, and ovarian cancer

Lipoid-cell tumor: adrenocorticoid tumor of ovary; ovarian hypernephroma; luteoma; masculinovoblastoma (Merivale and Forman; Rottino and McGrath)

Liver-cell carcinoma: hepatocellular cancer; malignant hepatoma

Lymphoma: malignant neoplasms of the lymphatic and reticuloendothelial tissues: appear as solid tumors

Lymphosarcoma: lymphocytoma; lymphoblastoma; lymphocytic reticulosarcoma/reticulum-cell sarcoma; reticulosarcoma; reticulum-cell lymphosarcoma; stem-cell lymphoma; clasmatocytic lymphoma

Magnetic resonance imaging: imaging technology allowing detection of small neoplasms in areas of high bone content

Malignant ciliary epithelial tumor: medulloepithelioma

Malignant hydatidiform mole: chorioadenoma destruens

Malignant nonchromaffin paraganglioma: alveolar soft-part sarcoma; malignant granular cell myoblastoma

Malignant synovioma: synovioma (Smith); synovialoma; synovial sarcoma; mesothelioma of joints; sarcomesothelioma; malignant angiofibroma

Mediastinoscopy: use of mediastinoscope for visual examination of the mediastinum through a suprasternal incision

Medicine: study of the cause and treatment of human disease, including the healing arts dealing with diseases which are treated by a physician or surgeon

Melanosis: abnormally dark pigmentation of various tissues; in oncology,the condition of cachexia by widespread melanoma metastasis

Melanuria: excretion of dark urine due to the presence of melanin or other pigments

Meningioma: psammoma (Virchow); dural endothelioma (Golgi, Ribbert); arachnoidal fibroblastoma (Mallory, Penfield); meningioblastoma (Oberling); tumor of the meninges

"Mesodermal mixed tumors" of the uterus: malignant mesenchymoma; mesenchymal sarcoma (Ober and Tovell); adenosarcoma (Sophian); dysontogenetic tumor (McFarland); malignant mixed Müllerian neoplasm (Krupp et al.)

Metastasis: transfer of the causal agent (cell or microorganism) of a disease from a primary focus to a distant one through the blood or lymphatic vessels; in oncology, a secondary neoplasm is derived from the primary malignant neoplasms by the seeding of neoplastic cells

Metastatic spread: via lymphatics, including thoracic duct; bloodstream; transcoelomic metastasis-serous membranes, i.e. ovarian tumor development; implantation on epithelial surfaces; metastasis of teratomas; metastasis of stroma

"Mixed tumors" of salivary glands: composite tumors; polymorphic adenomas; adenomes metaplastic polymorphs; enclavomas

Morphogenesis: transformation involved in the growth and differentiation of cells and tissue; also known as topogenesis

Multi-modality therapy: application of several types of therapy simultaneously or consecutively to prohibit the progression of primary neoplasms and their spread

Multiple enchondromatosis: dyschondroplasia

Multiple-endocrine-adenoma syndrome: polyendocrine adenomas; pluriglandular adenomatosis; adenomatosis of endocrine glands familial endocrine adenomatosis

Multiple myeloma: mollities ossium (McIntyre, 1850); myelogenous pseudoleukemia (Zahn, 1885); Kahler's disease (1889); senile osteomalacia (Marchand, 1896); plasma cell myelosarcoma; myeloma; plasma cell myeloma; plasmacytoma

Multiple osteochondromatosis: diaphysial aclasis (Keith); hereditary deforming dyschondroplasia

Mutagen: an agent that raises the frequence of mutation above the spontaneous rate

Myxoma: myxosarcoma

Neoplastic metabolism: aberrant changes of normal metabolism during cancer development

Neoplasm: actively growing tissue composed of cells which have undergone an abnormal type of irreversible differentiation; a cellular tumor that may either be benign or malignant

Nephroblastoma: Wilms' tumor of kidney, adenosarcoma; embryonal nephroma, "mixed" tumor of kidney; embryonic adenosarcoma

Neurilemoma: neurolemmoma; Schwann-cell tumor, Schwannoma

Neuroblastoma (Wright): sympathicoblastoma

Neuron-specific enolase (M): isozyme of enolase found in neuronal tissue and in endocrine cells of the neuroendocrine system; present in large amounts in all types of neuroendocrine tumors

Nodular fasciitis: subcutaneous pseudosarcomatous fibromatosis; proliferative fasciitis

Nuclear imaging: highly sensitive technique important for the detection and characterization of brain tumors

Organic Chemistry: study of the composition, reactions, and properties of carbon compounds except CO, CO_2, and certain ionic compounds. The majority of chemical carcinogens are organic compounds.

Organ-specific treatment: treatment specific for one or several types of neoplasms, e.g. mammography

Organ transplantation: implantation of an organ in one of two ways: 1) homogenous transplantation: transfer of an organ from an organism of one species to another of the same species; 2) heterogenous transplantation: transfer of an organ from an organism of one species to another of a different species

Osteoclastoma: giant cell tumor; myeloid sarcoma; tumeur a myeloplaxes

Osteosarcoma: osteogenic sarcoma; osteoblastic sarcoma

Ovarian carcinoma antigen (M): monoclonal antibody-identified tumor marker for ovarian cancer and possibly other epithelial cancers

Oxyphilic adenoma: oncocytoma

Paleontology: science dealing with the study of prehistoric forms of life through the study of plant and animal fossils. This science is essential for understanding of such facts as the first phylogenetic appearance of parent tissues of neoplasms and the sequence of neoplasms found in fossils.

Papillary carcinoma: carcinoma characterized by finger-like outgrowths

Papilloma: growth pattern of benign epithelial tumors in which the proliferating epithelial cells grow outward from a surface accompanied by vascularized cores of connective tissue to form a branching structure

Paraneoplastic syndromes: remote effects constituted by the tumor through elaboration of soluble factors and humoral substances influencing the ability of the host to function normally; i.e. ectopic hormone production as in Cushing's syndrome and hypercalcemia

Parosteal osteosarcoma: parosteal osteoma (Geshickter and Copeland); juxtacortical osteogenic sarcoma (Jaffe and Selin); parosteal osteogenic sarcoma (Dwinne et al.)

Particle beam radiation therapy: method of treatment to increase the rates of local and regional control of malignant neoplasms based on improved physical dose distributions achievable with protons, He ions, heavy ions, and pions

Pathology: branch of biological science dealing with the nature of disease through study of its causes, processes, and effects, together with the associated alterations of structure and function; and the laboratory findings of disease, as distinguished from clinical signs and symptoms

Peritoneoscopy: see celioscopy

Pheochromocytoma: chromaffinoma

Photodynamic sensitizers: light absorbing chemicals (i.e. hematoporphyrin derivative (Hpd)) that are essential components of photoreactions leading to the inactivation of biologic systems in cancer therapy

Phytopathology: branch of biological science which investigates plant diseases

Pinealoma: atypical teratoma of the pineal body

Pineoblastoma: pinealoblastoma

Pineocytoma: pinealocytoma

Polyp: nonspecific term signifying tissue growth of a mucous membrane which may be an inflammatory lesion or a true tumor; two types exist: (a) pedunculated polyp – mass of tissue attached to an organ by a freely movable, narrow stalk or pedicle; (b) sessile polyp – mass of tissue attached by a broad base

Polyposis: presence of multiple polyps, usually occurring in the gastrointestinal tract

Primary tumors of coelomic surfaces: mesotheliomas

Progressive recurring dermatofibroma: dermatofibrosarcoma protuberans

Prostatic acid phosphatase* (M): glycoproteins used in the radioimmunoassay to evaluate the progression of localized prostate cancer or the response to therapy of patients with metastatic disease

Radiation sensitizers and protectors: chemical compounds (hypoxic cell sensitizers and sulfhydryl compounds) that interact with reactive species during irradiation to aid in the repair of initial radiochemical lesions

Radiotherapy: treatment of radiosensitive neoplasms by radiation, e.g. testicular neoplasms

Rehabilitation: restoration, following cancer treatment, of ability to function in a normal or near normal manner

Reticulum-cell sarcoma: reticulosarcoma; reticulum cell lymphosarcoma; stem cell lymphoma; clasmatocytic lymphoma

Retinoblastoma: neuroblastoma retinae; glioma retinae; neuroepithelioma of the retina; ependymoma retinae

Reversible toxic changes during carcinogenesis: reversible structural and metabolic changes of tissue undergoing neoplastic transformation during the onset of neoplastic development; similar to the process of ischemia

Rhabdoblastic sarcomas: rhabdosarcomas

Sarcoma: nonepithelial malignant neoplasm deriving from connective, muscle, or nervous tissues

Seborrheic keratosis: Verruca senilis; pigment-forming papilloma; basal cell papilloma

Second primary cancers: Primary neoplasm appearing in a patient who had earlier developed another primary tumor of differing histology

Seminoma: spermatocytoma; embryoma; embryonal carcinoma with lymphoid stroma; large cell carcinoma testis; germinoma

Solid alveolar carcinoma: medullary carcinoma; solid carcinoma with amyloid stroma

Solitary osteochondroma: solitary osteocartilaginous exostosis

Subependymal astrocytoma: subependymal glomerate astrocytoma, subependymoma

Subependymal giant-celled astrocytomas: tuberose sclerosis (syn. astrocytome sousependymaire to gross cellular fusiforms, (Roussy and Oberling, 1931))

Subependymoma: subependymal glomerate astrocytoma (Boykin et al., 1954); subependymal astrocytoma (French and Bucy, 1948)

Syringocystadenoma papilliferum: superficial hidradenoma

T-cells: lymphocytes produced in the thymus

Testicular adenocarcinoma of infancy: orchioblastoma; endodermal sinus tumor; yolk-sac tumor; infantile embryonal carcinoma

Thoracoscopy: examination of the pleural cavity with an endoscope

Transcatheter management: management of a neoplasm by applying chemotherapy with a catheter

Treatment administration: administrative handling of the treatment of cancer patients

Tumor: (a) widely used term for a neoplasm as a new growth of tissue, serving no function; (b) a swollen or distended part of the body, or as used in paleontology of a fossil, such as a skull or bone; (c) sometimes also used for a genus specific phylogenetic condition of bones and known as pachyostosis; (d) in botany and phytopathology, used for a gall

Tumor markers *: enzymes, isoenzymes, and hormones (precursors and small active peptides included) associated with various types of cancers

Tumor spread: direct spread

Tumors of the meninges: psammoma; dural endothelioma; arachnoidal fibroblastoma; meningioblastoma (see also meningioma)

Tumors of specialized gonadal stroma (Mostofi): androblastoma (Teilum); Sertoli-cell tumor (Collins and Symington); granulosa theca cell tumor of testis

Ultrasound: ultrasonic waves (frequency 20,000 Hz), used in medical diagnosis, surgery, and therapy

Unknown primary: condition in which secondary metastatic deposits develop from primary neoplasms of unknown location

Unusual types of metastasis: metastasis which occurs less common as by unusual distribution on epithelial surfaces, or in an unusual way of direction as from the center of the body to its periphery (metastasis to a big toe) or to a rarely metastasized organ (tongue)

Virology: science dealing with the study of viruses and in oncology with oncogenic viruses

Zoology: scientific study of the taxonomy, behavior, and morphology of animal life also a basic science of comparative oncology

Xanthogranulomatous pyelonephritis: foam cell granuloma; renal xanthomatosis

---

*(M) = tumor marker

INDEX